Acute Care and Emergency Gynecology

A Case-Based Approach

Acute Care and Emergency Gynecology

A Case-Based Approach

Edited by

David Chelmow
Leo J. Dunn Professor and Chair,
Virginia Commonwealth University School of Medicine, Richmond, VA, USA

Christine R. Isaacs
Associate Professor and Director, General Obstetrics and Gynecology Division, Medical Director of Midwifery Services,
Virginia Commonwealth University School of Medicine, Richmond, VA, USA

Ashley Carroll
Assistant Professor, Department of Obstetrics and Gynecology,
Virginia Commonwealth University School of Medicine, Richmond, VA, USA

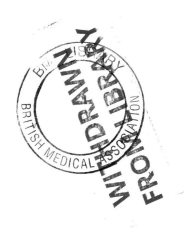

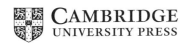

CAMBRIDGE
UNIVERSITY PRESS

University Printing House, Cambridge CB2 8BS, United Kingdom

Cambridge University Press is part of the University of Cambridge.

It furthers the University's mission by disseminating knowledge in the pursuit of education, learning and research at the highest international levels of excellence.

www.cambridge.org
Information on this title: www.cambridge.org/9781107675414

© Cambridge University Press 2015

First published 2015

Printed in the United Kingdom by Bell and Bain Ltd

A catalogue record for this publication is available from the British Library

Library of Congress Cataloguing in Publication data
Acute care and emergency gynecology : a case-based approach / edited by David Chelmow, Christine R. Isaacs, Ashley Carroll.
       p. ; cm.
Includes bibliographical references and index.
ISBN 978-1-107-67541-4 (Paperback)
I. Chelmow, David, editor.   II. Isaacs, Christine R., editor.
III. Carroll, Ashley, editor.
[DNLM: 1.   Female Urogenital Diseases–Case Reports.   2.   Critical Care–Case Reports.   3.   Emergency Treatment–Case Reports.
WJ 190]
RG158
618.1025–dc23   2014015828

ISBN 978-1-107-67541-4 Paperback

....

Contents

Contents

Contents

Contributors

Tod C. Aeby MD MEd
Department of Obstetrics, Gynecology and Women's Health, University of Hawaii John A. Burns School of Medicine, Honolulu, HI, USA

Melanie D. Altizer MD
Department of Obstetrics and Gynecology, Carilion Clinic/Virginia Tech-Carilion School of Medicine, Roanoke, VA, USA

Ronan A. Bakker MD
Department of Obstetrics and Gynecology, Virginia Commonwealth University School of Medicine, Richmond, VA, USA

Meghann E. Batten MSN CNM
Department of Obstetrics and Gynecology, Virginia Commonwealth University School of Medicine, Richmond, VA, USA

Anita K. Blanchard MD
Department of Obstetrics and Gynecology, University of Chicago Medical Center, Chicago IL, USA

Brian Bond MD PharmD
Department of Obstetrics and Gynecology, Tufts Medical Center, Boston, MA, USA

Megan A. Brady MD
Department of Obstetrics and Gynecology, Virginia Commonwealth University School of Medicine, Richmond, VA, USA

Saweda A. Bright MD
Department of Obstetrics and Gynecology, Virginia Commonwealth University School of Medicine, Richmond, VA, USA

Ellen L. Brock MD MPH
Department of Obstetrics and Gynecology, Virginia Commonwealth University School of Medicine, Richmond, VA, USA

Amy Brown MD
Department of Obstetrics and Gynecology, Virginia Commonwealth University School of Medicine, Richmond, VA, USA

Ashley Carroll MD
Department of Obstetrics and Gynecology, Virginia Commonwealth University School of Medicine, Richmond, VA, USA

Jori S. Carter MD MS
Department of Obstetrics and Gynecology, Virginia Commonwealth University School of Medicine, Richmond, VA, USA

Frances Casey MD MPH
Department of Obstetrics and Gynecology, Virginia Commonwealth University School of Medicine, Richmond, VA, USA

Weldon Chafe MD
Department of Obstetrics and Gynecology, Virginia Commonwealth University School of Medicine, Richmond, VA, USA

David Chelmow MD
Department of Obstetrics and Gynecology, Virginia Commonwealth University School of Medicine, Richmond, VA, USA

Jessica M. Ciaburri DO
Department of Obstetrics and Gynecology, Virginia Commonwealth University School of Medicine, Richmond, VA, USA

Stephen A. Cohen MD
Department of Obstetrics and Gynecology, Virginia Commonwealth University School of Medicine, Richmond, VA, USA

Adrianne M. Colton MD
Department of Obstetrics and Gynecology, Virginia Commonwealth University School of Medicine, Richmond, VA, USA

PonJola Coney MD
Department of Obstetrics and Gynecology, Virginia Commonwealth University School of Medicine, Richmond, VA, USA

Jennifer A. Cross MD
Department of Obstetrics and Gynecology, Virginia Commonwealth University School of Medicine, Richmond, VA, USA

Julie Zemaitis DeCesare MD
Department of Clinical Sciences, Florida State University College of Medicine, Pensacola, FL, USA

Layson L. Denney MD
Department of Obstetrics and Gynecology, Virginia Commonwealth University School of Medicine, Richmond, VA, USA

Megan L. Evans MD MPH
Department of Obstetrics and Gynecology, Tufts Medical Center, Boston, MA, USA

Nicole S. Fanning MD
Department of Obstetrics and Gynecology, Virginia Commonwealth University School of Medicine, Richmond, VA, USA

Tanaz R. Ferzandi MD MA
Department of Obstetrics and Gynecology, Tufts Medical Center, Boston, MA, USA

Katie P. Friday MD
Department of Women's and Infants' Services, Medstar Washington Hospital Center, Washington, DC, USA

Nancy D. Gaba MD
Department of Obstetrics and Gynecology, George Washington University School of Medicine and Health Sciences, Washington, DC, USA

Rajiv B. Gala MD
Department of Obstetrics and Gynecology, Ochsner Medical Center/University of Queensland-Ochsner Clinical School, New Orleans, LA, USA

Andrew Galffy MD
Department of Obstetrics and Gynecology, University of Connecticut Health Center, Farmington, CT, USA

Adrienne L. Gentry DO
Department of Obstetrics and Gynecology, Carilion Clinic/Virginia Tech-Carilion School of Medicine, Roanoke, VA, USA

Edward J. Gill MD
Department of Obstetrics and Gynecology, Virginia Commonwealth University School of Medicine, Richmond, VA, USA

Philippe Girerd MD
Department of Obstetrics and Gynecology, Virginia Commonwealth University School of Medicine, Richmond, VA, USA

Meredith Gray MD
Department of Obstetrics and Gynecology, Carilion Clinic/Virginia Tech-Carilion School of Medicine, Roanoke, VA, USA

Amy Hempel MD
Department of Obstetrics and Gynecology, Virginia Commonwealth University School of Medicine, Richmond, VA, USA

Audra Jolyn Hill MD
Department of Obstetrics and Gynecology, Cleveland Clinic, Cleveland, OH, USA

Chris J. Hong MD MSEE
Department of Obstetrics and Gynecology, Virginia Commonwealth University School of Medicine, Richmond, VA, USA

Kathryn A. Houston MD
Department of Obstetrics, Gynecology and Reproductive Sciences, University of California, San Francisco, San Francisco, CA, USA

Patricia S. Huguelet MD
Department of Obstetrics and Gynecology, University of Colorado School of Medicine, Aurora, CO, USA

Warner K. Huh MD
Department of Obstetrics and Gynecology, University of Alabama at Birmingham, Birmingham, AL, USA

Jordan Hylton DO
Department of Obstetrics and Gynecology, Virginia Commonwealth University School of Medicine, Richmond, VA, USA

Christine R. Isaacs MD
Department of Obstetrics and Gynecology, Virginia Commonwealth University School of Medicine, Richmond, VA, USA

Alison F. Jacoby MD
Department of Obstetrics, Gynecology and Reproductive Sciences, University of California, San Francisco, San Francisco, CA, USA

Isaiah M. Johnson MD
Department of Obstetrics and Gynecology, Carilion Clinic/Virginia Tech-Carilion School of Medicine, Roanoke, VA, USA

Nicole W. Karjane MD
Department of Obstetrics and Gynecology, Virginia Commonwealth University School of Medicine, Richmond, VA, USA

Emily E. Landers MD
Department of Obstetrics and Gynecology, University of Alabama at Birmingham, Birmingham, AL, USA

Susan M. Lanni MD
Department of Obstetrics and Gynecology, Virginia Commonwealth University School of Medicine, Richmond, VA, USA

Eduardo Lara-Torre MD
Department of Obstetrics and Gynecology, Carilion Clinic/Virginia Tech-Carilion School of Medicine, Roanoke, VA, USA

Lee A. Learman MD PhD
Department of Obstetrics and Gynecology, Indiana University School of Medicine, Indianapolis, IN, USA

Nikola Alexander Letham DO
Department of Obstetrics and Gynecology, University of Connecticut, Farmington, CT, USA

Rachel K. Love MD
Department of Obstetrics and Gynecology, Virginia Commonwealth University School of Medicine, Richmond, VA, USA

Richard Scott Lucidi MD
Department of Obstetrics and Gynecology, Virginia Commonwealth University School of Medicine, Richmond, VA, USA

Elisabeth McGaw MD
Department of Obstetrics and Gynecology, Virginia Commonwealth University School of Medicine, Richmond, VA, USA

Kimberly Woods McMorrow MD
Virginia Physicians for Women, Richmond, VA, USA

Christopher A. Manipula MD
Department of Obstetrics and Gynecology, Virginia Commonwealth University School of Medicine, Richmond, VA, USA

Kirk J. Matthews MD
Department of Obstetrics and Gynecology, Virginia Commonwealth University School of Medicine, Richmond, VA, USA

Michelle Meglin MD
Department of Obstetrics and Gynecology, Virginia Commonwealth University School of Medicine, Richmond, VA, USA

Megan Metcalf MD
Department of Obstetrics and Gynecology, Carilion Clinic/Virginia Tech-Carilion School of Medicine, Roanoke, VA, USA

Sarah H. Milton MD MS
Department of Obstetrics and Gynecology, Virginia Commonwealth University School of Medicine, Richmond, VA, USA

Gaby Moawad MD
Department of Obstetrics and Gynecology, George Washington University School of Medicine and Health Sciences, Washington, DC, USA

Christopher Morosky MD
Department of Obstetrics and Gynecology, The Hospital of Central Connecticut, New Britain, CT, USA

Lindsay H. Morrell MD
Department of Obstetrics and Gynecology, Virginia Commonwealth University School of Medicine, Richmond, VA, USA

Elizabeth L. Munter MD
Department of Obstetrics and Gynecology, Virginia Commonwealth University School of Medicine, Richmond, VA, USA

Erin L. Murata MD
Department of Obstetrics and Gynecology, University of New Mexico Health Sciences Center, Albuquerque, NM, USA

Amanda B. Murchison MD
Department of Obstetrics and Gynecology, Carilion Clinic/Virginia Tech-Carilion School of Medicine, Roanoke, VA, USA

Nguyet A. Nguyen MD
Department of Obstetrics and Gynecology, University of Alabama at Birmingham, Birmingham, AL, USA

Nan G. O'Connell MD
Department of Obstetrics and Gynecology, Virginia Commonwealth University School of Medicine, Richmond, VA, USA

Tony Ogburn MD
Department of Obstetrics and Gynecology, University of New Mexico Health Sciences Center, Albuquerque, NM, USA

K. Nathan Parthasarathy MD MS
Department of Obstetrics and Gynecology, The Reading Health System, West Reading, PA, USA

Thomas C. Peng MD
Department of Obstetrics and Gynecology, Virginia Commonwealth University School of Medicine, Richmond, VA, USA

Ashley Peterson MD
Department of Obstetrics and Gynecology, Tufts Medical Center, Boston, MA, USA

Sarah Peterson MD
Department of Obstetrics and Gynecology, Virginia Commonwealth University School of Medicine, Richmond, VA, USA

John G. Pierce Jr MD
Department of Obstetrics and Gynecology, Virginia Commonwealth University School of Medicine, Richmond, VA, USA

Amber Price MSN CNM
Department of Obstetrics and Gynecology, Virginia Commonwealth University School of Medicine, Richmond, VA, USA

Heidi J. Purcell MD
Department of Obstetrics and Gynecology, Baylor College of Medicine, Houston, TX, USA

Ronald M. Ramus MD
Department of Obstetrics and Gynecology, Virginia Commonwealth University School of Medicine, Richmond, VA, USA

Nicole Calloway Rankins MD MPH
Department of Obstetrics and Gynecology, Virginia Commonwealth University School of Medicine, Richmond, VA, USA

Fidelma B. Rigby MD
Department of Obstetrics and Gynecology, Virginia Commonwealth University School of Medicine, Richmond, VA, USA

Amanda H. Ritter MD
Department of Obstetrics and Gynecology, Virginia Commonwealth University School of Medicine, Richmond, VA, USA

Barbara L. Robinson MD
Department of Obstetrics and Gynecology, Georgia Regents University, Augusta, GA, USA

Danielle Roncari MD MPH
Department of Obstetrics and Gynecology, Tufts Medical Center, Boston, MA, USA

Lisa Rubinsak MD
Department of Obstetrics and Gynecology, Virginia Commonwealth University School of Medicine, Richmond, VA, USA

Jennifer Salcedo MD MPH MPP
Department of Obstetrics, Gynecology and Women's Health, University of Hawaii John A. Burns School of Medicine, Honolulu, HI, USA

Mary T. Sale MD
Department of Obstetrics and Gynecology, University of New Mexico Health Sciences Center, Albuquerque, NM, USA

Peter F. Schnatz DO
Department of Obstetrics and Gynecology, The Reading Health System, West Reading, PA, USA

John W. Seeds MD
Department of Obstetrics and Gynecology, Virginia Commonwealth University School of Medicine, Richmond, VA, USA

Kathryn Shaia MD MHA
Department of Obstetrics and Gynecology, Virginia Commonwealth University School of Medicine, Richmond, VA, USA

Karen Shelton RNC IBCLC
Sacred Heart Health System, Pensacola, FL, USA

Megan M. Shine MD
Department of Obstetrics and Gynecology, University of Alabama at Birmingham, Birmingham, AL, USA

Haller J. Smith MD
Department of Obstetrics and Gynecology, University of Alabama at Birmingham, Birmingham, AL, USA

Roger P. Smith MD
Department of Obstetrics and Gynecology, Indiana University School of Medicine, Indianapolis, IN, USA

Nancy A. Sokkary MD
Department of Obstetrics and Gynecology, University of New Mexico Health Sciences Center, Albuquerque, NM, USA

Reni A. Soon MD MPH
Department of Obstetrics, Gynecology and Women's Health, University of Hawaii John A. Burns School of Medicine, Honolulu, HI, USA

Aparna Sridhar MD MPH
Department of Obstetrics and Gynecology, David Geffen School of Medicine at UCLA, Los Angeles, CA, USA

Lilja Stefansson MD MS
Department of Obstetrics and Gynecology, Virginia Commonwealth University School of Medicine, Richmond, VA, USA

Laurie S. Swaim MD
Department of Obstetrics and Gynecology, Baylor College of Medicine, Houston, TX, USA

Chemen M. Tate MD
Department of Obstetrics and Gynecology, Indiana University School of Medicine, Indianapolis, IN, USA

Hong-Thao Thieu MD
Department of Obstetrics and Gynecology, Tufts Medical Center, Boston, MA, USA

Meredith S. Thomas MD
Department of Obstetrics and Gynecology, Tufts Medical Center, Boston, MA, USA

L. Chesney Thompson MD
Department of Obstetrics and Gynecology, University of Colorado School of Medicine, Aurora, CO, USA

Tiffany Tonismae MD
Department of Obstetrics and Gynecology, Carilion Clinic/Virginia Tech-Carilion School of Medicine, Roanoke, VA, USA

Angela M. Tran MD
Department of Obstetrics and Gynecology, Virginia Commonwealth University School of Medicine, Richmond, VA, USA

Breanna Walker MD
Department of Obstetrics and Gynecology, Virginia Commonwealth University School of Medicine, Richmond, VA, USA

Alan G. Waxman MD MPH
Department of Obstetrics and Gynecology, University of New Mexico Health Sciences Center, Albuquerque, NM, USA

C. Nathan Webb MD MS
Department of Obstetrics and Gynecology, Virginia Commonwealth University School of Medicine, Richmond, VA, USA

Valerie L. Williams MD
Department of Obstetrics and Gynecology, LSU Health Sciences Center, New Orleans, LA, USA

Sarah B. Wilson MD
Department of Obstetrics, Gynecology and Reproductive Sciences, University of California, San Francisco, San Francisco, CA, USA

Elizabeth M. Yoselevsky MD
Department of Obstetrics and Gynecology, Virginia Commonwealth University School of Medicine, Richmond, VA, USA

Amy E. Young MD
Department of Obstetrics and Gynecology, LSU Health Sciences Center, New Orleans, LA, USA

Preface

Gynecologic emergencies and urgent problems are common events in women's health care. While there are many available references covering such issues, nearly all are written as traditional textbooks. Many practitioners are more comfortable with case-based learning, and practically speaking, clinical problems present themselves as cases in the form of real patients.

Acute Care and Emergency Gynecology: A Case-Based Approach presents common gynecologic problems in a case-based format, promoting learning from clinical scenarios. Chapters are designed to be suitable as a reference when similar cases present in a busy clinical practice.

We chose approximately 100 gynecologic problems and illustrated our vignettes with pictures and images whenever possible. Cases were typically inspired by patients cared for by the authors, but have been modified to ensure patient confidentiality and maximize educational value. Most cases were chosen based on the likelihood of being frequently encountered, but to keep the book interesting, we also cover some more unusual and challenging cases. The cases largely fall into two categories. Some deal with the diagnostic evaluation of presenting complaints, while others focus on the management of specific diagnoses.

In writing the cases, we realized that there are many problems where clear evidence-based recommendations exist, and should be followed. Wherever high quality evidence-based guidelines exist, they are introduced and their application discussed. In instances where such guidelines do not exist, we present evidence for management when available, and carefully reasoned expert opinion where there is a lack of evidence to support clear recommendations. All discussions were prepared by first searching for existing guidelines, then performing a thorough literature search. By using this format, we were also able to cover many areas such as common incidental findings that are an everyday occurrence, but where little has been written.

The problems and diagnoses were chosen to capture the breadth of general obstetrics and gynecology practice, in addition to subspecialty areas including Urogynecology, Reproductive Endocrine and Infertility, Pediatric and Adolescent Gynecology, and Gynecologic Oncology. The cases were written to be of particular relevance to specialists in general obstetrics and gynecology, but are intended to be useful to anyone caring for women in urgent and emergency settings. We are very grateful to our extensive team of authors, many from the Virginia Commonwealth University School of Medicine and the Society for Academic Specialists in General Obstetrics and Gynecology (SASGOG).

A 45-year-old woman with heavy vaginal bleeding

Tod C. Aeby

History of present illness

A 45-year-old gravida 6, para 6 woman presents to the emergency department with a complaint of 2 days of heavy vaginal bleeding and passing clots. She is light-headed and short of breath. Previously she had regular but heavy periods. A few days prior to this bleeding episode she noted increasing pelvic pressure and a malodorous vaginal discharge.

Her past medical history is significant for recurrent anemia thought to be from abnormal uterine bleeding. Her surgical history is significant for a previous postpartum tubal ligation. She takes no medications.

Physical examination

General appearance: Well-developed, moderately obese woman in moderate distress
Vital signs:

Temperature: 38.1°C
Pulse: 120 beats/min
Blood pressure: 92/68 mmHg
Respiratory rate: 18 breaths/min
Oxygen saturation: 98% on room air

Abdomen: Soft with suprapubic tenderness to deep palpation, no guarding or rebound
Pelvic: Active vaginal bleeding and a large firm mass presenting at the vaginal introitus (Fig. 1.1). You are unable to do a speculum or bimanual examination
Laboratory studies:

Urine pregnancy test: Negative
WBCs: 21 000/μL (normal $3.8–11.2 \times 10^9$/L)
Hb: 4.8 g/dL (normal 11.6–15.1 g/dL)
Ht: 16.2% (normal 34.1–44.2%)

How would you manage this patient?

This patient clearly has a prolapsing submucous myoma complicated by severe anemia, hypovolemia, and likely infection. Her management requires immediate fluid resuscitation and correction of her anemia, in preparation for surgical removal of the myoma. With a 96% success rate, vaginal myomectomy in the operating room, under general or regional anesthesia, is the therapy of choice. Given her fever, elevated white blood cell count, and malodorous discharge, preoperative broad spectrum intravenous antibiotics are warranted.

The patient received aggressive fluid resuscitation, and was transfused four units of packed red blood cells. A second-generation cephalosporin was started 30 minutes before going to the operating room, where she was placed under general anesthesia. After she was prepped and draped, a single-tooth tenaculum was placed on the myoma and, while avoiding excessive downward traction, gentle torque was applied. The myoma moved easily through several rotations before detaching. Hysteroscopy was not possible due to the widely dilated cervix. Gentle sharp curettage was performed to assess the cavity and to obtain an endometrial sample. Hemostasis was adequate and the patient tolerated the procedure well. After recovery from anesthesia, she was asymptomatic and discharged following overnight observation.

Prolapsing submucous myomas

Uterine myomas are the most common tumors of the female reproductive tract, occurring in 20–40% of women [1]. Submucous myomas (those that lie just beneath the endometrial lining)

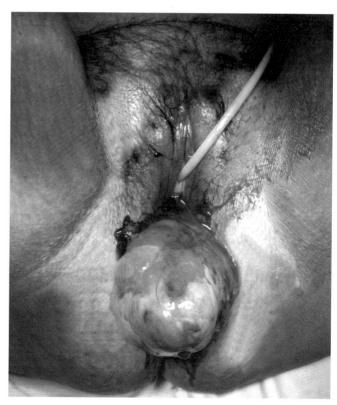

Fig. 1.1 Typical appearance of a prolapsing submucous uterine myoma.

Acute Care and Emergency Gynecology, ed. David Chelmow, Christine R. Isaacs and Ashley Carroll. Published by Cambridge University Press.
© Cambridge University Press 2015.

constitute about 5% of all leiomyomas and a small proportion will become pedunculated (suspended from a stalk) and be expelled from the uterus. The largest study looking at this issue found that about 2.5% of all myomas will prolapse through the cervix [2]. As the myomas prolapse, the stalk will be stretched and the blood supply compromised. Necrosis and secondary infections are common and, as in this patient, leads to the frequent complaint of a malodorous vaginal discharge. Other presenting symptoms include acute vaginal bleeding (59%), heavy and irregular vaginal bleeding (74%), uterine cramps (20%), pelvic pressure (15%), and, occasionally, urinary retention [2].

While in this patient the diagnosis of a prolapsed myoma was quite obvious, usually the myoma has only prolapsed through the cervix and will not be diagnosed prior to a vaginal exam. The differential diagnosis should include an endometrial polyp, a cervical or vaginal neoplasm, and an endocervical (Nabothian) cyst. Prolapsing polyps are the second most common finding and will typically have a soft texture and a ragged appearance, as opposed to the firm, smooth texture of a myoma. Necrosis and infection can make the gross appearance indistinct and the final determination requires pathologic analysis. Leiomyosarcomas are quite rare.

Imaging, such as a pelvic ultrasound, is occasionally useful to identify the presence of additional myomas. In some cases MRI can be used to confirm the diagnosis of a myoma and to localize and characterize the stalk to aid in selection and planning of a surgical approach [3].

Patients with suspected prolapsing myomas should be managed in the operating room with adequate anesthesia and the ability to respond to complications, particularly bleeding. Preoperative counseling should include discussion of rare complications, such as severe infection, excessive bleeding, uterine perforation, and an approximately 5% rate of conversion to hysterectomy. In the vast majority of cases, a simple vaginal myomectomy is the procedure of choice and consists primarily of grasping the myoma with a ring clamp or a single-toothed tenaculum and gently twisting until it is released. Occasionally, myomas may be broad based. These myomas typically do not rotate easily and visualization of the stalk is obscured. In these cases, the myoma may require morcellation (cutting the myoma into smaller pieces using a scalpel, electrosurgical loop, or bovie) to aid in removal. Broad-based pedicles may require clamping or suture ligation and laparoscopic endoloops may be helpful. Care should be

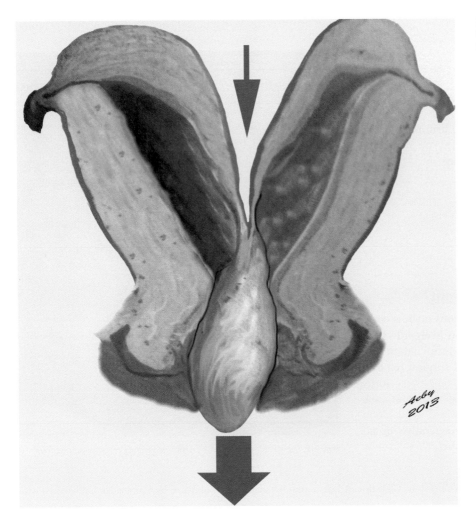

Fig. 1.2 Excessive downward traction can lead to uterine inversion, placing the fundus of the uterus at risk for rupture or perforation.

exercised when twisting the pedicle since lacerations of the uterus and even the bladder have been described when too much torque was applied to a broad pedicle. Additionally, excessive downward traction can lead to inversion of the uterus and subsequent rupture or perforation of the fundus during resection (Fig. 1.2). In the case of a broad pedicle, where firm traction is required for adequate exposure, consideration should be given to a combined laparoscopic and vaginal approach. If heavy bleeding develops or persists after the myoma has been removed, a Foley catheter with a 30-cc balloon can be inserted through the cervix and inflated until it tamponades the site of hemorrhage [4]. If the balloon has been placed and bleeding continues, ultrasound or laparoscopy should be used to rule out uterine rupture or perforation. At that point, hysterectomy may be required to control the hemorrhage.

Other surgical options for managing a prolapsed submucous myoma include hysterectomy via a vaginal, abdominal, or minimally invasive approach. If the prolapsing myoma is significantly distorting the lower uterine segment, removing the myoma separately may facilitate the procedure. However, due to the low morbidity and effectiveness of vaginal myomectomy, hysterectomy should be reserved for patients who fail an attempt at myomectomy or who have persistent bleeding after the procedure. Because the myomas are often necrotic, severe intra-abdominal infections have been reported following hysterectomy [2]. Thus, antibiotics sufficient to cover normal vaginal flora (in most cases a second-generation cephalosporin) should be started prior to the hysterectomy and continued until the patient is afebrile for at least 24 hours.

Following the myomectomy, the vast majority of women (80%) will have a normal or only slightly enlarged uterus and return to having regular menstrual periods. Some even become pregnant and go on to have a normal, term delivery. Cervical insufficiency has been reported, but there is inadequate published data with which to advise patients. Twenty percent of patients with successfully treated prolapsing myomas will require removal of additional myomas or a hysterectomy over the next several years. The tissue removed at vaginal myomectomy should be submitted to pathology to rule out malignancy. Routine gynecologic care should be sufficient follow-up for most patients.

Key teaching points

- Prolapsed submucous uterine myomas are relatively common.
- Presenting symptoms include vaginal bleeding, pain, pelvic pressure, malodorous vaginal discharge, and, occasionally, urinary retention.
- Vaginal myomectomy is a simple and highly successful method of treatment and should represent the first-line approach.
- During a vaginal myomectomy, avoid aggressive rotation and excessive downward traction.
- Following vaginal myomectomy, most women return to their normal menstrual cycle.
- As myomas are frequently necrotic and infected, preoperative broad spectrum prophylactic antibiotics are important.

References

1. Riley P. Treatment of prolapsed submucous fibroids. *S Afr Med J* 1982;62(1):22–4.

2. Ben-Baruch G, Schiff E, Menashe Y, Menczer J. Immediate and late outcome of vaginal myomectomy for prolapsed pedunculated submucous myoma. *Obstet Gynecol* 1988;72(6): 858–61.

3. Panageas E, Kier R, McCauley TR, McCarthy S. Submucosal uterine leiomyomas: diagnosis of prolapse into the cervix and vagina based on MR imaging. *Am J Roentgenol* 1992; 159(3):555–558. DOI: 10.2214/ ajr.159.3.1503024.

4. Golan A, Zachalka N, Lurie S, Sagiv R, Glezerman M. Vaginal removal of prolapsed pedunculated submucous myoma: a short, simple, and definitive procedure with minimal morbidity. *Arch Gynecol Obstet* 2004;271(1):11–13. DOI:10.1007/ s00404-003-0590-x.

A 29-year-old woman with a pelvic mass and altered mental status

Saweda A. Bright and Stephen A. Cohen

History of present illness

A 29-year-old gravida 0 African-American woman was transferred to a tertiary care hospital emergency department for management of cardiac arrest and altered mental status. Approximately two weeks prior, she had diarrhea, nausea, and vomiting, followed by a fall in the bathroom, which was presumed to be a syncopal event. She subsequently developed altered mental status with delusions and psychosis, which resulted in admission to the psychiatric ward at a community hospital. There, she was given several antipsychotic medications without any improvement in her symptoms.

When her clinical symptoms worsened, this prompted hospital transfer to a higher level of care. Upon transfer, she was tachycardic and had periodic episodes of sinoatrial arrest. She was transferred to the ICU for management, where she then experienced a generalized seizure. Her deteriorating symptoms prompted cardiology consultation and pacemaker placement for management of her cardiac arrhythmia. She ultimately required intubation and sedation.

The patient's past medical history was negative for any psychiatric, cardiac, or seizure disorders. Her past surgical history was notable for a right salpingo-oophorectomy three years ago with pathology confirming a mature cystic teratoma.

Physical examination in the ICU

General appearance: Thin, reclining, sedated woman
Vital signs:

Temperature: 37°C
Pulse: 77 beats/min
Blood pressure: 96/54 mmHg
Respiratory rate: 12 breaths/min on mechanical ventilation
Oxygen saturation: 100% on the ventilator
BMI: 14 kg/m^2

HEENT: Oral endotracheal tube in place, dysconjugate gaze, 2 mm pupils, sluggishly reactive to light
Cardiovascular: Pacemaker in place, native sinus rhythm apparent
Lungs: Clear to auscultation bilaterally
Abdomen: Hypoactive bowel sounds, soft, nondistended
Extremities: Palpable distal pulses, no cyanosis or edema
Neurologic: Clonus bilaterally, hyperreflexic
Laboratory studies:

Arterial blood gas, electrolytes, liver function, thyroid, and coagulation studies: All within normal limits

Lactate: Normal
HIV: Negative
RPR: Nonreactive
Toxicology screen: Negative
Lumbar puncture: Revealed evidence of aseptic meningitis with a prominence of lymphocytes

Imaging:

Chest radiograph: Showed endotracheal tube in the appropriate position
Head CT and head MRI: Both within normal limits
Cervical spine MRI: Unremarkable
EEG: No evidence of seizures, but did show findings thought to be consistent with encephalopathy
Abdominal/pelvis CT: Revealed a left adnexal complex cystic mass measuring 4.3 × 5.4 cm and noted to contain numerous internal calcifications and solid nodular components. A solid nodule was medially measured at 18 mm. These findings were suggestive of a cystic teratoma (Fig. 2.1)

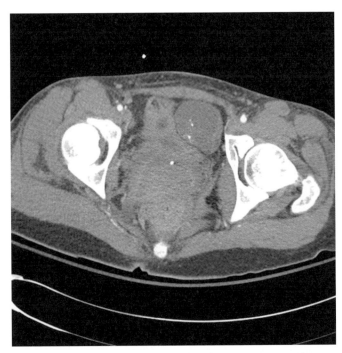

Fig. 2.1 CT of female pelvis. Arrow signifies left ovarian teratoma with numerous calcifications within a complex cystic ovarian mass.

Acute Care and Emergency Gynecology, ed. David Chelmow, Christine R. Isaacs and Ashley Carroll. Published by Cambridge University Press. © Cambridge University Press 2015.

How would you manage the patient?

The diagnosis is anti-*N*-methyl-D-aspartate-receptor (anti-NMDA-R) encephalitis. The ICU team suspected the diagnosis based on the patient's clinical presentation and course, and consulted the Gynecology team for surgical management. The diagnosis was based exclusively on clinical suspicion. The patient was taken to the operating room and underwent an exploratory laparotomy with left ovarian cystectomy to remove the pelvic mass (Fig. 2.2)

Surgical pathology confirmed a mature cystic teratoma containing brain tissue with brisk perivascular lymphocytic infiltrates that was thought to be related to the presence of circulating anti-NMDA-R antibodies. The final diagnosis was confirmed when the patient's serum NMDA-R antibody titer returned highly positive.

A multidisciplinary approach was used to care for the patient. In addition to the Gynecology team, the ICU team consulted Neurology, Infectious Disease, Endocrinology, Cardiology, Dermatology, Psychiatry, and Physical Medicine and Rehabilitation teams. The patient was treated with intravenous immunoglobulin, methylprednisolone, rituximab, and plasmapheresis. Her symptoms slowly reversed. She was transferred out of the ICU 29 days after her surgery. On that day, she was noted to be alert, interactive, and although not fully recovered clinically, trying to communicate.

The patient remained in the hospital for two months recovering from her acute events, followed by two months of care in a rehabilitation facility. Eight months following her initial presentation, she was being followed as an outpatient in the office and noted to have complete recovery.

Anti-NMDA-R encephalitis

Anti-*N*-methyl-D-aspartate-receptor (anti-NMDA-R) encephalitis was first described in the literature in 2007. The illness was originally diagnosed in women who presented with a

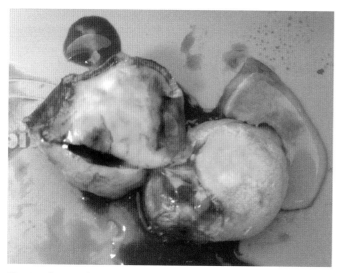

Fig. 2.2 Sectioned mature cystic teratoma with presence of brain tissue and sebum.

constellation of clinical findings, including severe neuropsychiatric symptoms, an ovarian teratoma, and autoantibodies targeting glutamate receptors, specifically NMDA-type receptors. NMDA receptors are ligand-gated cation channels located on the post-synaptic membranes that are responsible for synaptic transmission and plasticity. Antibodies binding to the NR1 subunit of the NMDA-R results in the characteristic symptoms associated with the syndrome [1].

The true incidence of NMDA-R encephalitis is unknown. Although initially described in women, the syndrome has also been described in children under the age of 18 years and men.

The clinical course occurs in several phases. Initially, there is a prodromal phase during which patients experience nonspecific flu-like symptoms. Patients may experience headaches, fevers, nausea, vomiting, diarrhea, fatigue, and upper respiratory symptoms. Within a couple weeks of these initial symptoms, patients develop psychiatric symptoms, which can include anxiety, insomnia, delusions, mania, hallucinations, or memory deficits. Patients are often initially evaluated by a psychiatrist and treated with antipsychotic medications during this phase. In the subsequent stage of the disease, patients experience decreased consciousness and may become unresponsive, as this patient did. They may alternate between periods of catatonia and agitation. They can experience lethargy, seizures, autonomic instability (hyperthermia, hypertension, hypotension, tachycardia, bradycardia) and dyskinesias, with orolingual-facial dyskinesias being most characteristic. Eventually, patients may go into status epilepticus or a comatose state. Patients frequently require ICU management. Interestingly, as patients respond to therapy, symptoms usually resolve in the reverse order of how they originally presented.

Dalmau and colleagues found that about 75% of patients with anti-NMDA-R encephalitis either completely recover or have mild sequelae [1]. The remaining patients were either severely disabled or died. Prognosis depends on early diagnosis and treatment.

The diagnosis of anti-NMDA-R encephalitis is made based largely on clinical suspicion from the presenting symptoms, with the addition of results from laboratory and radiologic studies supporting the diagnosis. Oftentimes, physicians must act based on clinical suspicion alone in order to provide life-saving care with removal of teratoma, as the results of antibody tests may take several weeks. The disease is frequently unrecognized due to its uniqueness among paraneoplastic syndromes, since it involves young women with primarily psychiatric symptoms and brain MRI findings that can be either normal or atypical [2]. In the initial paper documenting this disorder, Dalmau and colleagues noted that the time from development of neurologic symptoms to diagnosis of teratoma ranged from three weeks to four months [1]. Anti-NMDA-R encephalitis should be suspected in patients with unexplained psychiatric symptoms, especially with a flu-like prodrome, who then develop cardiac or respiratory compromise. If the diagnosis is suspected, a multidisciplinary approach should be employed. The most important diagnostic finding is the detection of anti-NMDA-R antibodies in the patient's serum or cerebrospinal fluid. The severity of symptoms correlates with the amount of anti-NMDA-R antibodies in circulation. Physicians may follow the antibody titers to help determine clinical response to therapy, as a decrease in titers correlates with clinical remission.

MRI of the brain is abnormal in about half of patients and, in those cases, will reveal T2 signal hyperintensity in the hippocampi, cerebellum, cerebral cortex, basal ganglia, or brain stem [1]. EEGs are abnormal in most patients showing nonspecific, slow, and disorganized activity with seizures. In catatonic patients, EEGs show slow, continuous, rhythmic activity in the delta-theta range [1]. Despite these EEG changes, patients usually do not respond to antiepileptic medications.

Cerebrospinal fluid analysis is abnormal in the vast majority of patients and may reveal moderate lymphocytic pleocytosis, normal or mildly elevated protein concentration, and oligoclonal bands. Brain biopsy is unnecessary for diagnosis because findings are usually normal or ambiguous.

About 60% of anti-NMDA-R encephalitis patients have coexisting tumors, with ovarian teratomas being the most common in women [3]. Testicular teratomas and small cell lung cancers have been found to be associated in men diagnosed with the illness. Pathologic reviews of the tumors have shown the manifestation of nervous tissue, which tests positive for anti-NMDA-R antibodies. Since the presence of teratomas appears to be related to anti-NMDA-R encephalitis and their timely removal affects the prognosis, patients should be screened for the presence of a teratoma with MRI, CT scan, or ultrasonography. Identification of a teratoma and subsequent removal is crucial to the prognosis; therefore, physicians should perform one of the aforementioned imaging modalities to identify a teratoma in patients with unexplained mental status changes and cardiac or respiratory compromise. It is important that physicians do not wait on the results of antibodies before surgical removal of the teratoma is performed.

Management of anti-NMDA-R encephalitis includes immediate supportive care. Patients with evidence of a teratoma should have the entire tumor removed as soon as possible. This may be accomplished with a cystectomy or an oophorectomy. Early removal is essential to patient recovery. First-line medical therapy consists of corticosteroids, intravenous immunoglobulin, and plasma exchange. Patients with an associated teratoma usually respond well to first-line therapy. Second-line therapy consists of rituximab and/or cyclophosphamide. Second-line therapy is recommended for patients without evidence of teratoma, patients who have delayed diagnosis, or patients who do not respond to first-line therapy within 7–10 days after tumor removal. To date, no standard algorithm for management exists, so a multidisciplinary approach is recommended to best care for patients.

In approximately 75% of cases, patients have substantial regression of symptoms, with the remaining 25% suffering from either severe neurologic deficits or death [3]. Relapses can occur in 20–25% of patients, usually those without teratoma. In these patients immunotherapy may be considered for up to one year after clinical recovery. Additionally, clinicians may consider periodic screening for ovarian teratomas for at least two years after clinical recovery. It is common for patients to experience amnesia and require rehabilitation, physical therapy, or psychotherapy. Even after initial signs of recovery, patients need to have continued supportive care as complete recovery may take years.

Key teaching points

- Anti-N-methyl-D-aspartate-receptor (anti-NMDA-R) encephalitis is a disease that affects mostly women. It most commonly presents with psychotic symptoms, autonomic instability, and ovarian teratomas.
- High clinical suspicion with early recognition, expedient tumor removal, and initiation of immunomodulatory therapy are crucial to patient recovery and survival.
- Final diagnosis is made by confirmation of anti-NMDA-R autoantibodies in the serum or cerebrospinal fluid.
- Therapy should be initiated based on high clinical suspicion, even if results of final diagnostic studies are still pending.
- First-line treatment involves immediate tumor removal, intravenous immunoglobulin, and corticosteroids.

References

1. Dalmau J, Lancaster E, Martinez-Hernandez E, et al. Clinical experience and laboratory investigations in patients with anti-NMDA-R encephalitis. *Lancet Neurol* 2011;10:63–74.

2. Dalmau J, Tuzun E, Wu H, et al. Paraneoplastic anti-N-methyl-D-asparate receptor encephalitis associated with ovarian teratoma. *Ann Neurol* 2007;61: 25–36.

3. Wandinger K, Saschenbrecker S, Stoecker W, et al. Anti-NMDA-receptor encephalitis: A severe, multistage, treatable disorder presenting with psychosis. *J Neuroimmunol* 2010;231:86–91.

Acute exacerbation of chronic pelvic pain in a 32-year-old woman

Lee A. Learman

History of present illness

A 32-year-old gravida 3, para 3 woman presents to your emergency department (ED) with a complaint of midline lower abdominal pain rated at 10 out of 10 on the pain scale. She has used extended-cycle birth control pills (84 days) to suppress her menstruation for 2 years since undergoing laparoscopic treatment for endometriosis. Yesterday, on her first pill-free day, she began to have vaginal bleeding and severe cramping pain. She's had no nausea, vomiting, dysuria, frequency, or urgency, and no change in her bowel habits. She is monogamous with her husband. Her other medical problems include irritable bowel syndrome, depression controlled with sertraline 50 mg daily, and fibromyalgia treated with gabapentin 900 mg daily.

She has had pelvic pain since menarche at age 12. At first she had pain the day before and during the first three days of her periods, with no pain on the lighter fourth and fifth days, and no pain between her periods. Later, during college, her pain worsened and eventually occurred during most of the month. She has undergone four laparoscopies in the last 10 years to excise or ablate endometriosis. The last procedure two years ago improved her menstrual pain for three months, but it gradually returned. Extended-cycle birth control pills have reduced her periods to just four per year, with some light days of spotting in-between. She continues to have daily pain requiring hydrocodone 10 mg/acetaminophen 325 mg, 2 pills every 6–8 hours, every day. When she has periods the pain becomes uncontrollable and she comes to the emergency room for additional medication.

Physical examination

General: Well-developed, well-nourished woman grimacing and holding her lower abdomen

Vital signs:

Temperature: 37.0°C
Pulse: 90 beats/min
Blood pressure: 128/76 mmHg
Respiratory rate: 18 breaths/min
Oxygen saturation: 100% on room air

Abdomen: Soft, no masses, lower abdominal/suprapubic tenderness without rebound or guarding, normal bowel sounds

External genitalia: Unremarkable

Vagina: No lesions; scant discharge

Cervix: Parous; scant blood

Uterus: Retroverted, tender, normal size, minimal mobility

Adnexa: Nontender; without masses

Laboratory studies: Urine pregnancy test: Negative

How would you manage the patient?

The patient has an acute exacerbation of chronic pelvic pain and endometriosis, which started on her first pill-free day after completing an extended-cycle pill pack. Her baseline pain is managed with opioid medication that is not providing adequate pain relief. Because her physical examination showed only midline lower abdominal and uterine tenderness in the setting of mild vaginal bleeding, a pregnancy test was performed. No other tests were ordered.

The patient was given ibuprofen 800 mg PO and a heating pad was placed on her lower abdomen. After 1 hour her pain level improved to a 6 out of 10 on the pain scale. She was discharged 1 hour later with a tolerable pain level of 4 out of 10 on the pain scale. Discharge instructions were to continue using heat and ibuprofen 800 mg every 6–8 hours, start her next contraceptive pill pack immediately, and see her primary care doctor within 2 weeks to discuss a continuous active pill regimen. She was advised to continue taking her medications for chronic pelvic pain, depression, and fibromyalgia on schedule.

Acute pain management for chronic pelvic pain

An American College of Obstetricans and Gynecologists (ACOG) Committee Opinion published in 2012 highlights the burden of prescription drug misuse or abuse, which in 2009 led to over 1.2 million ED visits, a greater number than the 974 000 ED visits from illegal drug abuse [1]. It can be challenging to determine whether a patient on prescription opioids coming to the ED with pain is demonstrating signs of drug abuse or has an acute cause of pain that is refractory to their usual analgesic regimen. It is prudent to first rule out acute causes.

As our patient had mild vaginal bleeding, midline lower abdominal cramping pain, and no signs of infection, peritonitis, gastrointestinal or urinary tract abnormalities, it is critical to exclude pregnancy. Additional evaluation is rarely warranted. Although urinalysis from a voided specimen could rule out an acute urinary tract infection, the timing of our patient's

Acute Care and Emergency Gynecology, ed. David Chelmow, Christine R. Isaacs and Ashley Carroll. Published by Cambridge University Press.
© Cambridge University Press 2015.

symptoms, concomitant bleeding, and pelvic examination findings favor a uterine source (dysmenorrhea). Without lateralizing signs and symptoms suggestive of an adnexal process or appendicitis, pelvic ultrasound or CT scanning would also not be warranted. These tests add cost and delay and, in the case of CT scanning, unnecessary radiation exposure.

This patient was not given parenteral opioids, which are commonly used in the ED while evaluation is underway for patients with acute pain. Because of the challenges of coping with chronic pain, patients who have a pain flare may seek care in the ED for rapid control of their pain rather than relying on nonopioid medications or other approaches. Although parenteral opioids may provide immediate relief, their benefits are not long-lasting, and at best provide a bridge to specific treatments aimed at the conditions causing the pain [2]. In this case it was possible to complete the history and physical examination without acute pain relief. However, short-term parenteral opioid treatment to aide evaluation of acute pain would be appropriate if needed.

For patients with acute pain from dysmenorrhea there are many effective treatments (Table 3.1). The application of heat to the lower abdomen can be as effective as acetaminophen or ibuprofen [3]. If heat alone is ineffective, nonopioid analgesics can be added or substituted. In our case the patient's baseline

Table 3.1 Selected treatment options for acute dysmenorrhea

Treatment	Regimen
Continuous low-level topical heat	Apply heated patch to lower abdomen
NSAIDS: • Ibuprofen • Mefenamic acid	 Up to 2400 mg daily in divided doses 500 mg initial dose and then 250 mg every 6 h
If dysmenorrhea is accompanied by heavy menstrual bleeding	
Oral contraceptives	OCs containing 35 µg ethinyl estradiol (and any progestin) taken 2–4 times daily will usually stop bleeding within 48 h, and then taper to 1 pill daily. To avoid nausea use an anti-emetic such as promethazine 12.5–25.0 mg PR
Progestins: • MPA • NET	 MPA 10–20 mg BID NET 5 mg 1–2 times daily
Transexamic acid (antifibrinolytic)	1300 mg TID (3900 mg daily) for up to 5 days until bleeding stops. Use if other treatments ineffective and patient not at increased risk for thrombosis

BID, two times daily; MPA, medroxyprogesterone acetate; NET, norethindrone; NSAIDs; non-steroidal anti-inflammatory drugs; OCs, oral contraceptives; PR, by rectum; TID, three times daily.

pain regimen includes 2600 mg of acetaminophen. Although up to 4 g acetaminophen per day is safe in patients without chronic liver disease, ibuprofen's prostaglandin inhibition makes it a better choice for dysmenorrhea [4]. Ibuprofen doses up to 3.2 g per day are safe for well-hydrated patients without renal insufficiency or a bleeding diathesis. For severe dysmenorrhea 800 mg every 6–8 hours is appropriate. In patients taking combined estrogen–progestin birth control pills, the bleeding that occurs during the placebo or pill-free period is not physiologic. It is the result of progestin withdrawal and can be minimized by the use of continuous hormonal contraception [5]. It is possible to resume active pill immediately, and even double the dose, to stabilize the endometrium and stop the bleeding. Our patient immediately received a heating pack and 800 mg of ibuprofen. Her pain improved within an hour, and was tolerable after another hour. She was discharged with instructions to start her next active pill pack immediately. Had her bleeding been heavier other interventions would have been considered, including higher doses of contraceptive pills, progestins, or antifibrinolytic agents (Table 3.1).

Prevention of future ED visits

Our patient was advised to follow-up with the doctor who prescribed her oral contraceptive pills to discuss switching from an extended cycle to a continuous regimen without pill-free periods. Other options can be discussed at that visit. In ambulatory management of patients with chronic pelvic pain and dysmenorrhea, the first step is to create therapeutic amenorrhea and ovarian suppression. Continuous hormonal contraception, gonadotropin-releasing hormone agonists, and danazol are highly effective treatments. The levonorgestrel intrauterine device (IUD) is also effective despite evidence it does not consistently suppress ovulation.

Patients taking opioid medication for chronic pelvic pain may also seek care in the ED for pain flares when they are not menstruating or ovulating. Avoiding these visits often requires the use by their prescriber of a treatment agreement that outlines the details of the doses of medications, the pharmacy filling the prescriptions, and requires that no other physician prescribe opioid medications for the patient. Patients who do not accept treatments to correct the underlying causes of pain or adjunctive treatments such as physical therapy, psychotherapy, or substance abuse counseling, can be dismissed from care. Before initiating opioid therapy, and periodically thereafter, it is important to screen patients for substance abuse using validated screening tools and, if indicated, with toxicology screening. In the United States, several states have established web-based prescription monitoring programs that collect all controlled substance prescriptions filled within their jurisdictions. Searches should be done at each office visit and ED visit to document patient adherence to their treatment agreements.

According to the US Centers for Disease Control and Prevention, between 2004 and 2008 the number of ED visits for nonmedical opioid procurement more than doubled. To decrease the numbers of patients making repeated ED visits for pain, several hospitals have established case management programs. One such program included narcotic restriction, nonnarcotic treatment regimens, medication restriction to one pharmacy and one provider, and referral to primary care providers and addiction specialists. To be eligible, patients needed to demonstrate ED overuse or other signs of drug-seeking or drug addiction. ED overuse was defined as three or more visits per month, two or more visits per month for two consecutive months, or greater than six per year. Comparing the year prior to enrollment to the year after enrolment, ED visits dropped by 77%, from 3689 to 852 [6].

Key teaching points

- Women with chronic pelvic pain who have acute pain should be evaluated for specific causes and not dismissed as medication-seeking.

- Diagnostic evaluation should be tailored to the patient's risk factors, history, and physical examination findings.
- Pain and bleeding during the placebo or pill-free segment of a birth control pill cycle are caused by progestin withdrawal and can be prevented using continuous hormonal contraception.
- Women with acute pain from dysmenorrhea should be treated acutely with heat, nonsteroidal anti-inflammatory medications (ibuprofen or mefenamic acid), and progestins or combined oral contraceptive pills to address the underlying cause of the pain.
- Frequent emergency department visits for pain can be reduced by use of case managers, narcotic restriction, nonnarcotic treatment regimens, "one pharmacy/one provider" restrictions, and appropriate referral to primary care providers and addiction specialists.

References

1. American Congress of Obstetricians and Gynecologists. Nonmedical use of prescription drugs. Committee Opinion No. 538. *Obstet Gynecol* 2012;120: 977–82.

2. Manterola C, Vial M, Moraga J, Astudillo P. Analgesia in patients with acute abdominal pain. *Cochrane Database Syst Rev* 2011, Issue 1. Art. No.: CD005660. DOI: 10.1002/ 14651858.CD005660.pub3.

3. Akin MD, Weingand KW, Hengehold DA, et al. Continuous low-level topical heat in the treatment of dysmenorrhea. *Obstet Gynecol* 2001;97(3):343.

4. Marjoribanks J, Proctor M, Farquhar C, Derks RS. Nonsteroidal anti-inflammatory drugs for dysmenorrhoea. *Cochrane Database Syst Rev* 2010, Issue 1. Art. No.: CD001751. DOI: 10.1002/ 14651858.CD001751.pub2.

5. Edelman A, Gallo MF, Jensen JT, Nichols MD, Grimes DA. Continuous

or extended cycle vs. cyclic use of combined hormonal contraceptives for contraception. *Cochrane Database Syst Rev* 2005, Issue 3. Art. No.: CD004695. DOI: 10.1002/14651858.CD004695. pub.

6. Masterson B, Wilson M. Pain care management in the emergency department: a retrospective study to examine one program's effectiveness. *J Emerg Nurs* 2012; 38(5):429–34.

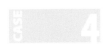

A 19-year-old woman with diabetes and hypertension requiring emergency contraception

David Chelmow

History of present illness

A 19-year-old gravida 1, para 1 woman presents to your urgent care clinic with complaint of a torn condom the prior evening. She has regular cycles. Her last menstrual period began two weeks ago. She is in a stable relationship with a single partner. They are using condoms as their birth control method, although irregularly. She has diabetes and chronic hypertension.

Due to lack of insurance and her other medical problems, she has had difficulty obtaining effective contraception. With her prior episodes of birth control failure, she took over-the-counter emergency contraception pills. She has done this several times in the last year, but is both worried about pregnancy and frustrated with the cost. She reports she is working while her partner completes college, and she hopes to have another child when he is employed and they have insurance.

Physical examination

General appearance: Well-developed, well-nourished woman appearing frustrated but in no apparent distress
Vital signs:

Temperature: 37.0°C
Pulse: 95 beats/min
Blood pressure: 142/90 mmHg
Respiratory rate: 16 breaths/min
Oxygen saturation: 100% on room air

Abdomen: Soft, nontender
External genitalia: Unremarkable
Vagina: Unremarkable, scant discharge
Cervix: Parous, no mucopurulent discharge
Uterus: Anteverted, nontender, normal size, mobile
Adnexa: Nontender, without masses
Laboratory studies: Urine pregnancy test: Negative

How would you manage this patient?

The patient had inadequately protected intercourse at midcycle. She has had recurring episodes of unprotected sex and contraceptive failure. She has not completed childbearing. She needs both emergency contraception to prevent unwanted pregnancy at present, and long-acting reversible contraception (LARC) to prevent pregnancy until she is ready to conceive. A copper intrauterine device (IUD) would safely and effectively meet both these needs.

Emergency contraception

This patient clearly needs emergency contraception. She has had a contraceptive failure at midcycle, which can have as high as a 25% risk of pregnancy. There are multiple options for emergency contraception (Table 4.1) [1]. Despite her medical comorbidities, she could use any of the available forms of emergency contraception. Recommendations for emergency contraception are outlined by the Centers for Disease Control and Prevention (CDC) in their "US selected practice recommendations for contraceptive use, 2013" [2] and their "US medical eligibility criteria for contraception use, 2010" [3]. The CDC's medical eligibility criteria are clear that, regardless of medical comorbidities, benefits likely exceed risks for each emergency contraceptive option, even use of combined (estrogen and progestin) hormonal contraception. This recommendation reflects the increased risks associated with continuing pregnancy in patients with comorbidities. Even with combined hormonal emergency contraception, the two doses required

Table 4.1 Options for emergency contraception

Option	Formulation
Progestin	Plan B One-Step® (1.5 mg levonorgestrel single dose)*
Ulipristal acetate	Ella® (ulipristal acetate 30 mg single dose up to 5 days after unprotected sex or birth control failure)
Combined oral contraceptives	One dose within 120 hours after unprotected intercourse and a second dose 12 hours after the first dose†
Copper intrauterine device (IUD)	ParaGard®

* Available over the counter to women over age 15 with proof of age. The package labeling states to use within 72 hours of unprotected sex, but it is still likely effective up to 120 hours.
† Per the Centers for Disease Control and Prevention's "US medical eligibility criteria for contraceptive use, 2010" [3], the FDA declared the following 22 brands of oral contraceptives to be safe and effective for emergency contraception: Ogestrel® or Ovral® (1 dose is 2 white pills); Levlen® or Nordette® (1 dose is 4 light-orange pills); Cryselle®, Levora®, Low-Ogestrel®, Lo/Ovral®, or Quasence® (1 dose is 4 white pills); Tri-Levlen® or Triphasil® (1 dose is 4 yellow pills); Jolessa®, Portia®, Seasonale®, or Trivora® (1 dose is 4 pink pills); Seasonique® (1 dose is 4 light blue-green pills); Empresse® (1 dose is 4 orange pills); Alesse®, Lessina®, or Levlite® (1 dose is 5 pink pills); Aviane® (1 dose is 5 orange pills); and Lutera® (1 dose is 5 white pills).

Acute Care and Emergency Gynecology, ed. David Chelmow, Christine R. Isaacs and Ashley Carroll. Published by Cambridge University Press.
© Cambridge University Press 2015.

for emergency contraception would be expected to have negligible risk, particularly when compared to those associated with long-term use for contraception in patients with medical comorbidities. This patient has appropriately used single-dose levonorgestrel emergency contraception in the past, which was Food and Drug Administration (FDA) approved and available without prescription for women 18 years of age and older when she used it. Related regulations are rapidly changing at the time of writing, and it is hoped that levonorgestrel emergency contraception will soon be available without prescription to women of any age. The FDA-approved single-dose levonorgestrel (Plan B One-Step®) is safe and effective, but unfortunately expensive, with retail prices typically in the $30–50 range. While it can be safely used as often as necessary, it is a poor substitute for an effective first-line birth control method.

This patient would also greatly benefit from effective LARC. She has no contraindications to any of the available methods [4]. The copper IUD (ParaGard® T380A) is particularly attractive in this situation as it is an effective option for LARC and is effective for emergency contraception. The Cochrane review [5] found limited data meeting inclusion criteria for their review. However, on the strength of seven nonrandomized studies included in their discussion, they quoted a 0.09% failure rate and explicitly stated that the copper IUD was the most effective method of emergency contraception, with the added benefit of long-term contraception. In comparison, the levonorgestrel regimen is 60–94% effective [1]. According to the Cochrane review, 80% of women who had their IUD placed for emergency contraception continued use of the IUD long-term [5]. A second systematic review also estimated a failure rate of 9% [6].

There are several barriers to use of the copper IUD for emergency contraception, with cost being the largest. Device and placement costs can be in excess of $500. Some patients have insurance that will cover the insertion and device. Under the Affordable Care Act, it should be available without copay. Some of these insurance companies will allow insertion without preapproval, while others have telephone preapproval processes that can be done while the patient waits. In other circumstances where the preapproval process is lengthy, it may not be possible to place the IUD for emergency contraception unless the patient is willing to pay. As emergency contraception in general appears to be most effective when administered as soon as possible after inadequately protected intercourse, if there is going to be a significant delay in obtaining the device or insurance preapproval, administration of pharmacologic emergency contraception would be advisable. For some patients without insurance coverage, anxiety related to potential pregnancy combined with accumulating costs from repetitive purchase of pharmacologic emergency contraception may make self-payment an acceptable option. Cost of the device and insertion is not dissimilar from the cost of pregnancy termination, and it is significantly lower risk. Alternatively, standard pharmacologic emergency

contraception could be provided, with a plan to initiate long-term reversible contraception as soon as possible. This option would be particularly appropriate for a woman who would strongly prefer a contraceptive implant or levonorgestrel-containing IUD, neither of which has been studied as emergency contraception.

The CDC's selected practice recommendations [2] are to place the copper IUD within five days of unprotected intercourse or suspected contraceptive failure, although they allow extending this as far as five days after ovulation in patients where the timing of ovulation can be determined. The CDC medical eligibility criteria [3] place only two limitations on copper IUD use for emergency contraception. First, it should not be used if the patient is already pregnant because of concerns about serious pelvic infection and septic spontaneous abortion. Second, caution needs to be exercised if placing for emergency contraception in the setting of rape. The criteria state that use is category 1 (no restriction) when the risk for sexually transmitted infection is low, but category 3 (risks usually outweigh benefits) when the risk is high. They provide no guidance as to how to make this determination in this setting, which would typically be associated with a high risk of sexually transmitted infection.

For this patient, the risk of pregnancy is not insignificant given the inconsistent use of condoms, and verifying a negative pregnancy test is important. The American College of Obstetricians and Gynecologists (ACOG) practice bulletin number 112 [1] states that administration of emergency contraception should not be delayed by pregnancy testing, but this statement was likely intended to refer to emergency contraception pills, which are unlikely to cause harm if administered to someone already pregnant. As placing an IUD in someone already pregnant poses a significant risk, verification of a negative pregnancy test is prudent for this patient.

In placing the device, consideration needs to be given to choice of the copper IUD as the long-term contraceptive method. There are several advantages of the copper IUD, including a low failure rate compared to nonlong-acting methods. Its major advantage compared to other long-acting reversible methods is its effectiveness for up to 10 years without change. This patient's plans are unlikely to require 10 years of contraception, but the device becomes cost effective relative to alternatives in a much shorter period of time. Removing the emergency contraceptive need from the decision, other LARC methods have some important advantages. In particular, the levonorgestrel IUD is chosen by many women because it decreases menstrual length and flow, and it is FDA approved as a treatment for heavy menstrual bleeding. For this patient, with otherwise normal menses, it would be expected that she would do well with the copper IUD.

The CDC's medical eligibility criteria [3] recommend that the copper IUD not be placed in the setting of high risk for sexually transmitted infection present at the time of method initiation. This patient does not appear to be at high risk. Thought about the relationship between IUD use and pelvic inflammatory disease (PID) has evolved. The ACOG practice bulletin number 121 [4] states: "There are no studies demonstrating an increased risk of pelvic inflammatory disease (PID) in nulliparous IUD users, and no evidence that IUD use is associated with subsequent infertility." The medical eligibility criteria list IUDs as category 2 for nulliparous and adolescent women, and ACOG encourages their use in these populations [4,7]. Despite her young age, the copper IUD is very appropriate for this patient. It is important not to place a copper IUD in an emergency contraception setting with intent of long-term use unless the patient meets the criteria for placement in an elective setting.

This patient underwent a physical examination as part of her evaluation. An examination is not necessary before administration of pharmacologic emergency contraception, which should be made available to patients with as few barriers as possible [1,2]. However, it is required to assess for mucopurulent cervicitis and uterine abnormalities prior to IUD placement [2], so an examination is appropriate here. Given her age, screening should be performed for chlamydia as per the US Preventative Services Task Force screening recommendations. Gonorrhea screening is also typically performed. The technique for placement of the IUD in emergency contraception setting is the same as when placed in a nonemergency setting.

Key teaching points

- Emergency contraception should be offered to anyone after unprotected intercourse not desiring pregnancy.
- Progestin-only and combined hormonal contraceptives, as well as the copper intrauterine device (IUD), are all safe and effective for emergency contraception.
- The Centers for Disease Control and Prevention's "US medical eligibility criteria for contraceptive use, 2010" [3] cite no medical conditions for which risks outweigh benefits for hormonal regimens for emergency contraception.
- The copper IUD is the most effective method of emergency contraception, with greater than 99% effectiveness, higher than the 60–95% effectiveness for the oral levonorgestrel regimen.
- Of the different methods for emergency contraception, only the copper IUD provides for long-term contraception.

References

1. American College of Obstetricians and Gynecologists. Emergency contraception. Practice Bulletin No. 112. *Obstet Gynecol* 2010;115: 1100–9.

2. Centers for Disease Control and Prevention. US selected practice recommendations for contraceptive use, 2013. *MMWR* 2013;62: 1–60.

3. Centers for Disease Control and Prevention. US medical eligibility criteria for contraceptive use, 2010. *MMWR* 2010;59:1–86.

4. American College of Obstetricians and Gynecologists. Long-acting reversible contraception: implants and intrauterine devices. Practice Bulletin No. 121. *Obstet Gynecol* 2011;118:184–96.

5. Cheng L, Che Y, Gülmezoglu AM. Interventions for emergency contraception. *Cochrane Database Syst Rev* 2012, Issue 8. Art. No.: CD001324. DOI: 10.1002/14651858.CD001324. pub4.

6. Cleland K, Zhu H, Goldstruck N, Cheng L, Trussel T. The efficacy of intrauterine devices for emergency contraception: a systematic review of 35 years of experience. *Hum Reprod* 2012;27:1994–2000.

7. American College of Obstetricians and Gynecologists. Adolescents and long-acting reversible contraception: implants and intrauterine devices. Committee opinion no. 539. *Obstet Gynecol* 2012;120:983–8.

Bleeding, pain, and fever four days after first-trimester termination

Erin L. Murata and Tony Ogburn

History of present illness

A 22-year-old gravida 1, para 0 woman presents to the emergency department with complaints of severe pelvic pain and fever to 38.3°C. She reports she underwent a surgical abortion at nine weeks' gestation at an outpatient clinic four days ago. She reports the procedure was uncomplicated and she recalls being given oral antibiotics prior to the procedure. She was well until she noted pelvic discomfort and a foul-smelling discharge two days ago. She has continued to have menstrual-like bleeding since the procedure. Her past medical history is unremarkable. She complains of nausea but no emesis. She has a prescription for birth control pills that she plans to start within the next week.

Physical examination

General appearance: Young woman in no acute distress
Vital signs:

Temperature: 38.5°C
Pulse: 102 beats/min
Respiratory rate: 18 breaths/min
Blood pressure: 100/55 mmHg
Oxygen saturation: 98% on room air

Abdomen: Soft, nondistended, tender to palpation in the suprapubic region, no peritoneal signs
Pelvic: External genitalia: normal
Vagina: Small amount of malodorous dark blood noted in vaginal vault
Cervix: Nulliparous appearing, small amount of blood in os
Uterus: Slightly enlarged, anteverted with moderate cervical motion and fundal tenderness
Adnexa: Moderate tenderness, no masses palpable
Laboratory studies:

WBCs: 14 200/μL
Ht: 36.0%

Imaging: Pelvic ultrasound showed an endometrial thickness of 2.7 cm consistent with retained tissue (Fig. 5.1a,b)

How would you manage this patient?

The patient has post-abortal endometritis with retained products of conception (POC). Patients with post-abortal endometritis should be treated with broad spectrum antibiotics. Treatment can be oral or intravenous depending on the severity of the infection and the patient's ability to tolerate oral medications. If retained POC are suspected on ultrasound, re-aspiration should be performed. This patient's ultrasound demonstrates a heterogeneous and thickened endometrium with normal appearing adnexa (not seen in Fig. 5.1a, b), raising concern for retained POC. There was no evidence of an abscess on her ultrasound.

This patient's symptoms and findings were consistent with endometritis with retained products. She did not appear severely ill but was complaining of nausea, so parenteral antibiotics were administered. The patient underwent an initial loading dose of intravenous antibiotics followed by uterine re-aspiration. The procedure can be performed in the outpatient or inpatient setting with electronic suction or a manual vacuum aspirator. Because of her nausea she was admitted overnight for hydration and continued observation. She did well overnight and was discharged home the next day to continue oral antibiotics (doxycycline 100 mg PO BID) for 14 days.

Post-abortal endometritis

Infection after first-trimester-induced abortion occurs with a reported frequency of 0.1–5.0% for first-trimester surgical termination, with most studies in the United States in the 0.1–2.0% range. The variation in reported frequency stems from differences in ascertainment of cases and definitions of infection among studies [1]. The incidence of retained POC following first-trimester abortion ranges from 0.29 to 1.96%.

Infection may manifest with pyrexia, pelvic pain or discomfort, persistent vaginal bleeding, and malodorous or purulent vaginal discharge. Findings on examination may include abnormal vital signs, including fever, tachycardia, and hypotension, as well as abdominal and pelvic tenderness, malodorous vaginal discharge, vaginal bleeding, cervical motion tenderness, and palpable tubo-ovarian abscess. Laboratory evaluation is typically limited to a complete blood count (CBC) and nucleic acid amplification tests (NAATs) for gonorrhea and chlamydia if the patient did not have them prior to the procedure. Vaginal, uterine, and blood cultures are not typically helpful and should not be obtained routinely. Imaging should include pelvic ultrasound as retained POC is a finding often associated with post-abortal infection. A thickened and heterogeneous endometrial stripe on ultrasound should raise suspicion for retained products. There are

Acute Care and Emergency Gynecology, ed. David Chelmow, Christine R. Isaacs and Ashley Carroll. Published by Cambridge University Press. © Cambridge University Press 2015.

(a)

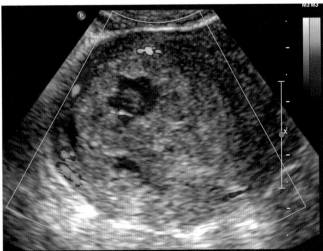

Fig. 5.1 (a,b) Retained products of conception.

(b)

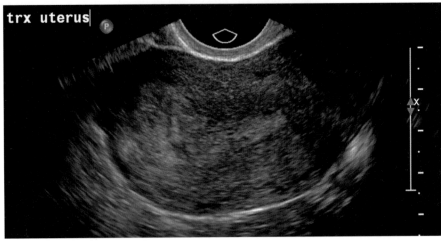

no definitive criteria for diagnosis of retained products on ultrasound. Hematometra or decidual tissue can have a similar appearance [2]. Additional imaging studies such as CT or MRI are not indicated unless pelvic abscess or other etiology, such as appendicitis or bowel injury with perforation, is suspected. In this case, the patient's examination is not consistent with a bowel injury as she had no peritoneal signs.

Genital tract infection following termination is usually polymicrobial with bacteria originating from the genital tract. Upper genital tract involvement is caused by ascending infection and can result in endometritis or pelvic inflammatory disease, while lower genital tract infection may manifest as vaginitis. Severe infection is rare after first-trimester abortion but can occur with the development of pelvic abscess, sepsis, or toxic shock syndrome. While endometritis typically presents with fever, pain, and bleeding, severe infection may present with bacteremia and hypotension with sepsis, or acute-onset cardiovascular collapse as in the case of toxic shock syndrome [3]. The patient with a pelvic abscess usually appears ill and will typically have findings on imaging.

Treatment of acute infection

Post-abortal infection should be treated promptly as it can progress to severe infection with the development of pelvic abscess or sepsis. In addition, there are associated long-term sequelae including increased risk of ectopic pregnancy, infertility, and chronic pelvic pain that may be diminished by timely treatment. In one large randomized trial, outpatient treatment appears to be as effective as inpatient treatment in resolution of disease as well as prevention of long-term sequelae [4]. This study excluded pregnant and post-abortal patients, but in the absence of data specific to such patients, a similar treatment approach may be utilized.

Treatment of the acute post-abortal infection should be guided by the patient's presentation and severity of infection. Uncomplicated infection may be treated with oral antibiotics if the patient is able to tolerate and comply with the regimen. Severe infection or patient inability to tolerate oral medication should prompt hospital admission and treatment with intravenous broad spectrum antibiotics.

Parenteral regimens

A. Cefotetan 2 g IV every 12 hours
OR
Cefoxitin 2 g IV every 6 hours
PLUS
Doxycycline 100 mg PO or IV every 12 hours

B. Clindamycin 900 mg IV every 8 hours
PLUS
Gentamicin loading dose IV or IM (2 mg/kg of body weight), followed by a maintenance dose (1.5 mg/kg) every 8 hours. Single daily dosing (3–5 mg/kg) can be substituted

Oral regimens

A. Ceftriaxone 250 mg IM in a single dose
PLUS
Doxycycline 100 mg PO BID for 14 days
WITH or WITHOUT
Metronidazole 500 mg PO BID for 14 days

B. Cefoxitin 2 g IM in a single dose and probenecid, 1 g PO administered concurrently in a single dose
PLUS
Doxycycline 100 mg PO BID for 14 days
WITH or WITHOUT
Metronidazole 500 mg PO BID for 14 days

* Adapted from Centers for Disease Control and Prevention [5].
 BID, twice a day; IM, intramuscularly; IV, intravenously; PO, *per os* (orally).

Patients with signs of sepsis require aggressive treatment with antibiotics and re-aspiration and may require fluid resuscitation and possibly pressors if hypotension develops. In the rare case of patients with toxic shock syndrome, treatment should be expeditious and aggressive with prompt fluid resuscitation, administration of pressors and broad spectrum antibiotics, and consideration of surgical intervention (e.g. hysterectomy). Patients with pelvic abscess may require percutaneous drainage or surgical intervention in addition to intravenous antibiotics.

Current antibiotic regimens for the treatment of post-abortal infection vary, but due to the polymicrobial nature of these infections, initial therapy should be broad spectrum. The regimens recommended by the Centers for Disease Control and Prevention [5] for treatment of pelvic inflammatory disease are appropriate for post-abortal infections. Recommended regimens are summarized in Table 5.1. Initial therapy for the uncomplicated patient should include parenteral cefoxitin (2 g + 1 g of probenicid) or ceftriaxone (250 mg) plus doxycycline 100 mg PO BID for a total of 14 days. Alternate oral regimens including the use of quinolones may not be as effective due to increased resistance. Patients who have worsening or persistent infection despite outpatient treatment, or who are unable to tolerate oral antibiotics, should be admitted for intravenous antibiotic therapy.

Parenteral treatment for severe infection or failed outpatient treatment includes doxycycline 100 mg IV BID with cefoxitin 2 g IV daily, or clindamycin 900 mg every 8 hours plus an aminoglycoside such as gentamicin at a dose of 1.5 mg/kg IV every 8 hours. Once the patient has stabilized and is improving, parenteral antibiotics may be discontinued and followed by a 14-day course of an acceptable oral antibiotic regimen such as doxycycline.

Retained products

In the patient with endometritis, if ultrasound suggests retained POC, uterine evacuation should occur promptly in conjunction with antibiotic administration. Thorough imaging, including Doppler assessment, is useful in the detection of retained products, but some cases may be missed. Consideration should be given to curettage in patients that fail antibiotic therapy, even if there is no evidence of retained products on ultrasound. If tissue is present in the cervical os, it should be removed. Patients with retained POC without symptoms of infection may be managed expectantly, medically with an uterotonic agent, such as misoprostol, or surgically.

Prevention of post-abortal infection

Appropriate equipment and technique will prevent most infectious morbidity [6]. Prophylactic antibiotics decrease the incidence of post-abortal infection and universal administration is more effective than risk-based or screen-and-treat approaches.

A meta-analysis published in the mid-1990s concluded that prophylaxis in all patients prior to induced abortion decreases the rate of infection by over 40%, is cost-effective, and should be universally employed [7]. As such, all patients undergoing surgical termination should receive prophylactic antibiotics prior to the procedure regardless of their risk factors. Though the optimal antibiotic and regimen has not been determined, tetracyclines and nitroimidazoles are effective. Doxycycline is the most common antibiotic utilized in the United States.

The American College of Obstetricians and Gynecologists (ACOG) recommends doxycycline 100 mg PO 1 hour before the procedure and 200 mg PO after the procedure, **or** metronidazole 500 mg PO BID for 5 days after the procedure [8]. The Society of Family Planning (SFP) recommends administering doxycycline within 12 hours of a surgical termination [9]. Taking the medication the night before the procedure is effective and may decrease the incidence of perioperative nausea and vomiting.

Contraception after abortion

Patients undergoing termination of pregnancy typically need effective contraception. It is acceptable, and it may be preferable, to place an intrauterine device (IUD) immediately after a surgical abortion [10]. There is no increase of expulsion or infectious complications and repeat unintended pregnancy may be decreased. If a patient with an IUD placed immediately after an abortion subsequently presents with an infection, the IUD may be left in place while antibiotic treatment is initiated. If the patient does not improve as expected, consideration should be given to removal of the IUD. In the patient with infection and retained products that requires re-aspiration, the IUD should be removed. In patients with retained tissue on imaging, but no evidence of infection, the IUD may be left in place and the patient treated expectantly or with medication.

Patients with post-abortal infection who are not using an effective contraceptive method should be counseled about their options. Except for the IUD, where insertion is contraindicated in the setting of acute infection, all methods can be initiated at this time including the implant, depot medroxyprogesterone acetate injection (Depo-Provera® CI), or combination hormonal methods.

Key teaching points

- Infection and retained tissue following first-trimester abortion is rare.
- Post-abortal infection should be treated promptly and with broad spectrum antibiotics.
- If retained tissue is present in the infected patient, re-aspiration should be performed. Re-aspiration is not necessary in the uninfected patient with retained tissue.
- In the uncomplicated patient, therapy may be performed as an outpatient.
- Effective contraception, including long-acting reversible contraception, should be offered to post-abortion patients.

References

1. Lichtenberg S, Grimes D. Surgical complications: prevention and management. In Paul M, Lichtenberg S, Borgatta L, eds. *Management of Unintended and Abnormal Pregnancy*. Chichester, UK, Blackwell Publishing Ltd, 2009, pp. 224–50.

2. Rahangdale L. Infectious complications of pregnancy termination. *Clin Obstet Gynecol* 2009;52(2):198–204.

3. World Health Organization. *Clinical Management of Abortion Complications: A Practical Guide*, 1994. Available at http://www.who.int/reproductivehealth/publications/unsafe_abortion/MSM_94_1/en/index.html.

4. Ness R, Trautmann G, Richter H, et al. Effectiveness of treatment strategies in women with pelvic inflammatory disease: a randomized trial. *Obstet Gynecol* 2005;106:573–80.

5. Centers for Disease Control and Prevention. *Sexually Transmitted Diseases. Treatment Guidelines, 2010. Pelvic Inflammatory Disease*, 2010. Available at http://www.cdc.gov/std/treatment/2010/pid.htm.

6. Meckstroth K, Paul M. First trimester aspiration abortion. In Paul M, Lichtenberg S, Borgatta L, eds. *Management of Unintended and Abnormal Pregnancy*. Chichester, UK, Blackwell Publishing Ltd, 2009, pp. 135–55.

7. Sawaya G, Grady D, Kerlikowske K, Grimes D. Antibiotics at the time of induced abortion: the case for universal prophylaxis based on a meta-analysis. *Obstet Gynecol* 1996;87:884–90.

8. American College of Obstetricians and Gynecologists. Antibiotic prophylaxis for gynecologic procedures. Practice Bulletin No. 104. *Obstet Gynecol* 2009;113:1180–9.

9. Society of Family Planning. Prevention of infection after induced abortion. *Contraception* 2011;83:295–309.

10. Centers for Disease Control and Prevention. US medical eligibility criteria for contraceptive use, 2010. *MMWR* 2010;59(No. RR-4):1–86.

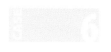

A 25-year-old woman requesting emergency contraception

Reni A. Soon and Tod C. Aeby

History of present illness

A 25-year-old gravida 0 woman presents to the urgent care clinic requesting emergency contraception (EC). She and her boyfriend had intercourse four days prior using a condom, which reportedly "broke." She states her last menstrual period (LMP) started approximately two weeks prior to today's visit. A friend told her about EC and so she came to the clinic as soon as possible. Her medical history is only significant for migraine headaches with aura. She denies any surgical history. She is on no medications. She smokes socially and drinks one or two alcoholic drinks per week. She is very stressed out about the possibility of getting pregnant.

Physical examination

General appearance: Normal, healthy woman who appears anxious
Vital signs: All within normal limits (BMI: 31 kg/m^2)
Laboratory studies: Urine pregnancy test: Negative

How would you manage this patient?

A copper intrauterine device (IUD) was recommended to her as the most effective method of EC. Since she declined this method [or if it had been unavailable], the next most effective method of EC was ulipristal acetate (UPA). She should be given a prescription or administered the 30 mg pill in the clinic and advised to either abstain from intercourse or to use condoms for the next 14 days (or until she gets her next menses, whichever comes first). She should also be counseled about the importance of initiating additional/alternative contraceptive methods as soon as possible.

Emergency contraception (Table 6.1)

Emergency contraception (EC) is available in four forms: the copper IUD, levonorgestrel emergency contraceptive pills (ECPs), UPA ECPs, and combination estrogen–progestin pills. There are almost no contraindications to EC, and EC should be considered for any woman presenting with a recent act of unprotected intercourse, or like in this case, a failed form of contraception.

ECPs are pills formulated specifically for use as EC and include UPA and levonorgestrel. UPA is a progesterone receptor modulator that has been shown to reduce the risk of pregnancy up to five days after unprotected intercourse. The mechanism of action of both UPA and levonorgestrel is the inhibition or delay of ovulation by interfering with the release of luteinizing hormone (LH) from the pituitary. The LH surge is required for ovulation to occur. While levonorgestrel cannot prevent ovulation once the preovulatory LH surge has begun [1], UPA has the additional benefit of preventing follicular rupture even after initiation of the LH surge [1]. This is believed to be the explanation for UPA's higher efficacy at preventing pregnancy, when compared to levonorgestrel, if the drug is given midcycle during ovulation, when a woman is most fertile.

If ECPs are obtained during the three- to five-day time period after unprotected (or underprotected) intercourse, UPA has again been shown to be more efficacious when compared to levonorgestrel [2]. Furthermore, data from two randomized trials of levonorgestrel and UPA suggest higher failure rates in obese women (BMI >30 kg/m^2) for both medications, but the risk of failure is greater with levonorgestrel, when compared to UPA [3]. Overall, it appears that UPA is more effective at preventing pregnancies, especially if the patient is obese or is in her midcycle. Both ECPs, levonorgestrel and UPA, are associated with slightly higher failure rates than the copper IUD [4].

UPA is available only by prescription in the United States (marketed under the brand name Ella®), and is available as a single 30 mg oral dose. Levonorgestrel can be taken as either two 0.75 mg oral doses (marketed as Plan B®) or one 1.5 mg dose (marketed as Plan B One-Step®). Generic equivalents for both are available. The label on the two-dose levonorgestrel formulations states to take the 0.75 mg tablets 12 hours apart. Research has shown, however, that the regimen is just as effective if taken as a single dose simultaneously [5], which eliminates the risk of noncompliance with the second dose. Plan B One-Step is available over-the-counter, and as of June 2013, there are no age restrictions to accessing this medication. The other formulations of levonorgestrel ECPs are "behind the counter," available without prescription to anyone aged 17 or older. A single treatment costs between $35 and $60, with generics being only slightly cheaper.

The combined estrogen–progestin (Yuzpe) [6] regimen can be created using conventional combination oral contraceptive pills and is taken in two doses. Each dose must contain at least 100 µg of ethinyl estradiol and 0.5 mg of levonorgestrel; therefore, depending on the pill formulation, each dose would consist of two to six pills. Like with other forms of EC, the first dose should be taken as soon as possible but within 120 hours of unprotected intercourse. The second dose is taken 12 hours later [5].

Although the combined estrogen–progestin regimen has not been compared to UPA specifically, it is considered to be

Table 6.1 A suggested approach to women requesting EC

What to assess?	Best choices for EC	Why?
Time since first act of unprotected or underprotected intercourse	If occurred between 3 and 5 days ago, consider copper IUD or UPA as best choices	Copper IUD and UPA are more effective than levonorgestrel, particularly if intercourse occurred >72 hours and <120 hours before administration of EC
Where in her menstrual cycle did the unprotected intercourse occur?	If occurred during most fertile time (near ovulation), consider copper IUD or UPA as best choices	Copper IUD and UPA are more effective than levonorgestrel, particularly when sex occurs during the most fertile time in the menstrual cycle
What is her BMI?	If she is obese (BMI $\geq$30 kg/m^2), consider copper IUD or UPA as best choices	Effectiveness of copper IUD is not affected by BMI. Effectiveness of UPA superior to levonorgestrel in obese patients
Can the patient access a prescription?	Yes: UPA No: Levonorgestrel regimens	Levonorgestrel regimens are available for "over-the-counter" access

BMI, body mass index; EC, emergency contraception; IUD, intrauterine device; UPA, ulipristal acetate.

less effective than both levonorgestrel (and thus UPA) in preventing pregnancy. It is also associated with more side effects such as nausea and emesis [5], and, for these reasons, the Yuzpe method should be a second-line choice for EC.

Routine use of anti-emetics before taking ECPs is not recommended; however, these medications may be considered, based on clinical judgment. If vomiting occurs within three hours of taking ECPs, another dose of ECPs should be taken and an anti-emetic should be added [7].

The US Medical Eligibility Criteria for Contraceptive Use (USMEC) does not list any medical conditions for which ECPs should be avoided [8], although it does not specifically address UPA as this medication was approved the same year the USMEC was released. Even medical conditions that may preclude the use of combined hormonal contraceptive methods for regular contraception (migraines with aura – as in our patient – cardiovascular disease, liver disease) are not contraindications for ECPs. The duration of use for the combined estrogen–progestin regimen as an EC is believed to be too short to incur a negative clinical impact despite a patient's medical comorbidities [8]. ECPs should, therefore, be offered to any woman who has had unprotected intercourse and does not desire pregnancy [5].

No clinical exams or testing need to be done prior to administration of ECPs [7]. However, because there is some evidence that BMI may affect the efficacy of levonorgestrel more so than UPA, the patient's weight may be an important consideration. Pregnancy testing is not necessary, as ECPs do not affect a pregnancy once implantation has occurred, and even high-dose oral contraceptives have not been shown to cause birth defects [7].

Because ECPs work by inhibiting or delaying ovulation, patients may be at risk for pregnancy later in the same cycle, and so regular contraception should be encouraged immediately. There is a theoretical concern that hormonal contraceptives could be affected by the antiprogestin activity of UPA. Therefore, in addition to advising regular contraceptive initiation, it is recommended that patients who take UPA abstain from intercourse or use condoms for 14 days after taking the pill [7]. For patients who take levonorgestrel-based EC, it is recommended that they abstain from intercourse or use condoms for seven days following EC use. They should also be encouraged to start a regular, reliable contraceptive method as quickly as possible [7].

Though our patient declined this option, the copper IUD is the most effective form of EC [4], and it can be inserted up to five days after the first act of unprotected intercourse that follows the onset of a woman's normal menstrual flow unless there is concern for pelvic inflammatory disease (PID) and/or purulent cervicitis [8]. If ovulation can be reasonably estimated (certain LMP and regular cycles), the copper IUD could be inserted more than five days after unprotected intercourse as long as it has not been more than five days after ovulation [7]. A recent systematic review of studies published over 35 years included over 7000 post-coital IUD insertions and found only 10 pregnancies, for a failure rate of 0.14% [4]. Not only is the copper IUD a highly effective form of EC, it has the added advantage of continuing to provide very reliable contraception for up to 10 years.

Because the mechanism of action of UPA is to inhibit or delay ovulation, our patient was counseled about the possibility that she may ovulate later in the cycle and that immediately starting an effective regular method of contraception is critical to preventing an unintended pregnancy. In addition to abstaining for the next 14 days, she decided that she would schedule an appointment with her gynecologist to obtain a contraceptive implant later in the week.

Key teaching points

- The copper intrauterine device (IUD) is the most effective method of emergency contraception (EC) and allows a woman to maintain long-acting reversible contraception.
- Emergency contraceptive pill (ECP) regimens include levonorgestrel pills, ulipristal acetate (UPA), and combined estrogen–progestin regimens.
- All EC can reduce the risk of pregnancy up to 5 days (120 hours) after unprotected or underprotected intercourse. BMI and ovulation timing should be taken into consideration when choosing an ECP

regimen as UPA (which requires a prescription) will be the more effective option.

- There are no contraindications to ECPs.

- The mechanism of action for ECPs is the delay of ovulation. Patients need to be advised that when using ECPs, regular contraception should also be initiated.

References

1. Gemzell-Danielsson K, Berger C, Lalitkumar PGL. Emergency contraception – mechanisms of action. *Contraception* 2013;87:300–8.

2. Glasier A, Cameron ST, Fine PM, et al. Ulipristal acetate versus levonorgestrel for emergency contraception: a randomized non-inferiority trial and meta-analysis. *Lancet* 2010;375:555–62.

3. Glasier A, Cameron ST, Blithe D, et al. Can we identify women at risk of pregnancy despite using emergency contraception? Data from randomized trials of ulipristal acetate and levonorgestrel. *Contraception* 2011;84:363–7.

4. Cleland K, Zhu H, Goldstuck N, Cheng L, Trussel J. The efficacy of intrauterine devices for emergency contraception: a systematic review of 35 years of experience. *Hum Reprod* 2012;27(7): 1994–2000.

5. American College of Obstetricians and Gynecologists. Emergency contraception. Practice Bulletin No. 112. *Obstet Gynecol* 2010;115(5): 1100–9.

6. Yuzpe AA, Percival Smith R, Rademaker AW. A multicenter clinical investigation employing ethenyl estradiol combined with dl-norgestrel as a postcoital contraceptive agent. *Fertil Steril* 1982;37:508–13.

7. Centers for Disease Control and Prevention. US selected practice recommendations for contraception use, 2013. *MMWR* 2013;62:1–60.

8. Centers for Disease Control and Prevention. US medical eligibility criteria for contraceptive use, 2010. *MMWR* 2010;59:1–86.

Persistent trichomonas infection

Lilja Stefansson

History of present illness

A 45-year-old black woman presents as an urgent walk-in appointment with complaints of vulvar itching and vaginal discharge. She reports that six months ago she had been sexually active one time with a new male partner and did not use a condom. She subsequently developed vaginal discharge several days after that event and was diagnosed with trichomonas at her local health department. She was given metronidazole 2 g PO, but she continued to have vulvar irritation and vaginal discharge. When she returned to the health department a second time, she was diagnosed with trichomonas once again and given a second course of metronidazole. Despite repeated treatment and no further sexual activity, she did not have complete relief of her symptoms. She reports that she has been seen multiple times in various urgent care clinics with treatments for "infections" including intramuscular ceftriaxone, oral doxycycline, and oral fluconazole, yet, her symptoms persist. She is very upset and wants "to know what is wrong."

The patient's past medical history is unremarkable. Her only surgeries are an appendectomy and a postpartum tubal ligation. She is a nonsmoker and does not drink alcohol. She works full time as a hair stylist. She adamantly denies having intercourse since her diagnosis of trichomonas and she is anxious about initiating any future intimate relationships due to her symptoms. Her review of symptoms is otherwise negative.

Physical examination

General appearance: Pleasant and cooperative woman who was tearful at times during the interview

Vital signs:

Temperature: 36.8°C
Pulse: 80 beats/min
Respiratory rate: 16 breaths/min
Blood pressure: 138/86 mmHg
BMI: 39 kg/m^2

Cardiovascular: Regular rate and rhythm
Respiration rate: Clear to auscultation with deep breaths
Abdomen: Obese, soft, nontender, nondistended
Pelvic:

Vulva: Erythematous around the introitus with excoriations. No lesions or ulcers

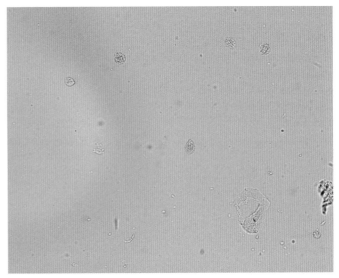

Fig. 7.1 Microscopic wet mount – motile unicellular, oval-shaped organisms with multiple flagella were visualized. (Courtesy of Aaron Hill, Virginia Commonwealth University School of Medicine.)

Speculum: Copious amount of green, frothy discharge, cervix mildly friable
Bimanual: No cervical motion tenderness, small, mobile anteverted uterus, no adnexal tenderness

Laboratory studies:

NAATs: Negative for chlamydia and gonorrhea
Microscopic wet mount (Fig. 7.1): Motile unicellular, oval-shaped organisms with multiple flagella are visualized. No clue cells, no hyphae, abundant white blood cells noted
Vaginal pH: >5.0

How would you manage this patient?

This patient has a persistent trichomonas infection despite being treated with the first-line therapy of metronidazole multiple times. Her treatment history suggests that she has a strain of *Trichomonas vaginalis* that has become resistant to metronidazole.

The patient was subsequently given 2 g tinidazole PO × 1 dose, but experienced only temporary and mild improvements of her symptoms. After a follow-up five-day course of metronidazole obtained suboptimal relief yet again, a trichomonas culture was collected and sent to the Centers for Disease Control and Prevention (CDC) for evaluation. Upon CDC

Acute Care and Emergency Gynecology, ed. David Chelmow, Christine R. Isaacs and Ashley Carroll. Published by Cambridge University Press. © Cambridge University Press 2015.

recommendations, she was given a prolonged course of tinidazole that alleviated her symptoms. A follow-up visit one month later revealed no motile trichomonads on wet mount microscopy. A repeat culture was negative and confirmed resolution of her infection.

Trichomonas vaginalis

Trichomonas vaginalis is one of the most common sexually transmitted infections worldwide. In the United States it has a prevalence of 3.1%, equating to approximately 7.4 million cases annually [1]. Trichomonas rates are higher in women than in men, with rates of 13–34% for women versus 3–17% for men [2]. Amongst women, there is a higher prevalence of infection in those from lower socioeconomic backgrounds and in African Americans. In these populations, rates are as high as 13%, whereas it is 1.3% in non-Hispanic white women [1–3].

Transmission of trichomonas occurs through sexual contact and results in symptoms such as vaginal discharge (classically green in coloration with frothy character), vaginitis, vulvar irritation, and pruritus. It is extremely rare that trichomonas is contracted through nonsexual means and there are only a few case reports, predominantly from third-world countries, which hypothesize transmission deriving from contaminated water supplies and the use of pit latrines. Trichomonads can live for more than three hours outside of the body if kept wet [4]. If a woman acquires trichomoniasis while pregnant, infection can lead to premature rupture of membranes, preterm labor, and low birth weight infants [1]. Currently, the CDC recommends treatment with nitroimidazoles (metronidazole and tinidazole) [3]. However, there is evidence of developing resistance to these medicines, which highlights the need for developing other treatment options.

Trichomonas infections are usually diagnosed by placing a sampling of vaginal or urethral discharge on a glass slide with normal saline (known as a wet mount), and then using light microscopy to identify motile, multiflagellated protozoans, as seen in Fig. 7.1. The specimens should be examined within 10 minutes of collection of the sample and preparation of the slide. This is a simple, inexpensive method of diagnosing an infection; however, the sensitivity is 51–65% and is examiner-dependent. The gold standard for diagnosing infection is by culture, with specificity at nearly 100% and sensitivity at 75–96%. Liquid-based Pap smears can also identify Trichomonas vaginalis infections that should be treated without warranting further testing. The specificity of this test is high at 98–100%, but it is important to emphasize that it should not be used as a screening test as sensitivity is low (73% in symptomatic patients and 44% in asymptomatic patients) [5].

Once trichomoniasis is diagnosed, treatment is generally accomplished with metronidazole 2 g PO × 1 dose, as this medication has been used since 1960. The newer drug, tinidazole, may be used as well (tinidazole 2 g PO × 1 dose) [3,6] (Fig. 7.2). If a patient is reexposed and reacquires trichomonias, repeating the basic treatment regimen should be adequate. If

---

Treatment pathway (Per CDC Guidelines)
Initial diagnosis:
Metronidazole 2 g PO x 1 dose
OR
Tinidazole 2 g PO x 1 dose
↓
If this fails and re-exposure is ruled out, then:
Metronidazole 500 mg PO BID x 7 days
OR
Tinidazole 2 g PO x 1 dose
↓
If this fails and re-exposure is ruled out, then:
Metronidazole 2 g PO daily x 5 days
OR
Tinidazole 2 g PO x 5 days
↓
If this fails and re-exposure is ruled out, then
CDC Consultation for *T. vaginalis* susceptibilities
(ph. 770-488-4115)

Fig. 7.2 Treatment pathway (per Centers for Disease Control and Prevention guidelines [3]).

the patient continues to have symptoms with confirmation of persistent infection and with verification that the patient has **not** been reexposed after the initial treatment, then the therapy needs to be modified as resistance to metronidazole must be considered. Low-level resistance (meaning that the isolate has a minimum lethal concentration of 50–100 μg/mL) to metronidazole is present in 2–5% of cases, and high-level resistance is rare (minimum lethal concentration >400 µg/mL) [1,3]. If the single-dose regimen does not succeed in curing the vaginal infection, then an increased dose should be administered, such as metronidazole 500 mg PO BID × 7 days [7]. It has been shown that a prolonged and increased dose of metronidazole can treat an infection that is refractory to the single-dose regimen [6]. If this prolonged metronidazole treatment does not succeed in eradication of the infection, then treatment should switch to tinidazole. Tinidazole has a longer half-life, is generally better tolerated by patients, and obtains higher concentrations in affected tissues [3,7]. In rare cases when symptoms persist despite all of these interventions, susceptibility testing may be required and this is possible through the CDC (contact number: 770–488–4115; website: http://www.cdc.gov/std) [3]. Despite widespread use, vaginal metronidazole gel is not recommended. This route is less than 50% effective when compared to the oral regimen, as it is unable to obtain therapeutic dosage levels in the urethra and vaginal mucosa. When prescribing nitroimidazoles, it is also important to counsel patients not to consume alcohol during the medical treatment and until 24 hours after completion of metronidazole, or until 72 hours after completion of tinidazole due to the risk of disulfuram-like side effects [3].

In the patient described in this case, a swabbed vaginal culture was eventually sent to the CDC after failing the standard single-dose metronidazole, a prolonged dosage, and then single-dose tinidazole therapy. Because of her high-resistance strain identified, her treatment regimen was adjusted based on the CDC recommendations obtained. In most cases, clinical follow-up is not necessary or recommended unless clinical symptoms persist.

Key teaching points

- Trichomonas is one of the most common sexually transmitted infections in the world, causing symptoms of vulvar irritation, pruritus, and a green, frothy discharge.
- First-line therapy for a trichomonas infection is a nitroimidazole, typically metronidazole 2 g PO × 1 dose.
- The clinician should ensure that the patient has complied with treatment and has not been reexposed before progressing to longer duration therapies or switching treatment regimens.
- Prolonged metronidazole or tinidazole treatment may be necessary for the treatment of refractory trichomonas infections.

References

1. Kirkcaldy RD, Augostini P, Asbel LE et al. *Trichomonas vaginalis* antimicrobial drug resistance in six US cities, STD surveillance network, 2009–2010. *Emerg Infect Dis* 2012; 18(6):939–43.

2. Bachmann LH, Hobbs MM, Sena AC et al. *Trichomonas vaginalis* genital infections: progress and challenges. *Clin Infect Dis* 2011:53(S3):S160–72.

3. Centeres for Disease Control and Prvention. *Sexually Transmitted Diseases Treatment Guidelines* 2006 (CDC Publication Vol. 55, No. RR-11), pp. 52–54. Atlanta: US Department of Health and Human Services. Also available online: http://www.cdc.gov/STD/treatment/2006/rr5511.pdf.

4. Crucitti T, Jespers V, Mulenga C et al. Non-sexual transmission of *Trichomonas vaginalis* in adolescent girls attending school in Ndola, Namibia. *PLoS One* 2011;6(1):e16310. Doi: 10.1371/journal.pone.0016310.

5. Lara Torre E, Pinkerton JS. Accuracy of detection of *Trichomonas vaginalis* organisms on a liquid-based Papanicolau smear. *Am J Obstet Gynecol* 2003;188(2):354–6.

6. Crowell AL, Sanders-Lewis KA, Secor WE. In vitro metronidazole and tinidazole activities against metronidazole- resistant strains of *Trichomonas vaginalis*. *Antimicrob Agents Chemother* 2003;47(4):1407–9.

7. Bosserman EA, Helms DJ, Mosure DJ et al. Utility of antimicrobial susceptibility testing in *Trichomonas vaginalis*-infected women with clinical treatment failure. *Sex Trans Dis* 2011; 38(10):983–7.

A 42-year-old woman with recurrent unexplained vaginitis symptoms

Chemen M. Tate

History of present illness

A 42-year-old gravida 2, para 2 woman presents to your office as an urgent consultation from her primary care physician for persistent symptoms of vaginitis not responsive to traditional therapy. The patient reports symptoms of vaginal dryness, burning with intercourse, an excessive amount of yellow discharge, and intermittent feelings of vaginal irritation for the past two years. She denies vaginal odor, does not douche, and is in a monogamous relationship with her husband who has had a vasectomy. She reports being tested for "everything" with only negative results. She has been treated multiple times with oral fluconazole, terconazole, and metronidazole by several providers with minimal or no relief. She has most recently been treated with boric acid suppositories, which only made her symptoms worse for a time. She reports regular menses and has no medical or surgical history. She takes no medications.

She is embarrassed by her symptoms and rarely enjoys intercourse because of the discomfort. She is concerned these issues are damaging her relationship with her husband and reports feeling hopeless and frustrated. She is "willing to try anything."

Physical examination

General appearance: Well-developed, well-nourished woman in no apparent distress

Vital signs:

Temperature: 37.0°C
Pulse: 97 beats/min
Blood pressure: 106/68 mmHg
Respiratory rate: 15 breaths/min

HEENT: Negative
Chest: Clear to auscultation
Cardiac: Regular rate and rhythm
Abdomen: Soft, nontender, no palpable masses
External genitalia: Unremarkable
Vagina: Erythematous mucosa, a yellowish discharge is noted, no ulcers or lesions
Cervix: Parous and without abnormality
Uterus: Anteverted, mobile, and nontender, normal size
Adnexa: Nontender, no masses palpated
Laboratory studies:

NAATs: Negative for chlamydia and gonorrhea

Candida/bacterial vaginosis/trichomonas DNA probe: Negative
HSV-1/2 serum IgG: Negative
Whiff test: Negative
Vaginal pH: 6
Wet prep: Many WBCs, amidst rounded-appearing epithelial cells with prominent nuclei, and an absence of lactobacilli. Negative for trichomonas, hyphae, or clue cells

How would you manage this patient?

This patient gives a history that is common for many types of vaginitis. She has dyspareunia, abnormal discharge, and vaginal irritation. On examination, she has clinical features of an inflammatory vaginitis but typical laboratory studies for infectious vaginitis (trichomoniasis, bacterial vaginosis, candidiasis, etc.) are all negative. Microscopy confirms an inflammatory process with the increased presence of white blood cells (WBCs) and shows signs of desquamation with the presence of immature epithelial cells or parabasal cells. While one might find many similarities with postmenopausal atrophic vaginitis, this patient is menstruating regularly and does not endorse any other symptoms of estrogen deficiency. This patient's combination of physical and microscopic findings are consistent with the diagnosis of desquamative inflammatory vaginitis or "DIV."

Desquamative inflammatory vaginitis

As in this patient, the diagnosis of desquamative inflammatory vaginitis (DIV) is clinical. The basic diagnosis involves a triad of dyspareunia, increased vaginal discharge, and inflammation, as evidenced by vaginal erythema and increased WBCs on wet prep [1]. Trichomoniasis, bacterial vaginosis, candidiasis, *Neisseria gonorrhoeae*, and *Chlamydia trachomatis* should also be excluded. The differential diagnosis also includes more rare causes of vaginitis such as erosive vulvar lichen planus, cicatrical pemphigoid, pemphigus vulgaris, and linear immunoglobulin A (IgA) disease. These diseases may show extra genital manifestations, such as oral or integumentary ulcerations, bullae, or erosions, and will likely be unresponsive to the therapy outlined in this case. Specific histopathology or immunofluorescence findings can also be seen on biopsy in these rare cases. Common histologic findings of vulvar erosive lichen planus include a well-defined band, composed primarily

Acute Care and Emergency Gynecology, ed. David Chelmow, Christine R. Isaacs and Ashley Carroll. Published by Cambridge University Press.
© Cambridge University Press 2015.

Table 8.1 Desquamative inflammatory vaginitis (DIV) treatment strategies

Medication	Instructions
Clindamycin 2% vaginal cream	Use nightly × 4 weeks. If incomplete response, continue and evaluate in 2–4 weeks, or switch to 10% hydrocortisone administered vaginally
10% Hydrocortisone vaginal cream or suppository*	Use nightly × 4 weeks. If incomplete response, continue and evaluate in 2–4 weeks or switch to clindamycin 2% vaginal cream
2% Clindamycin + 10% hydrocortisone compounded as a vaginal cream or suppository	Use nightly × 4 weeks. If incomplete response, continue and evaluate in 2–4 weeks
Maintenance therapy[†] (for recurrent or refractory cases)	Once or twice weekly 2% clindamycin or 10% hydrocortisone

* 10% Hydrocortisone cream is not commercially manufactured: 25 mg hydrocortisone rectal suppositories (Anusol®) can be more cost effective and can be administered vaginally as a substitute when compounding is not available.
[†] Maintenance therapy is dictated by patient symptoms. Therefore, patients can self-taper to a dosing frequency that maintains a symptom-free state.

of lymphocytes, at the dermoepidermal junction and liquefaction or signs of degeneration of the basal layer [2]. The autoimmune bullous disorders are primarily diagnosed by direct immunofluorescence (DIF) techniques. Deposition of antibodies, often IgG, IgA, or C3, are seen along the basement membrane zone in 80–100% of these cases [3].

The evaluation of all women with complaints of recurrent vaginitis should include a speculum examination, vaginal pH testing, and saline microscopy with further infection testing as indicated. Commercial DNA-based tests are available and can significantly improve the detection of bacterial vaginosis (45% vs. 14%) and *Candida* (11% vs. 7%), when compared to saline microscopy alone. The low sensitivity of microscopy as a diagnostic tool for trichomonas infections make it insufficient for the exclusion of this pathogen. WBCs, which are numerous in patients with DIV, can also make it very difficult to identify trichomonads on saline microscopy. Nucleic acid-based testing for trichomoniasis is now considered the gold standard and can be performed with testing for *N. gonorrhea* and *C. trachomatis* infection from a thin prep vial, endocervical swab, or urine sample. These testing modalities increase the accuracy of the diagnosis in settings where speculum examination and/or microscopy is/are unavailable or unfeasible. When there is suspicion for extragenital disease manifestations, ulcerative lesions, or unresponsiveness to therapy, biopsy for histopathologic evaluation should be considered [4].

It is not known whether DIV represents a sterile inflammatory vaginitis or is the result of an infectious agent. Therefore, treatment of DIV is targeted at resolution of inflammation and/or treatment of potential infectious organisms. There are no randomized control trials available to guide treatment and most available studies characterizing DIV involve small numbers of patients. The International Society for the Study of Vulvovaginal Disease (ISSVD) recommends treatment with clindamycin 2% vaginal cream and 10% hydrocortisone cream administered intravaginally [5].

There are several strategies that have been recommended by the ISSVD and have shown to be effective (Table 8.1). Duration of treatment seems to be an important factor that is common among all described treatment regimens, and should last four to eight weeks. It is generally recommended to treat for four weeks followed by a repeat pelvic examination and repeat microscopy [6]. If physical examination and microscopy findings are normal after four weeks, treatment can be considered complete. If inflammation is still present on physical examination or microscopy, treatment should be continued an additional two to four weeks depending on the clinical response. Some patients will not be able to stop treatment without relapsing and may need maintenance therapy with either topical clindamycin or hydrocortisone used once or twice per week. In more severe cases, a higher potency steroid such as clobetasol can be used during the initial treatment phase. A lower potency steroid such as hydrocortisone should be used for maintenance.

Unfortunately, patients may relapse at intervals of months to years later. Treatment should be approached in the same way and routine surveillance via microscopy during symptom-free intervals may be considered. As most women with DIV are nonmenopausal and in their thirties to mid-forties, vaginal estrogen is not part of the treatment and does not seem to improve symptoms. DIV does occur in postmenopausal women and should be considered if estrogen therapy does not resolve atrophic vaginitis, or in patients who have a large amount of purulent vaginal discharge.

To help diminish feelings of frustration and to encourage long-term follow-up and compliance, patients should be counseled that many types of vaginitis are recurrent and can require extended treatment durations or maintenance medications to control symptoms. Patients should also be counseled that a great deal of research still needs to be done regarding the cause of all types of recurrent vaginitis and that treatment regimens will continue to evolve. The patient in this case had significant improvement after a four-week treatment course, but ultimately required weekly clindamycin to maintain a symptom-free state.

Key teaching points

- Desquamative inflammatory vaginitis (DIV) is a form of vaginitis. The diagnosis involves a triad of dyspareunia, increased vaginal discharge, and inflammation as evidenced by vaginal erythema and increased white blood cells on wet prep.

- Other causes of vaginitis including trichomoniasis, bacterial vaginosis, and candidiasis must be ruled out.
- It is not known whether DIV represents a sterile inflammatory process, an infectious process, or some combination of both. Treatment is aimed at eliminating inflammation with intravaginal steroids and eliminating infection using intravaginal clindamycin.
- Treatment duration of four to eight weeks is usually required. Some patients will require weekly maintenance therapy with intravaginal clindamycin or steroid.

References

1. Sobel JD. Desquamative inflammatory vaginitis: A new subgroup of purulent vaginitis responsive to topical 2% clindamycin therapy. *Am J Obstet Gynecol* 1994;171(5):1215.

2. Simpson RC, Thomas KS, Leighton, P, Murphy R. Diagnostic criteria for erosive lichen planus affecting the vulva: An international electronic-Delphi consensus exercise. *Br J Dermatol* 2013;169(2):337.

3. Yali S, Pelivani N, Beltraminelli H, et al. Detection of linear IgE deposits in bullous pemphigoid and mucous membrane pemphigoid: A useful clue for diagnosis. *Br J Dermatol* 2011;165(5):1133.

4. Brown HL. Overview of vaginitis: office-based DNA testing. *The Female Patient* 2006;31(8 suppl):1–6.

5. International Society for the Study of Vulvovaginal Disease. *21st Biennial Conference on Diseases of the Vulva and Vagina.* Sept. 6–9, 2012. Available at www.ISSVD.org.

6. Sobel JD, Reichman O, Misra D, Yoo W. Prognosis and treatment of desquamative inflammatory vaginitis. *Obstet Gynecol* 2011;117;4:850.

A 30-year-old woman with vaginal itching

Lindsay H. Morrell

History of present illness

A 30-year-old gravida 2, para 2 woman presented with complaint of 3 days of vaginal pruritis and discharge. She describes the discharge as white and thick. She has not had symptoms like this before and has not used any over-the-counter medications to attempt to relieve her symptoms. She is sexually active with one partner and uses condoms irregularly. Her last menstrual period was seven days prior to presentation. She has a history of chlamydia five years prior, which was treated. She has no other history of sexually transmitted infections.

She has type 2 diabetes mellitus that is controlled with metformin. She takes no other medications. She has no other medical problems.

Physical examination

General appearance: Well-appearing woman in no apparent distress

Vital signs:

Temperature: 37.0°C

Pulse: 86 beats/min

Blood pressure: 133/68 mmHg

Respiratory rate: 18 breaths/min

Oxygen saturation: 100% on room air

BMI: 33 kg/m^2

HEENT: Unremarkable

Neck: Supple

Cardiovascular: Regular rate and rhythm without murmurs, rubs, or gallops

Lungs: Clear to auscultation bilaterally

Abdomen: Soft, obese, nontender, nondistended, no inguinal adenopathy

Pelvic:

Speculum: Thick lumpy white discharge coating vaginal sidewalls (Fig. 9.1), no cervicitis or mucopurulent discharge, no blood in vault

Bimanual: No cervical motion tenderness or adnexal masses, uterus small, mobile, anteverted

Extremities: No clubbing, cyanosis, or edema

Neurologic: Nonfocal

KOH prep: Was performed (Fig. 9.2). Saline wet mount did not show clue cells or trichomonads

Vaginal pH: 4.0

How would you manage the patient?

This patient had uncomplicated vaginal candidiasis. This patient was prescribed miconazole 4% cream intravaginally for 3 days. Her pruritis and vaginal discharge improved.

Vaginitis

Vaginitis is a common reason for seeking care. The differential diagnosis for a patient that presents with complaints of abnormal discharge includes trichomonas, vulvovaginal candidiasis, bacterial vaginosis, gonorrhea, chlamydia and physiologic discharge. Vulvovaginal candidiasis accounts for 17–39% of vaginitis [1], and it's estimated that 75% of sexually active women will have vulvovaginal candidiasis at least once in their lifetime [2]. The most common organism causing vulvovaginal candidiasis is *Candida albicans*, which causes more than 90% of cases [2,3]. The remaining 10% of cases are caused by

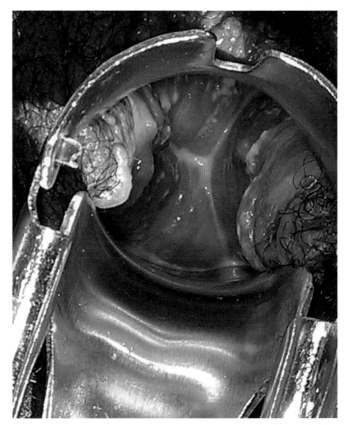

Fig. 9.1 Speculum examination of patient with symptomatic vaginal discharge. Note the thick white curd-like discharge adherent to the vaginal sidewalls.

Acute Care and Emergency Gynecology, ed. David Chelmow, Christine R. Isaacs and Ashley Carroll. Published by Cambridge University Press. © Cambridge University Press 2015.

Table 9.1 Treatment of uncomplicated *Candida vaginitis**

Drug	Formulation	Application
OTC intravaginal agents		
Butoconazole	2% Vaginal cream, 5 g	Intravaginally for 3 days
Clotrimazole	1% Vaginal cream, 5 g	Intravaginally for 7–14 days
	2% Vaginal cream, 5 g	Intravaginally for 3 days
Miconazole	2% Vaginal cream, 5 g	Intravaginally for 7 days
	4% Vaginal cream, 5 g	Intravaginally for 3 days
	100 mg Vaginal supp.	1 Supp. daily for 7 days
	200 mg Vaginal supp.	1 Supp. daily for 3 days
	1200 mg Vaginal supp.	1 Supp., once
Tioconazole	6.5% Vaginal ointment, 5 g	1 App. vaginally, once
Prescription intravaginal agents		
Butoconazole	2% Vaginal cream, single dose bioadhesive product, 5 g	Intravaginally for 1 day
Nystatin	100 000 U Vaginal tablet	1 Tablet daily for 14 days
Terconazole	0.4% Vaginal cream, 5 g	1 App. vaginally for 7 days
	0.8% Vaginal cream, 5 g	1 App. vaginally for 3 days
	80 mg Vaginal supp.	1 Supp. daily for 3 days
Prescription oral agent		
Fluconazole	150 mg Oral tablet	1 Tablet, single dose

* Modified from Centers for Disease Control and Prevention [4].
App., applicatorful; OTC, over-the-counter; sup., suppository.

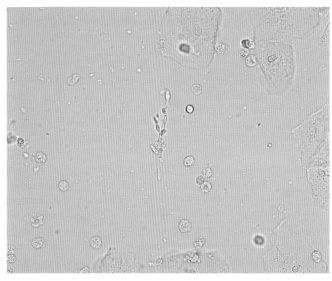

Fig. 9.2 KOH preparation from sample of discharge of patient with vaginal itching. Prominent hyphae consistent with *Candida vaginitis* is visible in the center of the image. (Image provided by Aaron Hill.)

nonalbicans *Candida* sp., most commonly *Candida glabrata*. More rare species include *Candida parapsilosis*, *Candida tropicalis*, and *Candida krusei* [2].

Signs and symptoms include pruritis, vaginal burning, dyspareunia, external dysuria and abnormal discharge. On physical examination, vulvar or vaginal erythema and edema, as well as fissures and excoriations may be present [4]. Speculum examination typically reveals thick white curd-like discharge that coats the vaginal sidewall and cervix. Symptoms and signs can vary significantly, and many patients do not have the classic curd-like discharge.

Mycolic diagnosis is made by collecting a sample of discharge during a pelvic examination and applying 10% KOH solution. Applying KOH solution results in lysis of epithelial cells and bacteria, making yeast more easily identifiable on the slide. A saline wet mount can also show yeast, though visualization may be more difficult. Microscopy shows budding yeast or branching pseudohyphae. Vaginal pH is typically normal (<4.5). The diagnosis is confirmed in a symptomatic patient by a KOH or saline wet mount that demonstrates yeast, hyphae, or pseudohyphae [4]. A yeast culture may be considered in a symptomatic patient with a negative wet mount and no other identifiable cause. Cultures can also useful in cases of candidiasis refractory to standard treatments. Cultures should be sent in asymptomatic women since yeast can be part of the normal vaginal flora in 10–20% of women [4]. A negative culture rules out yeast as a cause.

The Centers for Disease Control and Prevention (CDC) classifies *Candida* infections as complicated and uncomplicated [4]. Most cases of vaginal candidiasis are uncomplicated. Cases are typically considered uncomplicated if they are sporadic or infrequent, occurring three or less times in a year. Symptoms tend to be mild to moderate. In uncomplicated cases, patients are not immunocompromised and the organism causing the vaginitis is likely *C. albicans* [4]. Uncomplicated vaginal candidiasis typically responds well to topical azole therapy for treatment (Table 9.1). The recommended treatment of vulvovaginal candidiasis in pregnancy is topical azoles for seven days.

Cases are considered complicated if they are recurrent (four or more episodes per year), or the patient has severe symptoms. They often involve nonalbicans species. Vulvovaginal infections occurring in women with uncontrolled diabetes, debilitation, or immunosuppression are also classified as complicated. Complicated infections occur in less than 5% of women. Yeast culture should be sent in complicated infections to confirm the diagnosis and to assist in determining the treatment. While this patient had diabetes, it was well controlled and this was her first episode of candidiasis. Culture was not indicated, and management as uncomplicated candidiasis is appropriate.

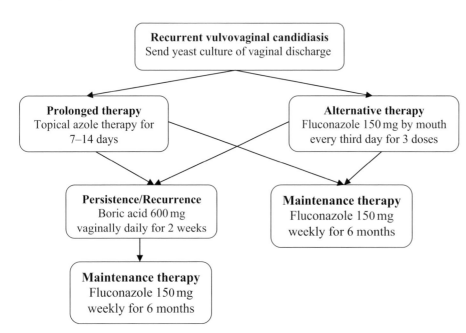

Fig. 9.3 Recurrent vulvovaginal candidiasis treatment algorithm. Choice of antifungal may be guided by the results of culture and sensitivities.

Treatment of nonalbicans candidiasis is less likely to respond to topical azole therapy [1]. Prolonged intravaginal therapy in combination with oral fluconazole is often recommended [1,4] (Fig. 9.3). Oral fluconazole 150 mg weekly for 6 months can be given for prevention of recurrent infections [5,6]. Fluconazole-resistant *C. albicans* infection has been increasing in incidence, likely due to the increase in prolonged use of fluconazole for recurrent infections [3]. The CDC recommends prolonged use of a nonfluconazole azole therapy for 7–14 days for treatment of resistant and recurrent nonalbicans infections [4]. According to a recent meta-analysis, nystatin and flucytosine, as well as several azole therapies including terconazole, intraconazole, clotrimazole, ketoconazole, buconazole, and miconazole as monotherapies may be efficacious [7]. In this situation, antifungal sensitivities may assist in determining which azole therapy to prescribe. An alternative to these therapies, 600 mg boric acid gelatin capsule intravaginally daily for 2 weeks, has shown success [7] and is recommended as treatment in cases of recurrence after prolonged use of azole therapy [4]. Despite its efficacy, boric acid can have more adverse effects compared to azole therapy. These adverse effects include a vaginal burning sensation (<10% of cases), watery discharge, and vaginal erythema [7].

Key teaching points

- Vulvovaginal candidiasis is a common cause of vaginitis with signs and symptoms including vulvar and vaginal erythema, pruritis, external dysuria, dyspareunia, and abnormal discharge.
- The majority of cases of vulvovaginal candidiasis are uncomplicated: infrequent or sporadic occurring three or less times per year, with mild to moderate symptoms. They are likely caused by *Candida albicans* and respond to topical azoles.
- Candidiasis is considered complicated if it recurs four or more times per year with severe symptoms. Complicated infections are often caused by nonalbicans candidiasis and occur in patients with immunosuppression, diabetes, or other severe illness.
- Culture can be helpful in recurrent vulvovaginal candidiasis or infections that are refractory to standard therapies.
- Boric acid 600 mg intravaginally daily for 2 weeks is the recommended treatment for refractory vulvovaginal candidiasis. Weekly fluconazole 150 mg for 6 months can be used for prevention in patients with recurrent vulvovaginal candidiasis.

References

1. American College of Obstetrics and Gynecology. Vaginitis. Practice Bulletin No. 72. *Obstet Gynecol* 2006;107:1195–206.

2. Sobal J. Vulvovaginal candidosis. *Lancet* 2007;369:1961–71.

3. Marchaim D, Lemanek L, Bheemreddy S, Kaye K, Sobel J. Fluconazole-resistant *Candida albicans* vulvovaginitis. *Obstet Gynecol* 2012;120(6):1407–13.

4. Centers for Disease Control and Prevention. *Sexually Transmitted Diseases Treatment Guidelines, 2010. Diseases Characterized by Vaginal Discharge.* Available at http://www.cdc.gov/std/treatment/2010/vaginal-discharge.htm#a3.

5. Rosa M, Silva B, Pines P, Silva F, Silva N, Silva F, et al. Weekly fluconazole therapy for recurrent vulvovaginal candidiasis: a systematic review and meta-analysis. *Eur J Obstet Gynecol Reprod Biol* 2013;167:132–6.

6. Sobel J, Wiesenfeld H, Martens M, et al. Maintenance fluconazole therapy for recurrent vulvovaginal candidiasis. *New Engl J Med* 2004;351:876–83.

7. Iavazzo C, Gkegkes I, Zarkada I, Falagas M. Boric acid for recurrent vulvovaginal candidiasis: the clinical evidence. *J Women's Health* 2011;20 (8):1245–55.

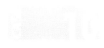

Sudden-onset left lower quadrant pain in a 21-year-old woman

Adrianne M. Colton

History of present illness

A 22-year-old female patient presents to the emergency department with acute onset of left lower quadrant pain. She was running when she suddenly developed sharp, stabbing abdominal pain that persisted despite rest. The patient denies fevers, chills, dysuria, diarrhea, or constipation. Upon further review of her history, she states that over the past month she has had episodes of abdominal pain that occur suddenly, are sharp and stabbing in nature, and resolve spontaneously. She is evaluated in the emergency room, where her physical examination was only remarkable for left adnexal tenderness and a fullness of the left adnexa on bimanual exam. A urine pregnancy test and urine dip are negative and no other labs are drawn. A transvaginal ultrasound was unremarkable with the exception of a slightly enlarged left ovary with a 5 cm simple cyst and no cul-de-sac fluid. She is treated in the emergency department with ibuprofen and her symptoms improve. She is discharged home with precautions to return for worsening pain.

She presents again to the emergency room approximately 24 hours later with similar complaints, though this time with nausea and vomiting. Her pain is now unrelieved by over-the-counter analgesics and she feels feverish.

Physical examination

General appearance: Woman who appears uncomfortable
Vital signs:

Temperature: 38.1°C
Pulse: 100 beats/min
Blood pressure: 122/74 mmHg
Respiratory rate: 20 breaths/min
Oxygen saturation: 100% on room air

Cardiovascular: Tachycardic, no peripheral edema
Lungs: Clear to auscultation bilaterally
Abdomen: Bowel sounds present in all four quadrants, left lower quadrant mildly tender to light and deep palpation, nondistended, no rebound or guarding
Genitourinary: Mobile anteverted uterus, no right adnexal tenderness or fullness, left adnexal tenderness with mass palpable in adnexa, mobile
Laboratory studies: Basic metabolic panel and CBC are within normal limits
Imaging: Transvaginal ultrasound confirms the same findings as seen on initial ultrasound, though this time with decreased intraovarian venous flow in the left ovary. Uterus of average size: 7 × 3 × 5 cm. Left ovary approximately 4 × 1.5 × 1.5 cm and right ovary approximately 7 × 10 × 7 cm, with a simple cyst with a single thin septation

Intravenous fluids and anti-emetics are administered.

How would you manage the patient?

This patient has ovarian torsion. She was taken to the operating room and underwent a diagnostic laparoscopy, which revealed an enlarged cystic left ovary that had undergone torsion (Fig. 10.1). Intraoperatively, the ovary was unwound along its vascular pedicle and ovarian venous outflow was restored. A cystectomy was performed. The patient had a routine postoperative course and was discharged on postoperative day 1. This diagnosis was made based on the patient's clinical picture detailing acute onset of sharp, unilateral abdominal pain, a history of intermittent resolution of the pain, and a transvaginal ultrasound that confirmed the presence of an enlarged left ovary with diminished intraovarian venous outflow.

Ovarian torsion

Ovarian torsion is the rotation of an ovary around its vascular and lymphatic pedicle that results in vascular compromise. It is the fifth most common gynecologic surgical emergency and most often occurs in the early reproductive years, but affects

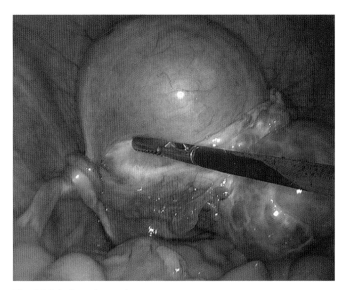

Fig. 10.1 Left ovarian torsion

Acute Care and Emergency Gynecology, ed. David Chelmow, Christine R. Isaacs and Ashley Carroll. Published by Cambridge University Press.

females of all ages [1,2]. In order to preserve ovarian function, prompt diagnosis and surgical management are imperative.

The average ovary is usually less than $6\,cm^3$ in volume in the premenopausal female and on average, less than $2.5\,cm^3$ at menopause [2]. It is supplied by both the ovarian artery and the adnexal branch of the uterine artery. When the ovary twists along its vascular pedicle it can cause complete absence or partial reduction in blood flow to and from the ovary, and if not recognized quickly, can result in necrosis of the ovary and ultimate loss of function [2]. Rates of adnexal torsion are increased in conditions that increase the size of the ovary including hemorrhagic cysts, cystadenomas, hyperstimulation, or tumors, benign or malignant [3]. Additionally, pregnant women are at increased risk of experiencing adnexal torsion, which may be a result of increased ovarian size due to an enlarged corpus luteal cyst or increased laxity of ligaments [3]. In cases where there are significant adhesions, such as pelvic inflammatory disease or endometriosis, torsion is less likely as the ovary is often fixed in place and lacks mobility.

Diagnosis of ovarian torsion is often difficult and usually requires high clinical suspicion as symptoms can be vague. Many women will present with the acute onset of sharp localized pain in either the left or right lower quadrants. This pain may radiate to the flank, groin, thigh, or back [1]. It can either be constant or intermittent, particularly if the ovary undergoes torsion and then untwists periodically and spontaneously [1]. Vital signs are usually within normal limits, though some patients may have a low-grade fever indicating the possibility of adnexal necrosis [4]. A physical examination is usually unremarkable, though a tender adnexal mass may be appreciated on bimanual examination [3].

A transvaginal ultrasound can assist in making the diagnosis of adnexal torsion [2]. An ovary that has undergone torsion may swell due to poor venous outflow and lymphatic drainage, resulting in stromal edema displacing secondary follicles to the periphery of the ovary [2]. Doppler ultrasonography can help clarify the diagnosis by showing decreased flow of blood into and out of the ovary. However, due to the increased smooth muscle tone in arteries, the arterial supply to the ovary may appear uncompromised despite collapse of the relatively thin walls of the vein [2]. Additionally, if the adnexa is only periodically undergoing torsion, there may appear to be normal flow when ultrasound is performed. In some cases, MRI or CT scanning may help elucidate the diagnosis, particularly if the symptoms are chronic or subacute in nature. With CT scans, common features of adnexal torsion include identification of an enlarged ovary, smooth wall thickening of the adnexal mass, and fallopian tube thickening [2].

Ultimately, if clinical suspicion is high, the most prudent next step following transvaginal ultrasound is a diagnostic laparoscopy. Studies have shown that only 23–66% of cases are given the correct presurgical diagnosis of adnexal torsion [5]. The diagnosis is best made at time of surgery and is based on visualization of an ovary that has twisted around its pedicle. It may appear enlarged, edematous, or even necrotic. It is important to expeditiously restore normal anatomic orientation of the ovary to reestablish blood flow, thereby improving the chances that the ovary remains viable and ultimately improving future fertility in reproductive age patients [1]. Reducing the torsion may be all that is necessary to restore flow to the ovary, despite an initially necrotic appearance [2]. However, if the patient is postmenopausal, and reproductive ability is not a concern, bilateral oophorectomy would be the treatment of choice [2].

Key teaching points

- Risk factors for adnexal torsion include those conditions that cause an increase in the volume of the ovary to greater than 6 cm.
- Evaluation of a patient suspected of having ovarian torsion can include the use of transvaginal grayscale and color Doppler ultrasound. However, the absence of blood flow to and from the ovary is not necessary to make the diagnosis.
- Adnexal torsion is a gynecologic surgical emergency and recognition with high clinical suspicion is the key to making the diagnosis.
- Adnexal torsion is treated with expedient operative evaluation, usually by diagnostic laparoscopy, and untwisting of the vascular pedicle that has undergone torsion in order to to reestablish blood flow to the ovary.

References

1. Tandulwadkar S, Shah A, Agarwal B. Detorsion and conservative therapy for twisted adnexa. *J Gynecol Endosc Surg* 2009;1(1):21–6.
2. Chang H, Bhatt S, Dogra V. Pearls and pitfalls in diagnosis of ovarian torsion. *RadioGraphics* 2008;28(5): 1355–68.
3. Schraga, E. *Ovarian Torsion*. Available at http://emedicine.medscape.com/article/2026938-overview.
4. Houry D, Abbott JT. Ovarian torsion: A 15-year review. *Ann Emerg Med* 2001;38: 156–9.
5. Roche O, Chavan N, Aquilina J, Rockall A. Radiological appearances of gynaecological emergencies. *Insights Imaging* 2012;3(3): 265–75.

A 35-year-old woman with IUD string not visible

Michelle Meglin

History of present illness

A 35-year-old gravida 2, para 2 woman presents for an urgent visit 4 weeks after a levonorgestrel intrauterine device (IUD) insertion. She reports intermittent left lower quadrant pain and inability to palpate the IUD strings. She is concerned that she may no longer be protected from unplanned pregnancy. Her IUD insertion was performed six weeks after an uncomplicated elective repeat Cesarean delivery. Her uterus was noted to be retroverted at the time of insertion. The insertion was performed without difficulty. She had mild cramping and bleeding that resolved five days following insertion.

Her obstetric history is significant for two Cesarean deliveries at term. Her gynecologic history is unremarkable. She has no chronic medical problems and takes no medications. She has had no other surgeries.

Physical exam

General appearance: Woman in no apparent distress
Vital signs:

Temperature: 37.3°C
Pulse: 75 beats/min
Blood pressure: 125/85 mmHg
Respiratory rate: 16 breaths/min
Oxygen saturation: 100% on room air

Abdomen: Soft, nontender, nondistended
External genitalia: Normal
Vagina: Normal
Cervix: Normal appearing cervix, no IUD strings visualized, unable to tease string from endocervix with cytobrush
Uterus: Small, retroverted uterus, mobile, no tenderness
Adnexa: No masses or tenderness
Laboratory studies: Urine pregnancy test: Negative
Imaging: Transvaginal ultrasound revealed a normal appearing uterus and thin endometrial stripe without evidence of an IUD. A following pelvic x-ray noted an IUD in the left pelvis overlying the left inferior iliac bone (Fig. 11.1)

How would you manage this patient?

This patient has an extrauterine intrauterine device (IUD) that should be removed by laparoscopy or laparotomy [1,2,3]. She underwent laparoscopy and the IUD was noted to be enveloped in omentum in the left paracolic gutter (Fig. 11.2).

There was no evidence of uterine defect or stigmata from uterine perforation. The IUD was teased from the omentum and removed via a 5 mm port.

IUD string not visible

The use of IUDs for contraceptive and noncontraceptive indications is increasing in the United States. The copper IUD (ParaGard® T380A, Teva Women's Health, Inc.) is approved for 10 years of contraceptive use in the United States and has contraceptive failure rates similar to tubal ligation. The levonorgestrel IUD is a highly effective contraceptive method that is approved for five years of use in the United States and also has several noncontraceptive benefits [1]. The levonorgestrel IUD effectively reduces blood loss in patients with heavy menstrual bleeding, adenomyosis, and uterine fibroids, and improves pain in patients with endometriosis and dysmenorrhea [4]. The levonorgestrel IUD may be used

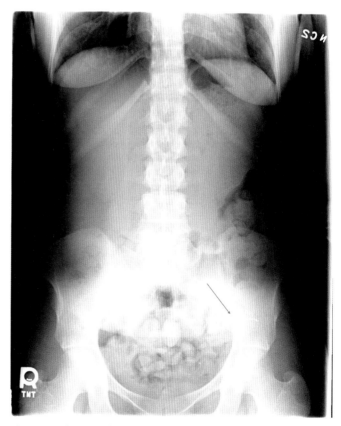

Fig. 11.1 Pelvic x-ray showing an extrauterine IUD in the left pelvis overlying the left inferior iliac bone. (Image provided by Steven Cohen, MD.)

Acute Care and Emergency Gynecology, ed. David Chelmow, Christine R. Isaacs and Ashley Carroll. Published by Cambridge University Press.
© Cambridge University Press 2015.

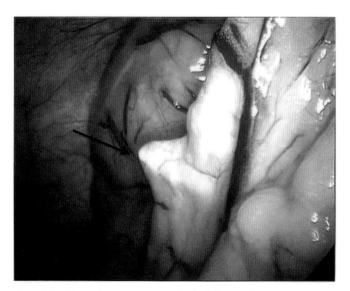

Fig. 11.2 IUD enveloped in omentum in the left paracolic gutter on laparoscopy. (Image provided by Steven Cohen, MD.)

to provide endometrial protection in patients on hormone therapy and tamoxifen and provide therapeutic progestin in women with endometrial hyperplasia [4].

Following IUD insertion many providers instruct patients to return for follow-up 4–12 weeks following insertion and instruct patients to periodically perform string checks [2,3]. However, according to the US Selected Practice Recommendations for Contraceptive Use, 2013 [5], there is insufficient evidence to recommend a routine follow-up visit after IUD insertion and it should not be required. Patients with IUD should be evaluated if they have problems or would like to change contraceptive method. Additionally, when a patient with an IUD returns for routine gynecologic care, providers should consider performing a pelvic examination to confirm the presence of IUD strings [5]. Possible explanations of nonvisible IUD strings include retraction of strings into the cervical canal, unrecognized expulsion of the IUD, pregnancy causing an enlarging uterus that draws the device upward, and partial or complete uterine perforation [6].

The incidence of inability to see IUD strings has been reported as 4.5–18.0% [6]. One study reviewed over 14 000 women who underwent IUD insertion (copper and levonorgestrel) and found that IUD strings were missing at 5% of routine follow-up visits [6]. In this study, 98.2% of the time the IUD strings had retracted into the cervical canal and the IUD was appropriately located in the uterus. Inadvertent expulsion occurred in 1.2% of cases and uterine perforation in 0.7% of cases [6]. In other studies, rates of expulsion range from 2 to 10% in the first year of use [1]. The perforation rate has been reported as 1 per 1000 insertions [1].

There are risk factors at time of IUD insertion that increase the risk of expulsion. IUD expulsion is more likely to occur if the insertion was difficult or performed by an inexperienced provider [6]. Expulsion rates are higher in adolescents and nulliparous women, but IUD use in these groups is US Medical

Eligibility Criteria for Contraceptive Use category 2 (advantages outweigh risks) [7]. Immediate postpartum insertion is associated with an expulsion rate up to 24%, but use in the immediate postpartum periods is still category 1 (no restrictions for use) for the copper IUD and category 2 for the levonorgestrel IUD [1]. Similarly, insertion of an IUD following a second-trimester abortion is category 2 due to a higher risk of expulsion [7]. The presence of risk factors for expulsion should not preclude recommending IUDs to these women.

Both uterine perforation and expulsion should be considered if the patient is pregnant. Uterine perforation should be considered when patients present with pain. Perforation may also be more likely when insertion is difficult, required cervical dilation, was performed by an inexperienced provider, in nulliparous women, and in women with prior Cesarean or retroverted or retroflexed uterus [6].

Several recent papers have proposed similar algorithms for management of missing IUD strings [6,8,9]. Initial evaluation of nonvisible strings typically involves attempts to visualize strings in the office. Strings can be retracted into the endocervical canal, and, in these instances, they can be visualized with an endocervical speculum or brought into view by probing the endocervical canal with a cytobrush or q-tip.

A pregnancy test should be performed if the strings cannot be found in the canal. If a pregnancy test is positive, an ultrasound should be performed to confirm an intrauterine pregnancy and to determine if the IUD has been retained in the uterus. Continuing a pregnancy with an IUD in utero increases the risk for miscarriage, septic abortion, preterm delivery, and chorioamnionitis; therefore, IUD removal is recommended if the IUD strings are visible or in the cervical canal. If the IUD strings are not visible or in the cervical canal then the IUD cannot be removed noninvasively and should remain in place [1].

If a pregnancy test is negative and the patient desires continuation of IUD use, then a transvaginal ultrasound should be performed. If transvaginal ultrasound confirms the IUD in the uterus (Fig. 11.3) and the patient desires continuation, then no further intervention is required. The IUD remains effective and, if the patient is otherwise happy with the IUD, then continuation should be encouraged [2,3,8]. Serial ultrasounds are not necessary and the IUD may be removed with an IUD hook at the usual time, or when conception is desired.

If a patient desires IUD removal and no strings are visible, the uterine cavity can be probed in the office with an IUD hook or forceps prior to ultrasound in the setting of negative pregnancy test [9]. If initial efforts to remove the IUD in the office are unsuccessful a transvaginal ultrasound is recommended to determine location of the IUD. If ultrasound is readily accessible, ultrasound can also be performed prior to attempts to instrument the uterus. If transvaginal ultrasound confirms the IUD in the uterus and the patient desires removal, further attempts at removal may be undertaken in the office. IUD

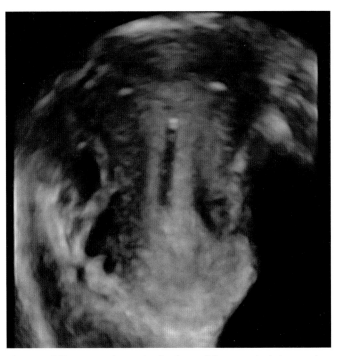

Fig. 11.3 IUD in situ at the uterine fundus on 3-D transvaginal ultrasound.

removal is often limited by poor pain control leading some to advocate for preparing the cervix with misoprostol or use of a paracervical block to facilitate removal in the office [8]. If this remains unsuccessful, the patient may be taken to the operating room for removal under anesthesia using an IUD hook or forceps. In rare cases, use of the hysteroscopy may be necessary.

If transvaginal ultrasound does not show the IUD in the uterus, as with our patient, one cannot assume the IUD has been expelled. An abdominal/pelvic x-ray is required to evaluate for extrauterine location of the IUD. Intraperitoneal adhesions, intestinal perforation, intestinal obstruction, and erosion into adjacent viscera have been reported when the IUD is left in the peritoneal cavity [2,3]. The American College of Obstetricans and Gynecologists (ACOG) and device manufacturers recommend removal of intraperitoneal IUDs via laparoscopy or laparotomy [1,2,3]. Removal of an intraperitoneal IUD is typically accomplished via laparoscopy. Laparoscopic forceps are used to grasp the IUD, scissors are used to lyse any adhesions and the IUD is removed via an accessory port. Occasionally, the location of the IUD is not apparent upon laparoscopic intra-abominal survey and the use of intraoperative x-rays may be helpful.

While patients are undergoing evaluation for missing IUD strings, they should be counseled to use back-up contraception since they are no longer receiving contraceptive benefit from their IUD.

Key teaching points

- Possible explanations for not being able to see intrauterine device (IUD) strings include retraction of strings into the cervical canal, IUD expulsion, pregnancy, and partial or complete uterine perforation.
- Many IUD strings may be retrieved from the cervical canal in the office by probing the endocervical canal with a q-tip or a cytobrush.
- Evaluation should include a transvaginal ultrasound followed by an x-ray if the IUD is not seen on ultrasound.
- If ultrasound confirms an intrauterine location, the IUD is effective and does not need to be removed.
- If ultrasound confirms that the IUD is not in the uterus, a pregnancy test should be performed and the patient should initiate another form of contraception immediately.
- Intraperitoneal IUDs can generally be removed by laparoscopy.

References

1. American College of Obstetricians and Gynecologists. Long-acting reversible contraception: implants and intrauterine devices. Practice Bulletin No. 121. *Obstet Gynecol* 2011;118(1):184–96.

2. Mirena levonorgestrel-releasing intrauterine system: full prescribing information [package insert]. Bayer HealthCare Pharmaceuticals Inc.; 2013.

3. ParaGard T380A intrauterine copper contraceptive: prescribing information and instructions for use [package insert]. FEI Products LLC; 2003.

4. American College of Obstetricians and Gynecologists. Noncontraceptive uses of hormonal contraceptives. Practice Bulletin No. 110. *Obstet Gynecol* 2010;115:206–18.

5. Centers for Disease Control and Prevention. US Selected practice recommendations for contraceptive use, 2013. *MMWR* 2013;62(RR-5): 1–46.

6. Marchi N, Castro S, Hidalgo MM, et al. Management of missing strings in users of intrauterine contraceptives. *Contraception* 2012;86:354–8.

7. Centers for Disease Control and Prevention. US medical eligibility criteria for contraceptive use, 2010. *MMWR* 2010;59(RR-4): 1–86.

8. Prabhakaran S, Chuang A. In-office retrieval on intrauterine contraceptive devices with missing strings. *Contraception* 2011;82:102–6.

9. Vilos GA, Di Cecco R, Marks J. Algorithm for nonvisible strings of levonorgestrel intrauterine system. *J Minim Invasive Gynecol* 2010;17(6): 805–6.

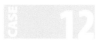
A 38-year-old woman with sudden-onset shortness of breath

Chris J. Hong and David Chelmow

History of present illness

A 38-year-old gravida 0 woman presents to the emergency department complaining of chest pain, difficulty breathing, and a blood-tinged cough that started suddenly several hours ago. She describes the pain as sharp, right sided, and worse with deep breaths. She denies any fevers, chills, nausea, vomiting, or pain radiating to her arms or jaw.

She returned last week to the United States after a month-long trip to South Korea. She has no significant past medical or surgical history. Family history is unremarkable. Her current medications include a multivitamin and a daily combined oral contraceptive pill containing 35 μg of ethinyl estradiol and 0.25 mg norgestimate, which she began taking 6 months ago. She denies any tobacco, alcohol, or illicit drug use.

Physical examination

General appearance: Woman with mild dyspnea and seeming uncomfortable
Vital signs:

  Temperature: 37.3°C
  Pulse: 104 beats/min
  Blood pressure: 122/76 mmHg
  Respiratory rate: 22 breaths/min
  Oxygen saturation: 93% on room air
  BMI: 37 kg/m^2
HEENT: Unremarkable
Neck: Supple, no masses
Cardiovascular: Tachycardic, regular rhythm, no murmurs, gallops, or rubs
Pulmonary: Increased respiratory effort, clear to auscultation bilaterally, no wheezes, rales, or rhonchi
Abdominal: Obese, bowel sounds active, nontender to deep palpation, no hepatosplenomegaly
Extremities: No swelling or tenderness, no visible cords
Laboratory studies:

  Urine pregnancy test: Negative
  CBC and basic metabolic profile: Within normal limits
Imaging:

  Twelve-lead ECG: Sinus tachycardia, no ischemic changes
  Chest x-ray: Unremarkable

What is the differential diagnosis?

The most likely differential diagnosis for the sudden-onset chest pain and shortness of breath in a 38-year-old woman on oral contraceptive pills includes pulmonary embolism, acute coronary syndrome/myocardial infarction (ACS/MI), Mallory–Weiss tear, and pneumothorax. ACS/MI is unlikely given the patient's age, negative medical and family history, and lack of ECG findings. Pneumothorax is unlikely given the patient's unremarkable chest x-ray, and a Mallory–Weiss tear is unlikely in the absence of vomiting.

How would you manage this patient?

This patient's history and physical examination are most consistent with a pulmonary embolism (PE), and as such, further diagnostic evaluation was required. She was placed on a cardiac monitor and 2 L oxygen, which improved her oxygen saturation to 98%. A computed tomography pulmonary angiogram (CTPA or "spiral CT") was performed (Fig. 12.1).

The patient has a large pulmonary embolus. Given the large size of the clot and her symptoms, she was admitted to the hospital and started on low-molecular-weight heparin and warfarin. The heparin was continued until she was therapeutically anticoagulated on warfarin. Oral contraceptive pills were immediately discontinued. Prior to initiating anticoagulation,

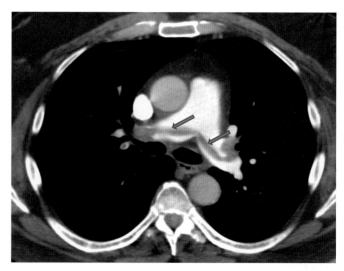

Fig. 12.1 CT of the chest from a 38-year-old female with saddle embolism. (Image provided by Kathyrn Olsen, MD.)

Acute Care and Emergency Gynecology, ed. David Chelmow, Christine R. Isaacs and Ashley Carroll. Published by Cambridge University Press.
© Cambridge University Press 2015.

blood was drawn to test for Protein S and C deficiencies, factor V Leiden mutation, antiphospholipid antibody, antithrombin III deficiency, prothrombin gene mutations, and lupus anticoagulant. All tests were negative. As the clot likely stemmed from her combined oral contraceptive use in conjunction with her obesity and recent immobility, a three-month course of anticoagulation was chosen. She was counseled on weight reduction and the need to avoid prolonged immobility. A levonorgestrel intrauterine device (IUD) was placed for contraception.

Venous thromboembolism

Risk factors for venous thromboembolism (VTE) include combined hormonal contraceptive use, age greater than 65 years, personal history of VTE, pregnancy and the puerperium, obesity, recent surgery, prolonged travel, and thrombophilia. The risk of VTE is increased up to fourfold among combined hormonal contraceptive users (3–9/10 000 woman-years) when compared with nonusers who are not pregnant and not taking hormones (1–5/10 000 woman-years). However, the risk of VTE with combined hormonal contraceptive use is still lower than the risk of VTE during pregnancy (5–20/10 000 woman-years) and the postpartum period (40–65/10 000 woman-years). Third-generation combined oral contraceptives were previously thought to carry significant risk compared to second-generation combined oral contraceptives, but recent studies are conflicting [1]. Twenty percent of patients with VTE have no identifiable risk factors at the time of presentation. This patient's risk factors for VTE include combined hormonal contraceptive use, recent immobilization, and obesity.

Patients suspected of having a PE can have their pretest probability for VTE determined by validated assessment tools such as the Wells Criteria and be stratified into low, moderate, and high probability groups. Pulmonary Embolism Rule-out Criteria (PERC) rules may be applied to patients with low pretest probabilities to clinically exclude the presence of PE; a negative test gives a probability of less than 2% for the presence of PE. This patient is PERC positive due to estrogen use, tachycardia, oxygen saturation less than 94%, and hemoptysis. Therefore, she requires diagnostic evaluation for PE [3].

Confirmatory tests for VTE include D-dimer testing, CTPA, Ventilation/Perfusion (V/Q) scans, and lower extremity Doppler testing. Use of D-dimer testing should be restricted to excluding VTE in patients with a low pretest probability. D-dimer testing was not performed for this patient as she was already at high probability for PE. CTPA is the diagnostic modality of choice with sensitivity and specificity ranging from 83 to 100% and 86 to 100% respectively. V/Q scans are second-line imaging studies, typically used for patients with a contraindication to CTPA such as allergy to contrast, kidney failure, or inability to obtain intravenous access. Pulmonary angiography was once considered the gold standard to diagnose PE, but is rarely used today due to the invasiveness of the test and the availability of CTPA. Lower extremity Doppler studies can

play a role in the evaluation of VTE. A patient with a positive Doppler study for deep vein thrombosis (DVT) and pulmonary symptoms can be presumed to have PE and can be managed accordingly. However, a negative study does not rule out PE. Here, CTPA confirmed the presence of PE.

Usual treatment for VTE includes anticoagulation with unfractionated or low-molecular-weight heparin and warfarin. Thrombolytics may be considered in patients with extensive DVTs involving the iliac and femoral veins as well as in patients with massive PEs. Inferior vena cava (IVC) filters may be placed in patients with contraindications to medical management or in patients with recurrent DVTs [2]. As this patient was hemodynamically stable, she was treated with low-molecular-weight heparin while initiating warfarin to therapeutic doses. An IVC filter was not indicated given this was her first VTE event.

Once VTE is confirmed, further evaluation for underlying coagulopathy may be performed. As some parts of the laboratory evaluation are altered by anticoagulation, laboratory studies should be drawn prior to initiation of such therapy. The evaluation typically includes Protein S and C deficiencies, factor V Leiden mutation, antiphospholipid antibody, antithrombin III deficiency, prothrombin gene mutations, and lupus anticoagulant. The presence of an underlying hypercoagulable state may require long-term anticoagulation. Routine screening for these disorders is not recommended prior to starting combined hormonal contraception due to the rarity of the conditions and the high cost of screening. A thrombophilia workup was ordered and found negative in this patient. As the VTE likely stemmed from her combined oral contraceptive use in conjunction with her obesity and recent immobility, a three-month treatment course of anticoagulation was recommended. She was counseled on modifiable risk factors including weight reduction and the need to avoid prolonged immobility.

Combined hormonal contraceptives are contraindicated in patients with a history of a VTE. However, due to the overall increased risk of VTE during pregnancy, effective contraception is advised in this patient. Although combined hormonal contraceptive use is associated with up to a fourfold increase in risk of VTE in a nonpregnant female, that absolute risk of VTE is still lower than women in the pregnant and puerperium state. As in other patients, long-acting reversible contraception (LARC) methods are preferred. Recommendations for contraceptive management in a patient with VTE are outlined by the Centers for Disease Control and Prevention (CDC) in their "US medical eligibility criteria for contraceptive use, 2010" [3]. These guidelines recommend the discontinuation of combined hormonal contraceptives in any patient with acute VTE or history of VTE regardless of current anticoagulation therapy or predisposing factors. In patients with DVT or PE, progestin-only contraceptive pills, depot medroxyprogesterone acetate injections, etonogestrel implants, and levonorgestrel or copper IUDs are all acceptable alternatives, and are category 2 (advantages of the method generally outweigh the theoretical or proven risks). This patient was instructed to discontinue combined oral contraceptives and she chose to initiate the levonorgestrel IUD, which may also help prevent heavy menstrual bleeding while the patient is anticoagulated.

Key teaching points

- The diagnostic evaluation and management of venous thromboembolism (VTE) in a female taking combined hormonal contraceptives is the same as patients with VTE from any other cause. Risk factors for VTE include combined hormonal contraceptive use, age greater than 65 years, personal history of VTE, pregnancy and puerperium, obesity, recent surgery, prolonged travel, and thrombophilia.
- Twenty percent of patients with VTE have no identifiable risk factors at presentation.

- Patients diagnosed with VTE are typically evaluated for: Protein S and C deficiencies, factor V Leiden, antiphospholipid antibody, antithrombin III deficiency, prothrombin gene mutations, and lupus anticoagulant.
- Patients who have VTE while taking combined hormonal contraceptives should discontinue use. Alternative safe methods include progestin-only contraceptive pills, depot medroxyprogesterone acetate injections, etonogestrel implants, and the levonorgestrel and copper intrauterine devices (IUDs).
- Although combined hormonal contraceptive use is associated with up to a fourfold increased risk of VTE, this absolute risk of VTE is still lower than that of women in the pregnant and puerperium state.

References

1. American College of Obstetricians and Gynecologists. Risk of venous thromboembolism among users of drospirenone-containing oral contraceptive pills. Committee Opinion No. 540. *Obstet Gynecol* 2012;120: 1239–42.

2. Fesmire FM, Brown MD, Espinosa JA, et al. Critical issues in the evaluation and management of adult patients presenting to the emergency department with suspected pulmonary embolism. American College of Emergency Physicians. *Ann Emerg Med* 2011;57:628–52.

3. Centers for Disease Control and Prevention. US medical eligibility criteria for contraceptive use, 2010. *MMWR* 2010;59:1–86.

Vaginal bleeding in a 75-year-old woman

K. Nathan Parthasarathy and Peter F. Schnatz

History of presenting illness

A 75-year-old gravida 4, para 1-1-1-2 woman presents to her gynecologist with 2 days of vaginal spotting. She has had vulvar pruritus and mild dysuria for the past two years. She has noticed a thin white discharge on and off for the past five weeks. Her husband died suddenly two years ago and she resumed vaginal intercourse four days ago with a new partner. She has been using condoms for protection against sexually transmitted infections.

She denies trauma, fever, night sweats, unexplained weight gain or loss, epistaxis, gingival bleeding, bruising, urgency, frequency, nocturia, or incontinence. She does not use any douches, deodorants, or soaps in her vagina and wears comfortable loose fitting clothing.

Past medical history is significant for a left-sided ductal breast cancer, successfully treated with a 5-year course of tamoxifen 20 years earlier. Annual gynecologic examinations have been performed without any concerns noted. She has no history of diabetes. She takes no medications and has never used hormonal therapy, soy, or herbal supplements. Surgical history is significant for a dilatation and curettage. Family history is significant for a mother with a hip fracture at age 56. She denies tobacco, alcohol, or nonprescription drug use.

Physical examination

General appearance: Well-nourished woman who appears her stated age and who is in no acute distress

Vital signs:

Temperature: 37.0°C
Pulse: 80 beats/min
Blood pressure: 130/90 mmHg
Respiratory rate: 18 breaths/min
BMI: 21.0 kg/m^2
Weight: 111 lb
Height: 61 inches

HEENT: Unremarkable

Neck: Supple, no neck or supraclavicular lymphadenopathy

Cardiovascular: Regular rate and rhythm without murmurs, rubs, or gallops

Lungs: Clear to auscultation bilaterally

Breast: Examination revealed symmetry with no skin or nipple changes. There is a 4-mm scar on the left breast

Abdomen: Soft, nontender, nondistended, without rebound. There are normal bowel sounds

Pelvic:

Examination showed multiple external healing vulvar excoriations, sparse pubic hair, absence of labia minora, nonmoist labia majora, and everted urethral mucosa. A two-finger breadth introital width and a shortened vaginal depth are noted
Bimanual examination: Revealed an anteverted uterus that is nontender, the size of a small orange. Ovaries were barely palpable, with no evidence of any masses
Speculum examination: Revealed an opaque thin pink discharge and a parous cervix. Blood was present on the cervix. Vaginal skin was nonrugated, shiny, erythematous, and friable. A minimal amount of blood was noted from multiple patchy vaginal wall and cervical abrasions

Rectal: Examination revealed normal tone with a paucity of stool and no masses

Extremities: No abnormalities or edema

Neurologic: Examination was nonfocal

Laboratory studies:

Vaginal pH: 7.1
NAATs: Tests for gonorrhea and chlamydia were collected
Vaginal microscopy: Revealed no evidence of *Candida*, trichomonads, or clue cells by KOH and saline wet preparation testing. The vaginal smear revealed an increased proportion of parabasal cells with a decreased proportion of superficial cells
Urinalysis: Obtained on a midstream clean catch. Revealed a large quantity of blood, with an absence of nitrites or leukocyte esterase

Imaging:

Transvaginal ultrasonography: Demonstrated an endometrial thickness of 3 mm, no polyps, and no leiomyoma
Color-flow Doppler: Demonstrated no flow in the subendometrium

How would you manage this patient?

The patient has symptomatic vulvovaginal atrophy (VVA). A vaginal smear revealed an increased proportion of parabasal (immature) squamous epithelial cells having enlarged nuclei with a background of inflammatory exudates and amorphous, roundish, basophilic debris (Fig. 13.1). Her *Neisseria*

Acute Care and Emergency Gynecology, ed. David Chelmow, Christine R. Isaacs and Ashley Carroll. Published by Cambridge University Press. © Cambridge University Press 2015.

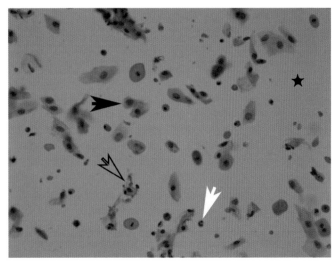

Fig. 13.1 Atrophic vaginitis in liquid-based preparation (LBP). Note dissociated parabasal cells (black arrow), degenerated parabasal cells (open arrow) and polymorphonuclear leukocytes (white arrow) in a relatively clean background (star) typical of a LBP.

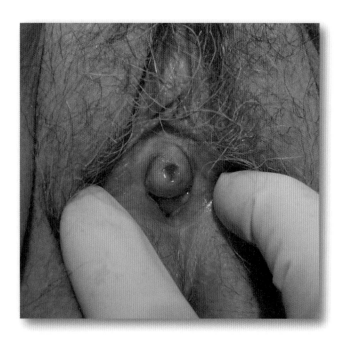

Fig. 13.2 This photograph demonstrates introital stenosis (<2 finger breadths) with urethral eversion in a postmenopausal woman who is not taking any hormonal therapy. Involutional vulvar changes include poor skin turgor, and fusion of the labia majora and minora, in addition to sparse pubic hair. (From Freeman [3].)

gonorrhoeae and *Chlamydia trachomatis* tests were negative. She was started on an estradiol vaginal cream (17 beta-estradiol) 2 g every day for 2 weeks and then tapering to 1 g 2–3 times per week. A vaginal moisturizer was recommended and she was advised to use a personal water-based lubricant in addition to the barrier contraception she is currently using. She noted successful resolution of her symptoms.

Symptomatic vulvovaginal atrophy

Up to 40% of postmenopausal women experience symptomatic VVA [1]. VVA predisposes postmenopausal women to super-imposed infections of the vagina and urinary tract. The presence of atrophy-related sexual dysfunction often results in emotional and relational distress [1,2]. The vagina and urinary tract share a common embryologic origin and are both strongly estrogen-dependent, and are consequently prone to atrophic changes in the postmenopausal years [1,2]. While still referred to as VVA or atrophic vaginitis, discussions are underway about possible new nomenclature such as genitourinary syndrome of menopause (GSM). This term would convey that this common condition associated with menopause is a symptom complex that can involve the vulva, vagina, and lower urinary tract.

Genital-only presentations typically include dryness, pruritus, burning, dyspareunia, leukorrhea, vaginal discharge, bleeding, or pain. The initial symptom is frequently a noticeable decrease in vaginal lubrication, followed by urinary symptoms. While the highly estrogenized vagina typically develops symptoms first, urinary tract symptoms often include dysuria, frequency, hematuria, and urgency. Any use of perfumes, douches, soaps, panty liners, lubricants, and tight fitting clothing should be discussed as they are potential irritants that may cause or exacerbate the symptoms. Physical examination findings are very dependent on the degree of tissue atrophy, superimposed infections, and sexual activity. Physical findings can include

poor skin turgor, sparse pubic hair, fusion of the labia minora to the labia majora, and visible dryness (Fig. 13.2 [3]). Introital stenosis is present if two fingers cannot be inserted into the vagina on bimanual examination. Sexual intercourse can commonly cause traumatic median lacerations in the posterior fourchette and at the introitus. Speculum examination usually demonstrates poorly or nonrugated (smooth), pale, shiny, and thin vaginal epithelium that is susceptible to trauma from intercourse, pessaries, irritants, and infections. Intercourse, manipulation of a pessary, and vaginal examinations can all result in bleeding or spotting. Urethral caruncles and eversion of the urethral mucosa are common urinary findings. Incontinence can also cause or exacerbate vulvar dermatoses.

The differential diagnosis of bleeding in this age range should be based on the location of the visible bleeding. If the bleeding is confined to the vagina and does not appear to involve the cervix, then a thorough examination should be performed and VVA should be considered. If bleeding is present at the cervical os, then endometrial polyps, endometrial cancer, endometrial hyperplasia, cervical cancer, infections, and hemato- or pyometra should be considered. In many instances, the source will be unclear and it will be important to consider both VVA and uterine abnormalities as potential sources.

Suspected intrauterine sources should initially be evaluated with an endometrial biopsy or an ultrasound measurement of the endometrial thickness, with further evaluation as indicated [4]. The presence of contributing vaginitis can be assessed with vaginal pH along with KOH and saline wet-mount preparations, although interpretation may be limited by the bleeding [1,2]. As vaginal dryness, irritation, or discomfort in a postmenopausal woman is not always VVA, a full differential

Table 13.1 Differential diagnosis of vaginal dryness, irritation, or discomfort in a postmenopausal woman

Vaginal infections
- Sexually transmitted infections
- Human papillomavirus infection
- Bacterial infections
- Fungal infections including candidiasis
- Infestations including scabies
- Molluscum contagiosum

Trauma

Dermatitis and dermatosis:
- Allergic or irritant reactions to local agents (perfumes, deodorants, soaps, panty liners, spermicide, lubricants, tight clothing)
- Eczema
- Psoriasis
- Lichen planus, lichen sclerosis, lichen simplex chronicus
- Vulvovaginal atrophy (VVA)

Malignancy and dysplasia

Urogenital ulcers, fissures, and fistulas due to systemic disease (i.e. Crohn disease)

Vestibulodynia or vulvodynia

diagnosis (Table 13.1) should be considered and appropriately evaluated. Evaluation for bleeding can include cultures, biopsies, or empiric therapies. VVA is usually diagnosed clinically after considering and excluding other potential diagnosis.

In this patient, VVA was diagnosed based on her combination of history and physical findings. She had atrophic-appearing vaginal skin as evidenced by the nonrugated, smooth shiny appearance. She also had several visible friable bleeding areas in the vagina, which were noted immediately after resuming sexual intercourse. Given that blood was visible on her cervix in conjunction with a slightly enlarged uterus and prior breast malignancy, an endovaginal ultrasound examination was performed to rule out a concomitant, albeit much less likely, uterine source.

Topical estrogen is the ideal treatment for VVA. Estradiol intravaginal cream can be administered 1–4 g at night for 2 weeks and then tapered to 1 g 2–3 times per week. As VVA is likely to be a chronic problem, the patient should plan to continue the cream long term. Topical administration has a local effect with minimal systemic effects. Systemic estrogen is also an option, as it is effective for VVA, but it is usually reserved for patients having other problems related to hypoestrogenism. In patients with significant risk factors (like a history of breast cancer in the current patient), it should be reserved for significant quality-of-life indications, when other options have been considered, and after the risks and benefits have been discussed.

In a patient like this with a history of breast cancer, topical intravaginal estrogen would be an option after appropriate counseling if VVA was her only symptom and nonhormonal options had been considered. Risks would be anticipated to be extremely low given the length of time she has been disease-

free and the minimal, if any, systemic absorption with low-dose vaginal estradiol. For women with a history of an estrogen-sensitive cancer, like the patient in the current case, consultation with the patient's oncologist could be considered. It would be prudent to use one of the lowest-dose therapies available, like the 17 beta-estradiol vaginal tablet, which has been shown to result in serum estradiol concentrations between 4 and 9 pg/mL. This level decreases the longer the patient is on therapy and is less than the average concentration found in most postmenopausal women [5].

Vaginal preparations are first-line therapy for women without systemic symptoms. They are frequently administered as creams, which can be messy and require some dexterity to insert. An alternate and equally efficacious treatment is a low-dose intravaginal hormone-releasing ring or tablets [2,6]. Both provide local estrogen, and the ring can also be worn during sexual intercourse. High-dose vaginal preparations should be avoided unless the patient has systemic symptoms, particularly severe hot flashes.

Systemic hormonal therapy (oral or transdermal) and ospemifene are options for women who prefer not to use a vaginal preparation. Systemic estrogen may be preferred for younger postmenopausal women with vasomotor symptoms, early menopause, bone loss, or other concerns related to estrogen deficiency. Ospemifene, a new systemic selective estrogen receptor modulator (SERM), has been approved for moderate to severe dyspareunia from VVA. Ospemifene is currently the only SERM approved for dyspareunia secondary to its vaginal effects. In the extension of the initial study of safety and efficacy, no venous thromboembolic events or endometrial pathology were noted through one year after the start of the drug. Vasomotor symptoms, however, are a likely side effect [7]. Lasofoxifene, another SERM not yet approved in the United States, has been shown to improve the vaginal pH and the vaginal maturation index (VMI) with a decreased incidence of breast cancer. Bazedoxifene (BZA) combined with conjugated estrogen (CE) has also been shown to improve the vaginal pH and the VMI. BZA/CE, classified as a tissue-selective estrogen complex (TSEC), has recently been approved by the Food and Drug Administration (FDA) [7,8].

Intravaginal DHEA is sold as a non-FDA-approved supplement and is thought to have a positive impact on VVA due to its effect on the estrogen and androgen receptors. Topical testosterone has also been investigated, but a lack of data precludes an ability to recommend its use for VVA at the current time [7].

Nonhormonal options are also available and can be helpful in any woman with VVA. They are particularly important for women with contraindications to hormonal therapy or for women preferring not to take prescription therapies. There are many lubricants, creams, and moisturizers that can help with local symptoms. A water-, silicone-, or oil-based lubricant can be suggested for symptomatic treatment of dryness related to intercourse. These personal moisturizers and lubricants typically require frequent reapplication but can ease sexual discomfort [2,7,9]. The benefits of regular sexual intercourse should be stressed in patients that have partners. In addition to increasing pliability and elasticity of the vaginal mucosa, sexual arousal stimulates the endogenous lubrication potential of the vagina and may increase vascularity [1,7]. Barrier contraception is essential for decreasing sexually transmitted infections for those who are not in a mutually monogamous relationship. For those women who are not in a sexual relationship, it is important to ask if they would like to preserve their capacity for sexual activity. If so, they should be informed about the benefits of self-stimulation, vibrators, and dilators as a means of maintaining vaginal size and flexibility during times when they do not have a partner.

Key teaching points

- Vaginal dryness can be an early indicator of decreased estrogen.
- Vaginal dryness, soreness, dyspareunia, or bleeding after intercourse should raise concern for symptomatic vulvovaginal atrophy (VVA).
- A concomitant urinary tract infection and vaginitis should be promptly evaluated and treated appropriately.
- Treatment with an estrogen cream, tablet, or ring should be considered if no contraindications exist. Otherwise, nonhormonal options should be considered. Systemic hormonal therapy may be preferred if there are no contraindications, especially if the patient has vasomotor symptoms or other indications for hormonal therapy.
- The addition of a moisturizer or lubricant should be considered for dyspareunia.
- Sexual intercourse, self-stimulation, vibrators, and dilators can promote the elasticity of the vagina and its potential for self-lubrication.
- If dyspareunia is not markedly improved by the use of estrogen, other causes such as vestibulodynia and vulvodynia should be considered. Also, consider other potential sources of vaginal bleeding, such as uterine pathology, especially if the etiology of bleeding is unclear.

References

1. Bachmann GA, Nevadunsky NS. Diagnosis and treatment of atrophic vaginitis. *Am Fam Physician* 2000;61:3090–6.

2. North American Menopause Society. *Menopause Practice: A Clinician's Guide*, 4th edn. Mayfield Heights, OH, North American Menopause Society, 2010.

3. Freedman M. Vaginal pH, estrogen and genital atrophy. *Menopause Management* 2008;17(4):9–13.

4. American College of Obstetricans and Gynecologists. *Committee Opinion. The Role of Transvaginal Ultrasonography in the Evaluation of Postmenopausal Bleeding.* No. 440, August 2009 (reaffirmed 2013). Available at http://www.acog.org/~/media/Committee%20Opinions/Committee%20on%20Gynecologic%20Practice/co440.pdf?dmc=1&ts=20120516T2213422403.

5. Eugster-Hausmann M, Waitzinger J, Lehnick D. Minimized estradiol absorption with ultra-low-dose 10 microg 17beta-estradiol vaginal tablets. *Climacteric* 2010;13:219–27.

6. Ballagh SA. Vaginal hormone therapy for urogenital and menopausal symptoms. *Semin Reprod Med* 2005;23:126–40.

7. North American Menopause Society. Position statement: Management of symptomatic vulvovaginal atrophy: 2013 position statement of the North American Menopause Society. *Menopause* 2013;20(9):882–902.

8. US Pharmaceuticals. *Duavee. Last revised 15 November 2013.* Available at www.medlibrary.org/lib/rx/meds/duavee-2/.

9. Marshall DD, Iglesia C. A guide to lotions and potions for treating vaginal atrophy. *OBG Management* 2009;21(12):29–37.

A 60-year-old woman with severe vulvar itching and an ulcer

Alan G. Waxman

History of present illness

A 60-year-old postmenopausal white woman, gravida 2, para 2 presents with an exacerbation of intense vulvar itching and burning. The symptoms have been present intermittently for the past 11 years, but until a few months ago, they presented only a mild annoyance. Recently, the itching has become constant and more intense. She has been able to tolerate the itching during the day. At night, however, the itching is so bad that she finds herself scratching in her sleep. She has found sexual relations increasingly difficult, and in the past two months has been unable to attempt to have intercourse. She denies recent changes in weight, vaginal discharge, and she does not douche or use feminine hygiene products. She wears cotton underwear and denies recent changes in soaps or detergents. Further review of symptoms is notable only for seasonal rhinitis, which is not currently bothering her.

The patient reports that she has seen her primary provider for these symptoms and has been to various urgent care clinics as well. She has been treated with both oral and vaginal medications for "yeast infections," and has also been prescribed vaginal metronidazole. She has also tried a number of over-the-counter treatments without success. Her nurse practitioner recently started her on estrogen cream. Most of these medications have given her transient relief, but the symptoms ultimately return.

Her past medical history is notable for osteoporosis, and her only surgery is the repair of a torn left rotator cuff 10 years prior. Her current medications are limited to estrogen vaginal cream, which she uses twice weekly, a weekly bisphosphonate, a daily multivitamin, calcium and a baby aspirin.

She reports having had two vaginal deliveries, the first with midline episiotomy. Menopause was at age 52, and she denies vaginal bleeding since. Her most recent cervical screening tests were negative for intraepithelial lesion or malignancy and negative for high-risk human papillomavirus (HPV) DNA.

She is a married, recently retired middle school social studies teacher. She does not smoke. She drinks alcohol twice a week with dinner.

Physical examination

General appearance: Well-developed, well-nourished woman who appears her stated age
Vital signs: All within normal limits. BMI: 24 kg/m^2
Skin: No lesions noted on scalp, face, extremities, chest, trunk, or buccal mucosa

HEENT: Normal
Chest: Clear to auscultation
Cardiac: Regular rate and rhythm, no murmurs or gallops
Abdomen: Soft, nontender, no masses
Lymph nodes: None palpable
External genitalia: Diminution of the labia minora bilaterally with the left narrowed and the right largely absent. The skin of the labia minora and inner labia majora is shiny and white with evidence of excoriation in the interlabial fold. There is a 1 cm ulcer on the left. The ulcer is tender with slightly raised, distinct white margins and a nonfriable base (Fig. 14.1)
Introitus: The introitus is narrow but accepts a Pederson speculum with some discomfort

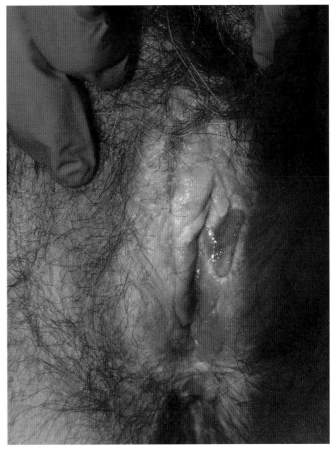

Fig. 14.1 The ulcer is tender with slightly raised, distinct white margins and a nonfriable base.

Acute Care and Emergency Gynecology, ed. David Chelmow, Christine R. Isaacs and Ashley Carroll. Published by Cambridge University Press.
© Cambridge University Press 2015.

Vagina: The vaginal mucosa appears pink and well rugated, consistent with topical estrogen use. The vaginal discharge is a creamy white and minimal in quantity. The cervix appears multiparous and without lesions

Uterus and adnexa: Because of the narrowness of the introitus, bimanual examination can only be performed with one finger. A rectovaginal examination facilitates outlining the uterus, which is unremarkable. No adnexal masses are appreciated

Laboratory studies:

Vaginal discharge: pH 4.2
Wet mount: Epithelial maturation and lactobacilli consistent with vaginal estrogen use. No yeast, trichomonas, or clue cells seen

How would you manage this patient?

The gross appearance is consistent with a clinical diagnosis of lichen sclerosus. The ulcer, while not uncommon in this setting, clearly poses a cause for concern of a secondary diagnosis. A biopsy is necessary to rule out malignancy. This was performed in the office setting with local anesthesia and a 4 mm Keys punch biopsy at the margin of the ulcer, including the ulcer floor. Biopsy of the margin is important to include both epidermis and dermis, which will be absent in the ulcer, itself.

The patient was started on clobetazol propionate ointment 0.05% with instructions to use a thin application twice a day for one month, tapered to once a day for a month, then on alternate days for two weeks followed by twice a week. Her itching largely resolved within the first two weeks of treatment. By six weeks the ulcer was completely healed. This patient's biopsy report confirmed lichen sclerosus with no evidence of malignancy.

This patient's topical steroid regimen was ultimately changed to use of a less potent steroid, triamcinolone ointment 0.1% used 2–3 times a week to reduce the incidence of flares. She manages the occasional episode of recurrent itching with a short course of clobetazol.

The patient is scheduled for semi-annual vulvar examinations to look for the development of plaques, ulcers, or other lesions that might require repeat biopsy to rule out vulvar intraepithelial neoplasia or malignancy.

Lichen sclerosus

Lichen sclerosus occurs in both men and women. It is, however, more common in women, and it is most commonly seen on the genitalia. It has a bimodal age distribution peaking in times of low estrogen, notably in postmenopausal women in the fifth and sixth decades, but also not infrequently in prepubertal girls [1]. It is an inflammatory disorder with a presumed autoimmune etiology. The exact pathophysiology remains unknown. The condition is associated with autoimmune thyroiditis, pernicious anemia, alopecia areata, and vitilago. There is a familial predisposition with an increased incidence in siblings and twins, but the inheritance pattern is not fully understood [1].

The spectrum of skin changes seen in lichen sclerosus ranges from isolated to confluent white patches, and from thickened appearing skin to thinned crinkled parchment-like skin. It may involve the labia minora and majora alone or demonstrate a classical keyhole shape extending around the anus. Longstanding lichen sclerosus may create a thickened yellowish or dull gray coloration in the labia and interlabial folds. Patients may experience a spectrum of symptoms ranging from nothing, to tingling and slight burning of the skin, to intense itching and burning as with the patient illustrated in this case. Chronic scratching and rubbing can create ecchymoses, excoriations, and ulcerations. Repeated scratching may thicken the epidermis resulting in adjacent lichen simplex chronicus, a condition of skin lichenification and swelling from chronic scratching. The "scratch–itch–scratch" cycle set up by lichen simplex chronicus can exacerbate and prolong the already intense itching of lichen sclerosis. Progression of the lichen sclerosis can result in loss of the architecture of the vulva with resorption or agglutination of the labia minora including the clitoral hood. In advanced cases, agglutination of the labia may lead to urinary retention requiring surgery. Such progression, however, is not an inevitable development in women with lichen sclerosus, and the disease in some patients may be limited to small white patches on the labia that continue without further progression. However, it is a chronic condition that will have recurrences and remissions throughout the patient's life. The diagnosis is made clinically and confirmed with biopsy.

Histologically, the epidermis thins with or without hyperkeratosis or parakeratosis and there is flattening of the rete ridges. A pathognomonic feature is a band of dermal homogenization with an underlying inflammatory infiltrate that is predominantly lymphocytic (Fig. 14.2).

Lichen sclerosus responds very well to class 1 super potent steroids such as clobetazol propionate 0.05%. A common regimen used in the United States starts with twice daily applications as described in this case. There are no randomized clinical trials recommending one regimen over another. The British Association of Dermatologists guidelines recommend application once nightly for four weeks, tapering to alternate nights for four weeks and then twice weekly [2]. The steroid should be tapered to avoid a steroid rebound effect but may be restarted for recurrence of symptoms. Topical testosterone was widely used in the past, but has not been shown to have the efficacy of the super potent corticosteroids [2,3]. The potential for steroid toxicity may be reduced by limiting the steroid to a thin layer application and limiting the amount given to the patient. A 30 g tube should last 3 months.

While comfort measures are based on expert opinion, most clinicians advise empiric measures to protect the sensitive skin that is easily subject to contact dermatitis, allergic reactions, and irritation from excess moisture. Specifically patients

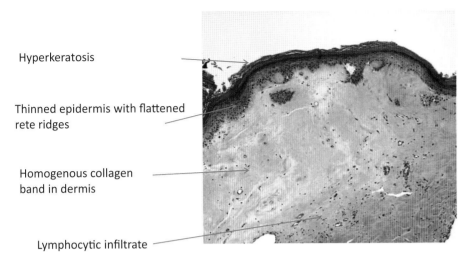

Fig. 14.2 Histology of lichen sclerosis.

Hyperkeratosis

Thinned epidermis with flattened rete ridges

Homogenous collagen band in dermis

Lymphocytic infiltrate

should be urged to avoid detergents or soaps with scents, and to consider using water alone to clean the vulva. A bland emollient may be used on the skin after bathing, and cotton underwear (or no underwear) should be encouraged, especially at night while sleeping. Many patients find warm soaks or use of cold gelpacks soothing and helpful to provide relief for the itching. In addition, patients may be started on hydroxyzine 50 mg at bedtime to relieve the itching and to help with sleep.

Squamous cell carcinoma is a rare cancer with an incidence of 1.5 cases per 100 000 women [1]. However, lichen sclerosus is present and adjacent to about 60% of all vulvar squamous cell cancers [1,4]. The squamous cell carcinoma associated with lichen sclerosis is HPV negative, and is associated with vulvar intraepithelial neoplasia, differentiated type. It has been estimated that the lifelong risk of a woman with lichen sclerosis to develop vulvar carcinoma is approximately 5% [1,4]. Long-term follow-up is therefore very important once the diagnosis of lichen sclerosis has been made. Most authorities recommend reevaluation of the patient every six months

looking specifically for new plaque-like lesions, white raised lesions, erythematous lesions, papillary tumors, ulcerations, or unexplained pain. Biopsies should be taken very liberally with any new clinical findings.

Key teaching points

- Lichen sclerosus presents most commonly with chronic, severe vulvar pruritis.
- While the diagnosis of lichen sclerosus is made clinically, biopsy confirmation should be obtained.
- Super potent topical corticosteroids are the mainstay of treatment for lichen sclerosus.
- Vulvar examination at six-month intervals is recommended for women with lichen sclerosus because of the elevated risk of vulvar squamous cell carcinoma carcinoma.
- Any new or different appearing lesion should be biopsied.

References

1. Murphy R. Lichen sclerosus. *Dermatol Clin* 2010;28:707–15.
2. Neill SM, Lewis FM, Tatnall FM, et al. British Association of Dermatologists' guidelines for the management of lichen sclerosus 2010. *Brit J Derm* 2010;163:672–82.
3. Ching-Chi C, Kirtschig G, Baldo M, et al. Systematic review and meta-analysis of randomized controlled trials on topical interventions for genital lichen sclerosus. *J Am Acad Dermatol* 2012;67(2):305–12.
4. Gutierrez-Pascual M, Vincente-Martin FJ, López-Estebaranz JL. Lichen sclerosus and squamous cell carcinoma. *Acts Dermosifilogr* 2012;103(1):21–8.

Urinary retention in a 19-year-old woman

Amanda B. Murchison and Megan Metcalf

History of present illness

A 19-year-old gravida 0 woman presents complaining of 3 days of worsening vulvar pain and vaginal discharge. The pain is bilateral and "burning." She reports dysuria, which has become more severe, and she is now unable to void. She has no hematuria, frequency, or urgency. She was last able to void eight hours ago.

She is currently sexually active and reports that she entered a relationship with a new partner approximately two weeks ago. She is not using any birth control. She denies fever or chills but reports increasing lower abdominal pain over the past four hours. She has no significant past medical or surgical history. She takes no medications.

Physical examination

General appearance: Well-developed, well-nourished, young woman appearing uncomfortable and tearful

Vital signs:

Temperature: 36.7°C
Pulse: 93 beats/min
Blood pressure: 116/79 mmHg
Respiratory rate: 18 breaths/min
Oxygen saturation: 98% on room air
BMI: 23.9 kg/m^2
Weight: 135 lb

Cardiovascular: Regular rate and rhythm with no murmurs

Lungs: Clear to auscultation

Abdomen: Some tenderness to palpation of suprapubic region

External genitalia: Bilateral swollen labia, which were erythematous with numerous coalescing ulcerative lesions (Fig. 15.1). Labia are tender to touch

Urethra: Urethral meatus appears normal

Vagina: Patient unable to tolerate speculum or bimanual exam

Voiding trial: Patient unable to void

Laboratory studies:

Urine pregnancy test: Negative
WBCs: 5500/μL
Hb: 13.3 g/dL
Ht: 39.8%
Platelets: 245 000/μL

How would you manage this patient?

The patient appears to be having a first clinical episode of genital herpes simplex virus (HSV) infection. Given the severity of the outbreak, the patient has significant discomfort and swelling which has led to urinary retention. Management of this patient included performing polymerase chain reaction (PCR) testing from the vulvar ulcerations to confirm the diagnosis. Given the clinical appearance, treatment should be initiated for presumed HSV while the results were pending.

Primary management was directed at relieving her urinary retention and controlling her pain. A Foley catheter was placed after the application of lidocaine jelly to the urethral area. Given the severity of the pain, she was admitted for pain control with intravenous narcotics. The patient was started

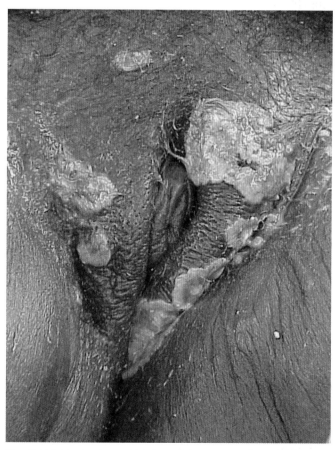

Fig. 15.1 Labia showing multiple herpetic lesions secondary to HSV-2. (Photograph provided by Steven Cohen, MD.)

Acute Care and Emergency Gynecology, ed. David Chelmow, Christine R. Isaacs and Ashley Carroll. Published by Cambridge University Press. © Cambridge University Press 2015.

on acyclovir and recommended sexually transmitted disease testing, which she accepted. As the patient could not tolerate a speculum exam, urine nucleic acid amplification tests (NAATs) were sent for gonorrhea and chlamydia. The patient was discharged home on hospital day 2 once her pain was under better control. The Foley catheter was left in place at the time of discharge and was removed at a follow-up visit two days later. She completed a 10-day course of acyclovir. PCR testing of the vulvar lesion returned positive for HSV-2. The likelihood of recurrence was discussed with the patient, and she was started on suppressive therapy.

Genital herpes simplex virus

Genital herpes simplex virus (HSV) infection is the most prevalent cause of ulcerative genital disease. Both HSV-1 and HSV-2 can cause genital herpes. Serologic surveys show that 26% of women of reproductive age and older are seropositive for HSV-2. However, HSV-2 prevalence underestimates the overall prevalence of genital herpes as outbreaks associated with HSV-1 are becoming more frequent [1]. The mean incubation period is one week. The virus enters the body via direct contact of epidermal cells with secretions or mucosal surfaces from an infected individual. The classic clinical presentation includes clusters of painful vesicles and ulcerations [1,2]. Pain, itching, dysuria, vaginal or urethral discharge, and inguinal adenopathy are the most common presenting symptoms [2]. The first clinical episode is defined as the first presentation of genital herpes and can be caused by HSV-1 or HSV-2. Primary first episodes refer to patients who were previously seronegative for HSV, while nonprimary first episodes refers to a first clinical infection in a patient who has preexisting antibodies to the other HSV type [3]. Primary infections are typically more severe than recurrent or first episode nonprimary infections. They may be associated with systemic symptoms like generalized flu-like complaints and can also be complicated by neurologic involvement.

Diagnosis has traditionally been made using a viral culture. This test is specific but lacks sensitivity and has been shown to have a false negative rate as high as 25% for primary infection and 50% for recurrences. PCR testing is becoming more widely available and has increased sensitivity [1]. The specimen should be obtained from the lesion base or vesicular fluid. According to the Centers for Disease Control and Prevention (CDC), serologic studies for type-specific antibodies for HSV-1 and 2 should be considered in the setting of a clinical suspicion for HSV with a negative virologic test [4]. This patient has a first clinical episode, which was confirmed by PCR testing. It could be either a primary or nonprimary outbreak, as she had extremely severe local symptoms, but no systemic symptoms. As the management is determined by symptoms, it is not necessary to determine whether the outcome is primary or nonprimary.

This patient's main issues are her pain from her lesions, and consequent urinary retention. The urinary retention is likely a result of pain and induration surrounding the urethra. It may be secondary to the dysuria caused by urine irritating the ulcerated skin and the patient's need to avoid this pain. In this situation, topical lidocaine jelly applied to the vulva prior to voiding may be of some benefit. Other things that might be of value in cases of urinary retention include having the patient try to void while taking a warm bath or shower, which allows the urine to minimize contact with the herpetic lesions. Use of a peribottle to spray warm water on the perineum while voiding can also be attempted. Relaxation techniques such as having the patient blow into a glass of water with a straw while sitting on the commode may help relax the pelvic muscles. There is no published evidence for any of these things, but they are all low risk and inexpensive.

If the patient is still unable to void, placement of a Foley catheter is necessary until the pain and swelling resolves enough for the patient to be able to void. Catheter placement can be difficult given patient pain and swollen anatomy. Lidocaine jelly should be applied to the urethra for a few minutes prior to insertion of the catheter. Use of a pediatric catheter with a smaller diameter or a catheter that is more rigid such as a latex-free or coude catheter may make placement easier. Pain medication should be given, including intravenous sedation if necessary. Patients usually get substantial relief once the bladder begins draining.

The catheter should be left in place until the lesions have begun to crust and pain decreases. If the bladder has become overdistended (usually defined at $\geq$600 mL of urine for at least 24 hours) then the patient may benefit from keeping the catheter in place for 2–3 days prior to attempting a voiding trial to allow restoration of bladder tone in addition to healing of the lesions. Our patient did require Foley catheter placement, which was kept in place for three days. The patient was successfully able to void once it was discontinued. At the time of catheter removal, the patient still had crusting HSV lesions that required approximately two more weeks to completely resolve. Primary lesions can last 2–6 weeks with new lesions continuing to form over the first 10 days [2]. Placement of a urethral catheter by itself does not necessitate hospitalization. Patients can receive leg bag training and manage the catheter at home while the lesions heal.

The patient's other main problem was pain from the lesions. Extensive ulceration of the vulva and vagina puts the patient at risk for bacterial superinfection. If superinfection develops, the patient may also need to be treated with an antibiotic. Frequent sitz bathing can provide pain relief and decrease the likelihood of superinfection. Pain medication with nonsteroidal anti-inflammatory drugs or oral narcotics can be helpful. For extremely severe infections, parenteral narcotics may be briefly necessary, as they were in this patient.

Antiviral medications are helpful in the management of both first clinical episode and recurrent genital herpes outbreaks. Table 15.1 lists recommended treatment regimens for both. Although resolution of outbreaks is hastened by antiviral treatment, it does not eradicate latent virus or affect the long-

Table 15.1 Recommended treatment regimens for genital herpes based on the 2010 CDC guidelines *

Recommended regimens	
First clinical episode of genital HSV	Acyclovir 400 mg PO TID for 7–10 days
	Acyclovir 200 mg PO 5 times a day for 7–10 days
	Valacyclovir 1 g PO BID for 7–10 days
	Famciclovir 250 mg PO TID for 7–10 days
Recurrent episodes	Acyclovir 400 mg PO TID for 5 days
	Acyclovir 800 mg PO BID for 5 days
	Acyclovir 800 mg PO TID for 2 days
	Valacyclovir 500 mg PO BID for 3 days
	Valacyclovir 1 g PO daily for 5 days
	Famciclovir 125 mg PO BID for 5 days
	Famciclovir 1000 mg PO BID for 1 day
Suppressive therapy	Acyclovir 400 mg PO BID
	Valacyclovir 500 mg PO QD
	Valacyclovir 1 g PO QD
	Famciclovir 250 mg PO BID

Adapted from Centers for Disease Control and Prevention [4].
BID, twice a day; CDC, Centers for Disease Control and Prevention; HSV, herpes simplex virus; PO, *per os* (orally); QD, every day; TID, three times a day.

term disease process [3]. This patient was administered a 10-day course of acyclovir, which likely shortened the duration and severity of her symptoms. The earlier the antiviral is started in the course of an outbreak, the greater the improvement.

Recurrence of genital herpes occurs in many patients with a symptomatic first episode. Episodes are more frequent in HSV-2 infected individuals than in those with HSV-1. Recurrent genital herpes can be managed with either episodic (at the time of a recurrent outbreak) or suppressive (daily prophylactic) therapy [1,4]. Recurrent outbreaks are typically milder than first episodes, with fewer lesions and less viral shedding [2]. Episodic treatment (Table 15.1) has been shown to decrease the duration of recurrence symptoms including pain, lesion persistence, and viral shedding. Given that this was the patient's first episode and was with HSV-2, episodic therapy would be a reasonable approach.

Suppressive therapy prevents 70–80% of recurrent episodes. It is a good option for patients with: (1) frequent outbreaks; (2) HSV-susceptible partners; or (3) psychosocial difficulty in coping with outbreaks. Breakthrough recurrences while on suppressive therapy are infrequent and typically short in duration. Suppressive therapy also markedly decreases viral DNA shedding, translating into a 48% reduction in sexual transmission to a susceptible partner. Studies show many patients prefer suppressive therapy [1,4]. Our patient was having difficulty coping with the new diagnosis of genital herpes. This difficulty, combined with the severity of her outbreak, led to her decision for suppression.

When a patient is diagnosed with a sexually transmitted infection she should be counseled both about the infection and how it might affect her current or future partners. Patients with a diagnosis of genital herpes should be encouraged to discuss this diagnosis with their partner(s). Patients should be informed that transmission of genital herpes to a partner can be decreased by taking the following measures: (1) refraining from sexual activity during prodromal symptoms or when lesions are present; (2) consistent use of male, latex condoms; and (3) daily use of antiviral therapy by the infected partner [4]. Many patients will experience feelings of anxiety, loneliness, and decreased self-worth as our patient did. Through educating patients, physicians can help empower patients to take an active role in managing this disease [2].

Key teaching points

- Urinary retention can occur during an episode of genital herpes due to pain or induration surrounding the urethra.
- Placement of a urinary catheter may be necessary.
- Placement of a urinary catheter may require application of lidocaine jelly and supplemental pain medication.
- Antiviral medications should also be given for outbreaks severe enough to cause urinary retention.
- Primary genital herpes infections are typically more severe than recurrent infections. They may be associated with generalized flu-like symptoms and can also be complicated by neurologic involvement.

References

1. American College of Obstetricians and Gynecologists. Gynecologic herpes simplex virus infections. Practice Bulletin No. 57. *Obstet Gynecol* 2004;104:1111–17.

2. Beauman JG. Genital herpes: a review. *Am Fam Physician* 2005;72(8): 1527–34.

3. Sen P, Barton SE. Genital herpes and its management. *BMJ* 2007;334(7602): 1048–52.

4. Centers for Disease Control and Prevention. Sexually transmitted diseases treatment guidelines, 2010. *MMWR* 2010;59(RR-12): 1–116.

Recurrent herpes infection in a 28-year-old woman

Breanna Walker

History of present illness

A 28-year-old woman presents to an outpatient general gynecology clinic with complaints of vaginal burning and pain. Symptoms have been present for three days. She initially noticed a tingling sensation that later developed into burning and pain. She finds it hard to urinate due to the symptoms. She denies any vaginal discharge. She had a subjective low grade temperature last night but otherwise is afebrile. She was diagnosed a few years ago with herpes but thinks this feels different. She is sexually active and in a monogamous relationship with her boyfriend of three months. Her last menstrual cycle was one week prior with a history of regular cycles. She has a copper intrauterine device (IUD) in place and has never been pregnant before. She is otherwise healthy and taking no medications.

Physical examination

Vital signs:

Temperature: 37.0°C
Pulse: 81 beats/min
Blood pressure: 118/73 mmHg
Respiratory rate: 16 breaths/min

HENNT: Unremarkable

Cardiovascular: Normal rate, regular rhythm

Respirations: Nonlabored respirations, clear to auscultation

Abdomen: Soft, nontender, nondistended, no rebound or guarding

Genitourinary:

External vulvar area with ulcerated lesions in the posterior forchet bilaterally, significantly tender to touch
Speculum examination: No internal lesions, normal appearing cervix with IUD strings in place
Bimanual examination: Limited secondary due to tenderness of the vulva but otherwise unremarkable

Extermities: No edema or tenderness

Laboratory studies:

Urine pregnancy test: Negative
Urine dip: Negative

How would you manage this patient?

This patient has a recurrent genital herpes outbreak. Her primary history of herpes simplex virus (HSV) makes this the most likely diagnosis. A viral culture was obtained and confirmed the diagnosis. She was treated with acyclovir for her current outbreak. The dose of acyclovir is different for recurrent herpes infection than a primary infection. Many different regimens could be used but in this case, she was given 800 mg PO twice a day for 5 days. Suppression therapy versus episodic therapy for future outbreaks was discussed with the patient at length. She opted for episodic therapy and was provided with a prescription with instructions to initiate therapy immediately following the first prodromal symptoms. She should return to clinic for a general health examination or if she needs a refill on her antiviral medication. If she needs frequent treatments for outbreaks, she may prefer suppressive therapy.

Recurrent episodes of herpes simplex virus

Herpes simplex virus (HSV) infection is a sexually transmitted infection that causes genital ulcers and cannot be cured. Genital infections can be caused by either HSV-1 or HSV-2, but generally HSV-2 is thought to be more associated with genital infections. An outbreak generally starts with prodromal symptoms of vulvar itching, burning, or tingling followed by the appearance of a blister. The skin overlaying the blister will break and an ulcer will be present [1]. The ulcer associated with HSV is typically painful which distinguishes it from syphilis which is painless. The HSV-2 serology is present in about 26% of women in the United States but only 10–25% of those patients have had a clinical outbreak of herpes [2]. Black women have the highest prevalence of the disease at 48% [1]. Women will typically have four recurrences in the first year following a HSV-2 primary outbreak [2]. This is more than HSV-1, which on average has about one recurrence per year.

The diagnosis of HSV is a clinical diagnosis but it can be confirmed with a viral culture or HSV polymerase chain reaction (PCR) [2]. The culture is widely available and best obtained by using the swab in the base of an ulcer. In a recurrent infection the culture can have a false negative rate of 50% [2]. Most labs require the specimen to remain cold during transport but this should be confirmed with the lab the provider is using. PCR testing differs from culture in that it is more sensitive for the detection of the virus and leads to less false negative results; however, it is more costly. Testing for the antibodies to HSV-1 and HSV-2 may also be helpful in distinguishing a primary versus recurrent infection, because it takes at least two weeks following an infection before the antibodies can be detected. These assays detect the glycoproteins of the antibodies to HSV-1 or HSV-2 with a high specificity [3].

Treatment for HSV should be initiated prior to confirming the diagnosis (Table 16.1). Symptomatic treatment can be

Acute Care and Emergency Gynecology, ed. David Chelmow, Christine R. Isaacs and Ashley Carroll. Published by Cambridge University Press.
© Cambridge University Press 2015.

Table 16.1 Treatment for herpes simplex virus (HSV)

First episode

Acyclovir	400 mg TID for 7–10 days
Acyclovir	200 mg 5 times daily for 7–10 days
Famciclovir	250 mg TID for 7–10 days
Valacyclovir	1 g BID for 7–10 days

Episodic treatment of recurrence

Acyclovir	400 mg TID for 5 days
Acyclovir	800 mg BID for 5 days
Acyclovir	800 mg TID for 2 days
Famciclovir	125 mg BID for 5 days
Famciclovir	1 g daily for 1 day
Valacyclovir	500 mg BID for 3 days
Valacyclovir	1 g daily for 5 days

Daily suppression

Acyclovir	400 mg BID
Famciclovir	250 mg BID
Valacyclovir	0.5–1.0 g daily

BID, twice a day; TID, three times a day.

obtained with topical anesthetics and narcotics. Acute treatment of the outbreak with antiviral therapy should be recommended. Antiviral medication reduces pain, viral shedding, and the length of the episode [2]. Multiple regimens are available on the Centers for Disease Control and Prevention (CDC) website [1]. Acyclovir is generally available for the lowest cost but requires frequent dosing. A once-daily regimen is valacyclovir 1 g daily for 5 days, which may help with patient compliance but is more expensive. Following treatment for this acute episode the patient should be given a prescription for antiviral therapy that she can fill and use without a clinic visit. For future outbreaks antiretroviral therapy should be started when she first starts to have prodromal symptoms. Most patients will be able to recognize the prodromal symptoms and delaying treatment until the diagnosis can be confirmed is not recommended [2].

Following treatment of the acute episode, this patient may benefit from daily suppression, but this is a decision that the provider would make with the patient. Daily suppression reduces transmission between partners by 48% and prevents 80% of recurrences [4]. If the patient's serologic studies returned as HSV-1, it would be less likely that she would have recurrences; therefore, daily suppression would be less beneficial [2]. In patients who have more than four to six episodes a year, daily suppression should be recommended. Regimens for daily suppression include acyclovir 400 mg BID or famciclovir 250 mg BID [1].

The patient should be counseled regarding the risk to future pregnancies. She should understand that she will need daily suppression at the end of pregnancy and that she should make any future providers aware of this diagnosis. The goal of daily suppression in pregnancy is to reduce the risk of episodes that would cause viral shedding during the intrapartum period [5]. The greatest risk for neonatal transmission occurs with active viral shedding at the time of delivery. In the event of an outbreak at the time of delivery, a Cesarean section should be performed to decrease transmission of the virus to the neonate. However, the rates of neonatal transmission for recurrent infections are overall low.

The patient also needs to be counseled regarding the sexual transmission of HSV. It is transmitted by direct contact and barrier methods are not completely effective at protecting the partner from acquiring the virus [1]. Viral shedding can be asymptomatic, but when lesions are present the viral shedding is the highest and sexual activity is strongly discouraged during this time [1]. Like any sexually transmitted disease, the patient should be counseled to notify her sexual partners so as to reduce the incidence of the disease. The partner may also desire testing to see if he is seropositive for the same type of HSV. If they are discordant, daily suppression should be recommended [2]. The diagnosis of HSV can be overwhelming and the patient would likely benefit from future visits to better understand how the diagnosis will affect her in the future.

Key teaching points

- Genital herpes simplex virus (HSV) can be both type 1 and type 2, but HSV-2 is most likely to cause recurrent episodes.
- Episodic treatment should be initiated when prodromal symptoms begin.
- Patients with frequent recurrences would likely benefit from daily suppression.
- The patient will likely need counseling both at diagnosis and in the future regarding the chronic nature of HSV and its implications on her sexual health.

References

1. Centers for Disease Control and Prevention. *Sexually Transmitted Diseases Treatment Guidelines, 2010. Diseases Characterized by Genital, Anal, or Perianal Ulcers.* Available at http://www.cdc.gov/std/treatment/2010/genital-ulcers.htm.

2. American College of Obstetricians and Gynecologists. Gynecologic herpes simplex virus infections. Practice Bulletin No. 57. *Obstet Gynecol* 2004;104:1111–17.

3. Ashley RL. Sorting out the new HSV type specific antibody tests. *Sex Transm Infect* 2001;77:232–7.

4. Corey L, Wald A, Patel R, et al. Once-daily valacyclovir to reduce the risk of transmission of genital herpes. Valacyclovir HSV Transmission Study Group. *N Engl J Med* 2004;350:11–20.

5. American College of Obstetricians and Gynecologists. Management of herpes in pregnancy. Practice Bulletin No. 82. *Obstet Gynecol* 2007;109:1233–48.

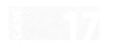

Vulvar infection and sepsis in a 42-year-old woman

L. Chesney Thompson

History of present illness

A 42-year-old gravida 2, para 2 woman presented to the emergency department with a history of several days of labial swelling and tenderness. She notes the discomfort was getting worse, which prompted her to seek medical care. She states her symptoms started from an "ingrown hair" after shaving. She does not describe any discharge or drainage. She thinks she may have a fever.

She is married and monogamous with no history of sexually transmitted infections. Her only surgery was a tubal ligation. She has type 1 diabetes and is on insulin therapy. She says her endocrinologist describes her control as "fair."

Physical examination

General appearance: Overweight woman appearing fatigued and lethargic

Vital signs:

Temperature: 37.7°C
Pulse: 90 beats/min
Blood pressure: 120/80 mmHg
Respiratory rate: 18 breaths/min
BMI: 38.1 kg/m²

Chest: Clear to auscultation bilaterally

Cardiovascular: Regular rate and rhythm

Abdomen: Soft, obese, with normal bowel sounds and no tenderness

Pelvic:

Right labia with a swollen area measuring 6 × 10 cm with mild erythema extending 10 cm to the mons with moderate tenderness to palpation. There appears to be generalized edema and induration without any discrete mass or pointing abscess. There is no inguinal adenopathy

Bimanual examination: Unremarkable. A marker was used to outline the erythema borders

Laboratory studies:

WBCs: 15 000/μL (normal 3500–12 500/μL), 75% neutrophils
Glucose: 185 mg/dL (normal <135 mg/dL)
CRP: 150 mg/L

The patient was presumed to have a vulvar cellulitis. She was admitted to the hospital given her poorly controlled diabetes and concerns for developing sepsis, and started on intravenous cefazolin. After 12 hours the patient required more narcotic pain medications for labial discomfort. Despite antibiotics, the erythema became more progressive and extended beyond the original inked boundary markings from her earlier examination onto the mons pubis. The patient noted marked tenderness with palpation and there was evidence of epithelial separation with bullae formation (Fig. 17.1).

Vital signs 12 hours after admission:

Temperature: 39.4°C
Pulse: 100 beats/min
Blood pressure: 110/60 mmHg
Respiratory rate: 22 breaths/min

How would you manage this patient?

The patient was diagnosed with necrotizing fasciitis. She was taken to the operating room for examination under anesthesia and debridement. The bullae was aspirated and the contents were sent for culture and gram stain. The subcutaneous tissue was incised, and the fascial layers were easily separated with blunt manipulation. There was a lack of bleeding consistent with tissue necrosis. The tissue was dissected further to the

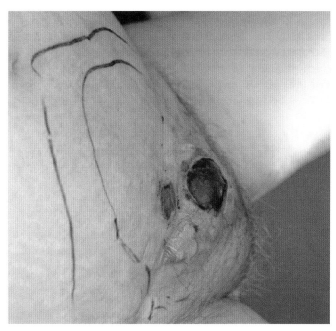

Fig. 17.1 Expanding erythema and bullae formation.

Acute Care and Emergency Gynecology, ed. David Chelmow, Christine R. Isaacs and Ashley Carroll. Published by Cambridge University Press.
© Cambridge University Press 2015.

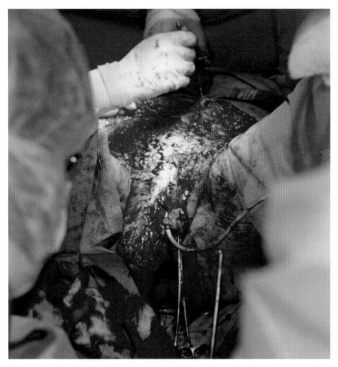

Fig. 17.2 Surgical debridement showing dissection of infected tissue and healthy underlying muscle.

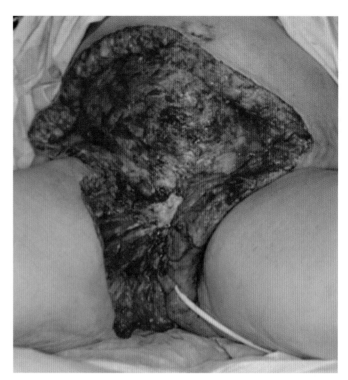

Fig. 17.3 Postoperative healing wound showing extent of dissection.

abdominal wall and lateral to the thighs until the bleeding and viable tissue was identified, and the underlying muscle layer appeared healthy and uninfected (Figs 17.2 & 17.3). The tissue removed was submitted for histologic evaluation. Antibiotic therapy was expanded to ampicillin, gentamycin, and clindamycin. The patient was recovered in the ICU with aggressive fluid resuscitation and blood glucose management. The tissue pathology revealed inflammation with necrosis and a perivascular inflammatory infiltrates, which was consistent with the diagnosis of necrotizing fasciitis. The gram stain and culture revealed beta-hemolytic streptococci and *Staphylococcus aureus*. The patient required additional debridement in the operating room on postoperative day 2 and responded to continued parenteral antibiotics and supportive care. She ultimately had a skin graft performed and recovered fully after a three-week hospital stay.

Necrotizing fasciitis

Necrotizing fasciitis is a soft tissue infection of the subcutaneous fat and fascia overlying the muscle layer. The blood supply to this area is sparse, which limits defense against infection. There are approximately 600–1200 cases of necrotizing fasciitis a year in the United States and they can involve any part of the body [1]. Morbidity and mortality are significant and dramatically increased with delay of initiating therapy. Recognized predisposing risk factors include diabetes, immune-compromised status, obesity, recent trauma or surgery, intravenous drug use, kidney disease, and peripheral artery disease.

The infection is generally an opportunistic process facilitated by diminished immunity and a breach of the integument. The inciting event can be surgery or minor trauma such as scratches or insect bites. There are two types, depending on the organisms involved. Polymicrobial infections are classified as type I, and infections caused by group A streptococcus or other beta-hemolytic streptococci are classified as type II. Type I infections may commonly include anaerobic species such as *Clostridia*, *Bacteroides*, or *Peptostreptococcus*. Additional bacterial species such as *Escherichia coli*, *Enterococcus*, and *Staphylococcus* may be involved. For this reason broad spectrum antibiotics are best utilized. Methicillin-resistant *Staphyloccus aureus* (MRSA) should also be considered, particularly when an abscess and purulent drainage is present.

A necrotizing fasciitis infection may spread over several days or progress more quickly, making the clinical presentation either indolent or rapid. Because the infection resides under the skin, the appearance of skin manifestations may lag behind the subcutaneous infection and destruction. The patient may initially have more pain and tenderness than expected based on visible findings. Initial erythema and cellulitis can be followed by more profound breakdown and necrosis of the skin with bullae formation. Nerve destruction may cause the affected area to become less tender and painful as the process evolves. Crepitus may be present if a gas-producing *Clostridia* species is involved.

As in our case, there may be little signs of sepsis early in the disease process. With progression, fever, tachycardia, and hypotension can develop. Necrotizing fasciitis should be suspected if cellulitis persists despite appropriate antibiotics.

Diagnostic evaluation should be primarily driven by history and physical findings in the context of risk factors, and may be augmented by laboratory testing. It is particularly important to suspect the diagnosis if vital signs begin to suggest systemic inflammatory response syndrome (SIRS) or sepsis. The white blood cell count is typically elevated and includes a left shift. C-reactive protein (CRP) is typically elevated. Creatinine kinase (CK) may be elevated particularly with muscle involvement (myonecrosis). Blood cultures are generally positive, but typically, results are not available when initial management decisions must be made. Wound culture and gram stain can be helpful for antibiotic management but are not available for initial management decisions. Recommendations for radiography using CT or MRI imaging have been suggested and may help establish the extent of the process, including whether there is muscle involvement or the presence of gas or an abscess. There is little evidence, however, to support its routine use, and patient management should not be significantly changed or delayed based on radiologic testing.

Initiating the treatment as early as possible is critical to the patient's survival, and morbidity and mortality increase with delayed intervention. The laboratory risk indicator for necrotizing fasciitis (LRINEC) assessment tool attempts to discern necrotizing fasciitis from less aggressive soft tissue infections [2,3]. A score is generated based on laboratory tests and vital signs. Based on a cutoff value, those at risk are candidates for more aggressive management including diagnostic imaging (if not previously utilized) or surgery. Another proposed preoperative measure to direct possible surgical intervention is needle aspiration of the leading edges of the infection with gram stain. If the gram stain is positive for organisms, surgery should be considered. An alternative is to make a small incision with local anesthesia and to use a finger to assess the lack of resistance to blunt dissection, degree of bleeding, and the appearance of "dishwater" pus. Recommendations have also been made to collect a biopsy for frozen section during this exam. Some clinicians feel the diagnosis is grossly apparent if all these findings are present, limiting the need for microscopic diagnosis. Most frequently, the diagnosis and decision to intervene are based on clinical suspicion.

Unfortunately, there are no well-designed studies and consequently no standardized protocols for the management of necrotizing fasciitis. Aggressive management is necessary. Surgical debridement is the mainstay of therapy. While broad spectrum antibiotics are essential, they will not be curative alone. Mortality rates approach 100% without surgery. Aggressive surgical and antibiotic therapy significantly reduces morbidity and mortality. Fluid resuscitation and hemodynamic support are also necessary. The goal of surgical therapy is to remove all of the infected, devitalized tissue until healthy viable tissue is reached. The area of debridement may be quite extensive, as in our case. Tissue should be sent for histology as well as gram stain, and cultures should be obtained from the wound. Antibiotics must provide broad spectrum coverage of gram-positive and negative bacteria as well as anaerobic organisms. A reasonable regimen would include penicillin for gram-positive organisms, gentamycin or a quinolone for gram-negative bacteria, and clindamycin for anaerobic coverage. Surgical debridement should be repeated as needed until the wound appears healthy with granulation tissue. Antibiotics may be withdrawn after the infection appears resolved. Small studies of intravenous gamma-globulin (IVIG) have not consistently demonstrated benefit. IVIG may be appropriate in cases involving streptococcal toxic shock. Hyperbaric oxygen therapy has received attention and support, but consistent evidence to promote its use is lacking. Management of these extremely sick patients requires interdisciplinary teams of surgeons with training in extensive debridement and skin grafting, and critical care specialists.

Key teaching points

- A high index of suspicion is key to early diagnosis of necrotizing fasciitis.
- Risk factors for necrotizing fasciitis include diabetes, immune compromise, obesity, recent trauma or surgery, intravenous drug use, kidney disease, and peripheral artery disease.
- Signs of necrotizing fasciitis may include: pain disproportionate to examination findings, deep tissue induration beyond the margins of skin involvement, painless or anesthetic areas, bullae or skin necrosis, crepitus, or findings of systemic inflammatory response syndrome (SIRS) or sepsis.
- Aggressive surgical debridement is essential to recovery and survival.
- Treatment requires broad spectrum antibiotics and aggressive management of medical comorbidities.

References

1. Trent JT, Kirsner RS. Diagnosing necrotizing fasciitis. *Adv Skin Wound Care* 2002;15:135–8.

2. Wong Khin LW, Heng KS, Tan KC, Low CO. The LRINEC (laboratory risk indicator for necrotizing fasciitis) score: A tool for distinguishing necrotizing fasciitis from other soft tissues infections. *Crit Care Med* 2004;32:1535–42.

3. Barie PS. The laboratory risk indicator for necrotizing fasciitis (LRINEC) score: Useful tool or paralysis by analysis? *Crit Care Med* 2004;32: 1618–19.

A 42-year-old woman with irregular bleeding

Alison F. Jacoby

History of present illness

A 42-year-old gravida 0 woman presents with a long history of irregular menstrual cycles. As a teenager her periods were unpredictable, occurring from every 16 days to every 6 months. In her twenties she was prescribed combined oral contraceptives (COCs). While she took them she had regular every 28-day cycles. At age 35, she discontinued COCs due to her tobacco use. In her late thirties she tried to become pregnant but was unsuccessful. For the last several years she has only had two to three periods a year. For the last six months she has been bleeding off and on without any pattern. Last month she bled for 20 days with the flow varying from light to heavy. She denies cramps or pelvic pain. She is sexually active without using a birth control method. She takes no other medications. She has not had surgery.

Physical examination

General appearance: A moderately obese woman in no apparent distress

Vital signs:

Temperature: 37.0°C
Pulse: 76 beats/min
Blood pressure: 138/88 mmHg
Respiratory rate: 14 breaths/min
BMI: 31 kg/m^2
Weight: 175 lb
Height: 63 inches

Abdomen: Soft, nontender, no palpable masses

External genitalia: Unremarkable

Vagina: Normal rugae, 3 cc dark red blood in vault

Cervix: Nulliparous, small amount of blood per os

Uterus: Normal size, anteverted, nontender, mobile

Adnexa: No palpable masses, nontender

Laboratory studies:

Urine pregnancy test: Negative
Hct: 36.7%

Biopsy: An endometrial biopsy was performed to evaluate the abnormal uterine bleeding. The endometrial cavity sounded to 8 cm. A moderate amount of tissue was obtained by making three passes with a 3-mm endometrial Pipelle®

Pathology report:

Diagnosis: Simple endometrial hyperplasia

Microscopic description: Mildly crowded endometrial glands with cystic dilation, infrequent mitoses, and no nuclear atypia

How would you manage this patient?

This patient has several risk factors for developing endometrial hyperplasia including obesity and prolonged exposure to unopposed estrogen. Her pattern of infrequent bleeding suggests chronic anovulation. Anovulatory cycles, most commonly associated with polycystic ovarian syndrome, lead to chronic estrogen stimulation of the endometrium, unopposed by the suppressive effects of progesterone. Simple endometrial hyperplasia can be treated with a variety of medications containing progestins such as COCs, medroxyprogesterone acetate (MPA) or a levonorgestrel-containing intrauterine device (LNG-IUD). Since the patient is older than 35 and smokes, COCs are contraindicated. Based on the side-effect profile of MPA and her desire for contraception, she chose the LNG-IUD. A follow-up endometrial biopsy was repeated three months later, and confirmed resolution of the hyperplasia. Although initially she continued to have frequent bleeding and spotting, this improved and was significantly better after the LNG-IUD had been in place for six months. In addition, she began working out with a trainer and meeting with a nutritionist and succeeded in losing 25 lb. She has also set a date to quit smoking.

Simple endometrial hyperplasia

Two classification systems exist for describing endometrial hyperplasia. The World Health Organization (WHO) system is the most widely used classification. It is based on the architectural pattern of the endometrial glands and the presence or absence of atypical nuclei [1]. The degree of gland crowding, or gland-to-stroma ratio, forms the basis for the terms simple and complex hyperplasia. The presence of nuclear atypia is the most important prognostic indicator for progression to endometrial cancer. The WHO system is useful because the categories correlate with the likelihood of progressing to endometrial cancer [2] (Table 18.1). It is limited by interobserver variability.

The endometrial intraepithelial neoplasia (EIN) system is used less often but has higher interobserver agreement [3]. This system divides endometrial changes into endometrial hyperplasia (EH) and EIN. Endometrium exposed to unopposed estrogen resulting in mildly crowded and branched glands would fall into the EH category, whereas endometrium with greater gland density and nuclear abnormalities would be

Acute Care and Emergency Gynecology, ed. David Chelmow, Christine R. Isaacs and Ashley Carroll. Published by Cambridge University Press. © Cambridge University Press 2015.

Table 18.1 Comparison of follow-up of patients with simple and complex hyperplasia and simple and complex atypical hyperplasia ($N = 170$)

	No. of patients	Regressed No. (%)	Persisted No. (%)	Progressed to cancer No. (%)
Simple hyperplasia	93	74 (80)	18 (19)	1 (1)
Complex hyperplasia	29	23 (80)	5 (17)	1 (3)
Simple atypical hyperplasia	13	9 (69)	3 (23)	1 (8)
Complex atypical hyperplasia	35	20 (57)	5 (14)	10 (29)

From Kurman et al. [2].

described as EIN. Based on the results of the endometrial biopsy, this patient would meet criteria for simple endometrial hyperplasia in the WHO classification.

The diagnosis of endometrial hyperplasia is most common in perimenopausal women between the ages of 50 and 54 years. Atypical endometrial hyperplasia and endometrial cancer are typically diagnosed a decade later. Hyperplasia is rarely detected in women younger than age 30. Abnormal uterine bleeding (AUB) is the most frequent presenting symptom. Occasionally, women with endometrial hyperplasia will present without AUB but will have abnormal endometrial cells on cervical cytology. Although this patient was younger than most women with endometrial hyperplasia, she was at increased risk due to many years of unopposed estrogen from anovulation and obesity.

The bleeding pattern of women with endometrial hyperplasia caused by anovulation is typically initially characterized by infrequent bleeding episodes followed by frequent and prolonged bleeding with varying amounts of flow. Initially, the bleeds are infrequent because without ovulation, a corpus luteum does not develop and the ovary does not produce progesterone. Without progesterone withdrawal, there is no trigger to initiate menses. The endometrium is exposed continuously to estrogen, leading to endometrial proliferation. Eventually, the fragile vascular endometrium begins to slough. The haphazard sloughing results in erratic and prolonged uterine bleeding.

The first step in evaluating women suspected of having endometrial hyperplasia is a pelvic examination. Important features to note are the size and mobility of the uterus and the presence or absence of an adnexal mass. All premenopausal women should have a urine or serum pregnancy test. A complete blood count can be helpful in women with prolonged bleeding or symptoms of anemia.

The next step in the evaluation of a woman with irregular bleeding is an endometrial biopsy performed in the office. This is the method of choice for diagnosing endometrial hyperplasia. Operating room procedures should be restricted to women who cannot tolerate an office biopsy, those with cervical stenosis preventing passage of the sampling instrument, and those with insufficient tissue on prior biopsies. There is no clear evidence that one method of endometrial sampling is superior to another [4]. The American College of Obstetricians and Gynecologists guidelines recommend that all women older than 45 years who present with suspected anovulatory uterine bleeding be

Table 18.2 Treatment options for simple endometrial hyperplasia without atypia

	Dose	Regimen
MPA	10 mg	Continuous: daily
MPA	10 mg	Cyclic: daily, 12–14 days/month
LNG-IUD	20 µg	
Combined oral contraceptives	Variable	Daily
Micronized progesterone	100–200 mg	Daily

LNG-IUD, levonorgestrel-containing intrauterine device (LNG-IUD); MPA, medroxyprogesterone acetate.

evaluated with endometrial biopsy [5]. Use of age 45 as the threshold is supported by evidence that the risk of endometrial hyperplasia and carcinoma is fairly low prior to age 45 and increases with advancing age. However, women like this patient, with risk factors for endometrial hyperplasia such as obesity and years of unopposed estrogen from chronic anovulation should undergo an endometrial biopsy regardless of their age.

Although a pelvic ultrasound can be useful for detecting the presence of uterine fibroids, endometrial polyps, and adnexal masses, it is not sensitive or specific for diagnosing endometrial hyperplasia. Regardless of the endometrial thickness, an endometrial biopsy is recommended for premenopausal women with AUB at risk for endometrial hyperplasia due to chronic anovulation.

Although the chance of developing endometrial cancer is very low for women with simple endometrial hyperplasia, treatment is warranted to reduce this risk and to regulate the bleeding. Since endometrial hyperplasia develops as a result of unopposed estrogen, most treatments consist of medications containing a progestin (Table 18.2). The two most common and effective progestin therapies for treating simple hyperplasia are oral MPA and the LNG-IUD. MPA at a dose of 10 mg daily can be prescribed in a continuous or a cyclic regimen for 3–6 months. When used cyclically, it is most effective to take it for at least 12 days each month. It is not unusual for women on MPA to experience side effects such as bloating, mood instability, depression, headaches, and irregular bleeding. Contraindications to progestin therapies include women with progesterone receptor-positive breast cancer or other hormone-sensitive malignancies.

Other progestin-containing treatment options include COCs, depot MPA 150 mg IM every 3 months, micronized progesterone 200 mg in a vaginal cream daily or cyclically, norethindrone acetate 5–10 mg daily or cyclically, and megestrol acetate 20 mg daily. Single-rod progestin implants containing etonogestrel (Nexplanon®, Implanon®) have not been studied for the treatment of endometrial hyperplasia. Nonhormonal treatment options shown to be effective for endometrial hyperplasia are gonadotropin-releasing hormone (GnRH) agonists or antagonists and danazol. Simple hyperplasia is treated medically. Hysterectomy is reserved for women who develop hyperplasia with atypia or women who have persistent AUB unresponsive to medical therapies.

Resolution of simple hyperplasia usually occurs within three to six months of treatment. An endometrial biopsy should be performed three months after initiating treatment. An endometrial biopsy can be performed with an IUD in place. If the hyperplasia has resolved then treatment can be discontinued; however, women with chronic anovulation benefit from ongoing progestin treatment. For women who stop taking a progestin, an additional biopsy should be performed three months later to confirm the hyperplasia has not recurred. If the hyperplasia persists or progresses while on therapy, then the progestin dose should be increased or the treatment changed to a different progestin.

For this patient, although the endometrial hyperplasia has resolved, she is at risk for recurrence off treatment since she has chronic anovulation. A LNG-IUD is a particularly good long-term option for her because it will provide a continuous low-dose of progestin to the endometrium and meet her contraceptive needs. Alternatives for long-term management for her include MPA, combined hormonal contraceptives (COCs, patch, vaginal ring), depot MPA, and etonogestrel implants. Of note, oral MPA is not a contraceptive while the other treatments are. Obese women should be encouraged to lose weight to reduce production of endogenous estrogens and to promote the resumption of ovulation.

Key teaching points

- Endometrial hyperplasia develops when the endometrium is exposed to unopposed estrogen for prolonged periods.
- Anovulation and obesity are common risk factors for simple endometrial hyperplasia.
- Medroxyprogesterone acetate (MPA) 10 mg daily and the levonorgestrel-containing intrauterine device (LNG-IUD) are well-tolerated effective treatments for simple hyperplasia.
- Endometrial sampling should be repeated three to six months after completing therapy to confirm resolution.
- Progestin should be continued for as long as chronic anovulation persists.

References

1. Scully RE, Bonfiglio TA, Kurman, et al. Uterine corpus. In *Histological Typing of Female Genital Tract Tumours*, 2nd edn. New York, Springer-Verlag, 1994, p. 13.
2. Kurman RJ, Kaminski PF, Norris HJ. The behavior of endometrial hyperplasia. A long-term study of "untreated" hyperplasia in 170 patients. *Cancer* 1985;56(2):403–12.
3. Mutter GL. Endometrial intraepithelial neoplasia (EIN): Will it bring order to chaos? The Endometrial Collaborative Group. *Gynecol Oncol* 2000;76:287–90.
4. Ben-Baruch G, Seidman DS, Schiff E, Moran O, Menczer J. Outpatient endometrial sampling with the Pipelle curette. *Gynecol Obstet Invest* 1994;37(4):260–2.
5. American College of Obstetricians and Gynecologists. Diagnosis of abnormal uterine bleeding in reproductive-aged women. Practice Bulletin No. 128. *Obstet Gynecol* 2012;120:197–206.

Persistent HSV in an HIV-positive woman

Jennifer A. Cross

History of present illness

A 43-year-old woman comes into your emergency room complaining of painful areas on her genital area. She states that they have been present for two months, but recently they have become very painful. She has had them before, but in the past they have not lasted this long. She is currently homeless and has been living under a bridge with several friends. You notice from previous hospital records that she is HIV positive and has had inconsistent follow-up. She is currently not taking any medications because "someone stole them." She admits to marijuana use and last used one week ago. She is sexually active with one male partner and they do not use condoms. She otherwise does not endorse any other medical problems and has had no prior surgeries.

Physical examination

General appearance: Alert woman in no acute distress that appears older than her stated age

Vital signs:

Temperature: 37.0°C
Pulse: 87 beats/min
Blood pressure: 105/67 mmHg
Respiratory rate: 16 breaths/min
Oxygen saturation: 100% at room air

Cardiovascular: Regular rate and rhythm

Respiratory: Lungs clear to auscultation bilaterally

Abdomen: Soft, nondistended, nontender

Genitourinary: Large ulcerative painful lesions covering most of her right and left external labia, smaller lesions located around her anal sphincter

Laboratory studies:

HIV viral RNA: >50 000 copies
Absolute CD4 count: 90 μL
HSV PCR: Positive

How should you manage this patient?

This patient is an HIV-positive patient with AIDS presenting with painful lesions on her vulva. The patient's care should revolve around identifying the causative agent responsible. She should be tested for all sexually transmitted infections as she is currently sexually active and having unprotected intercourse. In this case the patient is testing positive for herpes simplex virus (HSV) type 2 based on polymerase chain (PCR) testing.

This patient should be started on high-dose acyclovir with daily prophylactic acyclovir once the lesions resolve. A multidisciplinary approach should be used including Infectious Disease and Social Services.

Persistent HSV in an HIV-positive patient

Chronic herpes simplex virus (HSV), as seen in this patient, is defined by mucocutaneous genital lesions lasting greater than one month. Such lesions are found often in the human immunodeficiency virus (HIV)-positive population, and are commonly associated with declining CD4 counts and rising serum HIV RNA [1]. These atypical lesions have been identified since the outbreak of the HIV epidemic and were among the first opportunistic infections identified in the acquired immune deficiency syndrome (AIDS) population, especially in heterosexual females. Chronic HSV is an AIDS-defining illness as classified by the Centers for Disease Control and Prevention (CDC).

HSV-2 has been the subject of interest due to its global impact on health. The World Health Organization estimated the number of people living with genital herpes at 536 million worldwide in 2003. More women than men were affected, with a total of 315 million women affected globally [2]. This is especially important in the control of HIV spread due a two to threefold risk of acquiring HIV in those who are HSV-2 seropositive. HSV-2 is more prevalent in the HIV-positive population with 50–90% testing seropositive [3]. Active genital lesions and asymptomatic viral shedding have a fivefold increase in risk of HIV transmission per sexual contact for individuals not on highly active antiretroviral therapy (HAART).

The pathogenesis of HSV-2 impact on HIV disease transmission is multifactorial. First, mucosal disruption caused by HSV-2 provides a route for transmission. HSV infection also attracts CD4-positive lymphocytes to the infected area, the same host cells used by HIV. HSV-encoded proteins often increase the expression of HIV-encoded RNA [4]. Therefore, HIV RNA levels at the mucosal surface often exceed the amount in the serum of infected persons. These factors lead to increased HIV transmission even with lower HIV RNA levels.

The presentation of HSV in most patients who are HIV positive is similar to those who are immunocompetent, with most cases causing asymptomatic infections. However, prolonged and atypical infections can be seen including abnormal lesion locations, ulcers greater than 20 cm in diameter, and exophytic protrusions resembling malignancy or condylomas [5]. This can often lead to misdiagnosis or a delay in diagnosis. Reactivation of lesions is common, sometimes occurring more

Acute Care and Emergency Gynecology, ed. David Chelmow, Christine R. Isaacs and Ashley Carroll. Published by Cambridge University Press.
© Cambridge University Press 2015.

Table 19.1 Drug regimes for HSV in HIV-positive patients*

Daily suppressive therapy	Episodic treatment
Acyclovir 400–800 mg PO BID–TID	Acyclovir 400 mg PO TID × 5–10 days
Famciclovir 500 mg PO BID	Famciclovir 500 mg PO BID × 5–10 days
Valacyclovir 500 mg PO BID	Valacyclovir 1 g PO BID × 5–10 days

* Drug doses obtained from Centers for Disease Control and Prevention [6]. BID, twice a day; CDC, Centers for Disease Control and Prevention; HIV, human immunodeficiency virus; HSV, herpes simplex virus; PO, *per os* (orally); TID, three times a day.

than 12 times a year, with little healing time in between outbreaks. This can cause increased scarring, secondary infections with yeast or bacteria, and deep ulcerative painful lesions. Primary infections are usually more intense with persistent lesions, fevers, chills, and even dissemination causing encephalitis, hepatitis, and pneumonitis [1]. There are only a few such cases in the literature as most patients are already seropositive for HSV by the time they acquire HIV.

PCR and HSV cell culture remain the gold standard for diagnosis in the United States. PCR has a higher sensitivity and specificity for detecting HSV and is preferred. Viral culture sensitivity rapidly declines with chronic, nonhealing lesions but, if used, should be obtained from the base of the lesion [6]. As most cases of HSV are subclinical, type-specific serologic testing can be offered to patients especially if viral cultures are negative and HSV is suspected clinically.

Treatment of HSV in HIV-positive patients revolves around the use of HSV antiviral therapy including acyclovir, famciclovir, and valacyclovir (Table 19.1) [6]. Treatment should start as soon as possible and should not be delayed until the return of laboratory results. Doses and treatment duration are often increased from HIV-seronegative patients. Intravenous acyclovir 5–10 mg/kg every 8 hours can be used initially for severe infections [6]. Daily prophylactic HSV should be used in HSV-seropositive patients as it decreases the frequency and severity of outbreaks. However, antiviral therapy does not prevent asymptomatic shedding of viral particles in the genital area and, thus, transmission to sexual partners is a concern [4]. Patients must be counseled on the disease process and the possibility of transmission even without apparent vesicles or lesions.

Drug resistance to acyclovir is rare in the immunocompetent population but can occur in as many as 5% of cases in HIV patients. This should be suspected for persistent lesions or an increase in lesion size after 7–10 days of appropriately dosed antiviral therapy. Resistance can be diagnosed through plaque reduction assays, which rely on viral cultures [6]. If resistance occurs with acyclovir, it also confers resistance to valganciclovir and even famciclovir. Alternative therapies include foscarnet 40 mg/kg IV every 8 hours, or cidofovir 5 mg/kg IV given once weekly until lesions resolve. Topical agents include imiquimod and topical cidofovir. Transmission of resistance strains has not been documented in the literature. Resistance is often limited, with the wild-type acyclovir-sensitive strain predominating in an infected individual [3]. Therefore, treatment should be geared towards daily suppressive acyclovir, which has been shown to decrease the incidence of resistance in the future.

Management of HIV-infected persons should be focused on recognition and treatment of genital herpes. Although daily acyclovir treatment does not decrease the amount of asymptomatic shedding in HSV-2 seropositive individuals, it has been shown to decrease symptomatic ulcers and alter HIV disease progression for those not on HAART [3]. This has been theorized by noting that HIV viral DNA is unregulated in the serum of individuals with active HSV infections. Daily acyclovir treatment has been shown to decrease plasma levels of HIV RNA by as much as 35% over those not on treatment and who are also HSV seropositive. Vaccine research is underway for HSV given the large impact the virus has on HIV transmission [7].

For our patient, and for those who are HIV positive, disease prevention should be offered in the form of counseling for safe sex behaviors. Consistent condom use has been shown to decrease the risk of sexually transmitted infections by 80% [6]. It is important to inform your patient that HIV transmission and genital herpes transmission can still occur even when active lesions are not present. A multidisciplinary approach is ideal for treating HIV-positive patients. It is important to take into account social factors and easy access to medical care facilities when determining treatment options.

Key teaching points

- Genital herpes can affect disease progression; therefore, early initiation of antiviral therapy is imperative.
- Most individuals who are herpes simplex virus (HSV) seropositive do not have active lesions and have asymptomatic genital shedding. They are still able to transmit the disease without active lesions.
- Daily suppressive therapy with acyclovir decreases the frequency and severity of genital herpes outbreaks. It also decreases resistance to acyclovir in the future.
- A multidisciplinary approach should be used for all HIV-positive patients.

References

1. Baeten J, Celum C. *Herpes Simplex Virus and HIV-1.* HIV InSite Knowledge Base, 2006. Available at http://hivinsite.ucsf.edu/InSite?page=kb-05-03-02#S1X.

2. Looker K, Garnett G, Schmid G. An estimate of the global prevalence and incidence of herpes simplex virus type 2 infection. *Bull World Health Organ* 2008;86: 737–816.

3. Strick LB, Wald A, Celum C. HIV/ AIDS: Management of herpes simplex virus type 2 infection in HIV type 1-infected persons. *Clin Infect Dis* 2006;43(3):347–56.

4. Corey L, Wald A, Celum C, Quinn TC. The effects of herpes simplex virus-2 on HIV-1 acquisition and transmission: A review of two overlapping epidemics.

J Acquir Immune Defic Syndr 2004; 35(5):435–45.

5. Patel A, Rosen T. Herpes vegetans as a sign of HIV infection. *Dermatol Online J* 2008;14(4):6.

6. Centers for Disease Control on Prevention. *Diseases Characterized by Genital, Anal, or Perianal Ulcers. Sexually Transmitted Diseases.*

Treatment Guidelines 2010. Available at http://www.cdc.gov/std/treatment/ 2010/genital-ulcers.htm.

7. World Health Organization. *Initiative for Vaccine Research: Sexually Transmitted Diseases.* Available at http://apps.who.int/ vaccine_research/diseases/ portfolio/en/.

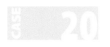

Incidentally discovered vaginal cyst in a 34-year-old woman

Roger P. Smith

History of present illness

A 34-year-old woman is referred for the evaluation of a cystic mass in her vagina. She recently became insured, and went to her local doctor earlier today for a routine pelvic exam. He was alarmed and requested urgent consultation. She had no symptoms. She has never had dyspareunia, intermenstrual bleeding, or any vaginal pressure or prolapse symptoms.

Physical examination

General appearance: Well-developed, well-nourished woman appearing concerned but in no apparent distress
Vital signs:

Temperature: 37.0°C
Pulse: 95 beats/min
Blood pressure: 142/90 mmHg
Respiratory rate: 16 breaths/min
Oxygen saturation: 100% on room air

Abdomen: Soft, nontender, with no organomegaly
External genitalia: Unremarkable
Vagina: A 4 × 5 cm cystic appearing structure is found on the left lateral vaginal wall beginning approximately 2 cm from the hymeneal ring and extending cephalward (Fig. 20.1). Scant discharge is present. Palpation of the mass confirms its cystic character and provides mild pelvic discomfort
Cervix: Parous, no mucopurulent discharge
Uterus: Anteverted, nontender, normal size, mobile
Adnexa: Nontender, without masses
Laboratory studies:

Urine pregnancy test: Negative
Microscopy of vaginal secretions was normal

How would you manage this patient?

The most likely diagnosis is a Gartner duct cyst. These generally require only reassurance, though if she develops dyspareunia symptoms, surgical excision of the cyst may be indicated.

Gartner duct cysts

Vaginal masses are relatively rare. It is likely that the actual prevalence is more common than recognized, since many are asymptomatic and therefore unnoticed and untreated [1]. Cystic masses in the vaginal wall may arise from either congenital (Gartner duct cysts) or acquired processes (epithelial inclusion cysts). Vaginal cysts are found in roughly 1 out of 200 women and are generally discovered from adolescence to the middle reproductive years. The differential diagnosis also includes urethral diverticula and loss of vaginal wall support such as cystoceles, enteroceles, and rectoceles [2].

Gartner duct cysts (Fig. 20.1) are blind pouches formed at the branching lower ends of the primitive mesonephric tubules. They may be single or multiple and seldom attain large size. They are typically 1–5 cm in diameter. When present, they are associated with slightly higher rates of upper genital tract

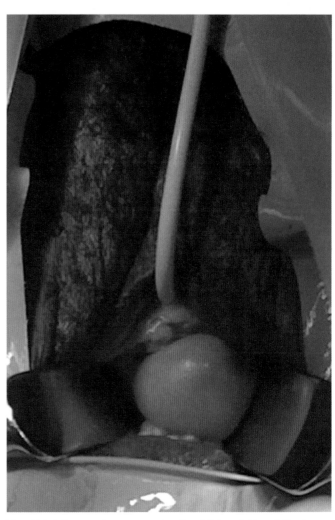

Fig. 20.1 A 5-cm cystic mass emerging from left lateral sidewall. Cyst is covered by normal appearing vaginal epithelium. (Image courtesy of Ashley Carroll, MD.)

Acute Care and Emergency Gynecology, ed. David Chelmow, Christine R. Isaacs and Ashley Carroll. Published by Cambridge University Press. © Cambridge University Press 2015.

malformations, as well as metanephric urinary anomalies such as ectopic ureter and ipsilateral renal hypoplasia [3].

Gartner duct cysts are generally asymptomatic. They may be associated with symptoms including a sense of vaginal fullness, dyspareunia, or difficulty with tampon insertion or retention (uncommon). Occasionally, a Gartner duct cyst can be large enough to occlude the vaginal canal and resemble a cystocele. In these extreme cases the patient may have pain, dyspareunia, bladder pressure, or even dystocia during parturition [4].

On physical examination, a Gartner duct cyst is generally found in the anterior lateral vaginal wall, while structural cysts (urethral diverticulum or loss of vaginal wall support) are generally seen in the midline of the anterior or posterior vaginal walls. Acquired cysts such as inclusion cysts represent over half of vaginal cysts and will generally be located distally in the vagina, typically at the site of previous obstetrical trauma. The cysts are typically 1–5 cm, and cystic with the base broadly embedded in the vaginal sidewall. The vaginal epithelium overlying the cyst may be normal appearing or attenuated. No solid components or nodularity should be present.

Biopsy is seldom needed to make the diagnosis. The cysts are lined by cuboidal epithelium, though the histologic architecture is extremely variable. The epithelial lining may consist of a single layer of cuboidal or high columnar epithelium, or either of these types may be stratified. Finding stratified epithelium generally suggests an inclusion (acquired) cyst. Imaging is not typically necessary for diagnosis. If the diagnosis is unclear, or excision of a large cyst is planned, MRI may be helpful to define anatomy, but is not routinely required. Ultrasonography is unlikely to adequately define the underlying anatomic relationships beyond what can be ascertained by physical examination alone.

Management generally consists of reassurance. Asymptomatic patients should be counseled that the cysts will almost certainly remain asymptomatic, and excision of an asymptomatic cyst is more likely to cause problems. Surgical excision is reasonable if the mass is symptomatic or its presentation is potentially consistent with a worrisome diagnosis. Excision should be done in an operating room. Care must be used in the excision of large cysts so that vaginal scarring and stenosis does not occur. Small cysts may be unroofed and marsupialized, though often small cysts that are the best candidates for such therapy actually do not require any intervention.

Key teaching points

- Lateral vaginal wall cystic structures are most likely to be of congenital (embryonic) origin and are benign.
- Most vaginal cysts are small and asymptomatic.
- No special workup or therapy is required for most patients.

References

1. Eilber KS, Raz S. Benign cystic lesions of the vagina: a literature review. *J Urol* 2003;170:717–22.

2. Smith, RP. *Netter's Obstetrics & Gynecology*, 2nd edn. Philadelphia: WB Saunders, 2009, pp. 269–70.

3. Dwyer PL, Rosamilia A. Congenital urogenital anomalies that are associated with the persistence of Gartner's duct: A review. *Am J Obstet Gynecol* 2006;195:354–9.

4. Arumugam AV, Kumar G, Si LK, Vijayananthan A. Gartner duct cyst in pregnancy presenting as a prolapsing pelvic mass. *Biomed Imaging Interv J* 2007;3(4):e46.

A 45-year-old woman with an enlarging pelvic mass

Alison F. Jacoby

History of present illness

A 45-year-old gravida 2, para 2 presents for a routine well-woman visit. She describes heavier and longer menstrual periods, but thought this was common for women her age. She does not experience any urinary symptoms or pelvic discomfort. She is sexually active with one male partner and denies dyspareunia. She had a tubal ligation at the time of her second Cesarean section. Her mother had a hysterectomy at age 42 for heavy bleeding. On her last pelvic examination two years ago, no mention was made of an enlarged uterus. She has no other medical problems.

Physical examination

General appearance: Well-developed, well-nourished woman in no apparent distress

Vital signs:

Temperature: 37.0°C
Pulse: 74 beats/min

Blood pressure: 128/72 mmHg
Respiratory rate: 16 breaths/min
Oxygen saturation: 100% on room air
BMI: 27 kg/m^2

Abdomen: Soft, nontender with a palpable mass extending from the pelvis to midway to the umbilicus, no hepatosplenomegaly

External genitalia: Unremarkable

Vagina: Unremarkable

Cervix: Parous, displaced anteriorly

Uterus: Bulky, mobile, nontender, 14-week size uterus with a prominent firm smooth mass filling the posterior cul-de-sac

Adnexa: Nontender, no masses

Laboratory studies:

Hb: 12.1 g/dL
Ht: 36.4%

Imaging: To evaluate the pelvic mass, a transabdominal and endovaginal pelvic sonogram is performed (Fig. 21.1).

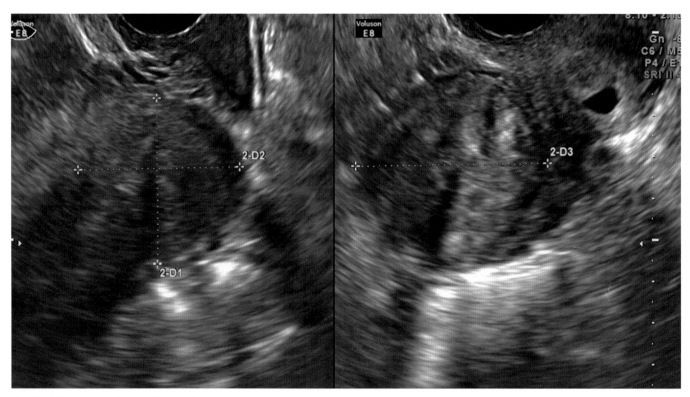

Fig. 21.1 Transvaginal ultrasound image of myoma.

Acute Care and Emergency Gynecology, ed. David Chelmow, Christine R. Isaacs and Ashley Carroll. Published by Cambridge University Press.
© Cambridge University Press 2015.

The uterus measures 14.3 cm in length, 8.9 cm in width, and 7.8 cm in anteroposterior (AP) dimension. A uterine myoma is identified along the posterior uterine body measuring 7.4 × 5.4 × 7.1 cm in diameter. There is displacement of the underlying endometrial cavity. The endometrium measures 8 mm. No free fluid is noted in the cul-de-sac. The left and right adnexa are unremarkable

How would you manage this patient?

The patient has a posterior intramural leiomyoma and increasingly heavy periods without anemia. Since her symptoms are manageable and her quality of life is not affected then expectant management is an acceptable approach. If her symptoms worsen over time then a number of treatment options are available to her including medical management of heavy bleeding, hysterectomy, myomectomy, uterine artery embolization, MR-guided focused ultrasound, and radio-frequency ablation.

Uterine leiomyomas

Uterine leiomyomas, commonly known as fibroids, affect 20–40% of premenopausal women. African-American women are at least three times more likely than white women to develop leiomyomas and to have more numerous and larger leiomyomas. Many leiomyomas are small and asymptomatic, but larger leiomyomas and those in specific locations can cause debilitating health problems. Common symptoms include heavy and prolonged menstrual bleeding, urinary frequency and urgency, dyspareunia, and pelvic pressure. The menstrual cycle typically remains regular and menstrual cramps are infrequent. Patients use terms like pelvic heaviness, pressure, and discomfort rather than pain. The only exception is during an episode of acute leiomyoma degeneration or infarction. When this occurs, women experience sharp, localized pain lasting from two to four weeks.

Leiomyomas are composed of a benign proliferation of smooth muscle cells and an abundant extracellular matrix of collagens, proteoglycans, and fibronectin. Estrogen, progesterone, and local growth factors stimulate the proliferation of the smooth muscle cells. There is no evidence that leiomyomas can transform into malignant sarcomas. Leiomyosarcomas are extremely rare with an incidence of 2–6 per 1000 cases of presumed leiomyoma. Therefore, when a premenopausal woman presents with typical symptoms and has characteristic ultrasound findings, the chance that the leiomyoma is benign is 99.4–99.8%.

The first tenet of leiomyoma management is that treatment is reserved for women with symptomatic leiomyomas that adversely affect their quality of life. Leiomyoma size and rate of growth are irrelevant if a woman is without symptoms. There is no evidence to support the long-held belief that rapidly growing leiomyomas in premenopausal women are at increased risk for leiomyosarcoma [1].

For women with symptomatic leiomyomas, the number of treatment options has expanded considerably in the last

20 years beyond that of hysterectomy and myomectomy. New procedures such as uterine artery embolization (UAE), magnetic resonance-guided focused ultrasound (MRgFUS) and radio-frequency thermal ablation (RFA) are examples of less invasive procedures.

Hysterectomy remains the most common treatment for leiomyomas because it provides guaranteed resolution of bleeding and eliminates the possibility of new leiomyoma growth. A number of factors, including uterine size, prior pelvic surgery, and a surgeon's expertise, dictate whether a hysterectomy can be performed via a laparotomy, laparoscopy, or transvaginally. Data have shown that the majority of women who undergo hysterectomy report improvement in health-related quality-of-life scores and rarely report adverse effects on their sexual function. However, hysterectomy has been associated with a greater likelihood for urinary incontinence and an earlier onset of menopause.

Myomectomy, a procedure in which leiomyomas are surgically removed, can be performed by laparotomy, laparoscopy, or hysteroscopy depending on the location, number, and size of the leiomyomas. Although rates of symptom improvement exceed 80%, the risk of persistent or recurrent ultrasound-documented leiomyomas is as high as 62%, and the risk for subsequent major surgery is 9% within 5 years after an abdominal myomectomy. The presence of multiple leiomyomas increases the risk for new leiomyoma growth [2]. Traditionally, myomectomy was reserved for women who desire future childbearing; however, recently women of all ages are choosing to conserve their uteri despite the chance for persistent symptoms and future leiomyoma development.

UAE, first described for the treatment of leiomyomas in 1995, has gained popularity in the United States and Europe. It is performed using conscious sedation, by an interventional radiologist, who introduces a catheter into a patient's femoral artery and uses real-time fluoroscopic imaging to guide it through the pelvic vasculature and into the uterine arteries. Small particles of polyvinyl alcohol, injected into each artery, adhere to form an obstruction to blood flow. With diminished perfusion, the leiomyomas become ischemic, leading to degeneration and involution. Patient selection is based on uterine size, leiomyoma size, and desire for future childbearing. Cases of ovarian failure and endometrial atrophy following UAE have been described; therefore, UAE should be used with caution for women who are pursuing pregnancy [3].

Observational studies have described the outcomes of more than 3000 patients who have undergone UAE. Overall, the mean reduction in leiomyoma size reported by individual studies ranged from 31 to 52%. Based on patient self-reports, 85–90% experience significant improvement in both bulk-related symptoms and menorrhagia following UAE. A recent Cochrane review of trials found that women who had UAE and women who had surgery were equally likely to be satisfied with their treatment [4]. However, the UAE group had significantly shorter hospital stays and a quicker return to daily activities. There were no differences in major

61

complication rates. However, within five years of UAE there was a five times increased risk of needing a surgical intervention.

MRgFUS is a promising technology that was approved by the Food and Drug Administration (FDA) for the treatment of leiomyomas in 2004. MRgFUS uses converging sound waves passing through the skin and internal structures to create a focus of intense heat within the targeted tissue. The high temperature results in protein denaturation, coagulative necrosis, and cell death. Dozens of "sonications" or pulses of sound energy are needed to ablate a leiomyoma.

For the duration of the 2–4-hour outpatient procedure, a woman lays prone with her abdomen positioned over the ultrasound apparatus and within the MR magnet. Pain control consists of narcotics, nonsteroidal anti-inflammatory drugs, and benzodiazepines. The recovery time is minimal with most women returning to full activities in one to two days. Outcome data is still limited to small observational studies with short follow-up. In a series of 130 women with symptomatic uterine leiomyomas treated with MRgFUS, at 3 and 12 months' follow-up, 86% reported symptom improvement and 13% reported no improvement [5].

The newest FDA-approved technique for treating symptomatic leiomyomas is RFA. In this procedure, patients undergo a diagnostic laparoscopy and an intra-abdominal sonogram to precisely map the size and location of the leiomyomas. A radio-frequency thermoablation needle is placed percutaneously into the center of the leiomyoma and several prongs are deployed to allow for ablation of the spherical mass. The target tissue is heated to 95°C. Complete ablation of a 4 cm leiomyoma takes 5 minutes. A series of overlapping ablations can be performed for larger leiomyomas. In several small observational studies, laparoscopic RFA successfully reduced leiomyoma volumes and improved mean health-related quality of life scores at 3, 6, and 12 months [6]. Recently, a prospective cohort study using transvaginal ultrasound-guided RFA was performed in 69 premenopausal women with symptomatic uterine leiomyomas. An improvement in menorrhagia occurred 1, 3, 6, and 12 months after the procedure.

A variety of minimally invasive procedures aimed at preserving the uterus and shortening recovery times have been introduced into the clinical arena. Although these techniques may prove to be effective, due to the small number of patients managed and the limited follow-up time, it is too soon to say whether they are comparable to the more established procedures such as hysterectomy and myomectomy.

Key teaching points

- Asymptomatic leiomyomas rarely need to be treated.
- Leiomyomas are benign in at least 99.4% of premenopausal women.
- Rapid growth is not associated with leiomyosarcoma and should not be used as a justification for recommending hysterectomy.
- Laparoscopic myomectomy, hysteroscopic myomectomy, and uterine artery embolization are the best-studied minimally invasive therapies for symptomatic leiomyomas, with significant improvement in menorrhagia and health-related quality of life, and infrequent complications.
- Magnetic resonance-guided focused ultrasound and radiofrequency ablation are FDA-approved procedures for symptomatic leiomyomas; however, additional outcomes data is needed before they should be widely adopted.
- Women who choose hysterectomy have high rates of satisfaction, sexual functioning, and health-related quality of life scores.

References

1. Parker WH, Fu YS, Berek JS. Uterine sarcoma in patients operated on for presumed leiomyoma and rapidly growing leiomyoma. *Obstet Gynecol* 1994;83:414–18.

2. Hanafi M. Predictors of leiomyoma recurrence after myomectomy. *Obstet Gynecol* 2005;105(4):877–81.

3. American College of Obstetricians and Gynecologists. Alternatives to hysterectomy in the management of leiomyomas. Practice Bulletin No. 96. *Obstet Gynecol* 2008;112: 387–400.

4. Gupta JK, Sinha A, Lumsden M, Hickey M. Uterine artery embolization for symptomatic uterine fibroids. *Cochrane Database Syst Rev* 2012, Issue 5. Art. No.: CD005073. DOI: 10.1002/14651858.CD005073.pub3.

5. Gorny KR, Woodrum DA, Brown DL et al. Magnetic resonance-guided focused ultrasound of uterine fibroids: review of a 12-month outcome of 130 clinical patients. *J Vasc Interv Radiol* 2011;22:857–64.

6. Garza Leal JG, Hernandez Leon I, Castillo Saenz L, Lee BB. Laparoscopic ultrasound-guided radiofrequency volumetric thermal ablation of symptomatic uterine leiomyomas: feasibility study using the Halt 2000 Ablation System. *J Minim Invasive Gynecol* 2011;18:364–71.

A 23-year-old woman with pelvic pain and fever

C. Nathan Webb

History of present illness

A 23-year-old gravida 1, para 1 woman presents to clinic with a month-long history of vague lower abdominal pain that has acutely worsened over the past several days. She initially had cramping, which progressed to a diffuse ache along with marked dyspareunia. She has felt feverish since yesterday but denies any rigors. She denies any nausea or emesis and has no dysuria or vaginal bleeding. She has scant vaginal discharge.

She had a levonorgestrel-releasing intrauterine device (IUD) placed last year and is happy with this method of contraception. Her menses have since diminished to a few days of spotting most months. She is unsure of her last menstrual period. She is sexually active with one male partner, most recently five days ago, and does not use condoms. She has no medical problems. She has never had surgery. She takes no medications. She had a single prior uncomplicated vaginal delivery.

Physical examination

General appearance: Well-nourished woman appearing moderately uncomfortable and tearful

Vital signs:

Temperature: 38.0°C

Pulse: 84 beats/min

Blood pressure: 108/74 mmHg

Respiratory rate: 16 breaths/min

Oxygen saturation: 100% on room air

Cardiovascular: Regular rate and rhythm, no murmurs, rubs or gallops, no peripheral edema

Chest: Clear to auscultation throughout

Abdomen: Soft, obese, nondistended, bilateral lower quadrants are moderately tender to light palpation without rebound or guarding, active bowel sounds, no flank tenderness

External genitalia: Unremarkable

Vagina: Scant white discharge, no lesions

Cervix: Mucopurulent discharge present at os (Fig. 22.1)

Bimanual exam: Cervical motion tenderness, normal-sized anteverted uterus moderately tender to palpation, right-sided adnexal fullness with moderate tenderness on palpation

Laboratory studies:

Saline microscopy of vaginal fluid: >25% clue cells, numerous leukocytes, no blood, yeast, or trichomonads

WBCs: 14 000/μL

NAATs: *Neisseria gonorrhoeae* and *Chlamydia trachomatis* tests sent

Urine pregnancy test: Negative

Urinalysis: Unremarkable

Imaging: A transvaginal ultrasound is obtained (Fig. 22.2)

How would you manage this patient?

This patient has pelvic inflammatory disease (PID). Immediate treatment is indicated. Since her symptoms are mild to moderate, outpatient therapy with an appropriate antibiotic regimen based on current Centers for Disease Control and Prevention (CDC) 2010 guidelines [1] is appropriate. Her IUD may be left in place. When treating PID with an IUD in

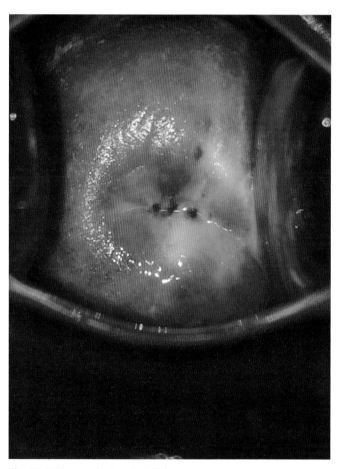

Fig. 22.1 Mucopurulent cervical discharge.

Acute Care and Emergency Gynecology, ed. David Chelmow, Christine R. Isaacs and Ashley Carroll. Published by Cambridge University Press.
© Cambridge University Press 2015.

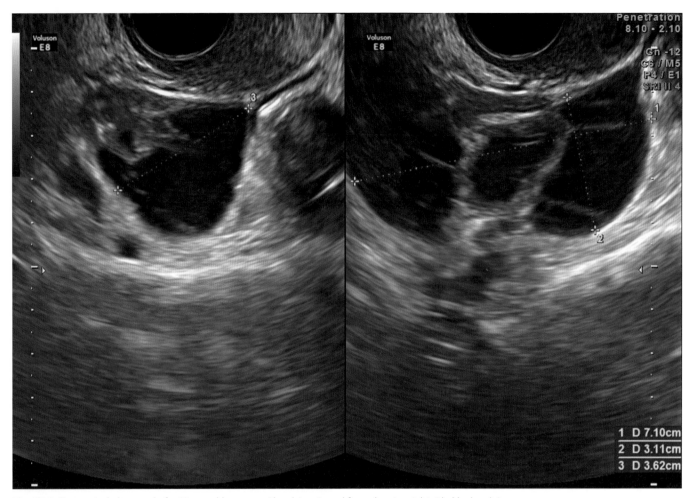

Fig. 22.2 Transvaginal ultrasound of a 23-year-old woman with pelvic pain and fever showing right-sided hydrosalpinx.

place, close follow-up within two to three days is essential. Consideration should be given to removal of her IUD should she fail outpatient treatment. Her partner should be examined and offered appropriate treatment for *N. gonorrhea* and *C. trachomatis*.

Pelvic inflammatory disease

Pelvic inflammatory disease (PID) is an ascending bacterial infection of the upper female genital tract characterized by inflammation of contiguous structures ranging from cervicitis, endometritis, and salpingitis to pelvic abscess formation and peritonitis. These infections are often polymicrobial and causative organisms include sexually transmitted bacteria such as *N. gonorrhea* and *C. trachomatis*, as well as endogenous vaginal anaerobes, enteric gram-negative rods, and genital mycoplasmas [1].

PID can have diverse and often subtle presentations, as seen in this patient whose infection likely began nearly one month ago, as suggested by her initial vague abdominal discomfort. These subtle and nonspecific findings often confuse the diagnosis of PID and delay treatment. This delay can have

serious consequences for women, since PID puts them at risk for tubal infertility, ectopic pregnancy, and chronic pelvic pain. Delay in treatment by as few as three days has been associated with a threefold increase in risk of these sequelae [2]. For this reason, the CDC has established a low threshold for diagnosing PID and recommends treatment of a presumptive diagnosis of PID even while the patient is being evaluated for other causes of her symptoms [1].

The diagnosis of PID is made with presence of pelvic or abdominal pain and either cervical motion tenderness, uterine tenderness, or adnexal tenderness on examination in any sexually active woman younger than 26 years or any woman with risk factors for sexually transmitted infections (STIs). Risk factors for STIs include prior history of STI and multiple sex partners. The lower threshold in younger women reflects both the increased incidence and greater need to protect fertility in these women. The specificity of the diagnosis is increased if these findings occur in the setting of additional signs of genital infection and inflammation (Table 22.1), several of which were demonstrated by this patient: cervical mucopurulence (Fig. 22.1), leukorrhea on saline microscopy of vaginal fluid; and evidence of a dilated, fluid-filled tube on ultrasound (Fig. 22.2).

Table 22.1 The CDC diagnostic criteria for PID*

Pelvic or lower abdominal pain in young (≤25 years) sexually active women or women with STI risk factors (prior STI, multiple sex partners) and one or more of the following
- Cervical motion tenderness
- Uterine tenderness
- Adnexal tenderness

Additional criteria to enhance specificity of diagnosis
- Oral temperature >38.3°C
- Cervical or vaginal mucopurulent discharge
- Saline wet mount of vaginal discharge demonstrating leukorrhea
- Elevated erythrocyte sedimentation rate
- Elevated C-reactive protein
- Verification of cervical infection with *Neisseria gonorrhoeae* or *Chlamydia trachomatis*

Most specific criteria for diagnosis of PID
- Endometrial biopsy demonstrating endometritis
- Transvaginal sonography or MRI showing thickened, fluid-filled tubes with or without free pelvic fluid or tubo-ovarian complex, or Doppler studies suggesting inflammation
- Laparoscopic confirmation of PID

* Adapted from CDC Guidelines 2010 [1].
CDC, Centers for Disease Control and Prevention; PID, pelvic inflammatory disease; STI, sexually transmitted infections.

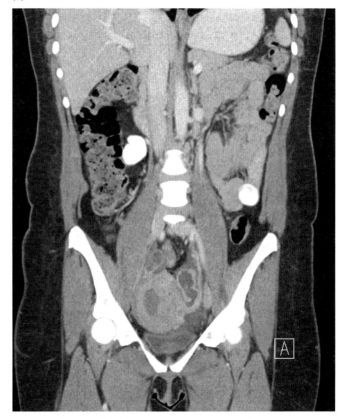

(a)

(b)

Fig. 22.3 Abdominal CT of a patient diagnosed with pelvic inflammatory disease and tubo-ovarian abscess. (a) Transverse and (b) coronal views.

Imaging is not always necessary. For this patient, imaging was obtained to further evaluate the adnexal fullness noted on examination. Imaging would also be reasonable in any patient with PID that does not improve with initial antibiotic treatment, who requires hospitalization, or whose physical examination is limited by habitus. Transvaginal sonography (TVUS) is readily available and rapidly obtained at the bedside in most practice settings. Because of its ready availability and ability to visualize tubal changes consisted with PID, TVUS is a good first choice for imaging. CT (Fig. 22.3a,b) is also useful, particularly when evaluating other diagnoses such as appendicitis or to guide percutaneous drainage of abscesses. MRI offers the greatest sensitivity and specificity of any imaging modality in diagnosing PID but is less practical given its high cost and limited availability in some settings.

Treatment of PID should be initiated at the time of diagnosis and be sufficiently broad to cover the most likely pathogens. At a minimum, all antibiotic treatment regimens should be effective against *N. gonorrhea* and *C. trachomatis*, regardless of cervical screening results since these tests are not predictive of upper genital tract infection. The CDC guidelines also recommend provision of anaerobic coverage because anaerobes have frequently been recovered from the upper genital tract of women with PID and several of these organisms can cause tubal damage with long-term effects on fertility [1]. The recommendations also allow supplemental coverage with metronidazole. Given valid concerns over the side effects of metronidazole and the consequent negative impact on

patient compliance, this additional coverage can be reserved for patients with bacterial vaginosis or pelvic abscesses [1,3].

For mild to moderate symptoms, outpatient management with oral antibiotics is appropriate and provides similar outcomes to parenteral therapy in rates of cure, risk of ectopic pregnancy, and future infertility (Table 22.2). It is important to reassess the patient within two to three days for compliance

Table 22.2 The CDC recommended outpatient antibiotic regimen for PID*

Ceftriaxone 250 mg IM in a single dose

Or cefoxitin 2 g IM and probenecid 1 g PO both given in a single dose

Or other parenteral third-generation cephalosporin (e.g. ceftizoxime or cefotaxime)

Plus:

Doxycycline 100 mg PO BID for 14 days

With or without:

Metronidazole 500 mg PO BID for 14 days

* Adapted from CDC Guidelines 2010 [1].
BID, twice a day; CDC, Centers for Disease Control and Prevention; IM, intramuscular; PO, *per os* (orally).

Table 22.3 Suggested admission criteria for women with PID

- Severe illness, nausea and vomiting, or high fever
- Unable to follow or tolerate outpatient oral regimen
- Inadequate clinical response to oral antibiotic therapy
- Pregnancy
- Presence of a tubo-ovarian abscess
- Surgical emergencies (e.g. appendicitis) cannot be excluded

* Adapted from CDC Guidelines 2010 [1].
CDC, Centers for Disease Control and Prevention; PID, pelvic inflammatory disease.

Table 22.4 Parenteral antibiotic regimens for PID

Regimen A

Cefotetan 2 g IV every12 hours

Or

Cefoxitin 2 g IV every 6 hours

Plus

Doxycycline 100 mg PO or IV every 12 hours

Regimen B

Clindamycin 900 mg IV every 8 hours

Plus

Gentamicin loading dose IV or IM (2 mg/kg body weight), followed by a maintenance dose (1.5 mg/kg) every 8 hours. Single daily dosing (3–5 mg/kg) can be substituted

Alternative regimen

Ampicillin/sulbactam 3 g IV every 6 hours

Plus

Doxycycline 100 mg PO or IV every 12 hours

* Adapted from CDC Guidelines 2010 [1].
CDC, Centers for Disease Control and Prevention; IM, intramuscularly; IV, intravenous; PID, pelvic inflammatory disease; PO, *per os* (orally).

and adequacy of clinical response to treatment. Recommended outpatient regimens consist of cefoxitin or a third-generation cephalosporin, typically ceftriaxone 250 mg IM OD along with doxycycline 100 mg PO BID for 14 days. The CDC guidelines also cite two studies using azithromycin 1 g orally once a week for 2 weeks as a substitute for doxycycline. The CDC guidelines recommend the addition of metronidazole 500 mg PO BID for 14 days if this regimen is employed [1]. The use of quinolones is no longer recommended for the treatment of PID due to the rising prevalence of quinolone-resistant *N. gonorrhea* [1].

The CDC has criteria for hospitalizing women with PID that should be applied combined with the provider's judgment of clinical severity (Table 22.3). These criteria include pregnancy, inadequate response to outpatient therapy, high fever, nausea, vomiting or poor tolerance of oral intake, inability to rule out surgical emergencies (e.g. appendicitis), and presence of an abscess. In the current case, the patient's symptoms are mild to moderate and she has no gastrointestinal complaints, making outpatient treatment a reasonable choice.

Recommended parenteral regimens include either cefoxitin or cefotetan, both cephalosporins with excellent anaerobic coverage, along with doxycycline (Table 22.4). Conversion to oral antibiotics may be considered after 24–48 hours of sustained clinical improvement and should be continued for 14 days.

If a pelvic abscess is identified, hospitalization for parenteral antibiotics and direct inpatient observation for at least 24 hours is recommended by the CDC. Any of the CDC-recommended parenteral regimens are appropriate; however, the effects of aminoglycosides are attenuated in low oxygen, acidic environments and may be less effective than cephalosporins in this setting [3]. The size of the abscess impacts success of antibiotic therapy and need for surgical drainage. Up to 60% or women with abscesses 10 cm or larger in diameter will fail to respond to antibiotics alone, so imaging is helpful when abscesses are suspected [4]. Drainage may be undertaken via laparotomy, laparoscopy, or percutaneously. Rupture of a tubo-ovarian abscess is a surgical emergency and must be suspected in women with PID progressing to sepsis. Surgical exploration, with drainage and excision of nonviable tissue may be necessary, which may require hysterectomy or salpingo-oophorectomy.

The presence of an IUD did not alter the management of PID in this patient. There is a small increase in risk of PID for the first three weeks after initiating IUD use, related to placement rather than presence of the device, but available data suggest retention of an IUD does not impact response to treatment for PID [5]. The decision to remove the device should be based upon clinical response to therapy or severity of initial presentation. If the device is left in place, close follow-up is vital. Presence of the endogenous anaerobe actinomyces is noted on cervical cytology in about 7% of IUD users. This likely represents colonization rather than infection and is not an indication for removal in asymptomatic patients. However, women with PID symptoms and a history of colonization should receive appropriate evaluation and treatment for actinomycosis and the IUD should be removed [6,7].

The examination and treatment of sex partners is recommended if sexual contact was within the preceding 60 days. Treatment should be given to the most recent sexual contact if this occurred more than 60 days prior to diagnosis. In both cases, treatment should cover both *N. gonorrhea* and *C. trachomatis* regardless of the cervical screening results in the affected women.

Long-term sequelae of PID include infertility, chronic pelvic pain, and ectopic pregnancy, all presumably from associated scarring of pelvic organs. The risks increase with number of recurrences, with infertility rates as high as 75% and ectopic pregnancy risk up to 14% after three or more episodes [8]. Chronic pain affects up to 30% of women after a single occurrence [3].

For this patient, strong clinical suspicion of PID in a young sexually active woman with pelvic pain and evidence of upper genital inflammation as well as a low threshold for treatment are key to proper management. A CDC-recommended antibiotic regimen was administered and further evaluation with imaging was performed based on examination findings. Clinical judgment was used to determine if her IUD could be left in place. Follow-up should include examination and treatment of

the patient's sex partner with antibiotics adequate to treat *N. gonorrhea* and *C. trachomatis.*

Key teaching points

- Pelvic inflammatory disease (PID) should be considered in any sexually active, reproductive-aged woman with pelvic pain.
- Early treatment of PID at the time of diagnosis improves long-term outcomes and should be started while alternate diagnoses are further evaluated.
- Mild to moderate PID can be treated as an outpatient.
- Clinical response to oral treatment should be assessed within 72 hours and the patient should be admitted for parenteral treatment if not improving appropriately.
- PID in intrauterine device (IUD) users may be treated without removing the device. Close follow-up is essential. Removal of the IUD is necessary in instances of treatment failure.
- Treatment regimens should follow the Centers for Disease Control and Prevention (CDC) sexually transmitted diseases treatment guidelines.
- Sex partners should be treated if contact was within the preceding 60 days.

References

1. Centers for Disease Control and Prevention. Sexually transmitted diseases treatment guidelines, 2010. *MMWR* 2010;59(RR-12):63–7.

2. Hillis S, Joesoef R, Marchbanks P, et al. Delayed care of pelvic inflammatory disease as a risk factor for impaired fertility. *Am J Obstet Gynecol* 1993;168:1503–9.

3. Soper DE. Pelvic inflammatory disease. *Obstet Gynecol* 2010;116:419–28.

4. Reed S, Landers D, Sweet R. Antibiotic treatment of tuboovarian abscess:

Comparison of broad-spectrum beta-lactam agents versus clindamycin-containing regimens. *Am J Obstet Gynecol* 1991;164:1556–62.

5. Grimes DA. Intrauterine device and upper-genital-tract infection. *Lancet* 2000;356:1013–19.

6. Tepper NK, Steenland MW, Gaffield ME, Marchbanks PA, Curtis KM. Retention of intrauterine devices in women who acquire pelvic inflammatory disease: A systematic review. *Contraception* 2013;87: 655–60.

7. American College of Obstetricians and Gynecologists. Long-acting reversible contraception: Implants and intrauterine devices. Practice Bulletin No. 121. *Obstet Gynecol* 2011;118: 184–96.

8. Weström L, Joesoef R, Reynolds G, Hagdu A, Thompson SE. Pelvic inflammatory disease and fertility. A cohort study of 1,844 women with laparoscopically verified disease and 657 control women with normal laparoscopic results. *Sex Transm Dis* 1992;19:185–92.

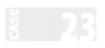
A 21-year-old woman with a new sexual partner

Elizabeth M. Yoselevsky and Christine R. Isaacs

History of present illness

A 21-year-old gravida 0 woman presents requesting contraception. She began a relationship with a new sexual partner approximately one month ago and admits to being inconsistent with using condoms. She has no active complaints. She has regular menstrual cycles and her last menstrual period began one week ago. She has no significant past medical history or prior surgeries. She takes no medications. She is currently a senior at the university. She drinks approximately six beers on the weekends and denies tobacco or illicit drug use.

Physical examination

General appearance: Well-developed, well-nourished, thin woman in no acute distress and cooperative

Vital signs:

Temperature: 37.0°C
Pulse: 80 beats/min
Blood pressure: 110/68 mmHg
Respiratory rate: 14 breaths/min
Oxygen saturation: 100% on room air

HEENT: Unremarkable
Cardiovascular: Normal S1, S2 without murmur
Lungs: Clear to auscultation bilaterally
Abdomen: Soft, nontender
External genitalia: Unremarkable
Vagina: Physiologic-appearing discharge
Cervix: Nulliparous, slight mucopurulent discharge from os. Small amount of bleeding elicited with gentle swabbing with a cotton-tip probe
Uterus: Anteverted, nontender, mobile
Adnexa: Nontender, no masses
Laboratory studies: Urine pregnancy test: Negative

What is your differential diagnosis and how would you manage this patient?

This patient has an asymptomatic mucopurulent discharge and is at risk for sexually transmitted infections (STIs) due to her age and inconsistent condom use. Because of this, she was advised to undergo screening for sexually transmitted diseases (STDs). The differential diagnosis for this presentation most commonly includes infection by *Chlamydia trachomatis* and *Neisseria gonorrhoeae*. Less likely causes include trichomoniasis or herpes simplex virus infection.

The patient was tested for gonorrhea and chlamydia and her chlamydia test returned positive. She was treated with 1 g of azithromycin given as a single dose in the office to ensure compliance. She was strongly advised to abstain from sexual intercourse for one week to reduce the risk of transmission and was advised to inform all of her recent sexual partners of the diagnosis and the need for their evaluation/treatment. She was started on oral contraceptives and counseled on the importance of consistent condom use for prevention of further STIs. She returned to the clinic three months later and had a negative test for reinfection.

Chlamydia cervicitis

Chlamydia trachomatis is the most commonly reported sexually transmitted pathogen with over 1.4 million cases reported in 2011. In the past 10 years, the incidence has been steadily increasing with the highest rates of infection found in women 15–24 years of age [1]. Cervicitis should be suspected when either a mucopurulent discharge is noted in the endocervical canal or if the cervix bleeds easily with manipulation or collection of specimens. While patients with chlamydia may experience urethritis, dysuria, abnormal discharge, or post-coital spotting, most women infected by *C. trachomatis* are asymptomatic. The sequelae of chlamydia cervicitis can be serious including pelvic inflammatory disease (PID), infertility, ectopic pregnancies, and chronic pelvic pain. These potential long-term complications make screening, recognizing, treating, and preventing chlamydial cervicitis imperative.

When a cervical examination reveals a mucopurulent discharge and/or easy bleeding as in the case of this patient, further testing should be performed to rule out chlamydial infections. Testing can be performed by a number of methods; however, nucleic acid amplification tests (NAATs) are the most sensitive and are Food and Drug Administration (FDA) cleared for endocervical swabs and urine samples. While cervical swab testing has a slightly higher sensitivity than urine testing, urine sampling avoids the necessity of an invasive pelvic examination and may provide a more feasible opportunity for screening. Before obtaining an endocervical specimen, a large swab should be used to remove all secretions and discharge from the cervical os. Once the cervix has been properly cleaned off, the cytobrush or swab provided by the test manufacturer should be inserted 1–2 cm deep into the endocervix and rotated at least 2 turns or for the length of time recommended by the test kit manufacturer. If using a

---

Acute Care and Emergency Gynecology, ed. David Chelmow, Christine R. Isaacs and Ashley Carroll. Published by Cambridge University Press. © Cambridge University Press 2015.

Table 23.1 The 2010 CDC treatment guidelines for *Chlamydia trachomatis* (in nonpregnant patients)*

Recommended regimens

Azithromycin 1 g PO in a single dose
or
Doxycycline 100 mg PO BID for 7 days

Alternative regimens

Erythromycin base 500 mg PO QID for 7 days
or
Erythromycin ethylsuccinate 800 mg PO QID for 7 days
or
Levofloxacin 500 mg PO OD for 7 days
or
Ofloxacin 300 mg PO BID for 7 days

* Centers for Disease Control and Prevention [4].
BID, twice a day; CDC, Centers for Disease Control and Prevention; OD, once a day; PO, *per os* (orally); QID, four times a day.

Table 23.2 The 2010 CDC treatment guidelines for *Chlamydia trachomatis* (in pregnant patients)*

Recommended regimens

Azithromycin 1 g PO in a single dose
or
Amoxicillin 500 mg PO TID for 7 days

Alternative regimens

Erythromycin base 500 mg PO QID for 7 days
or
Erythromycin base 250 mg PO QID for 14 days
or
Erythromycin ethylsuccinate 800 mg PO QID for 7 days
or
Erythromycin ethylsuccinate 400 mg PO QID for 14 days

* Centers for Disease Control and Prevention [4].
BID, twice a day; CDC, Centers for Disease Control and Prevention; OD, once a day; PO, *per os* (orally); QID, four times a day.

urine specimen to detect chlamydia, the first 10–30 mL of voided urine should be collected to test as greater amounts may dilute the sample and produce a false negative result [2].

When a patient presents with cervicitis, it is also important to assess the patient for signs of PID because cervicitis may be indicative of an upper genital tract infection, which requires different treatment and risks future sequelae. To diagnose PID, uterine tenderness, adnexal tenderness, or cervical motion tenderness must be present. Other concerning signs include fever greater than 38.3°C, mucopurulent discharge, many white blood cells in the cervical discharge, elevated erythrocyte sedimentation rate, or elevated C-reactive protein levels [3]. While data is limited regarding the incidence, many women with uncomplicated cervical infections already have subclinical upper-reproductive tract infections brewing. This makes obtaining a timely diagnosis essential for preventing future comorbidities.

As soon as a patient tests positive for chlamydia she needs to be treated. Treatment should follow the 2010 Centers for Disease Control and Prevention (CDC) treatment guidelines for STDs (Table 23.1) [4]. Healthcare providers are encouraged to observe the patient taking the first dose of treatment, when possible. First-line treatment includes azithromycin 1 g PO once or doxycycline 100 mg PO BID for 7 days. Both treatments are equally effective, but azithromycin is more ideal to ensure compliance as it is a single dose. If a patient is pregnant, azithromycin 1 g PO once is the preferred treatment. Amoxicillin 500 mg PO TID for 7 days is an acceptable alternative but understandably risks issues with compliance (Table 23.2) [4].

Patients who are treated for chlamydia cervicitis will require appropriate education following their infection. First, it is important to educate patients on the prevention of future STIs by employing consistent barrier method contraception such as male condoms. Secondly, healthcare providers should counsel patients on notifying all sexual partners from within the last 60 days about the infection. If the most recent sexual contact was greater than 60 days prior, that partner should still

be notified. Treating sexual partners minimizes the chances of reinfection in women. This is important because several studies have demonstrated that the risks of complications from infection increase with each subsequent reinfection [4]. Many states have laws that allow a healthcare provider the option of Expedited Partner Therapy (EPT), such that they may write an antibiotic prescription for the partner of an infected patient without seeing the partner in the clinic. The legal status of these regulations is constantly evolving and varies from state to state. The CDC's website (http://www.cdc.gov/std/ept/legal/default.htm) lists recommendations by state. A patient also needs to be counseled that he or she should wait seven days from the first dose of antibiotics before resuming sexual intercourse regardless of the treatment regimen.

The 2010 CDC guidelines do not recommend a test-of-cure for chlamydial infections in nonpregnant patients. Patients who test positive for chlamydia should be retested 3–12 months after treatment to confirm no evidence of reinfection or exposure from a new (infected) partner. Patients should only be tested sooner if therapeutic compliance is in question, symptoms persist, or reinfection is suspected. Pregnant women should undergo repeat testing to document chlamydial eradication (preferably by NAAT) three to four weeks after completion of therapy. These women should not only receive a test-of-cure but should also be retested again three months after treatment [4].

As most women infected by *C. trachomatis* are asymptomatic, it is important to annually screen age-appropriate and high-risk patients [3,4]. The current CDC recommendations are to screen all sexually active women aged 25 years or younger, or patients older than 25 years with risk factors. Risk factors include new or multiple partners, inconsistent condom use, and/or current or prior STD. These recommendations differ slightly from the United States Preventive Services Task Force (USPSTF) guidelines, which recommend annual screening in women age 24 years or younger [4]. Currently, there are no firm guidelines regarding screening sexually active males, but screening may be reasonable in settings with a high prevalence of the disease such as a correctional facility or STD clinic. The data has yet to support a comprehensive screening initiative for men because there has been no strong evidence that it will improve outcomes for women [4].

Key teaching points

- *Chlamydia trachomatis* is the most commonly reported sexually transmitted infection in the United States and its prevalence is highest in women ages 15–24.
- Chlamydia is asymptomatic in most cases, but may present as urethritis, dysuria, or post-coital spotting. There may be evidence of a mucopurulent discharge or a friable cervix.

- Sequale of chlamydia may include pelvic inflammatory disease, increased risk for ectopic pregnancy, infertility, and chronic pelvic pain.
- The Centers for Disease Control and Prevention (CDC) guidelines recommend that all sexually active women aged 25 years or younger (or older than age 25 with risk factors) should be screened for chlamydia annually. United States Preventive Services Task Force guidelines recommend that women 24 years of age or younger (or older and at increased risk) should be screened annually.
- Nonpregnant women should be tested for reinfection 3–12 months after treatment and pregnant women should undergo a test-of-cure 3–4 weeks after treatment.

References

1. Centers for Disease Control and Prevention. *Sexually Transmitted Disease Surveillance 2011.* Atlanta, US Department of Health and Human Services, 2012.

2. Centers for Disease Control and Prevention. Screening tests to detect *Chlamydia trachomatis* and *Neisseria gonorrhoeae* infections. *MMWR* 2002;51(RR-15):1–27.

3. Haggerty CL, Sami L, Gottlieb BD, et al. Risk of sequelae after *Chlamydia*

trachomatis genital infection in women. *J Infect Dis* 2010;201:S134–55.

4. Centers for Disease Control and Prevention. Sexually transmitted diseases treatment guideline 2010. *MMWR* 2010;59(RR-12):40–8.

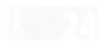

A 21-year-old woman with persistent pain and fever after treatment for PID

Nicole S. Fanning

History of present illness

A 21-year-old gravida 2, para 2 woman presented to the emergency department with a week of worsening right lower quadrant pain, subjective fevers, nausea, and emesis. One week prior she had been evaluated for similar symptoms and diagnosed with pelvic inflammatory disease (PID). Intramuscular ceftriaxone was administered at this time, and oral doxycycline was prescribed for 14 days. She was unable to keep her initial follow-up appointment and her worsening symptoms prompted her to seek care in the emergency department. She is a three cigarettes-a-day smoker and previously had a dilatation and curettage for an elective abortion.

Physical examination

General appearance: Awake, alert woman who is in no acute distress

Vital signs:

Temperature: 38.7°C
Pulse: 106 beats/min
Blood pressure: 111/58 mmHg
Respiratory rate: 16 breaths/min
Oxygen saturation: 99% on room air

Cardiovascular: Tachycardic

Pulmonary: Clear to auscultation bilaterally

Abdomen: Soft, nondistended, tender to palpation diffusely, worse in right lower quadrant, but with no rebound or guarding

Genitourinary:

Normal appearing cervix with mucopurulent discharge, positive cervical motion tenderness, normal-appearing vaginal mucosa

Bimanual examination: Limited mobility of a pelvic mass with significant tenderness and uterine deviation

Laboratory studies on admission:

Urine pregnancy test: Negative
WBCs: 26 700/μL (normal 3900–11 700/μL)
Hb: 12.8 g/dL (normal 12.0–15.0 g/dL)
Ht: 38.0% (normal 34.8–45.0%)
Platelets: 350 000/μL (normal 172 000–440 000/μL)
Cervical gonorrhea, chlamydia, trichomonas: Pending
Urinalysis: Specific gravity 1.08 and large blood

Imaging: CT scan of pelvis showed a large pelvic mass (10 × 10 × 8 cm) having solid and cystic aspects. Cystic components were defined as tubular; thus, interpretation was that of a tubo-ovarian abscess. A smaller fluid collection (7 × 3 cm) consistent with hemorrhage was also identified

How would you manage this patient?

This patient has a tubo-ovarian abscess (TOA), and thus was admitted to the inpatient Gynecology service where she was initiated on intravenous cefoxitin, doxycycline, and metronidazole in addition to intravenous morphine for pain control. After 48 hours of intravenous antibiotics she continued to be febrile with worsening pain. Thus, she was taken to the operating room for exploratory laparotomy. Intraoperative findings were consistent with purulent drainage upon entering the peritoneum and severely distorted pelvic anatomy. This included

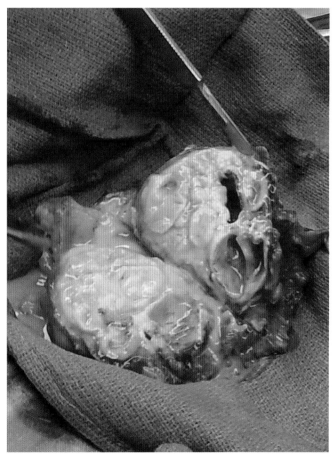

Fig. 24.1 Right tubo-ovarian abscess incised. This ovary contains loculations of purulent material.

Acute Care and Emergency Gynecology, ed. David Chelmow, Christine R. Isaacs and Ashley Carroll. Published by Cambridge University Press.
© Cambridge University Press 2015.

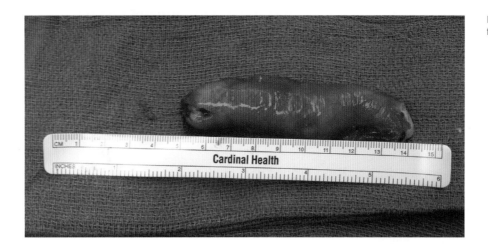

Fig. 24.2 Right fallopian tube. Tube is friable, fibrous, edematous, and has clubbed ending.

an extremely enlarged right ovary with multiple loculations of purulent drainage as well as an edematous, thickened, and fibrous right fallopian tube adherent to the uterus and ovary. Due to these findings, the right ovary and right fallopian tube were removed, and pathology was consistent with acute right-sided TOA and salpingitis (Figs 24.1 & 24.2, respectively). The patient was discharged to home on postoperative day 6 after an uncomplicated postoperative course. Discharge antibiotics included doxycycline and clindamycin orally to complete a total of 14-day course of antibiotics. She was seen one week following discharge, and was noted to be doing well. No anaerobic cultures were sent, but blood and urine cultures were without growth. Polymerase chain reaction (PCR) testing for gonorrhea and chlamydia returned negative.

Tubo-ovarian abscess

A tubo-ovarian abscess (TOA) is an inflammatory mass that involves the fallopian tube and ovary, and can also involve other pelvic structures such as bowel and bladder. A TOA is usually found as a complication of PID, and is a polymicrobial-ascending infection that involves the upper genital tract. It can also be associated with other intra-abdominal processes such as diverticulitis or appendicitis. Risk factors for developing a TOA are the same as those for PID, including age between 15 and 25 years, multiple sexual partners, and a prior history of PID. The long-term sequela of a TOA can be significant including infertility, ectopic pregnancy, and chronic pelvic pain. For abscesses that go undiagnosed and rupture the consequences can be severe, leading to sepsis and potential death.

A patient with a TOA will typically present with one or more of the following: pelvic pain, fever, vaginal discharge, nausea, and abnormal vaginal bleeding. Physical examination findings will be similar to that of a patient with PID, including tenderness to palpation of the cervix, uterus, or adnexa and mucopurulent cervical discharge. It may be possible to palpate a tender adnexal mass, but this is often limited due to patient discomfort. One should have a low threshold for imaging when a TOA is suspected in order to aid in diagnosis and management. The primary or preferable imaging modality is transvaginal ultrasonography, but transabdominal ultrasonography can be used as well as CT scans and MRI. Typical ultrasound findings are cystic structures, either uni- or multilocular with thickened walls with or without septae. Echogenicity of cystic contents are usually homogenous with ground-glass appearance [1]. A CT scan may be preferable in cases where the diagnosis is unclear and other etiologies need to be ruled out, such as appendicitis or diverticulitis.

Once TOA is diagnosed, parenteral antibiotics are the mainstay of treatment. Approximately 75% of all TOAs will resolve with parenteral antibiotics alone [2]. TOAs are polymicrobial infections with the most common pathogens being *Escherichia coli, Bacteriodes fragilis, Baceteroides* sp., *Peptostreptococcus, Peptococcus,* and aerobic *Streptococcus. Neisseria gonorrhoeae* and *Chlamydia trachomatis* are thought to lead to an ascending infection; however, they are rarely recovered from an abscess. It is pertinent, however, to routinely screen for *N. gonorrhea* and *C. trachomatis* before initiating treatment given that they are commonly encountered sexually transmitted infections. With these isolates in mind, the Centers for Disease Control and Prevention (CDC) recommends inpatient intravenous antibiotics for at least 24 hours with cefotetan 2 g IV every 12 hours or cefoxitin 2 g IV every 6 hours, plus doxycycline 100 mg PO or IV every 12 hours. For patients with a significant penicillin allergy, clindamycin plus gentamycin is recommended. Following initial parenteral treatment, the CDC then recommends continuation of treatment with oral clindamycin or metronidazole along with doxycyline for a total of 14 days of treatment to improve anaerobic coverage [3]. Use of clindamycin, metronidazole, and cefoxitin should be highly considered in treating a TOA due to their increased ability to penetrate an abscess wall [4].

If there is no clinical improvement after 48–72 hours of parenteral antibiotics, more aggressive treatment with surgery or drainage should be considered. Historically, a patient's response to parenteral antibiotics is dependent on the size of the abscess. Approximately 60% of abscesses greater than 10 cm will require surgical intervention, whereas 15% or less of patients with abscesses less than 4 cm will require surgical intervention [5]. Surgical approach to a TOA is based on the experience of the surgeon. Many surgeons prefer laparotomy due to the complexity of adhesions formation that may potentially involve the bowel. In cases where there is no evidence of rupture, laparoscopy may be a reasonable approach for the experienced surgeon, resulting in quicker recovery times and lower surgical morbidity. For those patients who have completed childbearing, a complete hysterectomy and bilateral salpingo-opherectomy may be a reasonable option, but for those younger patients a more conservative resection with removal of the necrotic and infected tissue only is appropriate.

Approach to drainage can be accomplished via ultrasound or CT guidance through the abdomen, vagina, rectum, or transgluteal. Studies have found that treatment of a TOA with drainage combined with antibiotics allowed patients to avoid surgery in a majority of cases and was associated with significantly shorter hospital stays and decreased morbidity [1,6]. Based on the findings of these reports, minimally invasive drainage may be an appropriate primary treatment along with antibiotic therapy, when available.

Key teaching points

- A tubo-ovarian abscess (TOA) is a usually found as a complication of pelvic inflammatory disease (PID), but can also be associated with other intra-abdominal processes such as diverticulitis or appendicitis.
- The long-term sequela of a TOA can be significant including infertility, ectopic pregnancy, and chronic pelvic pain.
- The primary or preferable imaging modality is transvaginal ultrasonography, but transabdominal ultrasonography can be used as well as CT scans and MRI.
- Approximately 75% of all TOAs will resolve with parenteral antibiotics alone.
- Reassessment and possibly escalation of care should occur within 48–72 hours of initiating antibiotics if no improvement occurs.

References

1. Gjelland K, Ekerhovd E, Granberg S. Transvaginal ultrasound-guided aspiration for treatment of tubo-ovarian abscess: a study of 302 cases. *Am J Obstet Gynecol* 2005;193(4):1323–30.

2. Soper D. Pelvic inflammatory disease. *Obstet Gynecol* 2010;116:419–28.

3. Centers for Disease Control and Prevention. *Sexually Transmitted Diseases Treatment Guidelines, 2010. Pelvic Inflammatory Disease.* Available at http://www.cdc.gov/std/treatment/2010/pid.htm.

4. Joiner KA, Lowe BR, Dzink JL, et al. Antibiotic levels in infected and sterile subcutaneous abscesses in mice. *J Infect Dis* 1981;143:487–94.

5. Jaiyeoba O, Lazenby G, Soper DE. Recommendations and rationale for treatment of pelvic inflammatory disease. Expert review in anti-infective therapy. *Expert Rev Anti Infect Ther* 2011;9(1):61–70.

6. Perez-Medina T, Heuras MA, Bajo JM. Early ultrasound-guided transvaginal drainage of tubo-ovarian abcesses: a randomized study. *Ultrasound Obstet Gynecol* 1996; 7(6):435–8.

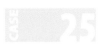

Acute vaginal and abdominal pain after defecation in a 79-year-old woman

Heidi J. Purcell and Laurie S. Swaim

History of preset illness

A 79-year-old gravida 5, para 5 white woman with multiple medical comorbidities presented to the emergency department with a sudden onset of severe vaginal and lower abdominal pressure after defecation one hour prior. She rated her pain at 10 out of 10 on the pain scale. Prior to this acute event, she was feeling well and in her usual state of health.

Review of her medical history revealed hypertension, hyperlipidemia, stable angina, and a remote history of a transient ischemic attack. Her surgical history is remarkable for a vaginal hysterectomy, anterior colporrhaphy, and transobturator sling uretheral suspension four months prior for a grade III cystocele, uterine prolapse, and stress urinary incontinence. Her surgery was uncomplicated, and her pathology was benign. She reports that she has had no medical/surgical restrictions since her postoperative examination two months ago. She denied a history of smoking or alcohol use. The patient's prior obstetrical history was significant for five uncomplicated spontaneous vaginal deliveries.

Physical examination

General appearance: Woman who appears her stated age and is in significant distress

Vital signs:

Temperature: 37.0°C
Pulse: 62 beats/min
Blood pressure: 151/69 mmHg
Respiratory rate: 24 breaths/min
Oxygen saturation: 96% saturation on room air
BMI: 22 kg/m²

HEENT: Unremarkable

Neck: Supple

Cardiovascular: Regular rhythm, without murmurs, rubs, or gallops

Lungs: Clear to auscultation bilaterally

Abdomen: Soft, without distension, severe tenderness to palpation in lower right and left quadrants, bowel sounds were not appreciated

Extremities: Warm, well perfused, nontender, without edema

Neurologic: Nonfocal. The patient was appropriately oriented

Genitourinary: Multiple loops of dark purple, edematous, and firm bowel protruding from vaginal introitus. The

remainder of gynecologic examination could not be accomplished secondary to protrusion of bowel and the patient's severe pain (Fig. 25.1)

Laboratory studies:

WBCs: 10 000/μL (normal 4000–11 000/μL)
Neutrophils: 82% (normal 40–74%)
Blood chemistries and coagulation studies: All within normal limits

How would you manage this patient?

The patient has vaginal cuff dehiscence with bowel evisceration. The patient's presentation was consistent with a bowel evisceration following a vaginal cuff dehiscence. After the

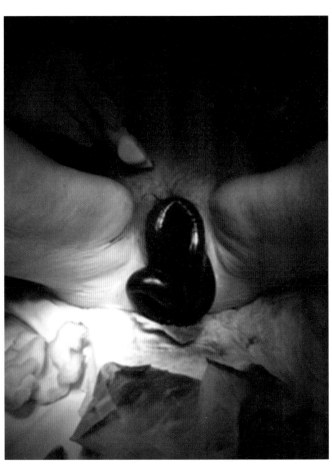

Fig. 25.1 Multiple loops of dark purple, edematous, and firm bowel protruding from vaginal introitus.

Acute Care and Emergency Gynecology, ed. David Chelmow, Christine R. Isaacs and Ashley Carroll. Published by Cambridge University Press. © Cambridge University Press 2015.

diagnosis had been established, general surgery was immediately consulted. Broad spectrum antibiotics were administered prophylactically. The patient was rapidly transported to the operating room where a triple lumen central line was placed. A midline vertical abdominal incision was performed to assess the anatomy from above and attempt to reduce the bowel back into the abdomen. As this could not be performed without risking bowel perforation due to the intraluminal distension and extensive necrosis of the eviscerated segment, a small bowel resection was performed via a vaginal approach. This was followed by an intra-abdominal bowel reanastomosis once the remaining bowel segments could be reduced through the vaginal cuff. The vaginal cuff was then repaired transvaginally with interrupted stitches of delayed absorbable suture. The patient tolerated the procedure well and was taken to the ICU for further recovery. She was ultimately discharged home on postoperative day 8 as she was tolerating a general diet and ambulating without difficulty. The patient was seen six weeks postoperatively and was noted to have made a full recovery with excellent healing of the vaginal cuff observed.

Vaginal cuff dehiscence

Vaginal cuff dehiscence (separation of the vaginal incision) is a rare yet potentially dangerous complication of a hysterectomy, especially when followed by bowel evisceration. Previous studies have estimated the incidence of cuff dehiscence to be 0.03–0.39%. A recent cohort study of 12 472 patients undergoing hysterectomy estimated the 10-year cumulative incidence of dehiscence after all modes of hysterectomy to be 0.24%. The incidence, however, is variable based on the route of hysterectomy. Cuff dehiscence is highest after total laparoscopic hysterectomy, with an incidence of 0.75%, followed by laparoscopic-assisted vaginal hysterectomy (0.46%), total abdominal hysterectomy (0.38%), and lowest with total vaginal hysterectomy (0.08–0.11%) [1].

Several factors have been identified which predispose a patient to cuff dehiscence after hysterectomy. These include increased parity, postoperative surgical site infection, postmenopausal status, vaginal trauma from intercourse or foreign body, presence of prolapse and pelvic floor disorders, history of vaginal surgery, previous radiation therapy, and tobacco use [2,3,4,5]. In this patient, her prior surgery, age, postmenopausal status, and medical comorbidities likely predisposed her to the event.

Prevention of dehiscence begins preoperatively by administering appropriate antibiotic prophylaxis and screening for vaginal infections in patients who are symptomatic prior to surgery. Good surgical technique is also important and should include minimizing the use of electrocautery along the colpotomy, and placing sutures at least 1 cm from the vaginal cuff edge while including full thickness of the vaginal epithelium and underlying supporting tissues. The studies regarding suture type and use of a running versus interrupted closure are inconclusive with some studies showing benefit to the use of a bidirectional barbed suture and others showing no difference [6]. Although not evidence based, most pelvic surgeons recommend pelvic rest and avoidance of heavy lifting for at least six to eight weeks postoperatively.

Diagnosis of vaginal cuff dehiscence primarily relies on physical examination with particular attention to key historical details. Dehiscence typically occurs within the first few months after surgery with a median time for occurrence of 1.5–3.5 months, but the time interval has been shown to range from 6 to 20 months [7,8,9]. After prompt diagnosis of the vaginal cuff dehiscence (and bowel evisceration in this case), the initiation of broad spectrum antibiotics with immediate surgical repair is paramount to preserve any viable bowel and to minimize patient morbidity. Vaginal cuff dehiscence without bowel evisceration may be repaired vaginally without an abdominal survey. In the case of more minor eviscerations, bowel replacement via the vaginal route followed by vaginal cuff closure may be considered if the eviscerated bowel segment has remained viable and non-edemetous. Because the patient in this case had eviscerated bowel that was necrotic, edematous, and essentially incarcerated outside of the vaginal introitus, a laparotomy was necessary to facilitate the surgical management and to inspect for any visceral injury.

Key teaching points

- Vaginal cuff dehiscence most commonly present within the first few months after vaginal surgery.
- The incidence of vaginal cuff dehiscence varies by route of hysterectomy, and is highest following total laparoscopic hysterectomy.
- Diagnosis is always clinical and relies on a thorough pelvic examination.
- Treatment consists of prompt broad spectrum antibiotic administration and surgical intervention.

References

1. Hur HC, Donnellan N, Mansuria S, et al. Vaginal cuff dehiscence after different modes of hysterectomy. *Obstet Gynecol* 2011;118(4):794–801.

2. Kowalski LD, Seski JC, Timmins PF, et al. Vaginal evisceration: presentation and management in postmenopausal women. *J Am Coll Surg* 1996;183(3):225–9.

3. Cardosi RJ, Hoffman MS, Roberts WS, Spellacy WN. Vaginal evisceration after hysterectomy in premenopausal women. *Obstet Gynecol* 1999; 94(5 Pt 2):859.

4. Chan WS, Kong KK, Nikam YA, Merkur H. Vaginal vault dehiscence after laparoscopic hysterectomy over a nine-year period at Sydney West Advanced Pelvic Surgery Unit – our experiences and current understanding of vaginal vault dehiscence. *Aust N Z J Obstet Gynaecol* 2012;52(2):121–7.

5. Hur HC, Guido RS, Mansuria SM, et al. Incidence and patient characteristics of vaginal cuff dehiscence after different modes of hysterectomies. *J Minim Invasive Gynecol* 2007;14(3):311–17.

6. Blikkendaal MD, Twinjstra ARH, Pacquee SCL, et al. Vaginal cuff dehiscence in laparoscopic hysterectomy: influence of various suturing methods of the vaginal vault. *Gynecol Surg* 2012;9(4):393–400.

7. Ramirez PT, Klemer DP. Vaginal evisceration after hysterectomy: A literature review. *Obstet Gynecol Surv* 2002;57:462.

8. Iaco PD, Ceccaroni M, Alboni C, et al. Transvaginal evisceration after hysterectomy: Is vaginal cuff closure associated with a reduced risk? *Eur J Obstet Gynecol Reprod Biol* 2006;125:134–8.

9. Siedhoff MT, Yunker AC, Steege JF. Decreased incidence of vaginal cuff dehiscences after laparoscopic closure with bidirectional barbed suture. *J Minim Invasive Gynecol* 2011;18: 218–23.

Tachycardia and vaginal bleeding in pregnancy

Kimberly Woods McMorrow

History of present illness

A 21-year-old gravida 2, para 1 woman at 14 weeks 0 days by sure last menstrual period presents with a 2-day history of lower abdominal cramping and vaginal spotting requiring her to wear a pad. She complains of some nausea which has been well controlled with odansetron. She has not yet received any prenatal care due to a lack of insurance. She is healthy and does not report any other medical problems. She delivered her first baby by Cesarean about a year ago for malpresentation. She denies a history of sexually transmitted infections and does not smoke, drink alcohol, or use illicit drugs.

Physical examination

General appearance: Anxious-appearing woman in no acute distress

Vital signs:

Temperature: 37.0°C

Pulse: 125 beats/min

Blood pressure: 111/55 mmHg

Respiratory rate: 16 breaths/min

Oxygen saturation: 99% on room air

Cardiovascular: Tachycardic, regular rhythm

Pulmonary: Lungs clear to auscultation bilaterally

Abdomen: Soft, nontender, uterus palpable three finger breadths above the umbilicus, absent fetal heart tones on Doppler

External genitalia: Unremarkable

Pelvic:

Speculum examination: Normal appearing cervix, minimal blood in vaginal vault, no discharge

Bimanual examination: Approximately 24–26 weeks' size nontender uterus, cervix closed, no cervical motion tenderness, no adnexal tenderness or masses

Laboratory studies:

WBCs: 6500/μL

Hb: 8.3 g/dL

Ht: 24.3%

Platelets: 293 000/μL

Thyroid-stimulating hormone: <0.01 mIU/mL

Quantitative beta-hCG: 2.8 million

Blood type: O positive

Imaging: Transvaginal ultrasound performed. Multiple vesicles noted throughout uterus. No intrauterine pregnancy noted. Unable to visualize ovaries bilaterally (Fig. 26.1)

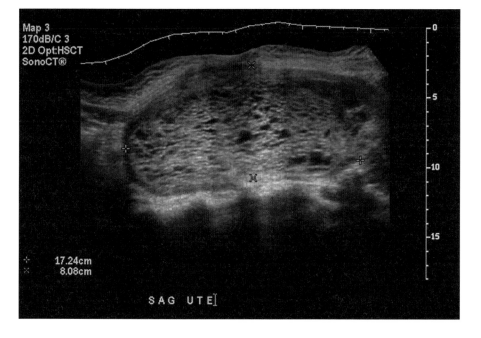

Fig. 26.1 Sagittal ultrasound image of the uterus. Note the vesicular pattern, characteristic of hydatidiform mole. (Image provided by Steven Cohen MD.)

Acute Care and Emergency Gynecology, ed. David Chelmow, Christine R. Isaacs and Ashley Carroll. Published by Cambridge University Press. © Cambridge University Press 2015.

How would you manage this patient?

The patient has a molar pregnancy. Her tachycardia is a result of hyperthyroidism induced by the extremely elevated beta-human chorionic gonadotropin (beta-hCG) level. She needs a suction dilation and curettage (D&C). Her tachycardia and hyperthyroid symptoms should resolve after treatment of the molar pregnancy. Following surgery, her quantitative beta-hCG levels need to be followed until they are negative and then continued to be followed to make sure they remain negative in order to rule out malignant post-molar gestational trophoblastic disease. She should be started on a reliable form of contraception and should be advised not to try to conceive again for at least six months after her hCG levels become negative.

Molar pregnancy

Hydatidiform mole is an abnormal pregnancy that classically shows vesicular swelling of the placental villi. The incidence varies throughout the world, but in the United States and Europe the incidence is approximately 0.6–1.1 per 1000 pregnancies. In Asia, the incidence is higher at 2–10 per 1000 pregnancies. Young women and women over age 40 are at an increased risk of molar pregnancy [1].

Hydatidiform moles may be classified as either complete or partial (Table 26.1). This patient has a complete mole. In a complete hydatidiform mole, the most common karyotype is 46,XX and usually occurs when a haploid sperm fertilizes an empty egg and duplicates. They are associated with diffuse villous edema and trophoblastic proliferation. A fetus is usually absent. In a partial hydatidiform mole, the most common karyotype is 69,XXY with an extra haploid set of chromosomes from the father. A fetus is often present as are fetal red blood cells. Villous edema as well as trophoblastic proliferation are only focal. Partial moles are very similar to and often diagnosed as a missed abortion [2].

Molar pregnancies are typically diagnosed in the first trimester of pregnancy. The most common symptom is vaginal bleeding. Other signs include uterine enlargement greater than the expected gestational age, absent fetal heart tone, cystic enlargement of the ovaries (theca lutein cysts), hyperemesis gravidarum, and an hCG level abnormally higher than what would be expected for gestational age. The diagnosis is

typically established using ultrasonography. Complete moles classically show a vesicular pattern on ultrasound [3].

This patient also showed signs of clinical hyperthyroidism induced by the excessively elevated hCG level. Clinical hyperthyroidism has been reported in up to 7% of patients with a complete molar pregnancy but is now less common due to earlier diagnosis secondary to widespread ultrasonography. These women may present with tachycardia, skin warmth, and tremor. Hyperthyroidism usually develops only in patients with extremely high hCG levels. Anesthesia or surgery may precipitate a thyroid storm; therefore, beta-blocking agents should be administered prior to induction of anesthesia [4].

The American College of Obstetricians and Gynecologists (ACOG) practice bulletin [3] recommends the following tests in patients who have a suspected hydatidiform mole: complete blood count with platelet count, clotting function studies, renal and liver function studies, blood type with antibody screen, hCG level, and chest x-ray. The preferred method of treatment in women who wish to preserve their fertility is suction D&C. After dilation of the cervix, the largest suction cannula that fits through the cervix should be used. Ultrasound guidance may sometimes be helpful to ensure that the uterus is completely evacuated. Oxytocin should be administered intravenously after dilation of the cervix and continued several hours post-operatively. Rh-negative patients should be given anti-D immune globulin after evacuation. For patients who do not wish to preserve their fertility, hysterectomy with ovarian preservation is acceptable. Medical induction of labor and hysterotomy are not acceptable management strategies because they are associated with increased blood loss and may increase the risk for subsequent malignancy.

After treatment, patients need to be monitored for the development of post-molar trophoblastic disease. The ACOG practice bulletin [3] recommends serial serum hCG assessments 48 hours after evacuation, every 1–2 weeks while elevated, and then at monthly intervals for an additional 6 months. Patients should use a reliable form of birth control during this period as a pregnancy may delay the diagnosis of post-molar trophoblastic disease. Post-molar malignant trophoblastic disease is diagnosed when hCG levels plateau or begin to rise in the weeks following molar evacuation. Approximately 20% of patients will develop post-molar trophoblastic disease following the evacuation of a hydatidiform mole. In patients who have undergone hysterectomy, the risk of trophoblastic disease still remains at approximately 3–5%. Patients who develop post-molar trophoblastic disease need to be treated with chemotherapy, most commonly methotrexate.

According to the ACOG practice bulletin [3], after six months of normal hCG levels, women may discontinue contraception and attempt pregnancy again. Women who have had a prior partial or complete mole have a 10-fold increase or 1–2% incidence of a second hydatidiform mole in a second pregnancy. Future pregnancies should be evaluated with an early ultrasound and any products of conception or placentas should be evaluated by pathology.

Table 26.1 Characteristics of complete and partial hydatidiform moles

Characteristic	Complete mole	Partial mole
Karyotype	46,XX or 46,XY	69,XXX or 69,XXY
Fetus	Absent	Present
Villous edema	Diffuse	Focal
Trophoblastic proliferation	Diffuse	Focal

Key teaching points

- Hydatidiform moles typically present with abnormal vaginal bleeding in the first trimester of pregnancy. Other signs include uterine enlargement greater than expected for gestational age, absent fetal heart tones, theca lutein cysts of the ovaries, hyperemesis gravidarum, and abnormally elevated human chorionic gonadotropin (hCG) level.
- Clinical hyperthyroidism is rare but may be present in cases where hCG is excessively elevated.
- The diagnosis is typically established using ultrasonography which classically shows a vesicular pattern.
- The treatment for molar pregnancy is evacuation of the uterus with suction dilation and curettage (D&C). Hysterectomy may be considered for patients who do not wish to preserve their fertility.
- Following treatment, hCG levels need to be monitored until they are negative and then for six months in order to evaluate for post-molar gestational trophoblastic disease.
- Post-molar gestational disease is diagnosed when beta-hCG plateaus or rises following molar evacuation and is treated with chemotherapy.

References

1. Smith HO. Gestational trophoblastic disease epidemiology and trends. *Clin Obstet Gynecol* 2003;46:541–56.

2. Lawler SD, Fisher RA, Dent J. A prospective genetic study of complete and partial hydatidiform moles. *Am J Obstet Gynecol* 1991;164:1270–7.

3. American College of Obstetricians and Gynecologists. Diagnosis and treatment of gestational trophoblastic disease. Practice Bulletin No. 53. *Obstet Gynecol* 2004;103:1365–77.

4. Walkington L, Webster J, Hancock BW, et al. Hyperthyroidism and human chorionic gonadotrophin production in gestational trophoblastic disease. *Br J Cancer* 2011;104:1665–9.

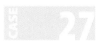

Vaginal spotting at eight weeks' gestation

Amanda B. Murchison and Melanie D. Altizer

History of present illness

A 19-year-old gravida 1 who is 8 weeks' pregnant by her last menstrual period, presents to the emergency department with a 1-day history of vaginal spotting. She reports that she had a positive home pregnancy test one week ago. Her periods are typically regular and she has not been using any form of contraception. She denies pelvic cramping, abdominal pain, or fever. She complains of mild nausea but no emesis. She reports that she was diagnosed with chlamydia one year ago and was treated with an antibiotic. She has no other medical problems and is not taking any medication.

Physical examination

General appearance: Well-appearing woman
Vital signs:

Temperature: 36.7°C
Pulse: 82 beats/min
Blood pressure: 116/72 mmHg
Respiratory rate: 16 breaths/min
Oxygen saturation: 100% on room air
BMI: 20 kg/m^2

Cardiovascular: Regular rate and rhythm with no murmurs
Lungs: Clear to auscultation
Abdomen: Soft, nontender, nondistended
External genitalia: Normal female external genitalia
Urethra: Urethral meatus appears normal
Vagina: Vaginal mucosa without lesions. There is a small amount of dark blood in the vaginal vault
Cervix: Cervix is without lesions and is closed
Uterus: Six to eight weeks' size with no tenderness
Adenxa: No adnexal tenderness or masses
Laboratory studies:

Quantitative hCG: 3600 mIU/mL
Hb: 12.6 g/dL (normal 12–16 g/dL)
Ht: 38% (normal 36–46%)
WBCs: 9500/µL (normal 4000–10 500/µL)
Platelets: 242 000/µL (normal 130 000–400 000/µL)
Blood type: A negative

Imaging: An ultrasound is performed. The uterus is anteverted and measures 12 × 8 × 9 cm. It contains an intrauterine gestational sac. Within the gestational sac is a yolk sac and a fetal pole measuring 8.4 mm, which is consistent with a gestational age of 6 weeks and 4 days. No fetal cardiac activity is present. Both ovaries are normal. There is no free fluid in the cul-de-sac (Fig. 27.1)

How would you manage this patient?

The patient has a missed abortion. An intrauterine pregnancy was identified on ultrasound with a fetal pole measuring 8.4 mm, but no cardiac activity was seen. This meets diagnostic

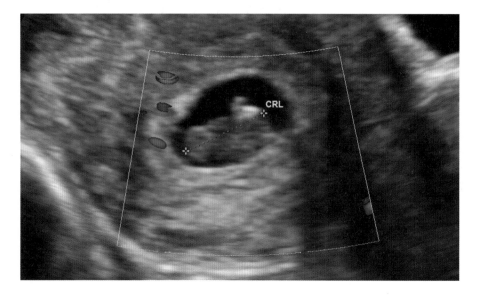

Fig. 27.1 Ultrasound.

Acute Care and Emergency Gynecology, ed. David Chelmow, Christine R. Isaacs and Ashley Carroll. Published by Cambridge University Press.
© Cambridge University Press 2015.

criteria for a missed abortion and no further testing is indicated. The patient was counseled on the options of expectant, medical, and surgical management and she chose medical management. She was given a prescription for misoprostol 800 μg to be placed vaginally and was instructed that the dose could be repeated in 48–72 hours if products of conception were not passed. In addition, a Rh-immunoglobulin injection was administered. She was scheduled for a follow-up appointment in four days. At that time she reported requiring two doses of misoprostol. She described heavy bleeding and cramping that lasted approximately four hours with passage of blood clots followed by bleeding similar to menstrual flow. She stated that her bleeding had been much lighter for the past 24 hours. A pelvic examination revealed a small amount of blood in the vaginal vault with a closed cervix and small uterus. A negative home pregnancy test two weeks later confirmed resolution of the pregnancy.

Missed abortion

Approximately 15–20% of clinically recognized pregnancies will end in an early pregnancy loss. If unrecognized pregnancies are included, this number increases to as high as 60% [1]. Patients who have a missed abortion may present with vaginal bleeding or pelvic cramping; however, it may also be diagnosed in an asymptomatic woman as an incidental finding on routine ultrasound. A physical examination finding of a uterine size less than expected for gestational age would raise suspicion for a missed abortion and an ultrasound would be prudent.

Making the diagnosis of a missed abortion may sometimes be possible in a single clinical encounter or may require subsequent follow-up with ultrasound or serum beta-human chorionic gonadotropin (beta-hCG) measurements. The American College of Radiology Appropriateness Criteria guidelines state that a missed abortion may be diagnosed when the mean gestational sac diameter is greater than or equal to 25 mm with no fetal pole, or when a fetal pole is present measuring greater than or equal to 7 mm but no cardiac activity is identified [2]. Our patient had a fetal pole measurement of 8.4 mm with no cardiac activity which met the guidelines for establishing a diagnosis of a missed abortion.

Successful management of a missed abortion requires complete evacuation of the uterus. Treatment options include expectant management, medical management, and surgical management. Not all management options will be appropriate for each patient, but when multiple options are appropriate, the patient should be counseled on the risks and benefits of each. The success of the approach depends on several factors including the presence of symptoms such a bleeding and cramping in addition to the gestational age of the pregnancy.

Expectant management is a reasonable option for women with a gestational age of 13 weeks or less, are hemodynamically stable, and without evidence of infection. The success rate varies from 25 to 76% within 4 weeks. The timing can be unpredictable, leading to patient anxiety [3]. It is important

that patients choosing this option understand that when the miscarriage happens there will be associated bleeding and cramping. Patients should be counseled that if heavy bleeding persists beyond 2–3 hours, they should be evaluated and may possibly need surgical intervention. Expectant management is associated with higher rates of incomplete miscarriage resulting in unplanned surgical intervention. Pelvic infections associated with miscarriage are low in all methods of management, but some studies show they are lower in patients who chose expectant management. Patients have greater success with expectant management when thorough counseling is provided about appropriate expectations regarding the length of time and symptoms.

Effective and safe medical therapy for missed abortion has afforded women new options for receiving active management in situations where surgical intervention is undesirable to the patient. Patients who choose medical management often want to avoid surgery but desire a more controlled time frame for passage of products of conception. This option should be discussed with patients who are hemodynamically stable and have no sign of a pelvic infection. The most commonly used medication is misoprostol, a prostaglandin E1 analog. It acts as an uterotonic that results in cervical softening and contractions that lead to expulsion of products of conception from the uterine cavity. The risk of a major complication from the use of misoprostol is rare. However, medical management of a missed abortion can result in incomplete passage of tissue resulting in hemorrhage that requires emergent surgical intervention. The most studied regimen has been misoprostol 800 μg vaginally once and repeated on day 3 if expulsion is incomplete [1]. A multicenter, randomized trial by Creinin et al. [4] showed that using this regimen in missed abortions of 10 weeks, 6 days' gestation or less (determined by crown rump length of ≤40 mm) resulted in a 71% success rate of pregnancy evacuation with the first dose of misoprostol and an 84% success if an additional dose was required and used. Many patients are comfortable placing the misoprostol vaginally, but a simple trick for patients that are less comfortable with this idea is to have them load the medication in a tampon applicator to assist with proper placement. Also consider prescribing a nonsteroidal anti-inflammatory drug (NSAID) or a small amount of narcotic pain medication when patients elect for expectant or medical management as passage of products of conception will be associated with moderate to severe cramping. Patients should be counseled to contact their physician if they experience heavy bleeding, consisting of soaking a menstrual pad every hour for 2 consecutive hours, or fever that persists beyond 24 hours. Misoprostol use can be associated with short-term elevations in temperature [1].

Some patients will elect for surgical management while others will require surgery as a result of failed expectant or medical management. Many patients experience anxiety associated with the uncertainty as to when they will start bleeding and how much discomfort will be associated with a miscarriage. Benefits of surgical intervention include a scheduled timing as well as potentially decreased amounts of bleeding and discomfort. Dilation and curettage also produces a surgical specimen for pathologic evaluation. Surgical management is usually accomplished by a suction dilation and curettage or dilation and evacuation. Risks of surgical management include complications from anesthesia, uterine perforation, intrauterine adhesion formation, cervical trauma, infection, and the risk of retained products. Prompt surgical intervention is the correct treatment when the patient is hemodynamically unstable or has evidence of infection (septic abortion) [5]. The use of ultrasound guidance during the procedure is optional, but no studies have been conducted determining its effectiveness in preventing uterine perforation or determining complete emptying of the uterine cavity.

There have been no randomized trials to define the optimal follow-up of patients after treatment for a missed abortion. Consider a follow-up visit in three to seven days after medical management and one to two weeks after expectant or surgical management. This visit may include a history, pelvic exam, and possibly an ultrasound to evaluate the uterine cavity.

Women who are Rh(D) negative and not sensitized should be given Rh(D)-immunoglobulin following surgical treatment or upon diagnosis of missed abortion when expectant or medical management is selected as the treatment option [6]. Gestations of 12 weeks or less can be treated with a dose of 50 μg. Pregnancies of greater gestational age should receive the standard 300 μg dose. There is no harm in using the larger dose at earlier gestation ages.

Key teaching points

- An intrauterine pregnancy should be seen by transvaginal ultrasound by the time the beta-human chorionic gonadotropin (beta-hCG) level is between 1000 and 2000 mIU/mL. This will vary by institution and is mostly dependent on the resolution of transvaginal imaging available.
- An early failed pregnancy diagnosis can be made when the mean gestational sac measurement is 25 mm or greater and no fetal pole is present.
- An early failed pregnancy diagnosis can be made when a fetal pole is present measuring 7 mm or greater but no cardiac activity is identified.
- Patients with a diagnosis of an early failed pregnancy who are hemodynamically stable, should be counseled on the options of expectant, medical, and surgical management.
- The most studied regimen of medical management for an early pregnancy failure has been misoprostol 800 μg vaginally repeated on day 3 if expulsion is incomplete.
- Patients who are Rh negative should be given Rh immunoglobulin at the time an early pregnancy failure is diagnosed.

References

1. Gariepy A, Stanwood N. Medical management of early pregnancy failure. *Contemporary Obgyn* 2013;**May**: 26–33.
2. Lane B, Wong-You-Cheong J, Javitt M, et al. ACR Appropriateness Criteria® first trimester bleeding. *Ultrasound Q* 2013;29(2):91–6.
3. Zhang J, Gilles JM, Barnhart K, et al. National Institute of Child Health and Human Development Management of Early Pregnancy Failure Trial. A comparison of medical management with misoprostol and surgical management for early pregnancy failure. *N Engl J Med* 2005;353(8): 761–9.
4. Creinin MD, Huang X, Westhoff C, et al; National Institute of Child Health and Human Development Management of Early Pregnancy Failure Trial. Factors related to successful misoprostol treatment for early pregnancy failure. *Obstet Gynecol* 2006;107(4):901–7.
5. Griebel C, Halvorsen J, Golemon T, Day A. Management of spontaneous abortion. *Am Fam Physician* 2005; 72(7):1243–50.
6. American College of Obstetricians and Gynecologists. Medical management of abortion. Practice Bulletin No. 67. *Obstet Gynecol* 2005;106:871–82.

Heavy bleeding after medical management of a missed abortion

Elizabeth L. Munter

History of present illness

A 30-year-old gravida 5, para 4 woman at 10 weeks' gestation presented to the emergency department with heavy vaginal bleeding and lightheadedness. She had been seen in the gynecology urgent care clinic earlier that day with light bleeding and lower abdominal cramping. An ultrasound was performed, which revealed an approximately eight-week-size intrauterine pregnancy without cardiac activity. She was informed of the diagnosis of a missed abortion, and was counseled on options and offered support. Management options were discussed with her, including expectant management, medical management with misoprostol, or surgical management with dilation and curettage (D&C). She elected to proceed with medical management and was given misoprostol 800 μg per vagina. A follow-up visit was scheduled two days later. Approximately 8 hours after placing the misoprostol, she noted her bleeding became significantly heavier and she soaked five sanitary pads over the hour prior to her arrival in the emergency department. Her past medical history was unremarkable. She had four prior spontaneous vaginal deliveries. A hemoglobin reading obtained at her initial prenatal visit 3 weeks prior was 12.1 g/dL.

Physical examination

General appearance: No acute distress, alert and oriented woman, though slow in answering questions

Vital signs:

Temperature: 36.6°C
Pulse: 122 beats/min
Blood pressure: 78/44 mmHg
Respiratory rate: 18 breaths/min
Oxygen saturation: 98% on room air

Cardiovascular: Tachycardic, no murmurs appreciated

Respiratory: Clear to auscultation bilaterally

Abdomen: Soft, nontender

Pelvic: Normal external genitalia. Speculum examination with multiple large clots and on estimated 200 mL of bright red bleeding during the brief exam. Cervix was 1 cm dilated. No obvious tissue was present at the os. Uterus was eight-week-size, mild tenderness on palpation. Adnexa nontender and without masses

Laboratory studies:

Hb: 6.4 g/dL (normal 12.0–15.0 g/dL)
Blood type: A positive

How would you manage this patient?

The patient has significant hemorrhage following misoprostol administration for a missed abortion. She has evidence of volume depletion with tachycardia, hypotension, and acute blood loss anemia. She needs stabilization with intravenous fluids and blood transfusion, and requires immediate D&C to control the bleeding.

Heavy bleeding after medical management of a missed abortion

Significant bleeding is a potential risk with any first-trimester pregnancy loss. Prompt recognition and management is critical. This patient already had tachycardia, hypotension, and a decrease in hemoglobin by the time she was evaluated, which was shortly after her heavy bleeding started, indicative of substantial blood loss. However, patients who present shortly after the onset of even life-threatening bleeding may show only some of these signs, or none at all. Young healthy women are frequently able to compensate systemic blood pressure and cerebral perfusion despite losing large amounts of blood. At some point, a critical volume is lost, and they then rapidly decompensate. Tachycardia is often the first sign of volume depletion and will typically be seen before the onset of hypotension or decrease in hemoglobin. Change in hemoglobin values frequently takes the longest to occur, and patients may have lost large amounts of blood volume prior to decreases in hemoglobin measurement. Acute-onset heavy bleeding in the setting of a normal hemoglobin level should not be ignored.

When heavy bleeding following medical management for a missed abortion is encountered, steps must first be taken to stabilize the patient, including establishing intravenous access and starting fluid resuscitation. Blood should be sent to the laboratory for complete blood count and type and screen. If blood loss is large enough that disseminated intravascular coagulation (DIC) is possible, coagulation studies including prothrombin time, partial thromboplastin time, and fibrinogen should be ordered. For presumed large blood loss, packed red blood cells should be ordered for possible transfusion. In the case of heavy bleeding with hemodynamic instability, the patient should have a uterine curettage performed emergently, with additional trained personnel present to assist in management of the hypovolemia.

Acute Care and Emergency Gynecology, ed. David Chelmow, Christine R. Isaacs and Ashley Carroll. Published by Cambridge University Press.
© Cambridge University Press 2015.

Isotonic crystalloid should be used for fluid resuscitation. Blood transfusion should be considered when symptoms such as lightheadedness or abnormal vital signs do not resolve with the initial fluid management. Decision for transfusion should be based on the estimated volume of blood lost, and should not be withheld based strictly on laboratory values. An unstable patient with a large clinical blood loss may still reflect a near normal hemoglobin value, as a sample drawn early in the hemorrhage will not reflect the ongoing amount of bleeding. Administration of fresh frozen plasma should be considered with significant transfusion, especially in the setting of abnormal coagulation studies. Massive transfusion protocols may be initiated if necessary.

Once the acute bleeding has resolved following curettage, the patient should be observed to ensure the bleeding does not resume. In most instances, the bleeding is caused by retained products of conception, and curettage corrects the bleeding. The patient should be discharged with an iron supplement to improve anemia. Otherwise, follow-up care is similar to other women undergoing curettage for an early pregnancy failure. Patients who do not desire pregnancy should be recommended contraception, as ovulation may resume as soon as two weeks following resolution of the pregnancy. Patients losing desired pregnancies should be offered support and grief counseling. Anti-D immune globulin should be administered to Rh-negative women. In instances of suction curettage for massive blood loss, consideration of pathologic analysis of the specimen may be appropriate to ensure molar pregnancy was not present.

While the amount of bleeding described in this case is unusual, it is a recognized complication with any management option. When a stable patient is initially diagnosed with a missed abortion, the management options include D&C, misoprostol, or expectant management. Misoprostol is a prostaglandin E1 analog that stimulates uterine contractions to promote expulsion of the uterine contents. Several regimens have been studied for missed abortion including 800 µg vaginally and 600 µg sublingually, with or without repeat doses. Efficacy rates for complete expulsion of uterine contents are approximately 80% [1]. Side effects may include vaginal bleeding, nausea, vomiting, and fevers.

Randomized trials comparing management of missed abortion have not individually been adequately powered to detect differences in catastrophic bleeding. However, data is available from a Cochrane review [2] and two additional randomized trials [3,4] not included in the systematic review. The Cochrane review [2] was updated in 2012 regarding medical management of spontaneous abortion. There was a single review concerning bleeding outcomes with misoprostol compared to D&C. The review identified a single study with 50 patients with no significant difference in post-treatment hematocrit identified. The Miscarriage Treatment (MIST) trial [3] was a randomized controlled trial conducted in Great Britain of missed or incomplete abortions prior to 13 weeks' gestation. It compared expectant management, medical management with misoprostol (800 µg per vagina), and surgical management with suction curettage. The primary outcome was confirmed gynecologic infection within 14 days; this was found not to be significantly different between any of the management options. One of the secondary outcomes was rate of blood transfusion. Four out of the 398 subjects who received misoprostol required transfusion, while none of the 402 subjects who underwent curettage did, though this difference was not statistically significant.

The Management of Early Pregnancy Failure Study was completed at multiple centers in the United States and published in 2007 [4]. The primary outcome was efficacy. The study was not powered to detect differences in bleeding; however, detailed information regarding bleeding was collected, including hemoglobin at baseline and 14 days following the intervention as well as daily bleeding diaries. There was a significant decrease in hemoglobin from baseline with misoprostol compared with curettage (–0.7 g/dL vs. –0.1 g/dL) and a significant increase in the percentage of subjects whose hemoglobin decreased by at least 2 g/dL (10.5% vs. 3.7%) and at least 3 g/dL (5.8% vs. 0.7%). Additionally, subjects who received misoprostol reported more days of bleeding following the intervention and were less likely to find the bleeding to be acceptable. Transfusions were given to 4 out of 488 women in the misoprostol group; none were required in the surgical group.

The above case certainly does not represent a typical outcome following misoprostol for missed abortion. Misoprostol is an appropriate management choice for many women with missed abortion, along with D&C or expectant management. The advantages of misoprostol can include faster time to resolution compared to expectant management while still avoiding a procedure, which some women prefer. Women should be counseled regarding the efficacy and possible side effects of misoprostol including longer duration of bleeding, and should be given instructions to present for evaluation in the case of brisk bleeding or light-headedness. Additionally, providers should be familiar with the appropriate course of action for heavy bleeding, as described above.

Key teaching points

- Acute-onset heavy bleeding in the setting of a normal hemoglobin level should not be ignored.
- In the case of heavy bleeding with hemodynamic instability, the patient should have a uterine curettage performed emergently, with additional trained personnel present to assist in management of the hypovolemia.
- In most instances, the bleeding is caused by retained products of conception, and curettage corrects the bleeding.
- Women should be counseled regarding the efficacy and possible side effects of misoprostol, including longer duration of bleeding, and should be given instructions to present for evaluation in the case of brisk bleeding or light-headedness.

References

1. American College of Obstetricians and Gynecologists. Misoprostol for postabortion care. Committee Opinion No. 427. *Obstet Gynecol* 2009; 113(2 Pt 1):465–8.

2. Neilson JP, Hickey M, Vazquez JC. Medical treatment for early fetal death (less than 24 weeks). *Cochrane Database Syst Rev* 2006, Issue 3. Art. No.: CD002253.

3. Trinder J, Brocklehurst P, Porter R, et al. Management of miscarriage: expectant, medical, or surgical? Results of randomised controlled trial (miscarriage treatment [MIST] trial). *BMJ* 2006;332(7552): 1235–40.

4. Davis AR, Hendlish SK, Westhoff C, et al. Bleeding patterns after misoprostol vs surgical treatment of early pregnancy failure: results from a randomized trial. *Am J Obstet Gynecol* 2007;196(31):e1–31.

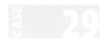

Abdominal pain and vaginal bleeding in a 24-year-old woman

Jessica M. Ciaburri

History of present illness

A 24-year-old gravida 2, para 1 woman presents to the urgent care clinic after she began having vaginal bleeding and pelvic pain the previous night. She comes with her partner and reports that she had a positive home pregnancy test approximately two weeks prior. She is tearful and asks, "Do you think I'm losing the baby?" She is a healthy adult with a benign past medical history and in the past carried a pregnancy to term without complications.

Her vaginal bleeding is similar to a heavy menstrual cycle and she is changing a pad every two hours. She has pain in the suprapubic region and describes it as a cramping sensation. The patient has not tried any over-the-counter pain relievers, as she was unsure if these would be harmful to her fetus. The review of systems is negative for fever or chills, nausea, vomiting, or dysuria.

Physical examination

General appearance: Alert-and-oriented woman who is tearful

Vital signs:

Temperature: 37.0°C
Pulse: 98 beats/min
Blood pressure: 110/65 mmHg
Respiratory rate: 18 breaths/min
Oxygen saturation: 100% on room air

HEENT: Unremarkable

Neck: Supple

Cardiovascular: Regular rate and rhythm without rubs, murmurs, or gallops

Lungs: Clear to auscultation bilaterally

Abdomen: Soft, nondistended, normal bowel sounds, tender to palpation in the suprapubic region without associated rebound or guarding

Pelvic:

Speculum: Moderate amount dark red blood and tissue/clot in vaginal vault
Bimanual: Cervix 1 cm dilated, no cervical motion tenderness, uterus ~8 weeks' size, anteverted, nontender, bilateral adnexa nontender

Extremities: No clubbing, cyanosis, or edema

Neurologic: Nonfocal

Laboratory studies:

Urine pregnancy test: Positive
Quantitative beta-hCG: 3500 mIU/mL
Hb: 11.0 g/dL (normal 12–16 g/dL)
Blood type and Rh: O negative
Urinalysis: Negative

How would you manage this patient?

This patient is experiencing a spontaneous abortion, defined as a loss of a pregnancy at less than 20 weeks without medical intervention – synonymous with miscarriage. Hemorrhage into the decidua basalis, followed by necrosis of the early pregnancy tissue, usually accompanies an early miscarriage. As the gestational sac and placental tissue detach from the uterine wall, contractions occur in an effort to expel the pregnancy tissue. With an incomplete abortion, the internal cervical os opens to allow passage of blood. The fetus and placenta may remain entirely in utero or may partially extrude through the dilated os. In addition to the above physical examination findings and laboratory values, imaging using transvaginal ultrasound will help to confirm the diagnosis and aid the clinician in helping the patient choose an appropriate management strategy (Fig. 29.1).

When choosing a treatment strategy, first and foremost the hemodynamic stability of the patient should be assessed. Signs such as hypotension, tachycardia, heavy vaginal bleeding, fever, or altered mental status necessitate immediate action on the part of the practitioner to begin fluid resuscitation, administer blood products and antibiotics as indicated, and transport the patient emergently to the operating room for definitive surgical management. In our patient, there is time to discuss treatment options to find the best management strategy to help her cope physically and emotionally with her loss. The approach to managing early pregnancy loss should be individualized, as current literature supports relatively equal efficacy of medical and surgical treatments [1].

A Cochrane review completed in November 2012 sought to review data from available randomized control trials comparing medical treatment with expectant care or surgery for incomplete abortion before 24 weeks. Twenty studies were included, encompassing 4208 women. Ultimately, it was determined that in pregnancies less than or equal to 13 weeks' gestation, success rates were high for all treatment options. The conclusion statement suggested that medical treatment

---

Acute Care and Emergency Gynecology, ed. David Chelmow, Christine R. Isaacs and Ashley Carroll. Published by Cambridge University Press. © Cambridge University Press 2015.

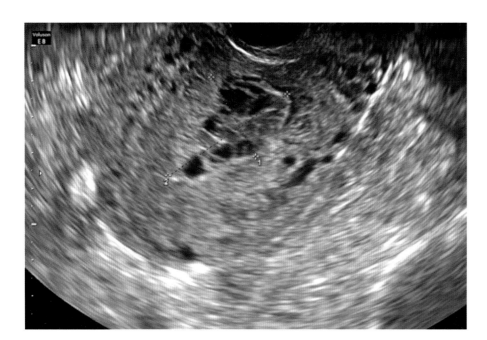

Fig. 29.1 Transvaginal ultrasound.

with misoprostol and expectant care are both acceptable alternatives to surgical evacuation given the availability of health service resources to support all three approaches [1].

Once a nonviable pregnancy has been identified, management focuses not only on the evacuation of products of conception but also on the patient's personal feelings about the pregnancy and beginning the grief process. Studies have documented that women who are given a choice in how to deal with their miscarriage have improved psychological health [2].

Expectant management

For women with incomplete abortions less than 12 weeks' gestation expectant management has been shown to have approximately a 50% success rate in various randomized control trials [1]. Expectant management is often a safe initial treatment option. The patient should be given precautions regarding signs and symptoms of infection (fever, chills, foul smelling vaginal discharge, severe abdominal pain) and hemorrhage (weakness, dizziness, heavy vaginal bleeding with clots, using one pad per hour) along with instructions to seek medical evaluation if these occur. A follow-up appointment should be scheduled for 10–14 days later to reassess [3].

Medical management

The most common choice for medical management of an incomplete abortion is the prostaglandin E1 analog, misoprostol. Study data has not clearly identified one misoprostol regimen or route to be superior to the others. Current accepted misoprostol regimens include a single dose of either 600 μg orally, 800 μg vaginally, or 400 μg sublingually [4]. Depending on the study, the success rates of completing the spontaneous abortion medically range from 71 to 99%. Misoprostol given by the vaginal route is generally preferred given that serum levels remain higher for a longer period of time, and uncomfortable gastrointestinal side effects including nausea, vomiting, and diarrhea are minimized. It is reasonable to prescribe a pretreatment dose of an anti-emetic. Patients should be counseled regarding expected side effects of bleeding and cramping pelvic pain. Passage of tissue should occur within 48–72 hours of medical therapy, and if this is unsuccessful, then surgical management is warranted [4].

Surgical management

In the past, surgical management of incomplete abortion with suction dilation and curettage was the gold standard. Surgical treatment is definitive and predictable, with a near 100% success rate in completing early pregnancy failures. But dilation and curettage is also invasive and carries additional risks, including uterine perforation, cervical laceration, hemorrhage, incomplete removal of pregnancy tissue, infection, and Asherman syndrome [3]. Surgical management is the recommended treatment course for gestations greater than or equal to 12 weeks. Antibiotic prophylaxis is needed to decrease infection risk. A common antimicrobial regimen is: Doxycycline 100 mg PO prior to procedure and 200 mg PO postprocedure. Broad spectrum antibiotic coverage is needed if a septic abortion is suspected.

Additional considerations

Within 72 hours of identifying a spontaneous abortion, Rh-negative women should receive a 50 μg dose of anti-D immune globulin (RhoGAM®). Following miscarriage as many as 5% of women will become isoimmunized without it [5]. It is important to provide a comforting environment for patients experiencing early pregnancy loss. It may be helpful to provide them with local resources for support groups and reputable websites such as the March of Dimes (www.march-ofdimes.com), which can help them through the grieving process. It is also essential to begin a dialogue about the patient's desire for future conception. Women under age 35 have approximately a 10% chance of spontaneous abortion with any given pregnancy; this is not increased after a single early pregnancy loss [3]. If desired an appropriate contraceptive should be initiated.

Key teaching points

- An incomplete abortion is defined by an open internal cervical os accompanied by vaginal bleeding. The fetus and placenta may remain in utero or partially extrude through the dilated os.
- If signs of hemodynamic instability or acute sepsis are identified in a patient with an incomplete abortion, urgent surgical management is indicated.

- In hemodynamically stable, afebrile women at less than or at 12 weeks' gestation, it is prudent to counsel the patient and allow her to choose between expectant, medical, and surgical management given the high success rates for completion of the abortion with all three treatment plans.
- Women choosing expectant management should be followed up in clinic within 10–14 days to determine whether or not the abortion has completed spontaneously.
- The preferred route for misoprostol administration is 800 μg placed vaginally. This route greatly decreases irritating gastrointestinal side effects.
- Surgical management with suction dilation and curettage is nearly 100% effective and is the recommended treatment modality for gestations greater than 12 weeks.
- Administration of RhoGAM to Rh-negative women experiencing a spontaneous abortion should be done within 72 hours to prevent isoimmunization.

References

1. Neilson JP, Gyte GML, Hickey M, Vazquez JC, Dou L. Medical treatments for incomplete miscarriage. *Cochrane Database Syst Rev* 2013, Issue 3. Art. No.: CD007223. DOI: 10.1002/14651858.CD007223.pub3.

2. Wieringa-De Waard M, Hartman EE, Ankum WM, et al. Expectant management versus surgical evacuation in first trimester miscarriage: health-related quality of life in randomized and non-randomized patients. *Hum Reprod* 2002;17(6):1638–42.

3. Puscheck EE, Lucidi RS. *Early Pregnancy Loss.* Available at http://reference.medscape.com/article/266317-overview.

4. Allen R, O'Brien BM. Uses of misoprostol in obstetrics and gynecology. *Rev Obstet Gynecol* 2009; 2(3):159–68.

5. American College of Obstetricians and Gynecologists. Prevention of Rh D alloimmunization. Practice Bulletin No. 4. *Obstet Gynecol* 1999;5:1–7. Reaffirmed 2010.

Unanticipated ultrasound findings at follow-up prenatal visit

Nikola Alexander Letham and Christopher Morosky

History of present illness

A 39-year-old gravida 5, para 3 woman presents to the emergency room 7 weeks after her last menstrual period with complaints of vaginal spotting and a positive pregnancy test at home 4 days ago. The patient also complains of fatigue and some mild nausea. She denies pelvic pain, cramping or recent trauma.

Her previous obstetrical history includes a preterm spontaneous vaginal delivery at 36 weeks followed by two term Cesarean deliveries, and then a first-trimester termination with dilation and curettage. Her medical and surgical histories are otherwise unremarkable.

This is an unplanned and undesired pregnancy. Her intention is to pursue termination. She also desires a reliable form of contraception, and is open to surgical sterilization.

Physical examination

General appearance: Alert woman who is in no apparent distress

Vital signs:

Temperature: 37.2°C
Pulse: 61 beats/min
Blood pressure: 113/74 mmHg
Respiratory rate: 18 breaths/min
Oxygen saturation: 100% on room air

Cardiovascular: Regular rate and rhythm without murmurs, rubs, or gallops

Lungs: Clear to auscultation bilaterally

Abdomen: Soft, nontender and nondistended, no guarding or rebound, normal active bowel sounds

Pelvic:

External genitalia: Normal appearing with no lesions or masses
Bimanual exam: Shows uterus 8-weeks' sized, anteverted, nontender, no pelvic masses
Speculum exam: Shows closed cervix, no lesions, a small amount of old dark blood is present in the vagina, no active bleeding

Laboratory studies:

Quantitative beta-hCG: 36 345 mIU/mL
Hb: 12.6 g/dL
Ht: 37.6%
Blood type: O positive

Imaging: A transvaginal ultrasound reveals a single gestational sac within the lower uterine segment with an hourglassing portion of the sac within the upper portion of the cervix (Fig. 30.1). Within the gestational sac is a single embryo measuring six weeks and five days by crown rump length measurement. Cardiac activity is present. The remainder of the endometrial stripe is thin and normal in appearance

How would you manage this patient?

The patient was discharged from the emergency room with the diagnosis of a threatened abortion. At her obstetrical follow-up appointment two days later, she underwent a repeat transvaginal ultrasound and the images confirmed the diagnosis of a cervical ectopic pregnancy.

In discussing the options for management, the patient elected to undergo hysterectomy. Her decision-making was guided by a desire to have the pregnancy terminated in a controlled setting in order to mitigate the risk of significant blood loss. This also accomplished her desired surgical sterilization.

The patient underwent an uncomplicated total abdominal hysterectomy. Histologic examination of the surgical specimen confirmed the diagnosis of a cervical pregnancy (Fig. 30.2). At her six week follow-up visit she was completely recovered and without complication.

Cervical pregnancy

Ectopic pregnancies account for approximately 2% of all pregnancies. The fallopian tube is the location of the majority (93–98%) of ectopic pregnancies. The remainder of ectopic locations can be divided between the cervix, interstitium, ovary, Cesarean section scar, or the abdomen. Cervical pregnancies account for less than 1% of all ectopic pregnancies. The frequency has been reported from 1 in 10 000 to 1 in 50 000 pregnancies [1]. The rate, however, is higher in patients undergoing in-vitro fertilization, where it accounts for up to 3.5% of ectopic pregnancies.

Due to their extremely low incidence, risk factors for cervical pregnancies have been difficult to determine. Two series found 50–70% of patients with cervical pregnancies have had a previous curettage [1,2]. Another very small series showed that 75% of the patients have had a previous Cesarean delivery [3]. Additional possible risk factors include Asherman syndrome and diethylstilbestrol (DES) exposure.

Acute Care and Emergency Gynecology, ed. David Chelmow, Christine R. Isaacs and Ashley Carroll. Published by Cambridge University Press.
© Cambridge University Press 2015.

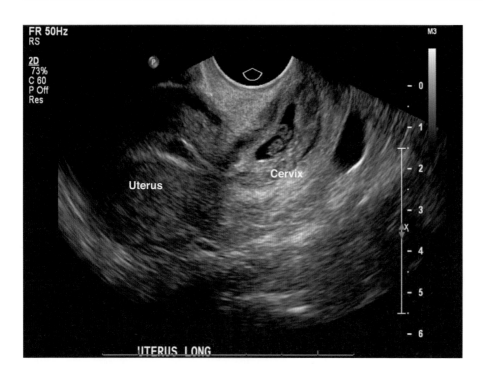

Fig. 30.1 Transvaginal ultrasound revealing a single gestational sac within the lower uterine segment with an hourglassing portion of the sac within the upper portion of the cervix.

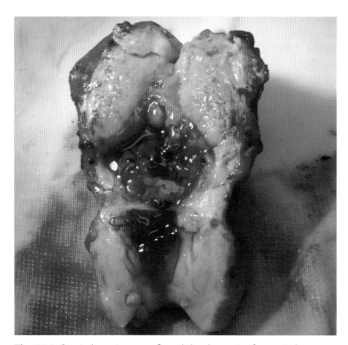

Fig. 30.2 Surgical specimen confirmed the diagnosis of a cervical pregnancy.

The presentation of a cervical pregnancy is fairly uniform, with 92% of patients presenting with vaginal bleeding, which is often painless. Thirty percent of women also experience abdominal cramping [1]. On speculum examination the cervical os is typically closed, but there may be dilation with products of conception visible. The differential diagnosis in this setting also includes a threatened, incomplete, or inevitable miscarriage. Any tissue in the cervix should not be

disturbed until an ultrasound evaluation of the cervix has been performed. Furthermore, products of conception in the lower uterine segment and cervix should not be disturbed in a setting that is not set up to handle significant acute hemorrhage. Patients should have emergent access to the operating room where aspiration and additional surgical measures can be performed if increased bleeding is encountered.

As in our patient, differentiating a cervical pregnancy from a threatened, incomplete, or inevitable abortion can be difficult. Ultrasound findings are the most important indicator of a cervical pregnancy. Ultrasound findings that are characteristic of a cervical ectopic pregnancy include:

1. A gestational sac or placenta in the cervix.
2. Doppler flow around the sac in the cervix.
3. An otherwise normal endometrial stripe.
4. An hourglass or figure of eight membranes, caused by ballooning of the cervix to accommodate the pregnancy.
5. A barrel-shaped cervix.

Any time there is fetal cardiac activity noted within the cervix, the diagnosis of a cervical pregnancy should be considered. Diagnosis by ultrasound is correct in nearly 90% of cases of cervical pregnancies. In cases where the diagnosis is unclear, further evaluation may be performed with MRI. In reviewing the ultrasound images of our patient, all of the above findings were present on her initial and follow-up ultrasounds.

Early correct diagnosis is extremely important. In an institutional review at McGill University, 12 cervical pregnancies were analysed [1]. Of the presenting patients, seven were initially misdiagnosed as threatened abortions, inevitable abortions, ruptured ovarian cysts, or an ectopic pregnancy. These misdiagnosed patients were treated primarily with curettage, laparotomy, or laparoscopy. All of the misdiagnosed patients encountered increased bleeding, resulting in four patients undergoing total abdominal hysterectomy and five patients receiving blood transfusions. Of the patients that were correctly diagnosed, none required a hysterectomy or a blood transfusion. These patients were successfully treated with methotrexate initially, followed by differing combinations of potassium chloride, uterine artery embolization, and curettage.

Treatment recommendations for cervical pregnancies are based upon case reports and small case series. The majority of the literature favors medical management for nonemergent cases of cervical pregnancies, particularly when the patient desires future fertility. Methotrexate is largely recommended, and when fetal cardiac activity is present concurrent feticide with intra-amniotic injection of potassium chloride (KCl) (1–5 mL of 20% solution) was found to greatly improve the efficacy of the methotrexate [3]. Transcervical injection of the KCl preparation, rather than injection through the cervical os, is recommended in order to decrease the risk of bleeding. Methotrexate has been administered intravenously, intramuscularly, and intramniotically. No clear difference in efficacy has been established between these treatment regimens, although no direct comparative date is available.

A review of available case reports of cervical pregnancies that were managed with various treatment regimens of methotrexate showed that the best candidates for medical management were those cervical pregnancies less than 9 weeks' gestation, with a beta-human chorionic gonadotropin (beta-hCG) level of less than 10 000 mIU/mL, and absent fetal cardiac activity [4]. After medical treatment, a decrease in the beta-hCG should be noticed on average within 14 days. Some authors use a cutoff of a 15% decrease, and if the cutoff is not met, a second dose of methotrexate may be given [3]. On average the beta-hCG values reached zero with a median of 68 days. The echogenic lesion in the cervical region will persist, and in a review it was noted to resolve with a median time of 86 days [4]. It is important to note that in the appropriately counseled patient who strongly desires a trial of medical management to avoid surgical intervention, the administration of methotrexate outside of these parameters is not unreasonable. These patients should understand that they are likely at a higher risk of failure for such medical management and may experience acute onset of heavy vaginal bleeding if the pregnancy tissue begins to abort vaginally.

For acutely hemorrhaging patients and those failing medical management, surgical intervention should be performed. Dilation and curettage has very limited success, with a high rate of hysterectomy (40–70%) as well as blood transfusion [1]. Recommendations vary and data is limited, but many authors recommend attempting to decrease blood flow to the uterus prior to attempting any form of instrumentation. Hemostatic options include uterine artery embolization, placement of a transvaginal cervical cerclage, or transvaginal ligation of the cervical branches of the uterine artery with suture [2,5,6]. Other suggestions are the placement of a Foley balloon or other hemostatic material within the cervix following curettage and the use of uterotonic or vasoconstricting agents.

Hysterectomy may be performed primarily or after failure of other treatments. Due to the increased vascular flow to the cervix, hysterectomy can also be complicated by significant bleeding. Hemostatic measures such as uterine artery embolization or hypogastric artery ligation have been used to limit the blood loss during hysterectomy for cervical pregnancies. Radical dissection of surrounding pelvic organs, such as the bladder and rectum, is occasionally required, and consideration should be given to preoperative consultation with pelvic surgical specialists. After being counseled about the option of medical management with methotrexate, our patient elected to undergo primary hysterectomy given her increased risks for failure (an elevated beta-hCG level and present fetal cardiac activity), as well as her desire to undergo sterilization.

In conclusion, cervical pregnancies are a rare manifestation of ectopic pregnancy. They are often misdiagnosed as spontaneous abortions or intrauterine pregnancies. In this setting, the risk of hysterectomy and transfusion is greatly increased when patients undergo dilation and curettage. Careful attention to specific ultrasound characteristics optimizes the proper early diagnosis of cervical pregnancies. Stable patients can be treated medically, with surgical management reserved for acutely hemorrhaging patients, those failing conservative management, and those who are poor candidates for medical management and not desiring future fertility.

Key teaching points

- Any pregnancy seen on ultrasound within the lower uterine segment should be viewed with suspicion for being a cervical pregnancy. Hourglass membranes and cardiac activity in the lower uterine segment should increase this suspicion.
- Misdiagnosis of a cervical pregnancy followed by dilation and curettage greatly increases the risk of emergency hysterectomy and the need for blood transfusion.
- In the stable patient with a cervical pregnancy, medical management should be the preferred course of treatment. Ideal candidates for medical management are those less than 9 weeks' gestation with a beta-human chorionic gonadotropin level below 10 000mIU/mL and absent fetal cardiac activity.
- Transcervical intra-amniotic injection of potassium chloride (KCl) can be performed in addition to methotrexate therapy when fetal cardiac activity is present.
- If surgical intervention is necessary there is a high risk of hemorrhage, and measures to prevent or manage such should be anticipated.

References

1. Vela G, Tulandi T. Cervical pregnancy: the importance of early diagnosis and treatment. *J Minim Invasive Gynecol* 2007;14(4):481–4.

2. Kim TJ, Seong SJ, Lee JH, et al. Clinical outcomes of patients treated for cervical pregnancy with or without methotrexate. *J Korean Med Sci* 2004; 19(6):848–52.

3. Hung TH, Shau WY, Hsieh TT, et al. Prognostic factors for an unsatisfactory primary methotrexate treatment of cervical pregnancy: a quantitative review. *Human Reprod* 1998;13(9):2636–42.

4. Song MJ, Moon MH, Kim JA, et al. Serial transvaginal sonographic findings of cervical ectopic pregnancy treated with high-dose methotrexate. *J Ultrasound Med* 2009;28(1): 55–61.

5. De La Vega GA, Avery C, Nemiroff R, et al. Treatment of early cervical pregnancy with cerclage, carboprost, curettage, and balloon tamponade. *Obstet Gynecol* 2007;109(2 Pt 2):505–7.

6. Nakao Y, Yokoyama M, Iwasaka T. Uterine artery embolization followed by dilation and curettage for cervical pregnancy. *Obstet Gynecol* 2008; 111(2 Pt2):505–7. DOI: 10.1097/01. AOG.0000286771.10377.4e.

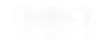

Early pregnancy spotting and an unusual ultrasound

Michelle Meglin

History of present illness

A 28-year-old gravida 3, para 1-0-1-1 woman presents to your clinic with a positive pregnancy test and vaginal spotting. Her gestational age is 10 weeks 2 days by sure last menstrual period. This is her first visit during this pregnancy. She reports intermittent vaginal spotting for the last two weeks but became alarmed today when it got heavier. She denies abdominal pain, nausea, vomiting, or urinary symptoms.

Her obstetrical history is significant for a term vaginal delivery and an early first-trimester spontaneous abortion. She has no medical or surgical history but reports an episode of pelvic inflammatory disease as a teenager. She smokes one pack of cigarettes daily. She lives two hours away from the hospital and does not have reliable transportation for clinic visits.

Physical exam

General appearance: Woman who is in no apparent distress
Vital signs:

Temperature: 37.0°C
Pulse: 85 beats/min
Blood pressure: 115/80 mmHg
Respiratory rate: 16 breaths/min
Oxygen saturation: 100% on room air
BMI: 27 kg/m^2

Chest: Clear to auscultation
Cardiovascular: Unremarkable
Abdomen: Soft, nontender, nondistended, no masses
External genitalia: Unremarkable
Vagina: One scopette of brownish blood, otherwise unremarkable
Cervix: External os closed, no active bleeding
Uterus: Anteverted, moderate tenderness to palpation, six to eight weeks' size, mobile
Adnexa: No masses, mild tenderness to palpation in the left adnexa, no tenderness on the right
Laboratory studies:

Beta-hCG: 18 000 mIU/mL
CBC: Normal
Liver function tests: Normal
Creatinine: Normal
Blood type: O positive

Imaging: Transvaginal ultrasound shows an empty uterine cavity with a large 4 cm gestational sac at the left cornua

surrounded by thin (<5 mm) myometrium, fetal cardiac motion noted. Normal appearing bilateral ovaries. No fluid in the posterior cul-de-sac (Fig. 31.1)

How would you manage this patient?

This patient has an interstitial ectopic pregnancy. Given her several relative contraindications to medical therapy including a gestational sac greater than 3.5 cm, cardiac motion, and concerns regarding compliance with follow-up due to her travel distance and lack of transportation, surgical management is most appropriate. She underwent a laparoscopic cornuostomy after injection of vasopressin (into the myometrium surrounding the pregnancy) without complication. She had an uneventful postoperative course and was discharged on postoperative day 1. Pathology confirmed products of conception. Beta-human chorionic gonadotropin (beta-hCG) levels were followed to zero.

Interstitial pregnancy

Interstitial pregnancy is a type of ectopic pregnancy in which implantation occurs in the interstitial portion of the fallopian tube, defined as the proximal portion of tube contained within the myometrium. This proximal portion of the fallopian tube lies within the muscular uterine wall and has greater distensibility compared to distal portions of the tube. Interstitial pregnancy is often confused with cornual pregnancy, which refers to a pregnancy within a uterine horn in a patient with a Mullerian anomaly [1]. Interstitial pregnancies account for approximately 2.5% of ectopic pregnancies [1].

Risk factors for interstitial pregnancy are similar to those for distal tubal pregnancies and include a history of prior ectopic pregnancy, sexually transmitted disease/pelvic inflammatory disease, tubal surgery, failed sterilization, use of assisted reproductive therapy (particularly in-vitro fertilization), and smoking [2]. Patients with an interstitial pregnancy typically present with abdominal pain and vaginal bleeding in the first trimester; however, the incidence of vaginal bleeding is less common than that with a distal tubal ectopic pregnancy [3]. While it was once thought that interstitial pregnancies presented and ruptured at later gestational ages due to the greater distensibility of the myometrium covering the interstitial segment of the fallopian tube, recent evidence suggests the average gestational age at diagnosis and rupture is 6.9–8.0 weeks, similar to distal tubal ectopic pregnancies [3]. Rupture of an interstitial pregnancy is associated with risk of severe

Acute Care and Emergency Gynecology, ed. David Chelmow, Christine R. Isaacs and Ashley Carroll. Published by Cambridge University Press. © Cambridge University Press 2015.

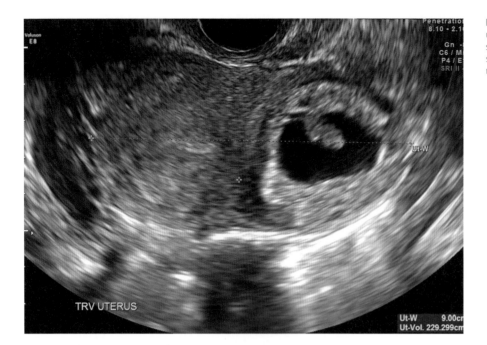

Fig. 31.1 Transvaginal ultrasound showing the uterine fundus in a transverse plan. The gestational sac is eccentric, separate from the endometrial stripe and surrounded by a thin layer of myometrium.

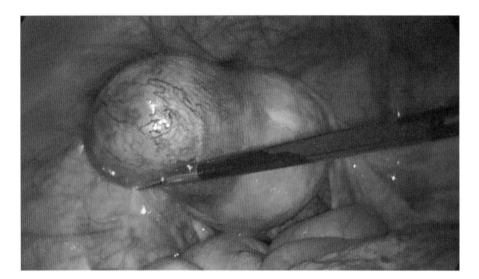

Fig. 31.2 Left-sided interstitial pregnancy on laparoscopy.

hemorrhage due to the potential larger size of the pregnancy and proximity to the uterine and ovarian arteries. In cases of severe hemorrhage, the mortality rate is as high as 2.5% making early diagnosis and management critical [3].

Early diagnosis of interstitial pregnancy has improved with the advent of high resolution transvaginal ultrasound and sensitive quantitative beta-hCG assays. Several ultrasonographic characteristics have been identified that help in diagnosing an interstitial pregnancy: an empty uterine cavity, an eccentric gestational sac, a chorionic sac at least 1 cm from the lateral edge of the uterine cavity, a thin (<5 mm) myometrial layer surrounding the gestational sac, and the "interstitial line" sign. The interstitial line sign describes an echogenic line extending from the lateral aspect of endometrial cavity that abuts the gestational sac. Occasionally, the diagnosis remains unclear by transvaginal ultrasound and is rather made intraoperatively with findings of a bulging pregnancy in the cornua, lateral to the fundus and round ligament (Fig. 31.2) [3].

Earlier diagnosis of interstitial pregnancy has led to alternatives to traditional management, which typically involved hysterectomy or cornual wedge resection via laparotomy. Nonsurgical treatment options include systemic methotrexate, local injection of cytotoxic agents, and, rarely, expectant management. Systemic methotrexate should be administered using one of the three treatment protocols used for distal tubal ectopic pregnancies: single-dose regimen, two-dose regimen, or a fixed multidose regimen [2]. To consider methotrexate management, patients must be hemodynamically stable without suspicion for a ruptured ectopic pregnancy, able to comply with follow-up surveillance, and without medical contraindications to consider methotrexate. Absolute contraindications to methotrexate therapy are breast-feeding, immunodeficiency, liver disease, blood dyscrasias, active pulmonary disease, peptic ulcer disease, known sensitivity to methotrexate, or other evidence of hepatic, renal or hematologic dysfunction. To evaluate for possible contraindications a complete blood count, creatinine and liver transaminases should be obtained. Relative contraindications where one should consider surgical management over methotrexate therapy are a gestation sac greater than 3.5 cm and fetal cardiac motion [2]. Case series have reported up to 80–94% success rates for treatment of interstitial pregnancy when using systemic methotrexate [3]. Low initial beta-hCG levels (<5000–9000 mIU/mL) is the strongest predictor of successful methotrexate management [1]. In the appropriately selected patient, systemic methotrexate is an appropriate first-line therapy [3].

Local injection of cytotoxic agents (most commonly methotrexate) under laparoscopic, ultrasound, or hysteroscopic guidance has been reported as an alternative treatment. From the limited data, local injection appears safe and effective compared with systemic methotrexate, but it is unclear if this method provides significant additional benefit to justify the procedure and cost. Expectant management of interstitial pregnancy should be reserved for the stable patient with spontaneously declining beta-hCG levels. These patients must be monitored closely for signs of rupture, and often requiring inpatient hospital monitoring [3].

Traditionally, surgical treatment of interstitial pregnancy involved a laparotomy to perform a cornual wedge resection, or hysterectomy since cases were often diagnosed after uterine rupture which lead to hemorrhage and significant uterine trauma. Surgical treatment remains the recommended therapy in cases of ruptured interstitial pregnancy and is also appropriate if there are contradictions to medical therapy (as in the case of our patient) including if patients are not agreeable to medical management or unable to comply with follow-up, if medical management fails (as evident by rising beta-HCG levels), or in patients who would not accept life-saving blood products (should subsequent rupture result in severe hemorrhage). Surgical excision can be performed via laparotomy or laparoscopy using one of several techniques such as cornuostomy, salpingostomy, and cornual resection. Cornuostomy involves removal of the pregnancy without removal of the surrounding myometrium via a linear incision in the myometrium overlying the pregnancy and extraction of the gestational tissue. Salpingostomy may similarly be performed at the site where the tube enters the fundus. Cornuostomy and salpingostomy are more suitable in cases of early, small (<4 cm) interstitial pregnancies. Cornual resection involves removes the interstitial pregnancy and surrounding myometrium and can be performed via laparoscopy in settings with appropriate resources and surgeon experience. Several methods to minimize blood loss have been described, the most common of which is injection of vasopressin into the myometrium surrounding the pregnancy. Transcervical evacuation of the pregnancy using a suction curettage under laparoscopic and ultrasound guidance has also been described in case series as an alternative surgical therapy [3].

Surveillance after medical treatment of interstitial pregnancy involves outpatient monitoring for signs/symptoms of rupture and observing beta-hCG levels to resolution as per methotrexate protocol guidelines [2]. Patients treated surgically with cornuostomy or salpingostomy remain at risk for persistent interstitial pregnancy due to suboptimal removal of all pregnancy tissue and should also have beta-hCG surveillance. In subsequent pregnancies patients with a prior interstitial pregnancy are at risk for recurrence and an early first-trimester ultrasound should be performed to identify pregnancy location. Additionally, it is recommended that patients with prior surgical management of interstitial pregnancy be delivered by Cesarean section at term due to reports of uterine rupture at the site of prior cornual excision [3].

Key teaching points

- Interstitial pregnancy is an uncommon type of ectopic pregnancy, but needs to be recognized early due the increased risk of severe hemorrhage and death.
- Diagnosis involves ultrasound findings of an empty uterine cavity, an eccentric gestational sac, a chorionic sac at least 1 cm from the lateral edge of the uterine cavity, a thin (<5 mm) myometrial layer surrounding the gestational sac, and the "interstitial line" sign.
- In asymptomatic, hemodynamically stable patients without contraindications, systemic methotrexate is an appropriate first-line therapy for treatment of interstitial pregnancy.
- Surgical management may be accomplished via laparoscopy or laparotomy with cornuostomy, salpingostomy, or cornual resection.
- Patients who have undergone medical or conservative surgical treatment should be followed until beta-hCG is undetectable due to the risks of interstitial rupture and/or persistent interstitial pregnancy tissue.

References

1. Chetty M, Elson J. Treating non-tubal ectopic pregnancy. *Best Prac Res Clin Obstet Gynaecol* 2009;23(4):529–38.

2. American College of Obstetricians and Gynecologists. Medical Management of Ectopic Pregnancy. Practice Bulletin No. 94. *Obstet Gynecol* 2008;111(6): 1479–85.

3. Moawad NS, Mahajan ST, Moniz MH, Taylor SE, Hurd MW. Current diagnosis and treatment of interstitial pregnancy. *Am J Obstet Gynecol* 2010;202(1):15–29.

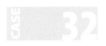

Undesired pregnancy in a 19-year-old woman

Megan L. Evans and Danielle Roncari

History of present illness

A 19-year-old woman presents after a home pregnancy test returned positive. The patient has been using condoms with her boyfriend for birth control but admits to inconsistent use. She does not remember when her last menstrual period was and reports her menses are usually irregular. She has occasional nausea, but overall feels well. The patient discloses that she is unsure she wants to continue the pregnancy and is interested in hearing her options for an abortion.

Physical exam

General appearance: Well-nourished woman who is nervous

Vital signs:

Temperature: 37.0°C
Pulse: 85 beats/min
Blood pressure: 110/76 mmHg

Cardiovascular: Regular, rate, and rhythm

Pulmonary: Clear to auscultation bilaterally

Abdomen: Soft, nontender, nondistended

Pelvic:

Cervix is normal appearing, no discharge or abnormal lesions visualized

Bimanual examination: Shows eight-week size anteverted uterus, no cervical motion tenderness, no adnexal tenderness

Laboratory studies:

Urine hCG: positive
Ht: 36.3%
Blood type: A positive

Imaging: Transvaginal ultrasound shows single intrauterine pregnancy with a fetal heart rate in the 150s. The crown–rump length correlates with a gestational age of eight weeks and three days

How would you counsel this patient?

You inform the patient that she is about eight weeks' pregnant. You then discuss all of her options for this pregnancy – continuing the pregnancy, adoption, and abortion. She informs you that she is firm in her decision to proceed with an abortion. You confirm that this is her decision and that she is not being coerced into making this decision.

At eight weeks' gestation, both the medication abortion and surgical abortion options are available to this patient. You review both procedures and their risks and benefits. After hearing all of her options, your patient elects to have an in-office vacuum aspiration. She likes the privacy and immediacy of this option as she is living with roommates and has school finals the following week. Her procedure was uncomplicated. In discussing contraception, she discloses that she does not desire pregnancy for at least two years and has trouble remembering to take contraceptive pills. She chooses a levonorgestrel intrauterine device (IUD). You are able to insert an IUD immediately after her procedure.

Epidemiology

Abortion is a common procedure in the United States. Each year, roughly half of all pregnancies in the United States are unintended, and 4 out of 10 of those pregnancies end by abortion [1]. By the time US women reach the age of 45, half have had an unintended pregnancy and one-third have had an abortion [2]. Over 60% of abortions occur before 9 weeks of gestational age, and 88% before 12 weeks of gestational age. Although late-term abortions are often the focus of restrictive legislation, only 1.5% of abortions occur at 21 weeks' gestational age or later [1].

More than half of all women who get an abortion are in their twenties, while 18% are teenagers. However, the rate of abortion is highest for women over age 40 (17.5/1000 women). Thirty-six percent of women who obtain an abortion identify themselves as non-Hispanic white, while 30% and 25% of women identify themselves as non-Hispanic black and Hispanic respectively. One-quarter of women have incomes between 100 and 199% of the federal poverty line while 42% have an income below the poverty line [2].

Like with our patient, the majority of women who have an abortion were using some form of contraception when they became pregnant, most often the oral contraceptive pill or male condoms. Seventy-six percent of pill users and forty-nine percent of condom users reported inconsistent use of these methods at the time of their unplanned pregnancy. Forty-six percent of women reported not using a contraceptive method when they became pregnant. This group of women perceived themselves at low risk for getting pregnant, had unexpected intercourse, or had concerns about using birth control [3].

Acute Care and Emergency Gynecology, ed. David Chelmow, Christine R. Isaacs and Ashley Carroll. Published by Cambridge University Press. © Cambridge University Press 2015.

Counseling

Patients who find themselves with an undesired or unplanned pregnancy often present to their primary care provider or obstetrician/gynecologist for counseling. Patients may be unsure of their options and are looking for guidance and information from their provider. If the provider has a moral objection to abortion or feels unable to provide accurate counseling, they should promptly refer the patient to a professional who is capable of counseling on all options.

Additionally, it is important that you, as her provider, and your clinical staff are familiar with your state's laws on abortion. For example, some states have parental consent laws, gestational age limits, or waiting periods where women must receive mandatory counseling at least 24 hours prior to obtaining an abortion.

There are many misconceptions about abortion. As part of the counseling, the provider should make it clear that abortion has not been shown to increase mental health problems, breast cancer, or infertility [4]. The patient should also be reassured about safety of the procedure. Less than 1% of all US patients have a major complication during their abortion. The earlier in the pregnancy that the procedure is performed, the lower the complication risk. Maternal mortality related to abortion is significantly lower than that associated with birth until approximately 20 weeks' gestation. Overall mortality is 0.567 per 100 000 abortions. This is in contrast to a live birth, which has a maternal mortality rate of 7.06 per 100 000 [5].

Discussion of contraception should also be incorporated into your abortion counseling. Patients should be offered all available methods of contraception for which they are eligible. Side effects, risks, benefits, and effectiveness of each method should be incorporated into this discussion. Long-acting reversible contraception (LARC), including IUDs and implants, has been shown to significantly reduce the risk of unintended pregnancy. LARC is safe, effective, and leads to higher contraceptive continuation than other methods. They can be inserted immediately after termination procedures, as done in this patient [6].

Abortion options

Accurate diagnosis of gestational age is necessary to perform either a medication abortion or a surgical abortion. This patient's gestational age was confirmed by ultrasound. The gestational age of the patient allows her to select either a medication abortion or surgical abortion.

Medication abortion

In the United States, medication abortion is typically offered up to 63 days of gestation with an effectiveness rate of 95–99%; it is slightly more effective at earlier gestational ages. Some centers have also begun offering medication abortion to 70 days' gestation [7,8].

The most common medication regimen in the United States involves two different medications. Typically, a patient will be given mifepristone, also known as RU-486, followed 24 to 48 hours later by misoprostol to complete the abortion [7]. The most commonly used dose of misoprostol is 800 μg. Misoprostol may cause strong uterine contractions, nausea, vomiting, diarrhea, and a low grade fever. If the regimen is successful, the vast majority of patients will pass the tissue within 24 hours. Alternatively, in settings where mifepristone is not available, patients can take up to 800 μg of misoprostol 24 hours apart to help expel the products of conception. Efficacy for this regimen ranges from 85 to 95% [7]. Risks of medication abortion are rare, but patients should be counseled on the risk of infection, heavy vaginal bleeding, and failure of the regimen or incomplete expulsion of products with the need for surgical aspiration.

Patients must have a follow-up visit to confirm completion of the abortion. Typical follow-up protocols involve a drop in beta-human chorionic gonadotropin (beta-hCG) levels of greater than 80% from the start of the procedure or an ultrasound [9]. Ongoing research is being done looking at alternative methods of follow-up. For patients with an ongoing pregnancy or retained pregnancy tissue, additional medication or instrumentation is typically offered.

Surgical abortion

The patient may also elect to have a surgical abortion. This procedure can be done in a clinic setting or in the operating room and is 98–99% effective in removing all products of conception. In the first trimester, the procedure can be done using either a handheld manual vacuum aspirator or electric suction. Some clinical settings may provide moderate sedation or general anesthesia; however, this procedure can be done safely and comfortably under local anesthesia with a paracervical block. Risks of the procedure are rare but include bleeding, infection, uterine perforation, retained products of conception, ongoing pregnancy, and cervical injury.

Prior to the procedure, it is important to confirm gestational age. If there is any uncertainty, the patient should have an ultrasound. A bimanual examination to confirm the uterine size and position should be performed. Accurate assessment of uterine size and position is essential in choosing the appropriate instruments and guiding the direction of instruments into the uterine canal. This assessment also helps to decrease complications during the procedure.

Either the manual vacuum aspirator or electric suction can be used to complete the procedure and usually requires only two or three passes into the uterine cavity to completely empty the uterus of all products. Rarely is a sharp curette needed to confirm all products of conception have been removed from the uterine cavity.

This manual vacuum aspirator or electric suction can also be used for missed or incomplete abortions, treatment of hematometra, endometrial sampling, and failed medication abortion.

Abortion providers

Although abortion is a legal procedure, the number of abortion providers has decreased in the United States. Between

1982 and 2005, the number of providers decreased by 38% and has recently reached a plateau. Unfortunately, 87% of US counties do not have an abortion provider and 35% of women between the ages of 15 and 44 live in those counties [10]. Sixteen percent of women have to travel between 50 and 100 miles to obtain abortion services, and an additional 8% of women have to travel greater than 100 miles [11]. Additionally, 80% of abortion clinics have reported at least one form of harassment, picketing being the most common [11].

Key teaching points

- Half of all pregnancies in the United States are unintended and 40% of those pregnancies will end by abortion. Of the women who reach the age of 45, one-third will have had an abortion.
- Most patients who seek abortions are between the ages of 21 and 24, are using contraception at the time of pregnancy, are already mothers, are living in poverty, and have a religious affiliation.
- Abortion is a safe and legal procedure; however, it is safer with earlier gestational ages.
- Patients below nine weeks' gestational age have the option for either a medication abortion or a surgical abortion.
- Abortion has not been linked to breast cancer, infertility, or mental health problems.

References

1. Finer LB, Zolna MR. Unintended pregnancy in the United States: incidence and disparities. *Contraception* 2011;84:478–85.

2. Jones RK, Kavanaugh ML. Changes in abortion rates between 2000 and 2008 and lifetime incidence of abortion. *Obstet Gynecol* 2011;117:1358–66.

3. Jones RK, Darroch JE, Henshaw SK. Contraceptive use among US women having abortions in 2000–2001. *Perspect Sex Reprod Health* 2002;34:294–303.

4. American College of Obstetricians and Gynecologists.Induced abortion and breast cancer risk. Committee Opinion No. 434. *Obstet Gynecol* 2009;113: 1417–18.

5. Grimes DA. Estimation of pregnancy-related mortality risk by pregnancy outcome, United States, 1991 to 1999. *Am J Obstet Gynecol* 2006;194:92–4.

6. American College of Obstetricians and Gynecologists. Long-acting reversible contraception: implants and intrauterine devices. Practice Bulletin No. 121. *Obstet Gynecol* 2011;118: 184–96.

7. American College of Obstetricians and Gynecologists. Medical management of abortion. ACOG Practice Bulletin No. 67. *Obstet Gynecol* 2005;106: 871–82.

8. Winikoff B, Dzuba IG, Chong E, et al. Extending outpatient medical abortion services through 70 days of gestational age. *Obstet Gynecol* 2012;120:1070–6.

9. Grossman D, Grindlay K. Alternatives to ultrasound for follow-up after medication abortion: a systematic review. *Contraception* 2011;83: 504–10.

10. Jones RK, Kooistra K. Abortion incidence and access to services in the United States, 2008. *Perspect Sex Reprod Health* 2011;43:41–50.

11. Henshaw SK, Finer LB. The accessibility of abortion services in the United States, 2001. *Perspect Sex Reprod Health* 2003;35:16–24.

A pregnant 37-year-old woman with lower left quadrant pain

Rajiv B. Gala

History of present illness

A 37-year-old female, gravida 2, para 1, presents to the emergency department with mild, left lower quadrant pain and vaginal spotting that started 2 hours prior to admission. Her last menstrual period was six weeks prior to presentation. A home pregnancy test was positive one week ago. The patient denies any fevers, chills, shortness of breath, or dizziness while walking. Her appetite has been normal and her last bowel movement was one day ago. She describes the pain as dull, colicky, and rated it at 3 out of 10 on the pain scale.

Her past medical history is significant for a tubo-ovarian abscess treated four months ago. Her past surgical history is negative. She has been married for four years and uses no contraception. She has no known drug allergies. Her only medication is a daily prenatal vitamin.

Physical examination

General appearance: Well-developed, well-nourished woman who is in mild discomfort but alert and oriented

Vital signs:

Temperature: 37.0°C
Pulse: 92 beats/min
Blood pressure: 110/72 mmHg
Respiratory rate: 16 beats/min
Oxygen saturation: 100% on room air
Height: 65 inches
Weight: 130 lb
BMI: 21.6 kg/m^2

Abdomen: Thin, soft, nontender, nondistended, no guarding, no rebound

External genitalia: Unremarkable

Vagina: Scant dark blood in posterior fornix

Cervix: Parous, closed, no active bleeding or passage of tissue

Uterus: Anteverted, mobile, normal size, mild tenderness on bimanual examination

Adnexa: Fullness in LLQ, mild discomfort with palpation

Laboratory studies:

Urine pregnancy test: Positive
Beta-hCG: 3241 mIU/mL
Blood group and Rh: B positive
Indirect Coombs: Negative
WBCs: 12 800/μL
Hb: 11.9 g/dL
Ht: 36.2%

Imaging: Transvaginal ultrasound shows uterus normal with endometrial thickness 6 mm, 3.4 cm left corpus luteum cyst with another mass adjacent to the ovary, no free fluid (Fig. 33.1)

How would you manage this patient?

The patient has a small unruptured ectopic pregnancy. The combination of beta-human chorionic gonadotropin (beta-hCG) above the discriminatory zone, absence of a visible intrauterine pregnancy, and presence of a suspicious adnexal mass makes ectopic pregnancy highly likely. Since the patient is hemodynamically stable, it is unlikely that the ectopic has ruptured and she is a candidate for either medical or surgical management.

The patient was thoroughly counseled on the risks and benefits of the different treatment options. Preservation of future fertility was a major priority for her and she decided to proceed with medical management using methotrexate. She received a single dose of 50 mg/m^2. The patient's serum beta-hCG levels dropped appropriately and became undetectable four weeks after her dose and she did not require any further treatment.

Small unruptured ectopic pregnancy

A pregnancy is ectopic when it implants anywhere other than the endometrial lining of the uterine cavity. While ectopic pregnancies most commonly occur in the ampullary portion of the fallopian tube, other less common sites of implantation include the ovary, cervix, interstitial portion of the fallopian tube, or the abdomen. Ectopic pregnancies are the leading cause of maternal death in the first trimester, primarily from severe hemorrhage after tubal rupture. Despite the fivefold increase in ectopic pregnancy rates from 1970 to 1992 [1], improved diagnosis and treatment has resulted in a 10-fold decline in the case fatality rate.

The classic triad of ectopic pregnancy symptoms is irregular vaginal bleeding, abdominal pain, and amenorrhea. Prior to rupture, the pain may be described as colicky, diffuse, or localized. Once the ectopic pregnancy ruptures, patients typically report sharp, diffuse pain likely from peritoneal irritation caused by the bleeding. Unfortunately, the classic symptoms are nonspecific and can be found with other disease processes in the differential diagnosis: ovarian torsion, hemorrhagic

Acute Care and Emergency Gynecology, ed. David Chelmow, Christine R. Isaacs and Ashley Carroll. Published by Cambridge University Press. © Cambridge University Press 2015.

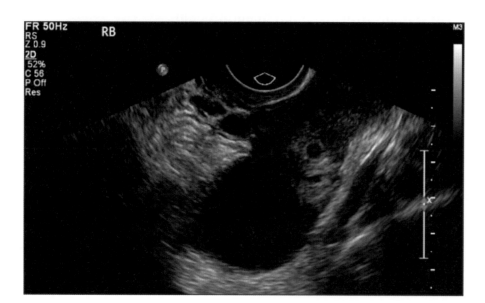

Fig. 33.1 Ultrasound image of left adnexa. 3.4 cm left corpus luteum cyst with another mass adjacent to the ovary.

corpus luteum cyst, salpingitis, or a threatened or spontaneous abortion. Consideration of ectopic pregnancy risk factors is important for a more timely and accurate diagnosis. The most common risk factors for ectopic pregnancy are a prior ectopic pregnancy, tubal surgery, prior pelvic inflammatory disease, smoking, and the use of assisted reproductive technology. It is not unusual for ectopic pregnancy to occur in patients without known risk factors. This patient's recent episode of pelvic inflammatory disease with tubo-ovarian abscess puts her at high risk.

Once an ectopic pregnancy is suspected and the patient is confirmed to be hemodynamically stable, a systematic approach using high resolution ultrasonography and serial serum beta-hCG measurements can be used to confirm the diagnosis. In normal pregnancies, the serum beta-hCG rises in a log-linear fashion until around 70 days after the last menstrual period. A normal intrauterine pregnancy should demonstrate a 53–66% increase in serum beta-hCG levels every 48 hours [2]. An inadequately rising serum beta-hCG only indicates an abnormal pregnancy, not its specific location. Pregnancies with inappropriately rising levels can be abnormal intrauterine pregnancies and are not necessarily ectopic gestations. Serum progesterone levels have been studied to aid in the diagnosis of ectopic pregnancies when the serum beta-hCG was inconclusive. The primary utility of serum progesterone levels is to help differentiate normal from abnormal pregnancies. A progesterone level of less than 5 ng/mL is consistent with an abnormal pregnancy and a value of greater than 20 ng/mL has a 95% sensitivity to identify a normal pregnancy. Serum progesterone levels have the same limitations as serial beta-hCG assays for determining location.

Transvaginal ultrasonography is highly effective at identifying intrauterine pregnancies. In normal intrauterine pregnancies, a gestational sac is usually visible by five weeks after the last menstrual period, a yolk sac appears between five and six weeks, and a fetal pole with cardiac activity is first detected around six weeks. When the date of the last menstrual period is uncertain, the serum beta-hCG levels can help define expected sonographic findings. The beta-hCG levels at which these landmarks typically occur can vary from institution to institution because of differences in ultrasound equipment and beta-hCG assays, and discriminatory levels should be determined for each institution. For most institutions, the serum beta-hCG discriminatory value is between 1500 and 2500 mIU/mL. The serum beta-hCG discriminatory value is higher when performing transabdominal ultrasonography. Inability to visualize a gestational sac above these values makes the likelihood of normal intrauterine pregnancy exceedingly small and should increase the suspicion for an ectopic pregnancy. Other ultrasound findings that can be seen with ectopic pregnancies include:

- Pseudogestational sac – one layer collection of sloughing decidua in the midline of the uterine cavity.
- Halo sign – thin hypoechoic area caused by subserosal edema in the fallopian tubes (Fig. 33.2).
- Ring of fire – placental blood flow within the periphery of a complex adnexal mass.

While the diagnosis of ectopic pregnancy was straightforward in this case, there are many times when the combination of beta-hCG level and ultrasound findings is not definitive. If the patient is hemodynamically stable and the pregnancy is desired, it is reasonable to repeat the serum beta-hCG and ultrasound in 48 hours to monitor for change, as there are scenarios such as multiple gestations where the ultrasound findings can lag behind the beta-hCG level. If the pregnancy was not desired or there is thought to be a very high likelihood of an ectopic pregnancy, uterine curettage can be performed. If trophoblastic tissue is obtained, an ectopic pregnancy has been effectively ruled out. If no trophoblastic tissue is obtained, ectopic pregnancy is extremely likely, and further treatment is indicated. Obtaining a

Table 33.1 Methotrexate treatment protocol for ectopic pregnancy*

	Single-dose protocol	Multidose protocol
Medication doses:		
Methotrexate	50 mg/m² BSA	1.0 mg/kg
Leucovorin		0.1 mg/kg
Serum beta-hCG collections	Days 1 (baseline), 4, 7	Days 0 (baseline), 1, 3, 5, 7
Need for repeat medication	• If serum beta-hCG does not fall by 15% from day 4 to 7 • If serum beta-hCG does not fall by 15% in 1 week	• If serum beta-hCG does not fall by 15% between days 0 and 1 • If serum beta-hCG does not fall by 15% between days 1 and 3 (after repeat doses)

Adapted from American College of Obstetricians and Gynecologists [6].
beta-hCG, beta-human chorionic gonadotropin; BSA, body surface area.

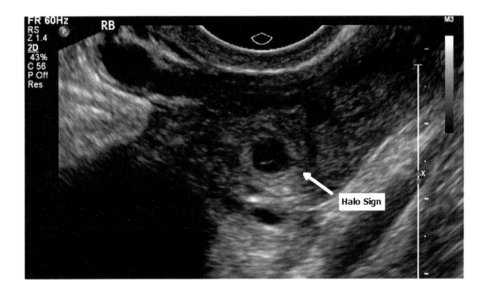

Fig. 33.2 Left corpus luteum cyst with adjacent ectopic pregnancy displaying halo sign.

definitive diagnosis can avert the use of methotrexate in nearly 40% of cases [3].

When patients are hemodynamically stable, a small unruptured ectopic pregnancy can be managed either medically or surgically. Expectant management with spontaneous resorption of an ectopic pregnancy should only be considered when the serum beta-hCG is less than 200 mIU/mL. Most patients prefer medical therapy using methotrexate. With methotrexate, rates of overall tubal preservation, tubal patency, repeat ectopic pregnancies, and future pregnancies are equivalent to surgical management [4]. Methotrexate works by inhibiting the binding of dihydrofolic acid to the enzyme dihydrofolate reductase, thereby arresting DNA, RNA, and protein synthesis. Since methotrexate targets rapidly dividing cells, side effects are mostly related to the gastrointestinal tract and bone marrow (ulcerative stomatitis, severe diarrhea, thrombocytopenia, and severe anemia). There are two intramuscular methotrexate protocols that have been well studied with similar success rates of between 67 and 93% (Table 33.1) [5]. The single-dose methotrexate protocol is the most widely used, in part due to patient convenience. Prior to

administration of methotrexate, a serum beta-hCG level, complete blood count, complete metabolic panel, blood type and Rh status, and liver function tests should be obtained. The patient is then administered 50 mg/m² body surface area of intramuscular methotrexate. Beta-hCG levels will usually continue to rise until day 4 after administration. A serum beta-hCG level should be obtained for comparison on days 4 and 7 following methotrexate administration. A decline by 15% or more between days 4 and 7 indicates an appropriate initial response, and patients should then have weekly serum beta-hCG levels drawn until they are undetectable. If there is less than a 15% decline between any weekly measurements, the patient is failing treatment and should receive an additional dose of methotrexate following the original protocol. An alternative multidose methotrexate protocol involves 1 mg/kg of methotrexate followed by a dose of leucovorin 24 hours later. If there is not a 15% drop in serial serum beta-hCG concentrations from days 0–1 or days 1–3, an additional methotrexate/leucovorin combination is given up to a maximum of four doses (Table 33.1 [6]). Proponents of the multidose protocol justify the more intense post-therapy monitoring because series suggest a better cure rate. Unfortunately, there has not been an adequately powered randomized trial comparing single and multidose therapy to confirm this difference.

Surgical treatment options include both laparoscopy and laparotomy, although laparoscopic treatment is preferred since there are shorter hospital stays, reduced blood loss, and shorter operating times. The two options for ectopic removal are salpingectomy (removal of the fallopian tube) or salpingostomy (preserving the fallopian tube). In the face of a normal contralateral fallopian tube, both techniques have similar subsequent intrauterine pregnancy rates. Salpingectomy would be preferred over salpingostomy if future fertility is not desired or there was complete tubal rupture. Compliance with serial serum beta-hCG after salpingostomy is important to monitor for incomplete eradication of trophoblastic tissue, as seen in 3–20% cases.

In this case, both treatment options were reviewed with the patient, as she was an appropriate candidate for either. She was a good candidate for medical therapy because she was asymptomatic and motivated enough to remain compliant with post-therapy surveillance. In addition, her chance of success was equivalent between medical and surgical options because the tubal diameter was less than 3.5 cm, no extrauterine fetal cardiac activity was present, and the serum beta-hCG was less than 5000 mIU/mL. Absolute contraindications to medical therapy include breast-feeding, alcoholism or liver disease, active pulmonary disease, peptic ulcer disease, and hepatic,

renal, or hematologic dysfunction [6]. All patients receiving medical therapy need to be counseled on the high likelihood of increased abdominal pain during the first few days after treatment. This pain is thought to be due to tubal distension caused by tubal abortion or hematoma formation. Typically acetaminophen is adequate for pain relief. An oral narcotic can be given if necessary, but, if substantial pain relief is needed, the patient should be evaluated for possible tubal rupture. The patient should be advised not to use folic acid supplements, nonsteroidal anti-inflammatory drugs, or alcohol while being treated with methotrexate. She should also avoid sunlight exposure, vigorous physical activity, and sexual activity.

Key teaching points

- The classic triad of symptoms for a patient with an ectopic pregnancy is irregular vaginal bleeding, abdominal pain, and amenorrhea.
- A uterine curettage in the face of a presumed ectopic pregnancy can confirm an abnormal uterine pregnancy in nearly 40% of cases.
- Hemodynamically stable patients with a small unruptured ectopic pregnancy can be managed medically with methotrexate or surgically via laparoscopy or laparotomy.
- Failure of medical therapy is defined as tubal rupture with massive intra-abdominal hemorrhage or lack of resolution after four doses of methotrexate.

References

1. Centers for Disease Control and Prevention. Ectopic pregnancy – United States, 1990–1992. *MMWR* 1995;44: 46–8.

2. Barnhart KT, Sammel MD, Rinaudo PF, et al. Symptomatic patients with an early viable intrauterine pregnancy: hCG curves redefined. *Obstet Gynecol* 2004;104:50–5.

3. Shaunik A, Kulp J, Appleby DH, Sammel MD, Barnhart KT. Utility of dilation and curettage in the diagnosis of pregnancy of unknown location. *Am J Obstet Gynecol* 2011;204(2):130.e1–6.

4. Hajenius PJ, Mol F, Mol BWJ, et al. Interventions for tubal ectopic pregnancy. *Cochrane Database Syst Rev* 2007, Issue 1. Art. No.: CD000324. DOI: 10.1002/14651858. CD000324.pub2.

5. Lipscomb GH, Givens VM, Meyer NL, et al. Comparison of multidose and single-dose methotrexate protocols for the treatment of ectopic pregnancy. *Am J Obstet Gynecol* 2005;192:1844–7; discussion 187–8.

6. American College of Obstetricians and Gynecologists. Medical management of ectopic pregnancy. Practice Bulletin No. 94. *Obstet Gynecol* 2008;111:1479–85.

Unruptured advanced ectopic pregnancy

Ellen L. Brock

History of present illness

A 32-year-old gravida 4, para 3 woman presented with right lower quadrant pain. Her last menstrual period was six weeks, five days ago, and she had a positive home pregnancy test six days ago. She describes the pain as cramping, with intermittent episodes of sharper pain of moderate severity. She reports nausea but no vomiting, and has a decreased appetite. She denies fever. She has no pain with urination or defecation, and bowel function has been normal.

Her only surgery was a Cesarean delivery for active phase arrest. She has no medical problems. She is a Jehovah's Witness. Her only medication is a prenatal vitamin.

Physical examination

General appearance: Woman is alert and oriented, appears uncomfortable but is in no acute distress

Vital signs:

Temperature: 36.8°C

Pulse: 72 beats/min

Blood pressure: 100/60 mmHg

Respiratory rate: 18 breaths/min

Abdomen: Soft, tenderness to palpation in right lower quadrant without rebound

Vulva: Normal

Vagina: Normal, no blood in vault

Cervix: Normal appearing, closed

Uterus: Upper normal size, slightly tender, more on the right side than left

Ovaries: Without palpable masses, right exquisitely tender to palpation

Laboratory studies:

Beta-hCG: 5622 mIU/L

WBCs: 10 200/µL

Hb: 12.6 g/dL

Imaging: An ultrasound image taken from the right cornual area is displayed in Fig. 34.1. The uterus measured normal size with a 15 mm endometrial stripe. There was a 1.2 × 1.5 × 1.0 cm pocket of cul-de-sac fluid. The left adnexa imaged normally

How would you manage this patient?

The patient has an advanced apparently unruptured ectopic pregnancy. The findings are concerning for a cornual pregnancy, but tubal or ovarian pregnancy are also possibilities. This patient has a high human chorionic gonadotropin (hCG) level, fetal cardiac motion, and a refusal to accept blood transfusions. Medical management is not appropriate for this patient. Our patient underwent laparoscopic salpingectomy and cornual resection. Findings at laparoscopy (Fig. 34.2) were

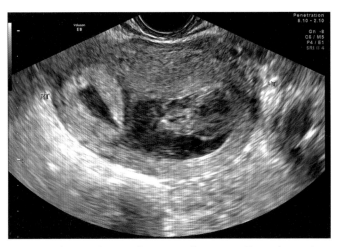

Fig. 34.1 Ultrasound image of an interstitial pregnancy. The endometrial stripe was seen entirely separate from the gestational sac and adjacent to the ovary. Note the thin rim of myometrium surrounding the gestational sac.

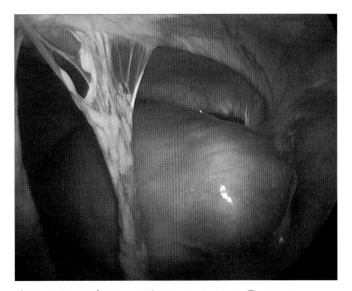

Fig. 34.2 Image of an interstitial pregnancy at surgery. The pregnancy appears as a bulge in the cornual region. The myometrium surrounding the pregnancy is obviously thinner than the remainder of the uterus.

Acute Care and Emergency Gynecology, ed. David Chelmow, Christine R. Isaacs and Ashley Carroll. Published by Cambridge University Press. © Cambridge University Press 2015.

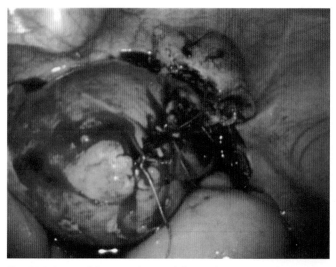

Fig. 34.3 Image of the cornual region following laparoscopic salpingectomy and cornual resection of the pregnancy shown in Fig. 34.2.

consistent with interstitial pregnancy, and cornual resection was performed. The cornual defect was sutured in two layers, and the final result is shown in Fig. 34.3. The patient was discharged home in good condition on the day of surgery.

Unruptured ectopic pregnancy

Advanced unruptured ectopic pregnancy can be found in the fallopian tube, uterine cornu, Cesarean scars, cervix, or ovary, and location has some bearing on the management. Taken as a group, advanced ectopic pregnancies have a higher failure rate with medical management than small ectopic pregnancies [1]. Factors which are associated with higher failure rates are increased level of hCG (with 5000 mIU/mL proposed as a cutoff point by several authors of case reviews), presence of embryonic cardiac activity and higher serum progesterone level. While methotrexate therapy has been effective in extra-tubal ectopic pregnancies, these pregnancies are associated with greater morbidity; and careful selection and counseling is required before medical therapy should be considered [2].

If this patient's pregnancy had been tubal, and if blood transfusions were an option should rupture occur, then we could reasonably offer her medical therapy to her. Methotrexate management is successful in approximately 90% of suitably selected patients. Failure rates for single dose methotrexate from 13 to 65% have been reported in patients with initial serum hCG levels above 5000 mIU/mL. While this range is too broad to be useful in counseling, it is clear that failure risk with single dose therapy is increased when initial hCG level exceeds 5000 mIU/mL [3], and that the presence of fetal cardiac activity roughly doubles the risk of failure [4]. Multidose therapy should be considered for patients with these findings where medical therapy is still being considered.

Multidose therapy for ectopic pregnancy consists of administration of methotrexate at a 1 mg/kg dose in alternating daily doses with leucovorin 0.1 mg/kg. Dosing is continued up to four doses each or until the hCG level falls by 15% from the prior value (checked on days 1, 3, 5, and 7). Approximately half of women will require fewer than four doses, and a rapidly rising hCG level following the second dose is considered treatment failure. The only randomized trial comparing multidose to single-dose therapy found them equally effective but excluded pregnancies with fetal cardiac motion and included patients with low hCG levels [4]. Larger retrospective reviews have concluded that multidose therapy is more effective in advanced pregnancies [5].

A hybrid two-dose regimen has been proposed in which methotrexate is administered in a 50 mg/m^2 dose on day 1, and repeated on day 7 and day 11 if there is a less than 15% decrease in hCG level between days 4 and 7. The two multidose regimens have not been compared in a randomized controlled trial.

Standard precautions and follow-up apply for patients with advanced unruptured ectopic pregnancy treated with methotrexate. RhoGam should be administered to Rh-negative women. Adequate compliance should be assured. Patients should avoid intercourse, should not take folic acid supplements, should not take aspirin or NSAIDs, and should not use alcohol. Stomatitis is a potential complication of multidose regimens and chlorhexidine mouthwashes are helpful. It is also recommended that patients delay conception for three months following medical therapy because of the potential teratogenicity of residual methotrexate.

Desire for future pregnancy need not alter choice of treatment. Success rates for future pregnancy do not differ between the two methods. The outcomes of tubal preservation, tubal patency, and subsequent intrauterine pregnancy are not significantly different when systemic methotrexate therapy is compared with salpingostomy [6].

Cost of therapy is a consideration. Published data are old, and may include practices such as a dilatation and curettage in patients planning to undergo medical therapy that are not always performed now. A cost–benefit analysis that takes into account pregnancy location, hCG level, single- versus multidose medical treatment regimens, and salpingostomy or salpingectomy would be useful but does not exist.

For our patient, medical therapy is not a reasonable option given her elevated risk of failure. This would be particularly risky in this patient, given her refusal of transfusion and inability to safely respond if her pregnancy ruptures. Surgery can be performed via laparoscopy or laparotomy, depending largely on operator expertise and experience. The techniques for surgical resection are similar regardless of approach, with cornual resection with or without salpingectomy being the most commonly used [7]. Regardless of approach, methods to minimize blood loss should be employed. These include injection of the myometrium just proximal to the pregnancy with a dilute vasopressin solution (10 U in 100 cc saline), placing sutures into the uterus and mesosalpinx just below the resection line, and careful use of energy sources to maximize coagulation during excision.

Care must be taken with the use of ultrasonic or electrical energy so that damage to the remaining myometrium is minimized.

Key teaching points

- Advanced ectopic pregnancy has a higher likelihood of failure with single-dose medical therapy, and multidose regimens should be considered in those patients opting for medical management.

- Medical management of extratubal ectopic pregnancies has been successfully undertaken, but decisions for medical management of these pregnancies should be considered in light of risk and morbidity of rupture, as well as other contraindications to medical management.

- Women with advanced tubal pregnancies who desire future fertility can be offered either medical or surgical management.

References

1. Medical Treatment of Ectopic Pregnancy: A Committee Opinion. American Society for Reproductive Medicine. *Fertil Steril* 2013;100: 638–44.

2. American College of Obstetricians and Gynecologists. Medical Management of Ectopic Pregnancy. ACOG Practice Bulletin No. 94. *Obset Gynecol* 2008; 111: 1479–85.

3. Menon S, Colins J, Barnhart K. Establishing a human chorionic gonadotropin cutoff to guide methotrexate treatment of ectopic pregnancy: a systematic review. *Fertil Steril* 2007; 87(3): 481–4.

4. Lipscomb G, McCord M, Stovall T, Huff G, Portera S, Ling F. Predictors of success of methotrexate treatment in women with tubal ectopic pregnancies. *N Engl J Med* 1999; 341: 1974–8.

5. Alleyassin A, Khandemi A, Aghahosseini M, Safdarian L, Badenoosh B, Hamed EA. Comparison of success rates in the medical management of ectopic pregnancy with single-dose and multiple-dose administration of methotrexate: a prospective randomized clinical trial. *Fertil Steril* 2006; 85(6): 1661–6.

6. Hajenius PJ, Mol F, Mol BWJ, Bossuyt PMM, Ankum WM, Van der Veen F. Interventions for tubal ectopic pregnancy. *Cochrane Database of Systematic Reviews* 2007, Issue 1. Art. No.: CD000324. DOI 10.1002/ 14651858.CD000324.pub2.

7. Moawad N, Mahajan S, Moniz M, Taylor S, Hurd W. Current diagnosis and treatment of interstitial pregnancy. *Am J Obstet Gynecol* 2010; 202(1): 15–29.

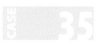

A 23-year-old pregnant woman with acute-onset abdominal pain and hypotension

Rachel K. Love and Nicole Calloway Rankins

History of present illness

A 23-year-old gravida 1 woman presents to the ultrasound clinic for a first-trimester dating ultrasound. By an unsure last menstrual period, she is approximately 10 weeks' pregnant. Her pregnancy thus far has been uncomplicated, with the exception of intermittent vaginal spotting for which she did not seek medical attention. Her past medical history is remarkable for asthma, and she has had no prior surgery. Her gynecologic history is significant for pelvic inflammatory disease at age 18, which was successfully treated on an outpatient basis.

The transvaginal ultrasound reveals a normal-sized anteverted uterus with no evidence of an intrauterine pregnancy. Her right adnexa contains a mass consisting of a gestational sac and fetal pole with cardiac activity (Fig. 35.1). At the end of her ultrasound appointment, she suddenly develops writhing abdominal pain and dyspnea. Immediate repeat ultrasound reveals a large fluid collection in the posterior cul-de-sac. She is urgently transported to the emergency department for further management.

Physical examination

General appearance: Well-nourished young woman in apparent distress from pain, diaphoretic

Vital signs:

Temperature: 36.0°C
Pulse: 95 beats/min
Blood pressure: 69/43 mmHg
Respiratory rate: 22 breaths/min
Oxygen saturation: 100% on room air

Respiratory: Increased respiratory rate, lungs clear to auscultation bilaterally

Cardiovascular: Mildly tachycardic, regular rhythm, no murmurs

Abdomen: Moderately distended, tender to light palpation in all four quadrants, rebound and guarding present

Pelvic: Deferred

Extremities: No edema, nontender

Laboratory studies:

Hb: 10.5 g/dL (2 days prior to presentation: Hb 13.5 g/dL)
Blood type: O positive

What is your diagnosis?

This patient has a ruptured ectopic pregnancy. Her diagnosis was made clinically based on the presence of peritoneal signs, hypotension, acute drop in hemoglobin concentration, and ultrasonographic evidence of hemoperitoneum in the setting of a known ectopic pregnancy.

How would you manage this patient?

This patient warrants rapid hemodynamic stabilization and prompt surgical treatment. She was placed on continuous vital sign monitoring, given two large bore intravenous catheters, and was administered a 2-L bolus of normal saline. A blood sample was sent for type and screen and complete blood count. She was consented for surgery and was emergently taken to the operating room where a diagnostic laparoscopy was performed. Findings during laparoscopy were significant for 2.5 L of blood in the peritoneal cavity, and a large right tubal pregnancy containing an intact fetus of approximately 9 weeks' gestation (Fig. 35.2). A laparoscopic right salpingectomy was performed using a laparoscopic vessel-sealing device without complications. Intraoperative hemoglobin was checked and returned to 7.2 g/dL. She was transfused 1 U of packed red blood cells in the recovery room for symptomatic acute blood loss anemia. Her hemoglobin on the morning of postoperative day 1 rose appropriately to 8.2 g/dL. She otherwise had an uncomplicated postoperative course and was discharged home on postoperative day 1. Prior to discharge she was counseled regarding ectopic pregnancy and the implications for future pregnancy. Surgical pathology confirmed products of conception.

Ruptured ectopic pregnancy

Ectopic pregnancy accounts for 1–2% of all pregnancies in the United States yet accounts for approximately 6% of all pregnancy-related deaths [1,2]. Although the incidence of ectopic pregnancy is becoming harder to estimate due to the number of cases treated as an outpatient, it still remains the leading cause of pregnancy-related mortality in the first trimester. Ninety-three percent of deaths associated with ectopic pregnancy are caused by hemorrhage [2]. Hence, it is imperative for the clinician to maintain a high index of suspicion for ectopic pregnancy in any sexually active reproductive-aged female presenting with abdominal pain and/or vaginal bleeding, and a urine pregnancy test should be obtained in the initial evaluation.

The risk factors for ectopic pregnancy are directly related to tubal damage and inflammation. These risk factors include prior ectopic pregnancy, prior tubal surgery, history of pelvic

Acute Care and Emergency Gynecology, ed. David Chelmow, Christine R. Isaacs and Ashley Carroll. Published by Cambridge University Press. © Cambridge University Press 2015.

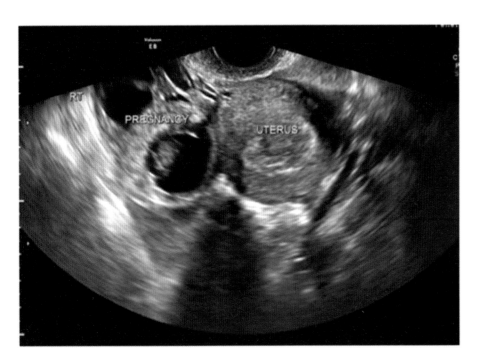

Fig. 35.1 Ultrasound findings with gestational sac and fetal pole in right adnexa.

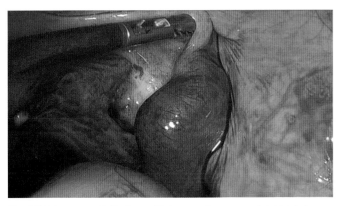

Fig. 35.2 Laparoscopic findings with hemoperitoneum and right tubal ectopic pregnancy.

inflammatory disease, *Chlamydia trachomatis* infection, and in utero diethylstilbestrol (DES) exposure [3].

Conversely, risk factors for tubal rupture in ectopic pregnancy are not as clearly outlined and are contradictory in retrospective cohort studies. In one retrospective cohort study of 693 ectopic pregnancies, tubal rupture was encountered more often in women with no history of ectopic pregnancy, and there was no correlation between serum beta-human chorionic gonadotropin (beta-hCG) levels and tubal rupture [4]. Furthermore, in 11% of the cases of tubal rupture, the beta-hCG level was less than 100 mIU/mL. In a French-population-based study, the following were identified as risk factors for tubal rupture: ovulation induction, beta-hCG levels exceeding 10 000 mIU/mL at the time ectopic pregnancy was suspected, never having used contraception, and a history of tubal damage in combination with infertility [5]. A case-control study conducted in Amsterdam identified no patient-related risk factors for severe intra-abdominal hemorrhage in women with tubal ectopic pregnancy (severe hemorrhage was defined as receiving transfusion of four or more units of packed red blood cells) [6]. However, the study did identify that substandard care was more often associated with cases of severe hemorrhage. Misdiagnosis, in which the provider incorrectly identified an ectopic pregnancy as an intrauterine pregnancy on transvaginal ultrasound, was the most common reason for substandard care in the women with severe hemorrhage. In summary, the results of the above studies illustrate a lack of consistent predictors for tubal rupture and severe hemorrhage, so providers must maintain an acute awareness for ectopic pregnancy. In cases of known ectopic pregnancy or pregnancies of unknown location, providers must counsel their patients on the signs and symptoms of tubal rupture and advise patients to seek immediate medical attention in such cases.

Most ectopic pregnancies occur in the fallopian tube, and the most common site of tubal implantation is the ampullary region. The rate of tubal rupture in ectopic pregnancy ranges from 18 to 34% [4,5]. Pregnancies implanted in the isthmic or ampullary regions tend to rupture earlier, while cornual and interstitial implantations tend to rupture later. Rupture is usually spontaneous, but may be precipitated by coitus or by bimanual examination. Clinical signs and symptoms of ruptured ectopic pregnancy may include abdominal pain with rebound tenderness, referred shoulder pain, cervical motion tenderness, hypotension, and tachycardia. Laboratory values assisting in the diagnosis of rupture are a low initial hemoglobin concentration or a rapidly decreasing hemoglobin concentration. In a ruptured ectopic pregnancy, transvaginal ultrasound will reveal fluid in the posterior cul-de-sac, and if the bleeding is severe, transabdominal ultrasound will display fluid in the subhepatic recess and the paracolic gutters.

Once the diagnosis of ruptured ectopic pregnancy is made, the treatment is urgent surgical intervention. Medical management with methotrexate is contraindicated in this setting. Initial stabilization measures in the case of massive hemoperitoneum or shock include obtaining two large bore intravenous catheters, intravenous fluid resuscitation with isotonic fluids, blood transfusion if necessary, administering supplemental oxygen, keeping the patient warm, and elevating the legs or placing the patient in Trendelenburg position.

Surgical treatment is accomplished by salpingectomy (removing the tube) or salpingostomy (incising the tube and removing the ectopic pregnancy tissue with conservation of the tube). Both salpingectomy and salpingostomy can be performed via laparoscopy or laparotomy. A Cochrane review of 35 studies analyzing the treatment for ectopic pregnancy found that laparoscopy was feasible and less costly than open surgery [7], and is generally the preferred approach. In cases of severe intraperitoneal hemorrhage, hemodynamic instability, or inadequate visualization at the time of laparoscopy, laparotomy may be warranted. Laparoscopic salpingostomy is less successful than open salpingostomy in the elimination of the ectopic pregnancy because of higher rates of persistent trophoblastic tissue, but long-term follow-up shows no difference in intrauterine pregnancy rates [7]. The decision to perform a salpingostomy versus a salpingectomy is often made by the provider at the time of surgery. Factors that may influence this decision include the extent of tubal damage, appearance of the contralateral fallopian tube, desire for future childbearing, prior ectopic pregnancy on the ipsilateral side as the current ectopic pregnancy, and surgeon skill. In cases where salpingostomy is performed, postoperative monitoring of beta-hCG levels is required as persistent trophoblastic tissue remains in the fallopian tube in 5–20% of women [8].

An important component of all ectopic pregnancy treatment is appropriate patient counseling. A prior ectopic pregnancy increases the risk for an ectopic with future pregnancy [3]; therefore, it is imperative that patients be counseled to present as soon as possible with future pregnancy recognition. Finally, if a patient is Rh negative, she should receive anti-D immune globulin as part of her treatment.

Key teaching points

- Ectopic pregnancy is the number one cause of maternal mortality in the first trimester, and hemorrhage from rupture accounts for greater than 90% of these deaths.
- Ruptured ectopic pregnancy is a gynecologic emergency that requires prompt diagnosis and surgical treatment.
- Beta-human chorionic gonadotropin (beta-hCG) levels have not been shown to consistently correlate with risk of tubal rupture, and tubal rupture can occur even when the beta-hCG level is low.
- Medical management with methotrexate is absolutely contraindicated in the setting of ruptured ectopic pregnancy.
- In general, laparoscopy is the preferred surgical approach for management. However, laparotomy may be needed in times of hemodynamic instability or inadequate visualization at the time of laparoscopy.
- Patients should be counseled regarding the importance of presenting for care as soon as possible after recognition of pregnancy in the future, as prior ectopic pregnancy increases the risk for future ectopic pregnancy.
- Patients with ectopic pregnancy who are Rh negative should receive anti-D immune globulin.

References

1. Centers for Disease Control and Prevention. Ectopic pregnancy – United States, 1990–1992. *MMWR* 1995;44;46–8.

2. Centers for Disease Control and Prevention. Pregnancy-related mortality surveillance – United States, 1991–1999. *MMWR Surveill Summ* 2003;52:1–9.

3. Ankum WM, Mol BW, Van de Veen F, Bossuyt PM. Risk factors for ectopic pregnancy: a meta-analysis. *Fertil Steril* 1996;65:1093–9.

4. Saxon D, Falcone T, Mascha EJ, et al. A study of ruptured tubal ectopic pregnancy. *Obstet Gynecol* 1997; 90:46–9.

5. Job-Spira N, Fernandez H, Bouyer J, et al. Ruptured tubal ectopic pregnancy: risk factors and reproductive outcome: results of a population-based study in France. *Am J Obstet Gynecol* 1999;180(4): 938–44.

6. van Mello NM, Zietse CS, Mol F, et al. Severe maternal morbidity in ectopic pregnancy is not associated with maternal factors but may be associated with quality of care. *Fertil Steril* 2012;97:623–9.

7. Hajenius PJ, Mol F, Mol BJW, et al. Interventions for tubal ectopic pregnancy. *Cochrane Database Syst Rev* 2007, Issue 1. Art. No.: CD0000324. DOI:10.1002/14651858.CD000324. pub2.

8. Barnhart KT. Clinical practice. Ectopic pregnancy. *N Engl J Med* 2009;361: 379–87.

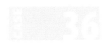

A woman with first-trimester vaginal bleeding

Valerie L. Williams and Amy E. Young

History of present illness

A 24-year-old woman presents to the emergency department complaining of vaginal bleeding. She reports a three-day history of vaginal spotting. She also complains of mild lower abdominal cramping, rated at a level of 4 on a scale of 0–10. She has been inconsistently taking oral contraceptive pills. She reports her last menstrual period was 10 weeks earlier. Her cycles were previously regular.

She has no prior pregnancies. She is otherwise healthy and has not had prior surgery. She takes no medications other than her birth control pills.

Physical examination

General appearance: Well-nourished, well-hydrated woman in minimal discomfort

Vital signs:

Temperature: 37.0°C
Pulse: 105 beats/min
Blood pressure: 95/55 mmHg
Respiratory rate: 18 breaths/min
Oxygen saturation: 98% on room air

HEENT: Unremarkable

Neck: Supple

Cardiovascular: Regular rate and rhythm without rubs, murmurs, or gallops

Lungs: Clear to auscultation bilaterally

Abdomen: Soft, nondistended, with tenderness to palpation in both lower quadrants without associated rebound or guarding. Bowel sounds present

Pelvic:

Speculum examination: Clotted blood in the vaginal vault obscuring the cervix. When blood was removed, the cervix appears closed
Bimanual examination: No cervical motion or adnexal tenderness. Uterus is eight-week size, mobile, and slightly tender to palpation. Cervix is closed on digital exam. Adnexa are not enlarged

Extremities: No clubbing, cyanosis, or edema

Neurologic: Nonfocal

Laboratory studies:

Hb: 9.1 g/dL
Blood type: B positive
Urine pregnancy test: Positive

Imaging: A pelvic ultrasound is obtained (Fig. 36.1a,b)

How would you manage this patient?

This patient has a threatened abortion. The ultrasound showed an intrauterine pregnancy with a crown rump length of 20 mm. Normal fetal cardiac activity was present, confirming viability. A quantitative beta-human chorionic gonadotropin (beta-hCG) was unnecessary given these ultrasound findings. Cervical nucleic acid amplification tests (NAATs) for gonorrhea and chlamydia were negative. The patient was reassured. A repeat ultrasound is unnecessary unless the patient has increased pain, a dilated cervical os, increased bleeding or passage of tissue, or an inability to obtain fetal heart tones with future assessments. The pregnancy was unplanned but desired. She was reassured that conception while taking oral contraceptive pills has no known adverse affects. Prenatal care was initiated and the patient had an uncomplicated pregnancy and delivery.

Threatened abortion

Threatened abortion refers to a viable intrauterine pregnancy with vaginal bleeding and a closed cervical os. Vaginal bleeding occurs in 15–25% of viable intrauterine pregnancies. The etiology is not fully understood, but bleeding may occur at the time of implantation or as the placenta expands (subchorionic hemorrhage) [1]. Bleeding is a presenting symptom of many early pregnancy complications including spontaneous abortion, molar pregnancy, and ectopic pregnancy. Spontaneous abortion is the spontaneous termination of a pregnancy prior to 20 weeks' gestation. It occurs by expulsion of products, failure of the embryo to develop, or death of the fetus in utero. Clinically, it can be categorized into threatened, missed, inevitable, incomplete, or complete abortion. Rapid diagnosis is important. Ectopic pregnancy must be ruled out as it can be life threatening. Early pregnancy loss is common and early confirmation allows the patient a broad range of management options under controlled circumstances. In addition to abnormal pregnancy, the differential diagnosis includes cervicitis, cervical lesions, polyps at the external cervical os, and a decidual reaction in the cervix.

Patients will typically present with vaginal bleeding and mild abdominal or pelvic pain and cramping. Physical examination findings may include an enlarged, minimally tender uterus, blood in the vaginal vault, and a closed cervical

Acute Care and Emergency Gynecology, ed. David Chelmow, Christine R. Isaacs and Ashley Carroll. Published by Cambridge University Press. © Cambridge University Press 2015.

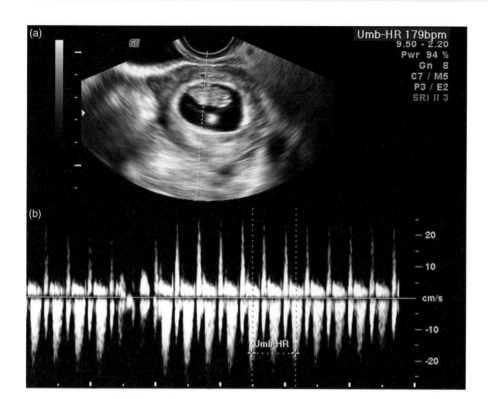

Fig. 36.1 Transvaginal ultrasound (a, top; b, bottom) from a 24-year-old pregnant female with vaginal bleeding.

os. A definite diagnosis cannot be made on clinical assessment alone. In a patient like this with bleeding but where her enlarged uterus and otherwise benign examination make ectopic unlikely, determination must be made as to the viability of the pregnancy and the presence of other explanations, particularly cervicitis. Evaluation would typically include cervical NAATs for gonorrhea and chlamydia, blood type determination, and an ultrasound. The Rh D antigen is present on fetal erythrocytes as early as 38 days' gestation. Rh-negative patients should receive anti-D immune globulin to prevent Rh isoimmunization. A dose of 50 μg is effective prior to 12 weeks. Ultrasound is the critical study for establishing the location, gestational age, and viability of a pregnancy.

In this patient, ultrasound clearly shows a normal embryo with normal fetal heart motion, indicative of a viable pregnancy. Ultrasound can confirm that a pregnancy is viable through observation of fetal heart rate activity, and earlier in pregnancy can confirm early pregnancy loss through failing to observe appropriate milestones. The first definitive sign of an intrauterine gestation is the gestational sac. It appears four to five weeks after the last menstrual period. It is characterized by a sonolucent center surrounded by two symmetrical, thick echogenic rings. This "double decidual sign" (Fig. 36.2) is the ultrasound correlate of a chorionic cavity surrounded by decidualized endometrium. Once a gestational sac is visualized, the mean sac diameter should grow 1 mm per day. A yolk sac appears by the time the mean sac diameter reaches 13 mm. It appears as a 2–6 mm, perfectly round, symmetrical structure

(Fig. 36.3). An embryonic pole appears around week 6 when the gestational sac reaches 20 mm. Fetal cardiac activity should be present at an embryo length of 4 mm. Once fetal cardiac activity is present, as it was in this patient, the risk of pregnancy failure is less than 5% [1,2]. These patients should be managed expectantly. Deviations from these normal milestones are indicative of early pregnancy failure. Some can be detected on a single ultrasound examination, others require serial examinations. Ultrasound findings that are diagnostic or highly suggestive of early pregnancy failure are listed in Table 36.1 [3].

There are no effective treatments for threatened abortion. Although often prescribed, there is no evidence to support bed rest to prevent spontaneous abortion in women with first-trimester bleeding [4]. Bed rest has both direct and indirect consequences. Immobilization in pregnancy potentially increases the risk for thromboembolism due to the hypercoagulable state of pregnancy. Other less direct harms include disruption of social relationships and loss of income. Progesterone has been prescribed in the past to support a potentially deficient endometrium for implantation. The quality of data to support this practice is poor and progesterone has not been shown to improve outcomes [5]. Reassurance should be given to the patient as bleeding can cause significant maternal anxiety. She should be counseled that bleeding in the first trimester is common and pregnancy loss after the presence of fetal cardiac activity is rare. Physical activity restrictions are unlikely to impact the final outcome. Routine prenatal care should be addressed including prenatal vitamins

Table 36.1 Guidelines for transvaginal ultrasonographic diagnosis of pregnancy failure in a woman with an intrauterine pregnancy of uncertain viability*

Findings diagnostic of pregnancy failure	Findings suspicious for, but not diagnostic of, pregnancy failure
Crown–rump length of ≥7 mm and no heartbeat	Crown-rump length of <7 mm and no heartbeat
Mean sac diameter of ≥25 mm and no embryo	Enlarged yolk sac (>7 mm)
Absence of embryo with heartbeat ≥2 weeks after a scan that showed a gestational sac without a yolk sac	
Absence of embryo with heartbeat ≥11 days after a scan that showed a gestational sac with a yolk sac	

* Adapted from Doubilet et al. [3].

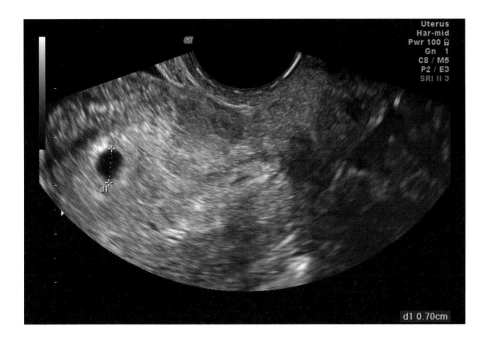

Fig. 36.2 Transvaginal ultrasound demonstrating an intrauterine gestational sac with a double decidual sign.

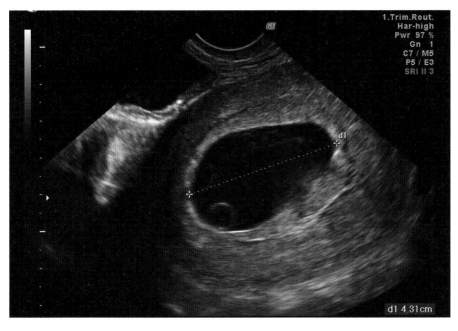

Fig. 36.3 Transvaginal ultrasound demonstrating an intrauterine gestational sac with a yolk sac.

and avoidance of tobacco and alcohol. This patient should be encouraged to establish prenatal care.

First-trimester bleeding is associated with an increased risk of spontaneous abortion. This risk is low if fetal cardiac activity is present on ultrasound. Risk factors associated with pregnancy loss include extremes of age (<20 or >35 years) and moderate to severe bleeding. First-trimester bleeding has also been associated with other adverse pregnancy outcomes. In a systematic review of viable pregnancies that had first-trimester bleeding, threatened abortion was associated with a significantly higher incidence of antepartum hemorrhage, preterm premature rupture of membranes, preterm delivery, intrauterine growth restriction, low birth weight, perinatal mortality, 5 minute Apgar score less than 7, and congenital anomalies [6]. These risks are low, however, and there is no data to suggest specific interventions to prevent these adverse events. First-trimester bleeding alone is not currently an indication for increased fetal or maternal surveillance.

Conception while taking oral contraceptive pills, as occurred in this patient, is not rare. There is no evidence that exposure in early pregnancy to combined hormonal contraception is associated with any adverse outcome [7] and bears no relationship to this patient's bleeding. The patient can be counseled that conceiving while taking combined hormonal contraceptives poses no risk to the fetus.

Key teaching points

- Vaginal bleeding is common in the first trimester. Every reproductive-age woman presenting with vaginal bleeding should be evaluated with a urine pregnancy test.
- In pregnant females with vaginal bleeding, a pelvic ultrasound is indicated to determine pregnancy location, gestational age, and viability. If fetal cardiac activity is present, the risk of pregnancy loss is low.
- Common ultrasound criteria to diagnose early pregnancy failure include a mean sac diameter (MSD) greater than 20 mm without a fetal pole or an embryo length greater than 4 mm without fetal cardiac activity.
- Once viability is documented, standard prenatal care should be initiated.
- Patients who have threatened abortions may have a slightly increased risk of other adverse pregnancy outcomes including antepartum hemorrhage, preterm premature rupture of membranes, preterm delivery, intrauterine growth restriction, and low birth weight.

References

1. Paul M, Lichtenberg S, Borgatta L, eds. *Management of Unintended and Abnormal pregnancy*. Chichester, Blackwell Publishing Ltd, 2009.

2. Perriera L, Reeves MF. Ultrasound criteria for diagnosis of early pregnancy failure and ectopic pregnancy. *Semin Reprod Med* 2008;26:373–82.

3. Doubilet PM, Benson CB, Bourne T, Blaivas M. Diagnostic criteria for nonviable pregnancy early in the first trimester. *N Engl J Med* 2013;369: 1443–51.

4. Aleman A, Althabe F, Belizan J, Bergel E. Bed rest during pregnancy for preventing miscarriage. *Cochrane Database Syst Rev* 2005;2:CD003576.

5. Wahabi HA, Fayed AA, Esmaeil SA, Al Zeidan RA. Progestogen for treating threatened miscarriage. *Cochrane Database Syst Rev* 2011;12:CD005943.

6. Saraswat L, Bhattacharya S, Maheshwari A, Bhattacharya S. Maternal and perinatal outcome in women with threatened miscarriage in the first trimester: a systematic review. *Br J Obstet Gynecol* 2010;117:245–57.

7. World Health Organization. *Medical Eligibility Criteria for Contraceptive Use*, 4th edn, 2009. Available at http://whqlibdoc.who.int/publications/2010/9789241563888_eng.pdf?ua=1.

Midcycle spotting and worsening menorrhagia

Patricia S. Huguelet

History of present illness

A 34-year-old gravida 3, para 3 woman presents complaining of heavy and irregular bleeding. She reports menarche at the age of 14, with regular menses until 1 year ago. At that time, she began having much heavier but regular periods. She describes heavy flow once a month, where she changes fully saturated tampons hourly. The bleeding is precipitated by breast tenderness, bloating, and cramping. Over the past three months, she has begun having three to four days of midcycle spotting. Her husband underwent a vasectomy after the birth of her third child two years ago.

She has no significant past medical or surgical history. Her gynecologic history is negative, including no history of sexually transmitted infections or abnormal cervical screening tests. She is sexually active without any other gynecologic complaints. She denies any significant weight changes, and a full review of systems was otherwise negative.

Physical examination

General appearance: Healthy-appearing woman, obese, and in no apparent distress

Vital signs:

Temperature: 36.9°C
Pulse: 78 beats/min
Blood pressure: 120/75 mmHg
Respiratory rate: 16 breaths/min
Oxygen saturation: 99% on room air
BMI: 31 kg/m^2

HEENT: Unremarkable

Neck: Supple without thyromegaly

Cardiovascular: Regular rate and rhythm, without rubs, murmurs, or gallops

Lungs: Clear to auscultation bilaterally

Abdomen: Soft, nondistended, active bowel sounds in all four quadrants, nontender without masses or hernias

Pelvic: Normal external genitalia; vagina notable only for physiologic discharge; cervix grossly normal; uterus slightly enlarged to six- to eight-week size, mobile, and nontender; no cervical motion or adnexal tenderness

Extremities: Normal

Laboratory studies:

Urine pregnancy test: Negative
Hb: 13.3 g/dL (normal 12.1–16.3 g/dL)
Ht: 38.1% (normal 35.7 – 46.7%)
Neisseria gonorrhoeae and *Chlamydia trachomatis* endocervical amplified probes: Negative

Imaging: Transvaginal ultrasound was performed (Fig. 37.1)

How would you manage the patient?

The patient has an endometrial polyp. Transvaginal ultrasound imaging demonstrates a nondescript, thickened endometrium, with heterogenous features suggestive of endometrial pathology.

Subsequent saline infusion sonohysterography (SIS) clearly delineates the presence of a circumscribed mass, including its size and location (Fig. 37.2).

The patient was counseled and underwent an uneventful operative hysteroscopy with polypectomy (Fig. 37.3).

Pathology confirmed a benign endometrial polyp without hyperplasia or malignancy. Endometrial curettings showed proliferative endometrium. After the procedure, the patient experienced several weeks of light, irregular bleeding, which progressively improved until her next menses. Thereafter, her menses were much lighter, and the intermenstrual bleeding resolved.

Menometrorrhagia and endometrial polyps

Structural abnormalities are frequent causes of abnormal bleeding, and of these, leiomyomas and endometrial polyps are the most common. Endometrial polyps are soft, fleshy intrauterine growths comprised of endometrial glands and fibrotic stroma, covered by a surface epithelium. In contrast, leiomyomas are benign smooth muscle neoplasms that typically originate from the myometrium. Endometrial polyps are common, occurring in 24–41% of women who have abnormal bleeding, and in about 10% of asymptomatic women. The prevalence of endometrial polyps increases with age [1]. Clinically, endometrial polyps have been associated with various bleeding patterns including heavy menstrual bleeding, intermenstrual bleeding, spotting, or postmenopausal bleeding. Despite these common complaints, most women with polyps are asymptomatic and many polyps are found as incidental findings.

While the majority of endometrial polyps are benign, some polyps may contain premalignant or malignant changes. Premalignant changes include hyperplasia, both with and without atypia. However, data regarding atypia is based on diffuse

Acute Care and Emergency Gynecology, ed. David Chelmow, Christine R. Isaacs and Ashley Carroll. Published by Cambridge University Press. © Cambridge University Press 2015.

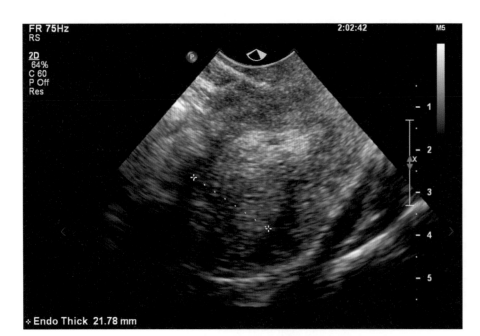

FR 75Hz
RS

2D
64%
C 60
P Off
Res

2:02:42   M5

— 1

— 2

— 3

— 4

— 5

❖ Endo Thick 21.78 mm

Fig. 37.1 Transvaginal ultrasound. (Images courtesy of William W. Brown III, MD.)

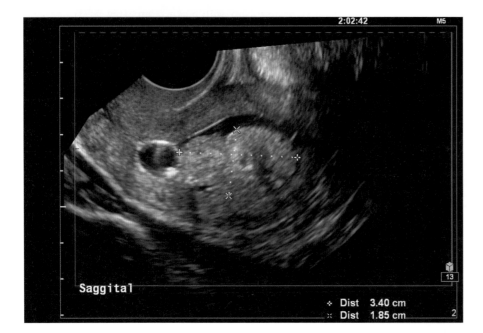

2:02:42   M5

13

Saggital

❖ Dist 3.40 cm
✕ Dist 1.85 cm   2

Fig. 37.2 Subsequent saline infusion sonohysterogram.

endometrial hyperplasia, not polyps. In studies of women with endometrial hyperplasia, the presence of atypia increases the risk of progression to neoplasia. Furthermore, in the presence of endometrial hyperplasia with atypia, the risk of occult malignancy approaches 40% [2]. In a recent systematic review, the prevalence of premalignant or malignant polyps was 5.42% in postmenopausal women, compared with 1.7% in reproductive-aged women. The prevalence of neoplasia within polyps in women with symptomatic bleeding was 4.15% compared with 2.16% of those without bleeding [3]. Based on data from these observational studies, symptomatic vaginal bleeding, hypertension, size greater than 1 cm, and postmenopausal status are all associated with an increased risk of endometrial malignancy [3,4,5].

In the setting of abnormal uterine bleeding due to endometrial polyps, the diagnostic goal is exclusion of hyperplasia and malignancy, followed by therapeutic intervention to correct the abnormal bleeding. For women struggling with infertility, restoring normal anatomy may also improve fertility outcomes.

The initial diagnostic evaluation should include pregnancy testing, followed by directed laboratory testing and imaging based on the clinical history. In an effort to create a universally accepted system of nomenclature to describe uterine bleeding abnormalities, a new classification system was introduced by

(a)

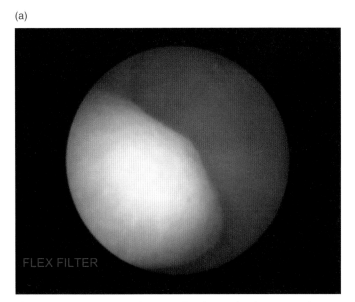

(b)

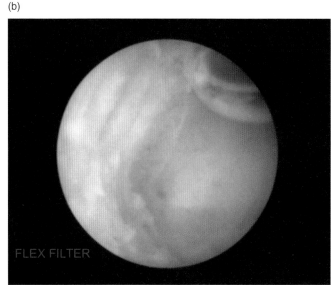

Fig. 37.3 Hysteroscopic confirmation of endometrial polyp at time of resection. (Images courtesy of William W. Brown III MD.)

the International Federation of Gynecology and Obstetrics in 2011 [6]. The new system is known by the acronym PALM-COEIN, which stands for polyp, adenomyosis, leiomyoma, malignancy and hyperplasia, coagulopathy, ovulatory dysfunction, endometrial, iatrogenic, and not yet classified. PALM refers to structural causes and COEIN to nonstructural causes.

When first approaching this clinical scenario, obtaining a detailed menstrual history is paramount, as it is important to establish whether the bleeding pattern is ovulatory or anovulatory [6]. In the absence of ovulation, bleeding will occur erratically, often without moliminal symptoms, suggesting a hormonal etiology and nonstructural causes (COEIN). Conversely, abnormal ovulatory bleeding strongly suggests an anatomic lesion (PALM), as was evident in our case presentation. Physical examination allows the physician to evaluate for vaginal and cervical lesions, as well as to assess uterine size and tenderness.

Once visible lesions have been ruled out, the next step involves assessment of the endometrial cavity. Various tools have been studied to determine their accuracy for detecting endometrial pathology. The preferred imaging study for the detection of focal endometrial pathology is SIS. In one study, 160 women suffering from menometrorrhagia were evaluated for the presence of endometrial pathology. All women underwent transvaginal ultrasound, followed by sonohysterography. The final diagnosis was established by diagnostic hysteroscopy and directed biopsy. In this study, the sensitivity and specificity for detection of endometrial polyps by transvaginal ultrasound was 65% and 75% versus SIS which was 93% and 94%, respectively (P<0.001). Transvaginal ultrasound resulted in false positive and false negative rates of 25% and 36.2%, whereas SIS resulted in only a 8.0% false positive and 5.4% false negative rate [7]. Doppler flow demonstrating a central feeding blood vessel further increases the specificity of both tests.

In this case scenario, the ovulatory bleeding pattern suggested an anatomic source. After physical examination ruled out a cervical problem, transvaginal imaging was ordered to evaluate for leiomyomas or polyps. The transvaginal ultrasound did not reveal any intramural pathology but did suggest heterogeneity within the endometrium. To better define the endometrial pathology, a saline infusion ultrasound was subsequently performed.

Transcervical resection is regarded as the optimal treatment of endometrial polyps [8]. Resection may be accomplished with various hysteroscopic instruments, including monopolar and bipolar resectoscopes utilizing radio-freqency energy, as well as newer devices that operate with a rotating mechanical blade. Choice of instrumentation depends primarily on provider preference, but does require careful attention to distension media and fluid deficit [9]. Hysteroscopy and polyp resection is generally performed under general anesthesia, but small endometrial polyps that don't require significant cervical dilation may be amenable to resection in the office setting under local anesthesia, with minimal discomfort to the patient. These procedures are generally considered safe, with low risk of complications depending on the approach. The most common complications associated with operative hysteroscopy include hemorrhage, cervical laceration, uterine perforation, and volume overload [9].

The treatment of asymptomatic polyps remains controversial because the risk of malignancy within these polyps is low and spontaneous regression may occur. Lieng and colleagues prospectively estimated the prevalence and 1-year regression rate of incidentally diagnosed endometrial polyps in women aged 40–45 years [10]. Women were randomly selected and underwent transvaginal ultrasound and SIS in order to estimate the prevalence of asymptomatic polyps in their population. Repeat imaging and hysteroscopy were then performed

12 months later. They discovered polyps in 12% of women with a spontaneous regression rate of 27% at 1 year [10]. Patients with incidental/asymptomatic polyp findings should thus be counseled regarding the risks and/or benefits of intervention versus expectant management given their clinical context.

The primary goals of treatment of symptomatic polyps are to relieve abnormal uterine bleeding and to rule out hyperplasia and malignancy, especially in women with risk factors for neoplasia. According to a recent systematic review by Nathani and Clark, polypectomy improved abnormal bleeding (range 75–100%), with follow-up ranging from 2 to 52 months [11]. In this clinical scenario, the patient was seen at her six-week postoperative visit where she reported resolution of her mid-cycle spotting, as well as decreased flow during her menses. She was advised that she did not require further follow-up, unless her abnormal bleeding returned.

Key teaching points

- Endometrial polyps are a frequent cause of heavy menstrual bleeding, intermenstrual spotting, or postmenopausal bleeding.
- Endometrial polyps are present in approximately 10% of asymptomatic women.
- The preferred imaging study for detection of an endometrial polyp is saline infusion sonohysterography (SIS). Doppler flow demonstrating a central feeding blood vessel further increases the specificity of the test.
- The risk of hyperplasia and malignancy within endometrial polyps is overall low but is increased in the postmenopausal patient. Treatment should be directed by patient symptoms and/or risk factors for malignancy.
- Hysteroscopic resection is the recommended treatment for endometrial polyps.

References

1. Clevenger-Hoeft M, Syrop CH, Stovall DW, et al. Sonohysterography in premenopausal women with and without abnormal bleeding. *Obstet Gynecol* 1999;94:516–20.

2. Sorosky, Joel. Endometrial cancer. *Obstet Gynecol* 2012;120: 383–97.

3. Lee SC, Kaunitz AM, Sanchez-Ramos L, et al. The oncogenic potential of endometrial polyps: A systematic review and meta-analysis. *Obstet Gynecol* 2010;116:1197–205.

4. Baiocchi G, Manci N, Pazzaglia M, et al. Malignancy in endometrial polyps: a 12-year experience. *Am J Obstet Gynecol* 2009;201:462.e1–e4.

5. Wang JH, Zhao J, Lin J. Opportunities and risk factors for premalignant and malignant transformation of endometrial polyps: management strategies. *J Minim Invasive Gynecol* 2010;17:53–8.

6. American College of Obstetricians and Gynecologists. Diagnosis of abnormal uterine bleeding in reproductive-aged women. Practice Bulletin No. 128. *Obstet Gynecol* 2012;120:197–206.

7. Kamel HS, Darwish AM, Mohamed SA. Comparison of transvaginal ultrasonography and vaginal sonohysterography in the detection of endometrial polyps. *Acta Obstet Gynecol Scand* 2000;79:60–4.

8. Lieng M, Istre O, Qvigstad E. Treatment of endometrial polyps: A systematic review. *Acta Obstet Gynecol Scand* 2010;89: 992–1002.

9. American College of Obstetricians and Gynecologists. Hysteroscopy. Technology assessment in obstetrics and gynecology No. 7. *Obstet Gynecol* 2011;117:1486–91.

10. Lieng M, Istre O, Sandvik L, et al. Prevalence, one-year regression rate, and clinical significance of asymptomatic endometrial polyps: cross-sectional study. *J Minim Invasive Gynecol* 2009;16:465–71.

11. Nathani F, Clark TJ. Uterine polypectomy in the management of abnormal uterine bleeding: A systematic review. *J Minim Invasive Gynecol* 2006;13:260–8.

A 40-year-old woman on tamoxifen therapy with a uterine mass

Megan A. Brady

History of present illness

A 40-year-old nulligravid Nigerian woman presented to the emergency room with two days of worsening abdominal pain. She describes the pain as severe and crampy. She denies constipation, diarrhea, nausea, or vomiting. Four years ago, the patient was diagnosed with breast cancer in Nigeria and underwent a left radical mastectomy, radiation, and chemotherapy. She has been on tamoxifen for the last three years. She has had three to four "periods" since chemotherapy. Her last episode of bleeding was two weeks ago. She often experiences hot flashes. She is not using contraception. She also has hypertension, for which she takes hydrochlorothiazide.

Physical examination

General appearance: Alert woman who is not in distress
Vital signs:

Temperature: 37.7°C
Pulse: 110 beats/min
Blood pressure: 139/85 mmHg
Respiratory rate: 14 breaths/min
Oxygen saturation: 99% on room air
Height: 165 cm
Weight: 180 lb
BMI: 30 kg/m^2

Cardiac: Tachycardic, no murmur
Pulmonary: Lungs clear to auscultation bilaterally
Breast: Absent left breast with post-surgical scarring
Abdomen: Soft, obese, diffusely tender to palpation, no rebound tenderness, normoactive bowel sounds
Genitourinary: Normal appearing external genitalia; vagina with scant clear discharge; cervix appears normal; bimanual examination significant for 12-week size, smooth, mobile, nontender uterus; adnexa nontender without appreciable masses
Laboratory studies:

Urine pregnancy test: Negative
WBCs: 4100/μL (normal 3900–11 700/μL)
Hb: 11.5 g/dL (normal 12–15 g/dL)

Imaging: The patient underwent a CT scan (Fig. 38.1a) which showed complex heterogenous fluid and soft tissue masses within the endometrial canal and uterus. An MRI was recommended given the CT findings (Fig. 38.1b). It showed a 9.6 × 5.7 × 4.9 cm multicystic mass protruding from the posterior fundus with lattice-like bands filling the entire endometrial canal. This was interpreted as consistent with endometrial hyperplasia, but mass with myometrial invasion cannot be ruled out

How would you manage this patient?

Since this finding was not a surgical emergency, the patient was discharged from the emergency room with narcotic analgesia and gynecology follow-up two days later. Office endometrial biopsy was attempted, but difficulty was encountered introducing the biopsy instrument through the cervix. False tracts were created during the attempted biopsy. Pathology of the specimen revealed no cervical or endometrial tissue.

The patient was scheduled for the operating room. Despite her age and likely ovarian insufficiency from her prior chemotherapy, she and her husband hoped for pregnancy, planning in-vitro fertilization with donor eggs if necessary. Fertility-sparing surgery was planned unless malignancy was diagnosed. She was consented for hysteroscopy with removal of the polypoid tissue and endometrial sampling, as well as possible diagnostic laparoscopy.

Hysteroscopy (Fig. 38.2) revealed a large mass of cystic appearing polyps, which were removed with multiple passes of uterine polyp forceps and a sharp curette. Laparoscopy was not performed as the intraoperative pathology from hysteroscopy provided an adequate diagnosis.

Pathology showed benign endometrial polyps with changes consistent with tamoxifen.

Gynecologic oncology consultants recommended that the patient stop tamoxifen and instead take anastrozole, an aromatase inhibitor. Anastrozole has not been associated with pathologic changes to the endometrium. Since her medication change, she has not had recurrence of bleeding and her breast cancer remains in remission.

Tamoxifen-induced changes of the endometrium

Tamoxifen use increases the risk of endometrial adenocarcinoma, as well as several other types of uterine pathology, particularly uterine polyps. Tamoxifen is a selective estrogen receptor modulator (SERM) used as adjuvant therapy for

Acute Care and Emergency Gynecology, ed. David Chelmow, Christine R. Isaacs and Ashley Carroll. Published by Cambridge University Press. © Cambridge University Press 2015.

(a)

(b)

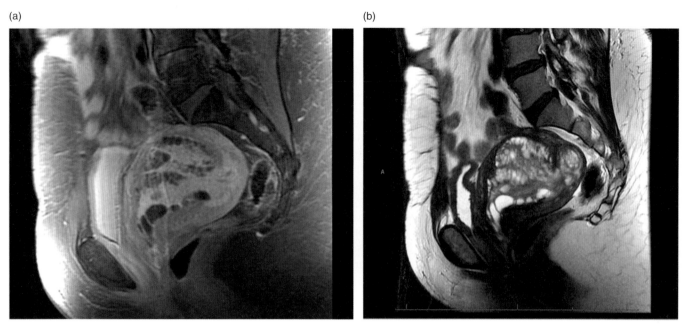

Fig. 38.1 CT (a) and MRI (b) images of uterine mass. (a) CT showed enlarged uterus with complex heterogenous fluid and soft tissue within the endometrial canal, as well as focal thinning of the posterior myometrium. (b) MRI showed a 9.6 × 5.7 × 4.9 cm multicystic mass protruding from the posterior fundus with lattice-like bands filling the entire endometrial canal.

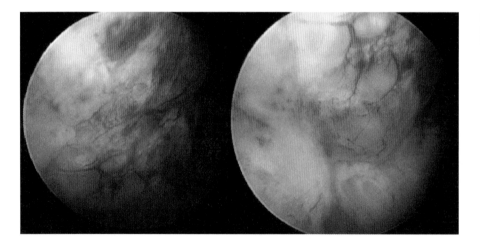

Fig. 38.2 Hysteroscopy findings. Note irregular, cystic appearing endometrium with scattered vascularities.

patients with estrogen receptor-positive breast cancer because of its anti-estrogen effects on breast tissue.

Effects on the endometrium are dependent on the presences or absence of endogenous estrogen. In postmenopausal women, tamoxifen has an agonist effect on the endometrium, while in premenopausal women, it acts as an antagonist. Although not well studied, adverse effects on premenopausal endometrium have not been documented [1]. The patient described, although age 40, has ovarian insufficiency from her prior chemotherapy, and is likely effectively menopausal as suggested by her hot flashes. The patient's bleeding episodes are probably from the uterine mass and unlikely to be menses.

Tamoxifen can stimulate proliferation of the postmenopausal endometrium, increasing risk for polyps, hyperplasia,

carcinoma, and sarcoma. The exact mechanism leading to these tissue changes is not well understood. Ten percent of women on tamoxifen will develop uterine pathology within five years leading to surgical evaluation [1]. Transvaginal ultrasound may show a thickened endometrium. However, no standard cutoff exists to define abnormal endometrial thickness in women on this medication [2]. Postmenopausal women on tamoxifen have a 2–3 times higher relative risk of developing endometrial cancer. This risk increases with treatment duration and dosage [3].

Tamoxifen-related endometrial changes have not been well described. One study describes patterns in almost 300 postmenopausal women on tamoxifen during a five-year treatment period at four tertiary care centers in Europe. Five dynamic patterns were characterized by transvaginal ultrasound, diagnostic hysteroscopy, and annual endometrial biopsy: atrophic, hypervascularized, cystic, endometrial polyp, and pattern suspicious for malignancy. The endometria of women in the study most commonly experienced the atrophic pattern in the first year, with the hypervascularized pattern seen most frequently in the second year of treatment. The cystic pattern was seen more frequently over time, mostly in the third and fourth years of treatment. Only eight of the patients in the study had a pattern suspicious for malignancy. Three of these patients had endometrial adenocarcinomas and one had papillary serous carcinoma [2].

The patient described was menopausal on tamoxifen with symptoms of vaginal bleeding and pain. Given their large size, the pain was thought to be from the polyps. Tissue diagnosis was necessary to ensure cancer was not present and as long as cancer was not present, removal of the polyps was necessary to resolve the patient's bleeding and pain. If the biopsy returned as a cancer, she would have undergone total hysterectomy and staging. Given the large mass on initial imaging, hysterectomy would have been a reasonable next step if she was not committed to preserving options for fertility. Given the benign pathology of the endometrial specimen at time of surgery, she discontinued tamoxifen and began taking anastrozole.

The American College of Obstetricians and Gynecologists states that, "In asymptomatic women using tamoxifen, screening for endometrial cancer with routine transvaginal ultrasonography, endometrial biopsy, or both has not been shown to be effective" [4]. Patients with endometrial polyps prior to tamoxifen initiation may be at higher risk for developing atypical hyperplasia so evaluation with transvaginal ultrasound or hysteroscopy before initiation of therapy may be reasonable [4]. Postmenopausal women on tamoxifen should have close follow-up. Although no routine surveillance should be performed, symptoms, especially vaginal bleeding, should be immediately evaluated. Premenopausal women on tamoxifen do not require additional surveillance besides routine care as this group has no known increased risk of uterine cancer. Tamoxifen has an important role in increasing survival of women with breast cancer, but increases the risk of endometrial pathology. Providers caring for women taking tamoxifen need to be aware of these risks to appropriately maximize benefits to the breast while minimizing risk to the endometrium.

Key teaching points

- Tamoxifen-induced endometrial changes are most often benign.
- Postmenopausal tamoxifen users have a 2–3 times greater risk of developing endometrial cancer than women not taking tamoxifen.
- The overall benefits from tamoxifen in patients with breast cancer outweigh the risks.
- Asymptomatic women on tamoxifen should not be screened for endometrial abnormalities with transvaginal ultrasound, endometrial biopsy, or hysteroscopy. Such screening may lead to unnecessary costly and invasive procedures without benefiting the patient.
- Postmenopausal women taking tamoxifen should be educated about the need for evaluation if they experience any vaginal bleeding or bloody vaginal discharge. These women should be fully evaluated with imaging, visualization of the endometrium with hysteroscopy, and endometrial sampling as necessary.

References

1. Kim HS, Jeon YT, Kim YB. The effect of adjuvant hormonal therapy on the endometrium and ovary of breast cancer patients. *J Gynecol Oncol* 2008;19:256–60.

2. Perez-Medina T, Salazar FJ, San-Frutos L, et al. Hysteroscopic dynamic assessment of the endometrium in patients treated with long-term tamoxifen. *J Minim Invasive Gynecol* 2010;18:349–54.

3. Dibi RP, Zettler CG, Pessini SA, et al. Tamoxifen use and endometrial lesions: hysteroscopic, histological, and immunohistochemical findings in postmenopausal women with breast cancer. *Menopause* 2009;16: 293–300.

4. American College of Obstetricians and Gynecologists. Tamoxifen use and uterine cancer. Committee Opinion No. 336. *Obstet Gynecol* 2006;107: 1475–8.

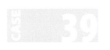

Small mass prolapsing from the cervix found on routine pelvic examination

John G. Pierce Jr

History of present illness

A 41-year-old, gravida 3, para 2-0-1-2, woman presents to the acute care clinic with vaginal itching. The itching has been present for three days, and is similar to episodes of bacterial vaginosis she has had in the past. She has regular periods lasting five days with some cramping. Her menses are heavier on days one and two of her cycle. She reports a normal Pap smear three years ago but recalls one abnormal Pap smear when she was in her early twenties.

She was divorced five years ago and is sexually active with one partner for the last year. She has no medical problems and had a bilateral tubal ligation after her last delivery at the age of 34. She takes no medications.

Physical examination

General appearance: Well-developed, well-nourished, pleasant woman

Vital signs:

Pulse: 88 beats/min
Blood pressure: 142/78 mmHg
Height: 66 inches
Weight: 155 lb

Neck: No thyromegaly

Lungs: Clear to auscultation bilaterally

Cardiovascular exam: Regular rate and rhythm with normal S1 and S2

Abdomen: Soft and nontender, no organomegaly

Pelvic: Normal external genitalia, vagina with scant discharge, cervix shows an approximate 1-cm round lesion at the external os (Fig. 39.1). Uterus is six weeks' size, nontender, and anteverted. There is no cervical motion tenderness. Adnexa are small and nontender

Vaginal pH: 4.5

KOH prep: No hyphae shown

Wet mount: Clue cells present, no trichomonads seen, positive whiff test

Laboratory studies: Urine pregnancy test: Negative

She clearly has bacterial vaginosis, for which you prescribe a seven-day course of oral metronidazole.

How would you manage the mass visible at the cervix?

The patient's mass is most likely an endocervical polyp. It was removed with a ring forceps in the emergency room at the time that it was seen, and sent for pathologic examination, which confirmed a benign endocervical polyp. Her vaginal symptoms resolved with her antibiotics. No mass was present at the time of her next well-woman visit.

Endocervical polyps are among the most common, benign neoplastic growths of the cervix. These lesions are overgrowths of benign endocervical stroma that are covered by epithelium. Most commonly, polyps are asymptomatic and found during a routine pelvic examination. They can be found as incidental findings on exams done for other reasons, as in this patient. Endocervical polyps can present with abnormal uterine bleeding, postcoital bleeding, or symptomatic vaginal discharge/leukorrhea. In this patient, the discharge was clearly bacterial vaginosis, and was unrelated to her polyp.

Typically, an endocervical polyp will appear as a single, red, smooth elongated mass protruding from the endocervical canal (Fig. 39.1). Multiple polyps occur occasionally. The majority of polyps are smooth, soft, and reddish purple to cherry red, varying in size from several millimeters to

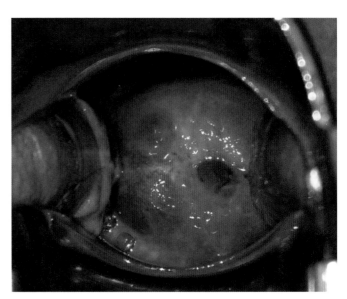

Fig. 39.1 Cervical lesion at the external os.

Acute Care and Emergency Gynecology, ed. David Chelmow, Christine R. Isaacs and Ashley Carroll. Published by Cambridge University Press.
© Cambridge University Press 2015.

2–4 cm. They can be "friable" and bleed when touched or exhibit some degree of inflammation and necrosis. The stalk can be of variable length and width and may arise from either the endocervical canal (endocervical polyp) or the ectocervix (cervical polyp). Endocervical polyps are much more common than ectocervical polyps.

Endocervical polyps are found more frequently in multiparous women in their forties and fifties and are rarely seen in prepubertal females. Besides being identified visually during a routine pelvic examination, some can be identified by cervical cytology findings. For example, evaluation for results showing atypical glandular cells may lead to the identification of an endocervical or endometrial polyp as the cause.

The differential diagnosis includes small prolapsing myomas, endometrial polyps, Nabothian cysts, retained products of conception, squamous papilloma, sarcoma, and cervical cancer. When the diagnosis is uncertain or if cancer is suspected, a biopsy should be performed. Pathologically, endocervical polyps are classified into six histologic types: adenomatous (80%), cystic, fibrous, vascular, inflammatory, and fibromyomatous.

The etiology of an endocervical polyp is thought to be from inflammation or an abnormal focal response to hormonal stimulation. A single enlarged endocervical villus can extend into the acidic vaginal environment initiating the metaplastic process [1]. Overall, an endocervical polyp is typically benign with the risk of dysplasia or malignancy typically less than 1% [2,3]. When stratified by age, symptoms, and cytology, there was no preinvasive disease or cancer in polyps of young, asymptomatic women with normal cervical cytology [4,5].

Polyps are typically removed when seen and the specimen sent for histologic evaluation. Unless they are extremely large or broad-based, they can be safely removed in the office or emergency room. The aim is to remove the entire polyp and stalk. The polyp should be grasped with either a ring forceps or uterine dressing forceps as close to the base of the polyp or stalk as possible. The forceps are then twisted repeatedly rotating the forceps 360° until the polyp twists off and is avulsed. The twisting of the stalk causes strangulation of the vessels supplying the polyp. The repeated twisting often leaves minimal bleeding at the base of the polyp or stalk. If needed, the base can be treated with chemical cautery (silver nitrate or ferric subsulfate), electrocautery, or cryocautery. Endocervical polyps can recur in 6–15% of cases [5,6]. In very unusual instances, the polyp may require excision in the operating room. Intolerance of the exam, heavier bleeding, or partial removal of the polyp may warrant removal in the operating room. Hysteroscopic-guided instruments can be used to excise a polyp deeper in the endocervical canal.

Although most endocervical polyps are benign, polyps should be sent for histologic evaluation. After the polyp is removed, the endometrium should be evaluated in women older than 35–40 years of age who presented with abnormal bleeding to rule out endometrial pathology. If the lesion was asymptomatic, the patient may be followed without performing endometrial sampling. Later, if the patient develops abnormal uterine bleeding, endometrial sampling should be performed.

Key teaching points

- Endocervical polyps are typically asymptomatic, varying in size from a few millimeters to 2–4 cm. They appear as small prolapsing masses at the endocervix.
- Polyps are found more commonly in multiparous patients.
- They are usually removed in the office with ring or uterine dressing forceps by grasping the polyp and twisting it repeatedly until avulsion occurs.
- The risk of dysplasia and cancer is less than 1%.
- Estimated recurrence rate is 6–15%.

References

1. Mayeaux E, Cox T, eds. *Modern Colposcopy Textbook and Atlas*, 3rd edn. Philadelphia, Wolters Kluwer, 2012.

2. Chin N, Platt AB, Nuovo GJ. Squamous intraepithelial lesions arising in benign endocervical polyps: a report of 9 cases with correlation to the Pap smears, HPV analysis, and immunoprofile. *Int J Gynecol Pathol* 2008;27(4):582–90.

3. Schnatz PF, Ricci S, O'Sullivan DM. Cervical polyps in postmenopausal women: Is there a difference in risk? *Menopause* 2009;16(3):524–8.

4. MacKenzie IZ, Naish C, Rees CM, Manek S. Why remove all cervical polyps and examine them histologically? *BJOG* 2009;116(8):1127–9.

5. Younis MT, Iram S, Anwar B, Ewies AA. Women with asymptomatic cervical polyps may not need to see a gynaecologist or have them removed: an observational retrospective study of 1126 cases. *Eur J Obstet Gynecol Reprod Biol* 2010;150(2):190–4.

6. Berzolla CE, Schnatz PF, O'Sullivan DM, et al. Dysplasia and malignancy in endocervical polyps. *J Womens Health (Larchmt)* 2007;16(9):1317–21.

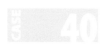

A 35-year-old woman with a painful vulvar mass

Philippe Girerd

History of present illness

A 35-year-old gravida 3, para 2, ab 1, woman presents to the emergency room with a week-long history of an increasingly painful swelling in her right labium majus. This began 10 days earlier with a punctate itchy lesion, which she thought was a spider bite. She reports having had scant bleeding, which she attributes to her scratching the area. A few days later she noticed redness spreading from the initial lesion and the formation of a tender nodule. She denies fever, malaise, or other systemic symptoms. She has never had anything like this before. She shaves her genital hair and has had a few small "pimple"-like lesions on occasion.

She is sexually active in a monogamous relationship. She reacts to sulfa drugs with itching and hives. She takes no other medications. She denies any medical problems.

Physical examination

General appearance: Healthy appearing woman who is in mild discomfort

Vital signs:

Temperature: 37.2°C
Pulse: 92 beats/min
Blood pressure: 116/74 mmHg
Respiratory rate: 16 breaths/min

HEENT: Unremarkable
Chest: Clear to auscultation
Heart: Regular rate and rhythm, no murmurs, rubs, or gallops
Abdomen: Soft, nontender, no rebound
Pelvic:

Erythema on the right labium majus extending superiorly 2 cm to the ipsilateral, lower mons (Fig. 40.1). The area is warm and slightly tender. There is a 2 cm moderately tender, fluctuant mass in the anterior portion of the right labium majus even with the level of the urethral opening. The area of the Bartholin's gland is soft and not involved. There is no crepitus or excessive tenderness. All integument appears viable and hyperemic with excellent capillary refill
Perineum and anus: Normal
Speculum examination: No speculum examination was performed at patient request due to pain
Bimanual examination: Within normal limits. The right vaginal sidewall was normal with no evidence of the process-spreading cephalad
Crural areas and thighs: Normal

How would you manage this patient?

The patient most likely has a vulvar abscess. Vulvar abscesses are frequently preceded by a history of pubic hair shaving or, less commonly, a spider bite or other vulvar trauma. She was treated in the emergency room with incision and drainage, placement of ribbon gauze in the wound, and local care with twice daily "sitz baths" in Epsom salts. At subsequent office visits, rapid resolution was observed and no antibiotics were necessary.

Vulvar abscess

This patient has labial swelling, erythema, tenderness, and warmth to touch over the affected area, which are classic signs of infection. When these findings are localized to an area with fluctuance, as in this case, abscess is likely. Since the

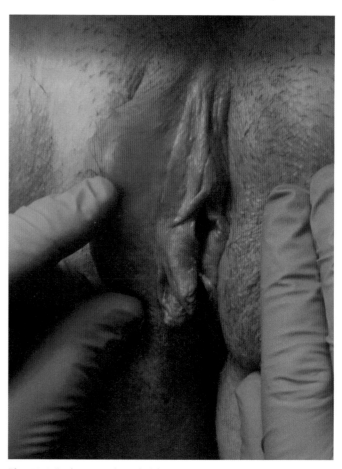

Fig. 40.1 Erythema on the right labium majus.

Acute Care and Emergency Gynecology, ed. David Chelmow, Christine R. Isaacs and Ashley Carroll. Published by Cambridge University Press. © Cambridge University Press 2015.

surrounding areas of this infection (upper mons, crura, buttocks, and thighs) show no signs of infection, cellulitis is not likely an important component here.

The distribution and location of this infection suggests involvement of *Staphyloccus aureus*. Streptococcal infections of the integument can also occur but generally cause cellulitis and are less likely to cause localized abscesses [1]. Skin abscesses are monoinfections resulting from *S. aureus* in up to 75% of cases [2]. The majority of vulvar abscesses are associated with methicillin-resistant *S. aureus* (MRSA) [3]. Interestingly, this can be a sexually transmitted disease [4]. Bartholin's gland abscesses are commonly polymicrobial. Vulvar abscesses originating in the skin and its appendages, however, are less often polymicrobial but may involve *Streptococci*, *Escherichia coli*, *Proteus*, *Klebsiella*, *Peptostreptococcus*, or *Bacteroides fragilis* [5].

There are two important diagnostic considerations. First, necrotizing infections can occur in the groin and external genitalia, are life threatening, and must be ruled out in patients with vulvar abscesses. Risk factors include diabetes, cancer, immune compromise, and poor nutrition. Features of necrotic infections include abnormal sensation, hyperesthesia (such as intense pain from a small stimulus), or, conversely, hypoesthesia or complete absence of sensation. Abnormal coloration spanning from pale grey to black is suggestive of necrosis and is typically accompanied by poor capillary refill. Second, infections arising in the epithelium must be differentiated from those arising in the Bartholin gland. Bartholin's gland cysts or infections require formation of a stoma to provide long-term drainage and prevent recurrence.

Treatment of skin abscesses can include local care, surgical intervention, and antibiotic therapy. Local care is usually directed towards smaller (2 cm or less) abscesses that show no signs of spread. Warm compresses or "sitz baths" with magnesium sulfate (Epsom salts) two or three times a day may be used. Although local care is usually effective, careful counseling and clinic follow-up is strongly recommended to allow early intervention in the event of a worsening abscess.

Incision and drainage (I&D) is often necessary with abscesses larger than 2 cm and for smaller abscesses that persist or appear to be "pointing." I&D involves making a small incision where the epithelium is thinnest. Loculations are sometimes encountered. If the lesion does not adequately decrease in size during the procedure, then a probe or hemostat may be introduced to break up loculations. Cultures of infected material should be obtained to document the presence of MRSA. A "wick" left in the incision will allow continued drainage of the abscess cavity. Plain ribbon gauze is preferred. Iodoform, peroxide or povidone have cytotoxic effects on cells involved in the healing process and should be avoided. Smaller, simpler abscesses may be drained in the office. Cases involving abscesses of 5 cm or more, significant cellulitis, or suspicion of deep involvement or necrosis should be done in an operating room setting. Follow-up should optimally include daily wick changes, which can be done by visiting nurses. Patients should be reexamined at an interval determined by the severity of the initial presentation and the response to treatment to assure resolution. Pain control requirements may range from oral nonsteroidal anti-inflammatory drugs to inpatient parenteral administration of narcotics.

Although local care or I&D can often clear smaller abscesses, antibiotics should be administered if the abscess is large or cellulitis is present. Since a high proportion of vulvar abscesses harbor MRSA, initial empiric antibiotic coverage should cover MRSA until cultures prove otherwise. Appropriate choices include trimethoprim/sulfamethoxazole (TMP/SMX), doxycycline or clindamycin [6]. Doxycycline would be a good choice for this particular patient due to her sulfa allergy. In most regions, MRSA is sensitive to tetracyclines and TMP/SMX. Sensitivity to clindamycin varies. Coverage for beta-hemolytic streptococcus with cephalexin or amoxicillin/clavulanate is appropriate when cellulitis is present.

Key teaching points

- A vulvar abscess should be treated as a methicillin-resistant *S. aureus* (MRSA) infection unless proven otherwise.
- Care must be exercised to correctly differentiate non-Bartholin's vulvar abscesses from Bartholin's abscesses as the treatment differs.
- All groin and vulvar abscesses must be evaluated carefully to rule out necrotizing infection.
- Outpatient treatment is possible in many cases of vulvar abscess.

References

1. Gabillot-Carré M, Roujeau JC. Acute bacterial skin infections and cellulitis. *Curr Opin Infect Dis* 2007;20:118–23.

2. Summanen PH, Talan DA, Strong C, et al. Bacteriology of skin and soft-tissue infections: Comparison of infections in intravenous drug users and individuals with no history of intravenous drug use. *Clin Infect Dis* 1995;20(2):S279–82.

3. Thurman AR, Satterfield TM, Soper DE. Methicillin-resistant *Staphylococcus aureus* as a common cause of vulvar abscesses. *Obstet Gynecol* 2008; 112(3):538–44.

4. Roberts, JR, McCawley L, Laxton M, Trumbo H. Genital community associated methicillin-resistant *Staphylococcus aureus* infection can be a sexually transmitted disease. *Ann Emerg Med* 2007;50: 93–4.

5. Kilpatrick CC, Alagkiozidis I, Orejuela FJ, et al. Factors complicating surgical management of the vulvar abscess. *J Reprod Med* 2010;55:139–42.

6. Liu C, Bayer A, Cosgrove SE, et al. Clinical practice guidelines by the Infectious Diseases Society of America for the treatment of methicillin-resistant *Staphylococcus aureus* infections in adults and children: Executive summary. *Clin Infect Dis* 2011;52:285–92.

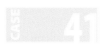

A 32-year-old woman urgently referred for a cervical mass noted on routine pelvic examination

Christopher A. Manipula

History of present illness

A 32-year-old gravida 0 woman presents to your office after being referred urgently by her primary care physician for a cervical mass. Her doctor noted the lesion while collecting a cervical cytology specimen during her annual exam. The patient is nervous and anxious because she is worried this could be cancer. She reports that her cycles continue to be regular, occurring every 28–30 days. Her last menstrual period began a week and a half ago. She denies any irregular bleeding, vaginal discharge, pain, or odors. She is married and has been taking oral contraceptives for the last five years. The patient's cervical cancer screening has always been normal including her testing one week prior, which was negative for both cytology and high-risk human papillomavirus (HPV). The patient has no other significant past medical, surgical, or family history. She does not smoke, and drinks alcohol only socially.

Physical examination

General appearance: Well developed, well-groomed, well-nourished woman who is mildly anxious

Vital signs:

Temperature: 37.0°C
Pulse: 85 beats/min
Blood pressure: 122/76 mmHg
Respiratory rate: 16 breaths/min
Oxygen saturation: 99% on room air
BMI: 24 kg/m^2

Head and neck: No palpable masses, no lymphadenopathy

Cardiovascular: Normal rate, no murmurs, rubs, or gallops

Respiratory: Clear to auscultation bilaterally, no wheezing, rales, or crackles

Abdomen: Soft, nontender, no scars or organomegaly

External genitalia: Unremarkable

Vagina: No discharge, no masses or lesions

Cervix:

Nulliparous, nonfriable cervix, no mucopurulent discharge. Two lesions noted on the cervix (Fig. 41.1). The first lesion is a translucent cyst located at the 12 o'clock position measuring approximately 5 mm in diameter. The second lesion is a yellowish, opaque cyst that is present at the 6 o'clock position measuring approx. 3 mm in diameter. The patient denies any pain or tenderness during the examination

Bimanual examination: The uterus is anteverted, nontender, symmetric and mobile. The adnexa were unremarkable. Both cysts are palpable and firm

Laboratory studies: Urine pregnancy test: Negative

How would you manage this patient?

These two lesions are consistent with Nabothian cysts. Nabothian cysts are benign mucus-filled lesions that can occur on the surface of the cervix. They usually do not cause any problems, and treatment is not necessary. A biopsy of the lesion is also not necessary when the clinical diagnosis is certain. It is important to reassure the patient that this is a common, benign, incidental finding that requires no intervention. The patient was instructed to continue with routine annual exams and was given reassurance.

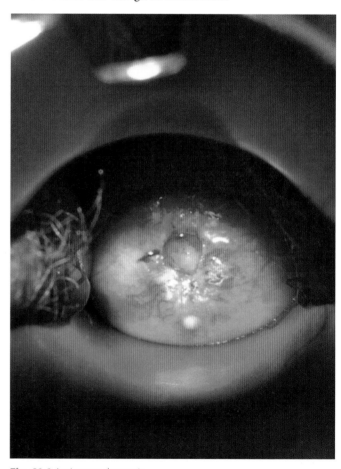

Fig. 41.1 Lesions on the cervix.

Acute Care and Emergency Gynecology, ed. David Chelmow, Christine R. Isaacs and Ashley Carroll. Published by Cambridge University Press. © Cambridge University Press 2015.

Nabothian cysts

Nabothian cysts are common incidental findings that are considered a normal feature of the adult cervix. They are named after the German anatomist Martin Naboth who described them in 1707, but they are also referred to as "mucinous retention cysts" or "epithelial cysts." Anatomically, the cervix is comprised of an endocervical canal and an outer cervical surface. The canal is lined with columnar epithelium and glands that secrete mucous. The outer cervical surface is comprised of squamous epithelium. These two areas meet at a transformation zone known as the squamocolumnar junction. Within the transformation zone, the columnar epithelium and glands may get covered by squamous epithelium. The endocervical glands will continue to produce mucus, but due to the covering and blockage by the squamous epithelium, the mucus is not released and a retention cyst or "Nabothian cyst" is formed.

Nabothian cysts can range in size from a few millimeters to as large as 3–4 cm [1]. There may also be multiple cysts on one cervix. Most commonly, Nabothian cysts are asymptomatic and typically encountered during routine gynecologic exams when the cervix is visualized. Occasionally, the cysts can become numerous and block the cervical os, making it difficult to obtain an endocervical specimen for cancer screening. Rarely, a woman may have complaints of fullness or pain due to an enlarged or multiple cysts. If this problem should arise, the cysts can be treated using electrocautery ablation or excision. Most patients with Nabothian cysts only need reassurance, as in the case of this patient. Currently, there are no medications for the treatment or prevention of Nabothian cysts.

The provider should be able to differentiate Nabothian cysts from other lesions of the cervix, both benign lesions and those with malignant potential. Approximately 3–9% of all fibroids originate anatomically from the cervix [1]. These masses tend to be a lot firmer than Nabothian cysts, and while most cervical fibroids are asymptomatic, they can occasionally cause dyspareunia, dysuria, menorrhagia, or dysmenorrhea. One way to determine the difference between a fibroid versus a Nabothian cyst is to make a small incision at the surface of the cystic mass/lesion. Nabothian cysts are mucus filled and will drain upon incising, while fibroids will appear solid. Adenomyosis can also involve the endocervical canal and form a mass that can protrude into the cervix [1]. A biopsy is necessary to confirm the diagnosis. Cervical polyps can also arise from the cervix and similarly, are often noted as an incidental finding during a routine exam. Patients may be asymptomatic, or may present with postcoital, intermenstrual, or postmenopausal bleeding. The etiology of cervical polyps is unknown, and most are benign. The incidence of malignancy is 1 in 1000, with malignancy being more common in postmenopausal women [1]. Excision or biopsy of any lesion is recommended when the diagnosis is uncertain or if malignancy is suspected.

When a Nabothian cyst is unusually large, it may cause an overall enlargement of the cervix that can be difficult to diagnose with visual inspection alone, and may raise concern for malignancy. Most cervical cancers are squamous epithelium in origin, but 20–25% can arise from the cells of the columnar epithelium [2]. Adenoma malignum is an adenocarcinoma of the mucinous type that can easily be mistaken for multiple Nabothian cysts because of its appearance [3]. These patients can similarly present with no symptoms, but are found to have an enlarged cervix with a cystic mass on routine exam. While Nabothian cysts tend to be more superficial, an adenoma malignum tends to invade deeper into the cervical stroma. If the patient has associated symptoms, such as pain or irregular bleeding, the diagnosis must be investigated further. Transvaginal sonography and MRI have been used to help differentiate benign versus malignant lesions. Nabothian cysts have a high T2 signal intensity on MRI versus adenocarcinomas, while adenocarcinomas have higher vascularity in the surrounding tissues that can be identified using sonography with Doppler imaging [4]. If malignancy is ever suspected, the patient should undergo a biopsy or excision.

The overwhelming majority of women with Nabothian cysts do not know that they have them. They are asymptomatic, incidental findings noted when patients present for well-woman check-ups or other gynecologic concerns requiring visualization of the cervix. For these women, reassurance is all that is required. Only rarely do Nabothian cysts require intervention for symptom relief or to confirm the diagnosis. Clinicians experienced in visualizing the cervix most often can make the clinical diagnosis with confidence and counsel patients accordingly as in this case.

Key teaching points

- Nabothian cysts are common benign lesions of the cervix that are often found during routine gynecologic examinations in asymptomatic women.
- Nabothian cysts require no treatment or intervention other than reassurance to the patient.
- There is currently no medical therapy for prevention of Nabothian cysts.
- Biopsy and/or drainage of a cyst may occasionally be necessary to confirm the diagnosis of a Nabothian cyst, particularly in patients presenting with associated symptoms of bleeding, pain, or an enlarged cervix.

References

1. Casey P, Long M, Marnach M. Abnormal cervical appearance: What to do, when to worry? *Mayo Clin Proc* 2011;86(2):147–51.

2. Seoud M, Tjalma W, Ronsse V. Cervical adenocarcinoma: Moving towards better prevention. *Vaccine* 2011;29:9148–58.

3. Sosnovski V, Barenboim R, Cohen HI, Bornstein J. Complex Nabothian cysts: A diagnostic dilemma. *Arch Gynecol Obstet* 2009;279:759–61.

4. Park S, Lee J, Lee Y, et al. Multilocular cystic lesions in the uterine cervix: Broad spectrum of imaging features and pathologic correlation. *AJR* 2010;195:517–23.

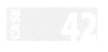

An 18-year-old woman with long-acting reversible contraception and new-onset bleeding

Jennifer Salcedo and Aparna Sridhar

History of present illness

An 18-year-old gravida 0 woman presents to your urgent care clinic with complaint of three days of moderate dark vaginal bleeding accompanied by mild pelvic cramping. She had a Nexplanon® (etonogestrel) contraceptive implant placed three months ago for long-acting reversible contraception after she had difficulty remembering to take oral contraceptive pills as prescribed. She has a long-term history of irregular menstrual cycles. She is uncertain of her last menstrual period, but believes it was a few weeks prior to the Nexplanon placement. Urine pregnancy testing performed in the office before the Nexplanon placement was negative.

Her past medical history is unremarkable. She takes no other medications. She has never had surgery. She is sexually active with a single partner.

Due to a recent change in insurance, she is unable to follow-up with her previous provider and wants reassurance that her current symptoms are normal before she leaves to travel for the summer.

Physical examination

General appearance: Well-developed, well-nourished woman who is in no distress
Vital signs:

Temperature: 37.0°C
Pulse: 86 beats/min
Blood pressure: 106/70 mmHg
Respiratory rate: 18 breaths/min
Oxygen saturation: 100% on room air

Extremities: Nexplanon rod palpable in left upper arm, approximately 8 cm proximal to the medial epicondyle in the intermuscular groove
Abdomen: Soft, nontender
External genitalia: Unremarkable without lesions
Vagina: Approximately 10 cc dark-appearing blood in the vault with one dime-sized clot. No mucopurulent discharge
Cervix: Closed without lesions. No cervical motion tenderness
Uterus: Fourteen-week size, mobile, mid-position, nontender
Adnexa: Nontender without masses

Laboratory studies:

Urine pregnancy test: Positive
CBC: Within normal limits
Blood type: O positive

Imaging: Transabdominal pelvic ultrasound shows a singleton intrauterine pregnancy consistent with 14 weeks and 1 day, posterior placenta without previa, cardiac motion present, uterus and cervix within normal limits, ovaries not clearly visualized, no adnexal masses seen, and no pelvic free fluid

How would you manage this patient?

The patient had a Nexplanon contraceptive implant placed a few weeks following her last menstrual period, prior to which she was irregularly using oral contraceptive pills. Inadequately protected intercourse took place prior to Nexplanon initiation, resulting in a pregnancy that was too early to be detected by the urine pregnancy testing performed in the office. The patient did not realize that her amenorrhea could be the result of pregnancy, given her history of irregular menstrual cycles and expectations for irregular bleeding with Nexplanon use. She now presents with a threatened abortion at 14 weeks' gestation, a complication unrelated to Nexplanon use. She needs referral for pregnancy options counseling and follow-up. Unlike an intrauterine device (IUD), the Nexplanon implant presents no threat to the ongoing pregnancy, and removal may be deferred to follow-up.

Implantable contraception

Nexplanon is a single-rod subdermal contraceptive implant containing a core of 68 mg of etonogestrel, a progestin, which is released over a period of 3 years. It is 4 cm in length and 2 mm in diameter. Nexplanon is a radiopaque second-generation version of the original etonogestrel implant, Implanon®, which was approved in the United States in 2006. It is distributed in a specially designed preloaded applicator and inserted under local anesthesia. All healthcare providers who provide Nexplanon insertion and removal must complete a formal training program administered by the device manufacturer [1]. Its primary mechanism of action is suppression of ovulation. It is the most effective method of reversible contraception, with a failure rate of 0.05% during the first year of use [2]. Its noncontraceptive benefits include improvement of dysmenorrhea and decreased pelvic pain related to endometriosis [3].

Acute Care and Emergency Gynecology, ed. David Chelmow, Christine R. Isaacs and Ashley Carroll. Published by Cambridge University Press.
© Cambridge University Press 2015.

Changes in menstrual bleeding patterns are common and may include amenorrhea, infrequent, frequent, or prolonged bleeding. However, Nexplanon users experience fewer mean bleeding and spotting days per cycle than women with natural menstrual cycles. Women with favorable bleeding profiles during the first three months of implant use are likely to continue such bleeding patterns, while those with unfavorable bleeding patterns have a 50% chance of those patterns improving. Women with lower body weight have fewer bleeding and spotting days with implant use than women with higher body weight [4]. The 1-year continuation rate for implant users is 84%, which compares favorably to the 67% annual continuation rate of oral contraceptive pill users [2].

According to the US Medical Eligibility for Contraceptive Use [5], use of the etonogestrel contraceptive implant by most women is category 1, meaning there are no restrictions for its use. There are few women for whom the theoretical risks of implant use are thought to outweigh the anticipated benefits. Such women include: those in whom ischemic heart disease or stroke begins or worsens during implant use; lupus and positive or unknown antiphospholipid antibodies; migraines with aura that begins or worsens during implant use; undiagnosed abnormal vaginal bleeding suspicious for malignancy; history of breast cancer in remission for at least five years; and severe liver disease or cancer. Implant use is only absolutely contraindicated for women with current breast cancer. There is no known harm to the woman, the course of her pregnancy, or the fetus if systemic progestin-only contraception (pill, injection, implant) is inadvertently used during pregnancy [5].

According to the US Selected Practice Recommendations for Contraceptive Use [6], a contraceptive implant can be inserted at any time when it is reasonably certain that the woman is not pregnant. A healthcare provider can be reasonably certain a woman is not pregnant if she lacks signs and symptoms of pregnancy and meets any of the following criteria: she is within seven days from the start of normal menses; has not has intercourse since the start of the last normal menses; has been correctly and consistently using a reliable method of contraception; is within seven days of a spontaneous or induced abortion; is within four weeks postpartum; or is exclusively breast-feeding and amenorrheic within six months of birth. In these circumstances, a pregnancy test is not required, but may be ordered based on clinical judgment. If a woman is not within five days of the start of her last menses, a back-up method of contraception, such as condoms, should be used for seven days following implant insertion [6]. In this case, at the time of Nexplanon insertion the provider

could not be reasonably certain the woman was not pregnant. If the decision had been made with the patient to proceed with Nexplanon insertion, the possibility of an early undetected pregnancy should have been discussed, and a plan made for follow-up pregnancy testing.

Urine pregnancy testing

Both qualitative urine pregnancy point-of-care (POC) tests used in medical settings and those purchased over-the-counter for home testing demonstrate wide variability in their sensitivity for detecting human chorionic gonadotropin (hCG). This variability is even more substantial when it comes to detecting the variants of hCG, such as hyperglycosylated hCG, that are common and variably excreted in early pregnancy [7]. POC tests demonstrate sensitivities of approximately 40–77% for detecting pregnancy the day of missed menses, and have been found to have lower sensitivities than available home tests [8]. Specifically, POC tests have poor sensitivity at hCG concentrations of 20–300 IU/L, and are correct only 50% of the time when evaluating urine with hCG in this range [9]. Home tests demonstrate a sensitivity of 55–100% in detecting pregnancy on the day of missed menses. At least 1 home pregnancy test has demonstrated the ability to detect 25% of pregnancies 6 days prior to missed menses and 74% of pregnancies 3 days prior to missed menses. However, it is important to note that at 6 days, 5 days, and 4 days prior to missed menses, only 29%, 40%, and 76% of pregnancies, respectively, have implanted and are releasing hCG [8]. In this case, the Nexplanon was likely placed during the woman's periovulatory period, during which time neither home nor POC pregnancy tests would be expected to detect the conception.

Key teaching points

- The Nexplanon implant is the most effective reversible method of contraception.
- Pregnancy should always be suspected in women who present with abnormal bleeding or pregnancy-related symptoms, even if the patient has a history of highly effective contraception use or sterilization.
- Qualitative urine pregnancy testing is inconsistently reliable until several days after missed menses.
- If a healthcare provider cannot be reasonably certain that a woman is not pregnant at the time of contraception initiation, emergency contraception should be offered, if appropriate, and a plan for follow-up pregnancy testing should be made.

References

1. American College of Obstetricians and Gynecologists. Long-acting reversible contraception: Implants and intrauterine devices. Practice Bulletin No. 121. *Obstet Gynecol* 2011;118:184–96.

2. Trussell L. Contraceptive failure in the United States. *Contraception* 2011;83:397–404.

3. Walch K, Unfried G, Huber J, et al. Implanon versus medroxyprogesterone acetate: effects on pain scores in patients

with symptomatic endometriosis – a pilot study. *Contraception* 2009;79:29–34.

4. Mansour D, Korver T, Marintcheva-Petrova M, Fraser IS. The effects of Implanon on menstrual bleeding

patterns. *Eur J Contracept Reprod Health Care* 2008;13(Suppl 1):13–28.

5. Centers for Disease Control and Prevention. US medical eligibility criteria for contraceptive use. *MMWR* 2010;59(RR-4):1–86.

6. Centers for Disease Control and Prevention. US selected practice recommendations for contraceptive use. *MMWR* 2013;62(RR-5):1–46.

7. Cervinski MA, Lockwood CM, Ferguson AM, et al. Qualitative point-of-care and over-the-counter urine hCG devices differently detect the hCG variants of early pregnancy. *Clinica Chimica Acta* 2009;406:81–5.

8. Cole LA. The hCG assay or pregnancy test. *Clin Chem Lab Med* 2012;50: 617–30.

9. Green DN, Schmidt RL, Kamer SM, et al. Limitations in qualitative point of care hCG tests for detecting early pregnancy. *Clinica Chimica Acta* 2013;415:317–21.

Cyclic pain after endometrial ablation

Ellen L. Brock

History of present illness

A 47-year-old married gravida 4, para 4 woman presents for an urgent visit due to severe pelvic pain worsening over the last 24 hours that has not responded to ibuprofen. Approximately 18 months prior she had undergone an endometrial ablation for menorrhagia, and she had been amenorrheic after the ablation until 3 months ago when she experienced a heavy painful menstrual bleed. Subsequently, she has had monthly menses accompanied by right-sided pain that was severe enough on one occasion to warrant an emergency room evaluation.

Her past medical history is unremarkable. Her obstetric/surgical history is significant for two prior vaginal deliveries followed by two Cesarean deliveries, with a tubal ligation performed during the second. She is on no medications, drinks alcohol socially, and works full time as a lawyer. Her review of symptoms is negative other than the pelvic pain as described.

Physical examination

General appearance: Alert-and-oriented woman appearing in mild distress

Vital signs:

Pulse 69 beats/min

Blood pressure: 131/69 mmHg

Respiratory rate: 16 breaths/min

BMI: 37 kg/m^2

Chest: Clear

Cardiac: Normal auscultation

Abdomen: Soft, no palpable masses, pain noted with palpation in the right lower quadrant

Pelvic:

External genitalia: Normal

Vagina: Normal

Cervix: Normal

Uterus: Upper normal size; uterine tenderness noted in both adnexal/cornual regions

Ovaries: Without palpable masses

Imaging: Transvaginal ultrasound shows a normal uterus with a small amount of fluid in the endometrial cavity. Adnexa appeared normal

How would you manage this patient?

Cyclic pelvic pain following endometrial ablation can be related to a central hematometra, a cornual hematometra, post-ablation tubal sterilization syndrome (PATSS) or endometriosis. This patient's history of a prior tubal ligation makes the diagnosis of PATSS more likely.

Because of this patient's new onset bleeding, she initially underwent a hysteroscopic examination to rule out malignancy. The cavity was contracted with no visible endometrium, and no endometrial tissue was identified in curettings. She continued to have severe debilitating pain and underwent laparoscopic hysterectomy with bilateral salpingectomies. At surgery she was found to have a normal appearing uterus and ovaries, and mildly dilated proximal tubal segments, consistent with the diagnosis of PATSS (Fig. 43.1).

Postoperatively the patient did well, and her pain completely resolved. Pathology confirmed intraluminal blood in the proximal tubal segments with acute and chronic inflammation.

Post-ablation tubal sterilization syndrome

Post-ablation tubal sterilization syndrome (PATSS) was initially described as a long-term complication following resectoscopic endometrial ablation. Subsequently, cases have been reported with all currently available types of global endometrial ablation devices (hot water balloon, free circulating hot water, bipolar radio-frequency array, cryoablation, and microwave ablation). Destruction of the endometrial surface results

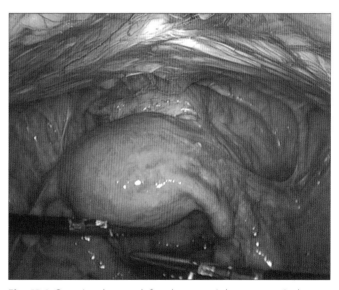

Fig. 43.1 Operative photograph from laparoscopic hysterectomy in the patient with post-ablation tubal sterilization syndrome. The proximal tubal stumps are moderately dilated, a finding that varies according to timing within the menstrual cycle.

Acute Care and Emergency Gynecology, ed. David Chelmow, Christine R. Isaacs and Ashley Carroll. Published by Cambridge University Press. © Cambridge University Press 2015.

in scarring and contracture of the endometrial cavity, producing an absolute or relative outflow obstruction. Because the cornual portion of the endometrium may be spared during an ablation procedure due to difficult access and thinness of the myometrium in that area, functioning cornual endometrium often persists. In the presence of an outflow obstruction, retrograde bleeding can occur with distention of the proximal fallopian tubal segment. The tube is occluded distally due to prior sterilization and, thus, the symptom of cyclic pain ensues. The cyclic pain of PATSS develops months to even years following endometrial ablation. The delay in presentation is thought to be related to the progression of endometrial scarring over many months following ablation, and the likelihood that outflow tract obstructions can develop months to years after the procedure [1].

PATSS occurs in approximately 10% of women undergoing endometrial ablation after a prior tubal sterilization, with reported incidences in various studies of up to 33%. It is not yet known whether PATSS occurs more or less frequently with global ablation devices than with resectoscopic or rollerball techniques. A recent Cochrane review of ablation complications showed no difference in the incidence of hysterectomy following ablations done with first- versus second-generation devices in the first five years following ablation, with a modest decrease in hysterectomy following global endometrial ablation after the first five years [2].

The diagnosis of PATSS can be difficult. Hematosalpinx may be visible in the proximal tubal stump if ultrasound imaging studies are performed during a woman's menses. Between menstrual cycles, however, the hematosalpinx may lessen significantly or may reabsorb altogether and may not be visible. T2-weighted MRI imaging can identify blood sequestered in the cornual and tubal regions. The diagnosis should be suspected whenever a patient with a prior history of a tubal ligation presents after ablation with new-onset unilateral or bilateral pelvic pain. The differential diagnosis will also include a central or cornual hematometra. Central hematometra can occur when there is occlusion of the lower uterine segment or cervix, with persistent functioning endometrium proximally. Cornual hematometra can occur when the proximal tubal segments and the distal endometrial canal are occluded, with persistence of functioning cornual endometrium. Adenomyosis can also be responsible for post-ablation cyclic pain. More rarely, adnexal abscesses or endometriosis have been reported following ablation, presumably due to either rupture or fistula formation of the proximal tubal stump.

The first patients presenting with PATSS were managed with attempts at relieving the outflow obstruction hysteroscopically, or by laparoscopic salpingectomy. However, many treatment failures have been reported for salpingectomy, leading most experts to recommend hysterectomy with salpingectomy as the treatment of choice [3]. Differentiating PATSS from central hematometra is important, since the latter can be

managed by dilatation of the cervix and drainage of the blood collection. Differentiation from other entities presenting as cyclic pain following ablation is less critical from a practical standpoint, as most of these women will require hysterectomy.

As the primary purpose of endometrial ablation is to avoid hysterectomy, it is desirable to find techniques to prevent endometrial contracture and outflow obstruction after ablation, or to use mechanisms of sterilization that carry less risk for PATSS development. Some authors have recommended a partial ablation technique, wherein either the anterior or posterior surface (but not both) of the endometrium is destroyed. The presence of intact endometrium on the opposite surface will theoretically prevent cavity obliteration due to scarring. This method has not been widely adopted, given the guaranteed persistence of menses and the primary use of global ablation devices in current practice. Other authors have advocated for methods of sterilization that occlude the tube at the cornu. All currently used laparoscopic tubal sterilization devices are recommended for use in the tubal midsegment only. Solutions would involve either laparoscopic salpingectomy for sterilization, or transcervical sterilization. Transcervical sterilization in a patient desiring ablation should be done at least three months prior to the ablation procedure to allow for the three-month hysterosalpingogram documentation of tubal occlusion.

As an alternative to endometrial ablation, the levonorgestrel intrauterine device (LNG-IUD) can also be an effective treatment for managing heavy menstrual bleeding. It has compared favorably with both systemic therapy and endometrial ablation. While the reduction in menstrual blood loss with the LNG-IUD is less than with ablation, there is no difference in effect on hemoglobin, and satisfaction rates with both methods are high [4].

This patient's tubal ligation was performed remote from her presentation with menorrhagia. Given her history of tubal ligation and her relatively young age, she had been counseled preoperatively about long-term sequelae of ablation, including PATSS. She had also been offered a LNG-IUD for management of her menorrhagia, but had declined.

Key teaching points
- Women with a history of a tubal ligation are at an estimated 10% risk for developing post-ablation tubal sterilization syndrome (PATSS) after an endometrial ablation.
- PATSS results when functioning cornual endometrium persists following ablation. In the presence of outflow obstruction, retrograde bleeding can occur with distention of the proximal fallopian tubal segment that has been occluded more distally by a prior sterilization procedure.
- Preoperative diagnosis of PATSS is difficult. Unless there is demonstrated central hematometra (which can be relieved

by cervical dilatation), women with cyclic pain after ablation will generally require hysterectomy for definitive management.

- There is insufficient evidence for recommending any specific ablation device or technique for decreasing the risk of PATSS.

References

1. McCausland A, McCausland V. Long-term complications of endometrial ablation: Cause, diagnosis, treatment, prevention. *J Minim Invasive Gynecol* 2007;12:399–406.

2. Lethaby A, Penninx J, Hickey M, Garry R, Marjoribanks J. Endometrial resection and ablation techniques for heavy menstrual bleeding. *Cochrane Database Syst Rev* 2013, Issue 8. Art. No.: CD001501. DOI: 10.1002/14651858.CD001501.pub4.

3. American College of Obstetricians and Gynecologists. Endometrial ablation. Practice Bulletin No. 81. *Obstet Gynecol* 2007;109(5):1233–48.

4. Lethaby A, Cooke I, Rees MC. Progesterone or progestogen-releasing intrauterine systems for heavy menstrual bleeding. *Cochrane Database Syst Rev* 2005, Issue 4. Art. No.: CD002126. DOI: 10.1002/14651858.CD002126.pub2.

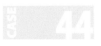

Positive hCG in a patient who reports no sexual activity for one year

Roger P. Smith

History of present illness

A 23-year-old gravida 3, para 3 woman presents to the emergency room (ER) with a 6-hour history of new-onset sharp right lower quadrant abdominal pain. Her last menstrual period was 26 days ago and was normal. The patient reports that she has not been sexually active with a male partner for the last year. The patient's pain began abruptly two hours before she arrived, while the patient was in her exercise class. It has grown steadily worse. She has noted mild nausea but no vomiting. Her bowel movements have been normal.

Past history reveals that she was raised on a farm with two other siblings and has generally been healthy. Menarche was at age 12 and her cycles have been regular and normal when she was not pregnant. Her last pregnancy delivered 16 months ago and was normal. She had a vaginal delivery. Her physician expressed concern that she bled more than normal after the delivery. She did not require blood transfusion.

Physical examination

General appearance: Well-developed, well-nourished woman appearing in mild distress

Vital signs:

Temperature: 37.0°C
Pulse: 75 beats/min
Blood pressure: 132/80 mmHg
Respiratory rate: 18 breaths/min
Oxygen saturation: 100% on room air

Abdomen: Soft, mildly tender in the right lower quadrant, with no organomegally

External genitalia: Unremarkable

Vagina: Normal. Scant discharge is present

Cervix: Parous. No mucopurulent discharge

Uterus: Anteverted, nontender, normal size, mobile

Adnexa: Moderately tender on the right side with diffuse fullness. No masses palpable on the left. Mild cervical motion tenderness is present but no rebound

Laboratory studies:

Serum beta-hCG: 180 mIU/mL
Microscopy of vaginal secretions with normal saline and KOH: Normal

Clinical course

The patient's pain gradually improved during the course of the evaluation in the ER, and was completely resolved by 10 hours after she presented. A urinary pregnancy test was negative. The patient was discharged. A follow-up serum beta-human chorionic gonadotropin (beta-hCG) level performed a week later was 200 mIU/mL. She reports the onset of vaginal bleeding four days after her ER visit, consistent with her normal menses.

How would you manage this patient?

The patient has falsely positive hCG testing due to heterophilic antibodies. Her resolved right lower quadrant pain was likely from a hemorrhagic corpus luteum cyst. Reassurance and education about the falsely positive serum pregnancy tests are all that are required. She should be instructed to inform all future healthcare providers of this problem, and the information should be included in her medical record [1].

False-positive hCG test results

The development of highly sensitive assays for proteins, such as hCG, has lead to diagnostic tests that can detect pregnancy even before the first missed period. Most of these tests use some form of intermediate antigen–antibody complex formation (sandwich assay) to detect the presence of the target protein, in this case hCG. Some individuals have circulating antibodies in their serum that interact with this process, the most common of which are heterophilic antibodies (Fig. 44.1) [2]. Heterophilic antibodies are human antibodies directed against the animal-derived antigens used in many immunoassays. These antibodies, most commonly against mouse or goat antigens, can create both false positive and false negative results. Two-site, noncompetitive immunoassays are particularly susceptible. In these assays, the target protein in the sample is bound to the antibody site, then a labeled detectable antibody is bound to the complex. The amount of labeled antibody is then measured, being directly proportional to the concentration of the target molecule. This type of assay is also known as a sandwich assay because the target protein is part of a "sandwich" with the other two components (Fig. 44.1). Heterophilic antibodies are typically not strong enough to interfere with competitive binding assays. Heterophilic antibodies are of particular importance clinically for their use in detecting Epstein–Barr virus, where immunoglobulin M (IgM) antibodies with an affinity for sheep and horse red blood cells are formed during the first few weeks of infection.

Heterophilic antibodies to mouse or goat proteins (like those used in many assays) are more common in people raised on farms or who work with animals on a regular basis.

Acute Care and Emergency Gynecology, ed. David Chelmow, Christine R. Isaacs and Ashley Carroll. Published by Cambridge University Press.
© Cambridge University Press 2015.

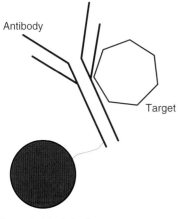

Antibody

Target

Detectable label

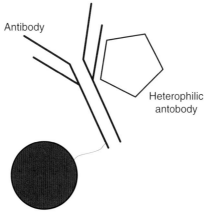

Antibody

Heterophilic antobody

Detectable label

Fig. 44.1 Immunoassays generally involve a two-step process in which an antibody is reacted with the sample to bond with the target protein. The unbound antibody is washed away and a detectable label (often another antibody or enzyme) is then bound to the insoluble antibody-target complex. The level of this detectable complex is then measured, reflecting the amount of the target originally present. Heterophilic antibodies can bind themselves to the antibody used in the test or can mimic the target agent, resulting in inaccurate or misleading results.

Heterophilic antibodies have caused falsely elevated results for other assays such as prostate-specific antigen, cancer antigen 125 (CA 125), and rapid HIV tests [3,4,5].

The size of the hCG molecule may vary in some individuals due to differences in the protein or carbohydrate structure of their hCG. This type of variability (microheterogeneity) can sometimes result in differences in the measured values delivered by different assays. Aberrant, biologically inactive forms, fragments of biologically active but metabolized hCG, or other hormones (historically follicle-stimulating hormone [FSH]), can cross-react with the assay process, resulting in inaccurately high or low values.

When a laboratory finding does not fit the clinical picture, the possibility of a testing error must always be considered. Because most of the heterophilic antibodies that can cause false results are not found in urine, urine pregnancy tests are much less susceptible to this kind of interference. When false positive serum pregnancy test from heterophilic antibodies is suspected, a simple urine pregnancy test can be performed to

confirm. A negative urine pregnancy test in the setting of substantially elevated serum hCG, and a clinical picture where true pregnancy is unlikely, can confirm that the positive test is false. In addition, heterophilic antibody interference does not change linearly with serial dilution, but a true result will, giving another way to help clarify the clinical suspicion of blocking antibodies. Consultation with the laboratory performing the test may also allow them to perform the test using alternative methods or to preabsorb the serum to remove the blocking antibodies before performing the assay.

Key teaching points

- Persistent low levels of human chorionic gonadotropin (hCG) detected in serum test that do not fit the clinical picture may be due to heterophilic antibodies.
- A negative urinary test for hCG in the face of unchanging serum levels should confirm the suspicion of cross-reactions with interfering antibodies.

References

1. American College of Obstetricians and Gynecologists. Avoiding inappropriate clinical decisions based on false-positive human chorionic gonadotropin test results. Committee Opinion No. 278. *Obstet Gynecol* 2002;100(5 Pt 1):1057–9. Reaffirmed 2013.

2. Check JH, Nowroozi K, Chase JS, et al. False-positive human chorionic gonadotropin levels caused by a heterophile antibody with the immunoradiometric assay. *Am J Obstet Gynecol* 1988;158:99–100.

3. Boscato LM, Stuart MC. Heterophilic antibodies: a problem for all immunoassays. *Clin Chem* 1988; 34(1):27–33.

4. Preissner CM, Dodge LA, O'Kane DJ, Singh RJ, Grebe SK. Prevalence of heterophilic antibody interference in eight automated tumor marker immunoassays. *Clin Chem* 2005; 51(1):208–10.

5. Spencer DV, Nolte FS, Zhu Y. Heterophilic antibody interference causing false-positive rapid human immunodeficiency virus antibody testing. *Clin Chim Acta* 2009; 399(1–2):121–2.

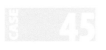

Recalcitrant severe vaginal discharge and odor

Amber Price

History of present illness

A 20-year-old gravida 1, para 0 woman presents for a problem visit at 11 weeks' gestation by sure last menstrual period. She reports common symptoms of pregnancy, but generally feels well. She reported that she was recently seen at a local emergency department (ED) for vaginal pain and odor, and was prescribed antibiotics for a diagnosis of bacterial vaginosis (BV) after the ED physician did a speculum exam. She reports that she finished the antibiotics two weeks ago, but states her symptoms have not improved and the odor has worsened. She describes the pain as constant vaginal "pressure," intermittently exacerbated by intercourse and urination. She reports two weeks of post-coital bleeding, which she thought was normal in pregnancy. She denies uterine cramping or loss of fluid. She reports that sexually transmitted disease testing done during the ED visit was normal. At the time of the ED visit, transvaginal ultrasound confirmed a viable intrauterine pregnancy with size measurements consistent with her stated last menstrual period dating. She is in a stable relationship with her partner of two years. She is happy about the pregnancy. She has not had any prior similar incidents. She denies any significant past medical or surgical history.

Physical examination

General appearance: Healthy woman, normal affect
Vital signs:

Temperature: 36.8°C
Pulse: 73 beats/min
Blood pressure: 119/68 mmHg
Respiratory rate: 18 breaths/min
Oxygen saturation: 100% on room air

Lungs: Clear to auscultation bilaterally
Cardiovascular: Regular rate and rhythm, no murmurs
Abdomen: Soft, nontender; fetal heart tones auscultated with Doppler at 158 beats/min above symphysis pubis; fundus palpable at symphisis
External genitalia: Unremarkable
Vagina:

Speculum exam: Marked odor, thick, cream colored, blood tinged discharge. No bleeding noted at the cervical os. Otherwise unremarkable
Bimanual examination: Revealed a hard object wedged tightly along the anterior vaginal wall, between the pubis symphysis and the right lateral fornix
Cervix: Closed, nulliparous

Uterus: Anteverted, nontender, 11–12 weeks' size, mobile
Adnexa: Nontender. Without masses
Laboratory studies:

Urine: Positive for 3+ leukocytes and trace blood. Negative for nitrites
Wet mount: Positive for clue cells. Negative for trichomonas and yeast
Chlamydia and gonorrhea cultures obtained and pending

How would you manage this patient?

Physical examination findings were consistent with a retained foreign body. With two fingers grasping the object and gentle manipulation, the object was removed and noted to be a pink plastic tampon applicator without the plunger. The open end of the applicator was towards the cervix and the closed end (crossed end, where the tampon ejects) was wedged in the vaginal tissue near the symphysis pubis. There was blood on the closed end of the applicator and marked blood tinged discharge and odor was noted with removal. The patient reported instant relief of her symptoms. The speculum examination was then repeated to allow visualization of the entire vagina, and revealed a small abrasion on the anterior vaginal wall at the site of the foreign body. The vaginal vault was cleared of discharge, blood, and debris with multiple scopettes.

Initially the patient was distraught, and reported being embarrassed. The patient was reassured and comforted. Upon questioning, she remembered using a tampon more than four months ago, but was very sure she removed the applicator and tampon. She stated she had never used a tampon before, and pulled the tampon out shortly after insertion because it did not feel right.

The foreign body alone is almost certainly responsible for her symptoms and no further testing is needed if her clinical course improves as would be expected. The foreign body was initially missed on speculum examination in the ED because the blades of the speculum obscured the object, and a bimanual examination was not performed. The patient was cautioned not to douche and to abstain from intercourse for a week in order to facilitate healing. She was told to report continued vaginal discharge or abdominal pain to her obstetric provider.

Foreign bodies

While true incidence is unknown, retained foreign body is common enough that it has its own International Classification of Diseases (ICD) code (ICD-9: 939.2 "Foreign body in

Acute Care and Emergency Gynecology, ed. David Chelmow, Christine R. Isaacs and Ashley Carroll. Published by Cambridge University Press. © Cambridge University Press 2015.

vulva or vagina"). The most common presenting symptoms are foul-smelling discharge and unusual vaginal bleeding. Occasionally urinary discomfort is reported. Commonly found objects include tampons and condoms, but the literature describes more unusual objects such as wooden sticks, deodorant sticks, balls, food, carpet remnants, paper clips, toilet paper, beads, and marbles [1]. Despite extensive searches, most medical literature on vaginal foreign bodies in adult women is isolated to specific case reports with unusual presentations. Research on the subject is largely limited to presentations in the pediatric patient.

Removal of objects may be done manually or with forceps. Forceps can be pierced through the finger of an examination glove, so that when the malodorous foreign body is extracted, the glove can immediately pulled over it to reduce the odor before it is discarded. Otherwise, the removed object should be placed immediately in a plastic bag, which should be promptly sealed. Upon complete removal, no further treatment is needed, unless significant vaginal injury is sustained, which can rarely require suturing to control bleeding or to repair anatomical defects [2]. While douching is discouraged, cleansing or rinsing the vagina with povidone-iodine (Betadine®) or warm saline after removal is not uncommon clinical practice [3]. Rarely, foreign bodies may cause systemic infection in immunocompromised individuals, or if the vaginal wall is disrupted. Generally, the cure for foreign body retention is prompt removal of the object once identified.

In some instances, objects may need to be removed using sedation or anesthesia in order to avoid pain. This may be particularly true of objects in the vagina of a child, or in an adult who is unable to tolerate a vaginal exam. In the case of retained foreign bodies found in children, the elderly, or patients who are incapacitated, it is important to investigate possible sexual abuse, and report possible cases to law enforcement as warranted. Rarely, a foreign body that has been retained for a period of time may cause erosion into the wall of the vagina and the object may perforate into the abdominal cavity. In these cases, secondary symptoms of abdominal infection may be present and abdominal imaging may be necessary for a complete diagnosis. Imaging may include ultrasound, MRI, CT scan, or an abdominal x-ray. MRI is the preferred technique for evaluating vaginal foreign bodies in young children [4] as MRI can detect nonmetallic objects missed by ultrasound and radiologic studies [5]. Vaginoscopy may also be necessary to fully visualize the entire vaginal canal.

After removal of the foreign body from our patient, her symptoms completely resolved and she went on to have an uneventful pregnancy.

Key teaching points

- In the presence of persistent vaginal odor, discharge and/or unusual bleeding, a thorough vaginal examination should be performed including a speculum examination and bimanual exam, with careful palpation to detect any foreign bodies.
- A foreign object in the vagina is not always found via speculum examination as the blades of the speculum may obscure direct visualization.
- Anesthesia may be necessary or appropriate to accomplish a complete examination in a patient who is unable to tolerate a bimanual office exam.
- Patients are typically unaware of the presence of a vaginal foreign body. Presentation is usually painless, with the most common complaints being recalcitrant odor, discharge and/or unusual vaginal bleeding.
- The cure for retained foreign object is removal of the object, typically manually or with forceps.

References

1. Esmaeili, M, Mansouri, A, Ghane, F. Foreign body as a cause of vaginal discharge in childhood. *J Pediatr* 2008;18(2):187–90.

2. Simon DA, Berry S, Brannian J, Hanson K. Recurrent, purulent vaginal discharge with long standing presence of a foreign body and vaginal stenosis. *J Pediatr Adolesc Gynecol* 2003;16: 361–3.

3. Stricker T, Narratil F, Sennhauser FH. Vaginal foreign bodies. *J Paediatr Child Health* 2004;40(4):205–7.

4. Kihara M, Sato N, Kimura N, et al. Magnetic resonance imaging in the evaluation of vaginal foreign bodies in a young girl. *Arch Gynecol Obstet* 2001;265(4):221–2.

5. Golan A, Lurie S, Sagiv R, Glezerman M. Continuous flow vaginoscopy in children and adolescents. *J Am Assoc Gynecol Laparosc* 2000;7(4):526–8.

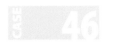

A 25-year-old woman with a painful vulvar mass

Nan G. O'Connell

History of present illness

A 25-year-old gravida 0 woman presents to the emergency department complaining of swelling and exquisite pain "down there." She had felt some soreness 2–3 days prior, but the symptoms acutely worsened 24 hours before her presentation. Her pain is exacerbated by sitting and walking. She denies fever, vaginal discharge, and dysuria. Her last menstrual period was two weeks ago. She is sexually active with the same partner for the past 10 months and uses an oral contraceptive. She was treated for chlamydia when she was 19 years old. She has never had symptoms like this before.

The patient's past medical history is notable for obesity. Her past surgical history is negative. She works as a nursing assistant and had to call in sick today because of her symptoms.

Physical examination

General appearance: Woman is obviously uncomfortable, ambulating slowly, and leaning to the left while seated on the stretcher

Vital signs:

Temperature: 36.9°C
Pulse: 90 beats/min
Blood pressure: 118/76 mmHg
Respiratory rate: 16 breaths/min

HEENT: Normal
Chest: Clear to auscultation
Cardiac: Regular rate and rhythm
Abdomen: Obese, nontender, no obvious masses
Pelvic: The lower aspect of the right labium majorum is swollen and very tender. Fluctuance of the mass is noted and the area is warm and erythematous. The mass measures approximately 5 × 6 cm. The left side appears normal. Gentle palpation of the mass reveals that it does not extend into the vagina (Fig. 46.1)

How would you manage this patient?

This patient has an abscess of the right Bartholin's duct. After local anesthesia, the abscess was incised and drained giving the patient immediate relief. To help prevent recurrence, a Word catheter was placed in the abscess cavity. The catheter was uneventfully removed in four weeks. The patient did well and remains symptom free.

Bartholin's abscesses

The Bartholins, or greater vestibular glands, are paired vulvar glands measuring approximately 0.5 cm in width, with a 2.5 cm duct that opens onto the vestibule at the 4 and 8 o'clock positions between the hymen and the labia minora. These glands produce very small amounts of mucus, which provides some moisture to the vulva but is not critical for sexual functioning. Unless diseased, the glands are not palpable and the ductal orifice is not usually visualized. The ducts, however, are prone to obstruction at their distal end due to the small size of the orifice. This obstruction in turn leads to cystic dilation of the duct. A Bartholin's abscess may arise from a secondarily infected Bartholin's cyst or, as with this patient, as a primary infection of the gland and duct. Gradual involution of the glands occurs with age; thus, a cyst or abscess in a woman aged over 40 should raise the suspicion of a possible cancer and warrant further investigation in the form of a biopsy or excisional procedure, particularly if there is fixation of the gland to the underlying tissues.

The diagnosis of a Bartholin's abscess is generally made by physical examination with the finding of a very tender, fluctuant mass at the lower aspect of the labia majora. The size of abscesses varies, but they may measure up to approximately 8 cm. The differential diagnosis includes vulvar abscesses, infected sebaceous cysts, hematomas, fibromas, lipomas, or hydradenitis suppurativa. A Bartholin's abscess is usually a polymicrobial infection. The more prominent organisms

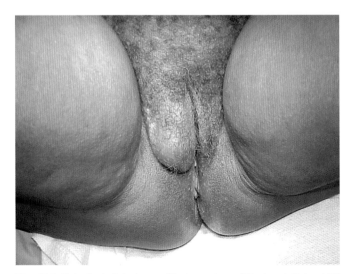

Fig. 46.1 Right Bartholin's abscess. (Photo courtesy of Stephen A. Cohen MD.)

Acute Care and Emergency Gynecology, ed. David Chelmow, Christine R. Isaacs and Ashley Carroll. Published by Cambridge University Press. © Cambridge University Press 2015.

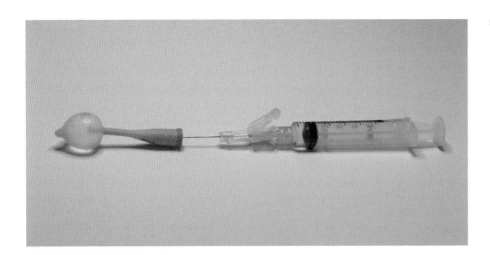

Fig. 46.2 Inflating the Word catheter.

cultured are *Escherischia coli, Staphlococcus aureas, Streptococcus faecalis, Bacteroidies* sp., *Peptostreptococcus* sp., *Neisseria gonorrhoeae*, and *Chlamydia trachomatis*.

The treatment described for this patient using the Word catheter is probably the most common treatment modality used in the outpatient setting in the United States. Drainage of the abscess will give immediate relief of the pain caused by the abscess; however, simple incision and drainage has a high rate of recurrent abscess formation. To prevent recurrence, the abscess can be drained through a linear incision and then a Word catheter can be placed to allow epithelialization and formation of a new, permanent orifice for the duct [1]. The Word catheter is small balloon-tipped catheter with a sealed end that can be inflated with saline or sterile water using a syringe and needle (Fig. 46.2).

Procedurally, after injection of a local anesthetic, a small incision is made with a scalpel on the inner aspect of the abscess near the hymenal ring. The purulent material is drained and when possible the abscess is probed to break up any loculations. The tip of the Word catheter is then inserted into the cavity and inflated with 2–3 mL of saline or sterile water. The end of the catheter can be tucked into the vagina for improved patient comfort. The Word catheter should be left in place for approximately four weeks to allow for complete fistulization. The patient can then be seen back in the outpatient setting where the balloon is deflated with a syringe (or by simply cutting the sealed end off) and the catheter easily removed. The major complication to this technique is premature expulsion of the Word catheter.

A Bartholin's abscess can also be ablated using a small silver nitrate stick inserted into the abscess cavity after incision and drainage. The area is covered with gauze and the patient returns in 48 hours to have the area cleaned to remove necrotic tissue and excess silver nitrate. This procedure has the advantage of being quick and easy to perform in the outpatient setting, but can cause pain and scarring.

Another option to manage a Bartholin's abscess is marsupialization. Marsupialization can be performed under local anesthesia in the outpatient office setting but, because it is a more involved procedure, most practitioners prefer to do it in an outpatient surgical setting. This procedure involves a 1.5–2.0 cm incision made in the abscess just outside the hymenal ring. The purulent material is drained from the abscess cavity, and the cyst wall is then grasped, everted, and sutured to the edge of the vestibular skin using interrupted absorbable sutures. This creates a new fistular tract to permanently drain the gland and minimize the chance of recurrence.

Finally, the entire Bartholin's gland and duct can be excised. This procedure is usually reserved for those patients who have failed other less invasive treatments as excision carries a much higher risk of complications including excessive bleeding, scarring, and dyspareunia. Because dissecting out the infected gland is more surgically involved, it should be performed in the operating room with appropriate anesthesia. This may be a preferred option in patients over age 40, as this excisional approach provides a specimen for histologic analysis.

Considering all treatment options, a systematic review in 2009 failed to identify the optimal treatment for a Bartholin's cyst or abscess, noting the lack of large, randomized controlled trials [2]. Given the lack of proven superiority of one procedure over another, the decision as to which technique to perform should be based on resources, patient history (especially a history of recurrent abscesses, which would favor marsupialization or excision), age of the patient, and provider experience [2].

The use of antibiotics for the treatment of Bartholin's abscesses is not routine. In most cases, the infection is polymicrobial and will resolve with abscess drainage without antibiotic therapy. However, the increased incidence of methicillin-resistant *Staphylococcus aureus* (MRSA) in vulvar abscesses [3] suggests that sending an aerobic culture is prudent. Patients considered at high risk for sexually transmitted infections should be screened for *N. gonorrhoeae* and *C. trachomatis* as well. Broad-spectrum antibiotic therapy should be considered for patients with surrounding cellulitis, fever, diabetes, or immunosuppression.

Key teaching points

- A Bartholin's abscess is a commonly encountered painful gynecologic condition, which can usually be treated in the outpatient setting with surgical incision and drainage.
- Because simple incision and drainage of a Bartholin's abscess is prone to recurrence, placement of a Word catheter or use of an ablative technique is recommended to prevent such recurrences.
- Antibiotic therapy is not routinely necessary but consideration should be given to screening for methicillin-resistant *Staphylococcus aureus* (MRSA), *Neisseria gonorrhoeae*, and *Chlamydia trachomatis*.
- Patients with a history of recurrent Bartholin's abscesses, or those who have failed multiple outpatient treatments, should be considered candidates for a marsupialization or an excisional procedure.

References

1. Word B. New instrument for office treatment of cyst and abscess of Bartholin's gland. *JAMA* 1964;190:777–8.

2. Wechter ME, Wu JM, Marzano D, Haefner H. Management of Bartholin duct cysts and abscesses: A systematic review. *Obstet Gynecol Surv* 2009;64:395–404.

3. Thurman AR, Satterfield TM, Soper DE. Methicillin-resistant *Staphylococcus aureus* as a common cause of vulvar abscesses. *Obstet Gynecol* 2008;112:538–44.

Acute abdominal pain two weeks after successful vaginal birth after Cesarean

Kathryn Shaia and Christine R. Isaacs

History of present illness

A 34-year-old gravida 2, para 2 woman presented to the emergency room with complaint of severe, acute-onset lower abdominal pain (described as 10 out of 10 on the pain scale) associated with severe nausea and vomiting. The patient notes that for the previous two days she had some intermittent lower abdominal pain, but was able to do her normal activities including caring for her newborn. The pain is now constant and stabbing, and she describes it "worse than any labor pains." She denied fevers, chills, or dysuria. She reported no flatus or bowel movements in over 36 hours.

Two weeks earlier she had a successful planned vaginal birth after Cesarean (VBAC). She presented in spontaneous labor and had a normal labor course with an epidural. Following three hours of pushing, she had an uncomplicated vaginal delivery with spontaneous delivery of the placenta. The patient's postpartum course was unremarkable and she was discharged home on postpartum day 2 with the usual precautions. At time of discharge, her abdominal examination noted a firm fundus at the level of the umbilicus with no other abnormalities.

Three years earlier she had undergone Cesarean delivery for second-stage arrest. She had no other prior surgeries. Her medical history was unremarkable. Her only medications were ibuprofen and a prenatal vitamin.

Physical examination

General appearance: Generally well-nourished and healthy woman but in marked distress

Vital signs:

Temperature: 37.0°C
Pulse: 100 beats/min
Blood pressure: 132/92 mmHg
Respiratory rate: 18 breaths/min
Oxygen saturation: 98% on room air

HEENT: Unremarkable

Neck: Supple

Cardiovascular: Regular rate and rhythm without rubs, murmurs, or gallops

Lungs: Clear to auscultation bilaterally

Abdomen: A well-healed Pfannenstiel surgical scar was noted in lower abdomen from the previous Cesarean. There was moderate distension throughout the lower abdomen with diffuse lower abdominal tenderness. Rebound and guarding was noted bilaterally. Bowel sounds were high-pitched. No palpable masses were appreciated, but examination findings were limited due to the patient's extreme discomfort

Pelvic: External genitalia normal. The uterus was firm, minimally tender and was palpable at the level of the pubic symphysis

Rectal: Normal tone. No masses

Extremities: No clubbing, cyanosis, or edema

Neurologic: Nonfocal

Laboratory studies:

WBCs: 15 200/μL (normal 3500–12 500/μL)
Neutrophils: 82% (normal 50–70%)
Hemoglobin and electrolyte levels were normal

Imaging: CT scan of the abdomen and pelvis was obtained (Fig. 47.1)

How would you manage this patient?

The patient has a strangulated hernia causing a small bowel obstruction. The abdominal/pelvic CT shows a midline ventral hernia through the rectus abdominis muscles in the lower abdomen/pelvis with small bowel findings concerning for a

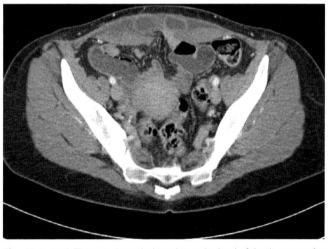

Fig. 47.1 Axial CT image through the pelvis at the level of the iliac crest after administration of intravenous and oral contrast.

Acute Care and Emergency Gynecology, ed. David Chelmow, Christine R. Isaacs and Ashley Carroll. Published by Cambridge University Press.
© Cambridge University Press 2015.

closed-loop obstruction. The arrows in Fig. 47.1 highlight the fascial defect revealing the closed loop of small bowel entering and exiting through the strictured area. There is no contrast visualized within the contained small bowel and surrounding colon, reflecting the obstructive process.

The general surgery service was consulted and the patient underwent emergent exploratory laparotomy with repair of an incarcerated ventral hernia and small bowel resection with primary reanastomosis. The abdomen was entered through the previous Pfannenstiel surgical incision until the incarcerated segment of small intestine was encountered. The fascia around the defect was widened and an end-to-end bowel reanastomosis was performed followed by fascial closure. There were no intraoperative complications. Surgical pathology confirmed small bowel with ischemic mucosa.

The remainder of the patient's postoperative/postpartum course was unremarkable. By postoperative day 3, she was tolerating a general diet, was afebrile, and met criteria for discharge.

Strangulated hernia and vaginal birth after Cesarean

An abdominal wall hernia is an abnormal protrusion of a peritoneal-lined sac through the musculo-aponeurotic covering of the abdomen. Umbilical and para-umbilical hernias are up to five times more common in women, and pregnancy is thought to be a significant risk factor. Things that increase the intra-abdominal pressure, such as intense muscular exertion, may produce a hernia by stretching the abdominal musculature. Obesity is another factor in hernia development as adipose tissue separates muscle bundles and weakens aponeuroses [1].

An incarcerated hernia is one that cannot be reduced. If the blood supply to the incarcerated bowel becomes compromised, the hernia is then described as strangulated, and the ensuing ischemia may lead to infarction, obstruction, and perforation [2]. A closed-loop obstruction indicates that a segment of intestine is obstructed both proximally and distally. In such cases, the accumulating gas and fluid cannot escape either proximally or distally from the obstructed segment. Closed-loop obstruction leads to a rapid rise in luminal pressure, rapid progression to strangulation, and is a surgical emergency.

Patients may present with nausea, vomiting, colicky abdominal pain, and obstipation. Vomiting is a more prominent symptom with proximal compared to distal intestinal obstructions [2]. On physical examination, marked abdominal distention is typically present, but may be absent if the obstruction is in the proximal small intestine [2]. Bowel sounds will initially be hyperactive and become hypoactive over time. Laboratory findings typically reflect intravascular volume depletion with an elevated blood urea nitrogen (BUN). Patients may have an increased lactate dehydrogenase (LDH)

due to bowel ischemia, and a mild leukocytosis is common [2]. In the setting of an acute abdomen, CT scanning is the test of choice as it can detect the presence of a closed-loop obstruction and strangulation [2]. If this patient's hernia had been reducible and lacked obstructive symptoms, her surgery may have been managed electively rather than emergently.

Incisional hernia formation through a Pfannenstiel incision after Cesarean delivery has reported rates from 0 to 3.1% [3]. Factors that significantly contribute to the development of an incisional hernia include a history of abdominal distension, intra-abdominal sepsis, wound infection or dehiscence, and postoperative fever. While there is limited data specific to hernia formation after Cesarean, one Nigerian study of 701 women who underwent Cesarean concluded that patient age, parity, and indication for Cesarean did not significantly influence the development of post-Cesarean incisional hernia formation [4]. The ability to generalize the results of this retrospective study conducted in a limited resource setting to settings with more extensive resources is uncertain.

The American College of Obstetricians and Gynecologists Practice Bulletin on VBAC recommends that a Trial of Labor after Cesarean (TOLAC) be offered to most women with a history of one prior low transverse Cesarean delivery [5]. Providers must weigh the risks and benefits of a TOLAC versus a repeat Cesarean while considering the patient's obstetrical issues and personal birth plans. This case describes an incarcerated hernia after VBAC, a rare complication that should not alter counseling expectant mothers about TOLAC. Our patient, having had a proper surgical repair of the ventral hernia, remains a good candidate for a future TOLAC.

Key teaching points

- Umbilical and para-umbilical hernias are up to five times more common in women, especially in those who are pregnant, obese, or undergoing physical strain.
- Postoperative abdominal distension, intra-abdominal sepsis, wound infection or dehiscence, and postoperative fever may contribute to incisional hernia formation.
- A patient with a strangulated hernia causing a small bowel obstruction may present with abdominal distention, vomiting, paroxysmal abdominal pain, and inability to pass flatus and stool. CT scan of the abdomen and pelvis is the imaging test of choice.
- Incisional hernia formation through a low transverse Pfannenstiel incision after Cesarean has reported rates from 0 to 3.1%. Patient age, parity, and indication for Cesarean section have not been shown to significantly influence the development of post-Cesarean incisional hernias.

References

1. Dabbas N, Adams K, Pearson K, Royale GT. Frequency of abdominal wall hernias: is classical teaching out of date? *J R Soc Med Sh Rep* 2011;2:1–6.

2. Tavakkolizadeh A, Whang EE, Ashley SW, Zinner MJ. Small intestine. In Brunicardi FC, Andersen DK, Billiar TR, et al., eds. *Schwartz's Principles of Surgery*, 9th edn. New York, McGraw-Hill, 2010. Available at http://www.accessmedicine.com.proxy.library.vcu.edu/content.aspx?aID=5017621.

3. Luijendijk RW, Jeekel J, Storm RK, et al. The low transverse Pfannenstiel incision and the prevalence of incisional hernia and nerve entrapment. *Ann Surg* 1997;225(4):365–9.

4. Adesunkanmiv ARK, Faleyimu, B. Incidence and aetiological factors of incisional hernia in post-Caesarean operations in a Nigerian hospital. *J Obstet Gynaecol* 2003;23(3): 258–60.

5. American College of Obstetricians and Gynecologists. Vaginal birth after previous Cesarean delivery. Practice Bulletin No. 115. *Obstet Gynecol* 2010;116: 450–63.

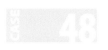

A 64-year-old woman with a simple ovarian cyst

John W. Seeds

History of present illness

A 64-year-old gravida 2, para 2 woman presented to the emergency department for left lower quadrant abdominal pain with a reported intensity of 8 out of 10 on the pain scale and an episodic pattern. The pain has worsened over the last three days. She also reports three days of constipation. She has no vaginal bleeding. She denies any urinary symptoms. She had no problems prior to the onset of the pain. She took acetaminophen without relief.

Her medical history was significant only for well-controlled hypertension. She has no prior surgeries. Her only medication was hydrochlorothiazide.

Physical examination

General appearance: Well-developed, well-nourished woman in moderate distress

Vital signs:

Temperature: 37.1°C
Pulse: 84 beats/min
Blood pressure: 130/85 mmHg
Respiratory rate: 16 breaths/min
BMI: 28 kg/m^2

HEENT: Unremarkable

Neck: Supple

Cardiovascular: Regular rate and rhythm without murmurs, rubs, or gallops

Lungs: Clear to auscultation bilaterally

Abdomen: Mild distension, left lower quadrant tenderness to direct palpation, no rebound, no adenopathy

Extremities: No clubbing, cyanosis, or edema

Neurologic: Nonfocal

Pelvic:

Speculum: Normal appearing vaginal discharge, mild atrophy
Bimanual: No cervical motion tenderness or distinct adnexal masses, uterus small, mobile, anteverted, mild tenderness in region of the left adnexa, generalized fullness consistent with stool

Rectal: Large amounts of stool in vault

Laboratory studies:

CBC and WBC: Normal
Blood chemistries: Normal

Imaging:

Pelvic ultrasound: Abdominal ultrasound showed right-sided ovarian mass. Vaginal ultrasound showed a 40-mm-average-diameter anechoic cystic mass in the right ovary with sharp margins and no internal septation or other complexity (Fig. 48.1).
Color Doppler: Examination of the ovary showed only minimal vascular activity at the margin of the cyst (Fig. 48.2)

Because of suspicion that her symptoms were from constipation, an enema was administered. She had a large bowel movement with complete resolution of all of her symptoms. Repeat pelvic examination was unremarkable.

How would you manage this patient?

The patient has a simple ovarian cyst, with characteristics that make the risk of ovarian cancer tremendously small. Given the location being contralateral to the pain, it was likely an incidental finding and not the cause of her symptoms, which were most likely from constipation. To provide further reassurance, a CA125 was drawn, which returned 5 U/mL (normal <35 U/mL). The patient was counseled on bowel regimens to prevent the recurrence of her constipation. She was counseled that the cyst was unlikely to be a problem, and had likely been present for some time. She had repeat ultrasound examinations in 6 and 12 months, which showed the cyst to be unchanged.

Simple ovarian cysts in the postmenopausal woman

The lifetime risk for ovarian cancer is 1 in 70, with about 15 000 deaths annually from this cancer [1]. Given this concern, for years a palpable ovary in a postmenopausal woman was an indication for surgery. Ovarian cancer is particularly concerning given the nonspecific symptoms of early development and spread. It is often diagnosed at a late stage with poor survival. While 90% diagnosed with stage I disease survive 5 years, only 20% of cases are stage I at diagnosis, and 65–70% are diagnosed at a late stage with only a 35–55% 5-year survival [1]. However, most adnexal masses in postmenopausal women are benign, such as serous cystadenomas [2,3]. Recent advances have given the ability to better differentiate benign from malignant masses.

Acute Care and Emergency Gynecology, ed. David Chelmow, Christine R. Isaacs and Ashley Carroll. Published by Cambridge University Press. © Cambridge University Press 2015.

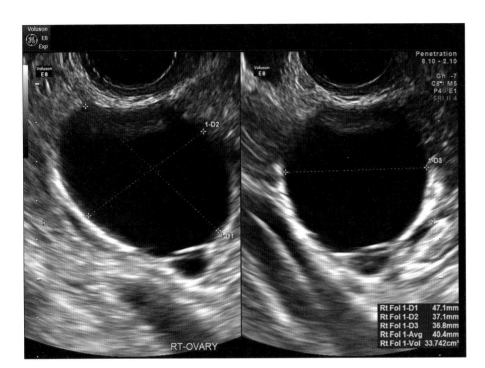

Fig. 48.1 These two orthogonal views of the ovary show the cyst to have no internal echos (anechoic or black) and no internal septae or solid components or marginal nodules.

Rt Fol 1-D1	47.1mm
Rt Fol 1-D2	37.1mm
Rt Fol 1-D3	36.8mm
Rt Fol 1-Avg	40.4mm
Rt Fol 1-Vol	33.742cm³

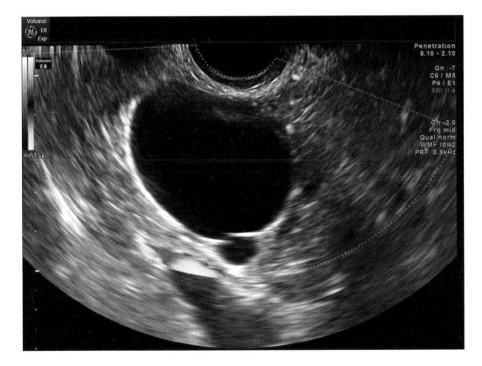

Fig. 48.2 This view of the cyst with color Doppler show few foci of vascular activity at the margin of the cyst.

Age is the most powerful risk factor for ovarian cancer with a median age at diagnosis of 63 years. A family history of breast cancer also increases risk. *BRCA1* carriers have a 60-fold increase in risk and *BRCA2* carriers have a 30-fold increase in risk [1]. Contrary to older thought, early ovarian cancer frequently does have symptoms. Unfortunately, the symptoms are nonspecific, and include increased abdominal size or bloating, abdominal or pelvic pain, or feeling full quickly or difficulty eating. These symptoms are common,

but patients with ovarian cancer tend to have them much more frequently and for longer periods of time [4]. This patient's symptoms, which were a single episode, likely from constipation, and completely resolved with treatment of her constipation, are not suspicious for ovarian cancer.

Screening for ovarian cancer continues to be widely studied and, to date, there are no effective screening tests. These studies have given significant information about the prevalence of adnexal masses in postmenopausal women. Bimanual examination is poor for detecting adnexal masses, with highly variable sensitivity related to the size of the tumor, examiner experience, and patient habitus.

Vaginal ultrasound, while widely available, is highly subjective and sensitivity varies by examiner experience. As a screening test, pelvic ultrasound has found the prevalence of adnexal cysts in the postmenopausal woman to be between 2.5 and 18%. Use as a primary screening test could be harmful as it could lead to unnecessary surgery if any adnexal cyst were considered an indication for surgery, while producing few early diagnoses of ovarian cancer [2]. Given the prevalence of ultrasound detectable adnexal masses in postmenopausal women, they are a frequent incidental finding on imaging studies done for other reasons, as in this patient. It can cause significant anxiety in the patient, and if not carefully managed, can lead to unnecessary intervention.

The ultrasound findings found in this patient are typical for a benign cyst [1]. Anechoic cysts with smooth walls, thin or absent septations, less than 10 cm in diameter, and absent solid components have a very low risk for malignancy [2]. The risk of malignancy in a cyst less than 10 cm, unilateral, unilocular, with no solid areas or papillary formations has been found to be 0–1%. Two-thirds of such masses were seen to resolve within 3 months, and the risk of malignancy is less than 0.1%.

CA125 may be helpful in further stratifying risk. While no major society has developed firm recommendations for the evaluation and management of simple cysts in postmenopausal women, many practitioners integrate CA125 into their assessment. CA125 is a serum protein elevated with virtually any process that disturbs the peritoneum, including ovarian cancer. While elevation of CA125 may be seen in over 80% of patients with epithelial ovarian cancer, it has been reported positive in only in 50% of stage I disease [5,6]. The reported sensitivity of CA125 in separating benign from malignant adnexal masses varies from 61 to 90% and the predictive value varies from 35 to 91%. It is rarely elevated in cancers other than epithelial [1]. CA125 appears to perform better in post-menopausal women. Any significant elevation of CA125 in a postmenopausal patient with an adnexal mass is very suspicious for malignancy and consideration of surgical intervention would be appropriate. Given the nonspecific nature of CA125, mild elevations are common, and need to be interpreted in the context of other clinical information. While some providers would be comfortable enough that the cyst in this patient was benign based on its ultrasound characteristics, use of CA125 provided additional reassurance.

Small asymptomatic simple cysts with thin or absent septations can be managed by observation. While no major society has specific guidelines for frequency of follow-up, repeat ultrasound at intervals of 6 and then 12 months is reasonable provided the cyst is stable or smaller on follow-up [2]. Some providers will repeat CA125 measurements as well. Aspiration is not recommended because cytology has shown poor sensitivity for the diagnosis of malignancy, the cyst will often recur, and if malignant, spillage of contents may increase the risk of spread [6]. Surgery is usually necessary if the patient develops symptoms, the CA125 rises, or new ultrasound findings of solid areas, excrescences, or ascites develop [1,2]. In this patient, long-term follow-up confirmed the stability of the benign cyst.

Key teaching points

- Simple ovarian cysts are found in up to 18% of postmenopausal women. The vast majority are resolved or unchanged in one year.
- If the cyst is anechoic, has sharp margins, few or no thin internal septa, no marginal nodularity or solid components, and is less than 10 cm in diameter, the risk of cancer is less than 0.1%.
- CA125 may be helpful for differentiating benign from malignant in postmenopausal women. If normal and the cyst is asymptomatic and appears simple on ultrasound, expectant management is appropriate. If elevated, surgery should be considered.
- Observation with vaginal ultrasound and serum CA125 at 6 and 12 months is appropriate for the management of postmenopausal women with asymptomatic simple cysts less than 10 cm.

References

1. American College of Obstetricians and Gynecologists. Management of adnexal masses. Practice Bulletin No. 83. *Obstet Gynecol* 2007;109:1233–48. Reaffirmed 2011.

2. Modesitt SC, Pavlik EJ, Ueland FR, et al. Risk of malignancy in unilocular ovarian cystic tumors less than 10 centimeters in diameter. *Obstet Gynecol* 2003;102:594–9.

3. Castillo G, Alcazar JL, Jurado M. Natural history of sonographically detected simple unilocular adnexal cysts in asymptomatic postmenopausal women. *Gynecol Oncol* 2004;92(3): 965–9.

4. American College of Obstetricians and Gynecologists. The role of the obstetrician–gynecologist in the early detection of epithelial ovarian cancer. Committee Opinion No. 477. *Obstet Gynecol* 2011;117:742–6.

5. Greenlee RT, Kessel B, Williams CR, et al. Prevalence, incidence, and natural history of simple ovarian cysts among women >55 years old in a large cancer screening trial. *Am J Obstet Gynecol* 2010;202(4):373.E1–9.

6. Nardo LG, Kroon ND, Reginald PW. Persistent unilocular ovarian cysts in a general population of postmenopausal women: Is there a place for expectant management? *Obstet Gynecol* 2003;102:589–93.

A 26-year-old woman with acute pelvic pain and free fluid in the pelvis

Isaiah M. Johnson and Adrienne L. Gentry

History of present illness

A 26-year-old gravida 1, para 1 woman presented to the emergency department with a chief complaint of abdominal and lower back pain. The patient reported a normal last menstrual period that had begun 21 days prior to presentation. The pain began two days prior to presentation and was confined to the left lower quadrant. The pain acutely worsened the day she presented for evaluation. The pain was described as constant and sharp. She rated the pain as 9 (on a scale of 1–10) and reported that it was not relieved by acetaminophen. She denied any other associated symptoms, such as fever, chills, nausea, vomiting, diarrhea, constipation, dysuria, urgency, or difficulty voiding.

She reported being sexually active with one partner. She uses condoms for contraception. She denies any past medical or surgical history. She takes no medications.

Physical examination

General appearance: Well-nourished woman in mild discomfort

Vital signs:

Temperature: 36.5°C
Pulse: 82 beats/min
Blood pressure: 119/65 mmHg
Respiratory rate: 16 breaths/min
Oxygen saturation: 100% on room air

Abdomen: Soft, no masses, normoactive bowel sounds, moderately tender to palpation in left lower quadrant, voluntary guarding present; no rebound tenderness, masses, or suprapubic tenderness

Musculoskeletal: No costovertebral angle tenderness

External genitalia: Unremarkable

Vagina: Nontender, with minimal vaginal discharge

Cervix: No lesions, no cervical motion tenderness or cervical discharge

Uterus: Anteverted, normal size, nontender, mobile

Adnexa: No masses or fullness appreciated, tender to palpation over left adnexa

Laboratory studies:

Urine pregnancy test: Negative
Leukocyte count: 8200/μL (normal 4000–10 500/μL) with no left shift
Hb: 13.2 g/dL (normal 12.0–16.0 g/dL)

Urinalysis: Negative for blood, nitrites, and leukocyte esterase
NAATs: For gonorrhea and chlamydia collected from cervix

Imaging: A transvaginal ultrasound was performed (Figs 49.1 and 49.2)

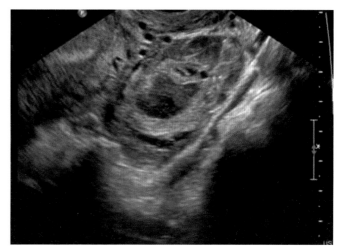

Fig. 49.1 Hemorrhagic ovarian cyst. High frequency transvaginal ultrasound imaging revealed a 3.3 × 2.6 × 2.1 cm mildly complicated cyst with low level internal echoes and slight wall thickening consistent with a hemorrhagic ovarian cyst.

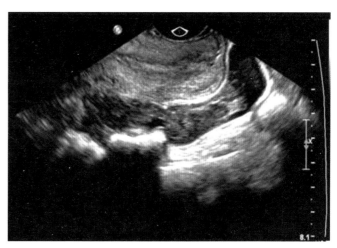

Fig. 49.2 Ruptured ovarian cyst. Fluid of mixed echogenicity is identified in the posterior cul de sac. In light of a negative pregnancy test and the finding of a hemorrhagic ovarian cyst, this is consistent with intra-abdominal bleeding following cyst rupture.

Acute Care and Emergency Gynecology, ed. David Chelmow, Christine R. Isaacs and Ashley Carroll. Published by Cambridge University Press. © Cambridge University Press 2015.

How would you manage this patient?

The patient has a ruptured hemorrhagic ovarian cyst. The transvaginal ultrasound revealed a $3 \times 3 \times 2$ cm, heterogeneous, complex left ovarian cyst (Fig. 49.1), as well as free fluid and heterogeneous material consistent with blood clots in the posterior cul-de-sac (Fig. 49.2). The free fluid in the cul-de-sac is consistent with rupture of the hemorrhagic cyst, leading to the patient's sharp pain. The patient's pain improved with intravenous analgesia, and she remained hemodynamically stable during the course of her evaluation. The patient was discharged from the emergency department with oral analgesia. A follow-up appointment a week later noted the patient's pain had completely resolved. A transvaginal ultrasound performed eight weeks later noted complete resolution of the cyst and free fluid.

Ruptured ovarian cysts

Ruptured ovarian cysts are a well-known cause of acute abdominal pain in women of reproductive age. The presentation of patients with ruptured ovarian cysts can vary greatly from an asymptomatic incidental finding to severe pain and hemodynamic instability depending on the nature of the ruptured cyst. The rupture of follicular or functional cysts or benign cystadenomas may be associated with minimal symptoms, as the serous or mucinous fluid released does not typically provoke a significant peritoneal inflammatory response. On the other hand, rupture of a dermoid cyst may result in a painful chemical peritonitis with long-term sequelae. Hemorrhagic ovarian cysts are usually associated with unilateral pain if unruptured, and more generalized lower abdominal and pelvic pain if rupture occurs causing the development of hemoperitoneum. The pain associated with a ruptured hemorrhagic ovarian cyst can persist for days to weeks while the hemoperitoneum is resorbed. This patient's presentation is consistent with a hemorrhagic corpus luteum with subsequent rupture and hemoperitoneum. She initially developed left lower quadrant pain due to bleeding into the corpus luteum and distention of the ovarian capsule. The pain acutely worsened after the cyst ruptured and hemoperitoneum developed.

Hemorrhagic ovarian cysts develop when vessels in the highly vascular corpus luteum are disrupted, resulting in hemorrhage into the ovary. If rupture of the cyst occurs, the resultant hemoperitoneum will cause significant peritoneal irritation and severe pain. Many patients will report intermittent, cramping pain for one to two weeks preceding this onset of acute severe pain, which is thought to reflect hemorrhage into the ovary and distention of the ovarian capsule prior to rupture [1]. Most ruptured hemorrhagic ovarian cysts occur on days 20–26 of the menstrual cycle [1]. While the majority of hemorrhagic ovarian cysts occur in reproductive age women, rupture and hemoperitoneum may develop in adolescents prior to the onset of menarche and recently menopausal women [1]. Interestingly, rupture of a hemorrhagic cyst occurs more frequently on the right side, which may be due to a protective effect of the rectosigmoid colon on the left ovary [1]. The quantity of blood loss may vary significantly, and massive hemorrhage may occur in patients with hereditary or acquired bleeding diathesis or on chronic anticoagulation [1,2].

High frequency transvaginal ultrasound imaging of the pelvis is the preferred method for imaging patients with suspected pelvic pathology or ovarian cysts [3]. The diagnosis of a ruptured hemorrhagic ovarian cyst is complicated by the significant variation in appearance based on the timing of imaging in relation to development of symptoms. Immediately following rupture, the fresh blood will appear as anechoic free fluid and a rounded well-defined heterogeneous ovarian mass may be identified [4]. As clots form in the peritoneal cavity, they will appear characteristically heterogeneous and may obscure visualization of the ovary or the hemorrhagic cyst. Hemorrhagic ovarian cysts may also mimic ovarian neoplasms, having fine linear echoes that may be mistaken for septations, or a retracted clot that may be interpreted as a mural nodule [4,5]. The ability of hemorrhagic cysts to mimic other gynecologic conditions such as dermoids, endometriomas, ovarian neoplasms, and ectopic pregnancies has caused some to refer to it as "the great imitator" [5]. CT imaging may be a useful adjunct to distinguish between cyst rupture and an inflammatory process.

As the presentation of a ruptured ectopic pregnancy and ruptured hemorrhagic ovarian cyst are similar, the initial testing must include a urine or serum assay for the beta subunit of human chorionic gonadotropin. A complete blood count to evaluate current hemoglobin levels, platelet count, and type and screen should also be ordered in patients presenting with suspected significant intrabdominal bleeding. Urinalysis should be ordered to evaluate for hematuria, which may suggest nephrolithiasis, and leukocytes, to evaluate for urinary tract infection. Adequate venous access should be obtained and fluid rescuscitation initiated.

Orthostatic vitals may be useful in evaluating the hemodynamic stability of younger patients, as significant hemoperitoneum may not result in tachycardia and has been associated with paradoxical bradycardia [6]. Hemodynamically stable patients with minimal free fluid and appropriate pain control may have outpatient management. This patient met these criteria and was managed as an outpatient.

Patients with moderate to large amounts of blood in the abdomen, anemia due to acute blood loss, signs of hemodynamic instability, or with uncertain diagnosis should be admitted for observation. Surgery is an appropriate option when there are signs of ongoing bleeding, or the diagnosis of cyst rupture is not certain and there is concern for other surgical emergencies such as appendicitis or ovarian torsion. In most cases, ovarian cystectomy and evacuation of hemoperitoneum may be accomplished laparoscopically. Oophorectomy should be reserved for cases where hemostasis cannot be achieved through cystectomy or there is a suspicion of other ovarian pathology.

Given the varied appearance of hemorrhagic ovarian cysts, repeat imaging with transvaginal ultrasound to document resolution of the cyst eight weeks after initial evaluation is reasonable in most patients. Combined oral contraceptives are not effective in hastening the resolution of ovarian cysts, but they may decrease the risk of developing new follicular or corpus luteal cysts [7]. Cases series have demonstrated that some women are a risk for developing recurrent ruptured cysts [1,4]. Women who are not attempting to conceive may benefit from the use of combined oral contraceptives as long as there are no contraindications.

Key teaching points

- Ruptured ovarian cysts are a common cause of acute pelvic pain and may be difficult to distinguish from pelvic

inflammatory disease, ovarian torsion, and ectopic pregnancy.
- Transvaginal ultrasound is the preferred method of imaging patients with acute pain and suspected ovarian pathology.
- Most patients with ruptured ovarian cysts may be managed conservatively and do not require surgical intervention.
- Urgent surgical intervention is indicated in unstable patients, massive hemoperitoneum, or if other surgical emergencies cannot be satisfactorily excluded.

References

1. Hallatt JG, Steele CH, Snyder M. Ruptured corpus luteum with hemoperitoneum: A study of 173 surgical cases. *Am J Obstet Gynecol* 1984;149(1) 5–9.

2. Gupta N, Dadhwal V, Deka D, Jain SK, Mittal S. Corpus luteum hemorrhage: rare complication of congenital and acquired coagulation abnormalities. *J Obstet Gynaecol Res* 2007;33(3): 376–80.

3. American College of Obstetrics and Gynecology. Management of adnexal masses. Practice Bulletin No. 83. *Obstet Gynecol* 2007;110(1): 201–14.

4. Baltarowich OH, Kurtz AB, Pasto ME, et al. The spectrum of sonographic findings in hemorrhagic ovarian cysts. *AJR Am J Roentgenol* 1987;148(5): 901–5.

5. Yoffe N, Bronshtein M, Brandes J, Blumenfeld Z. Hemorrhagic ovarian cyst detection by transvaginal sonography: the great imitator. *Gynecol Endocrinol* 1991;5:123–9.

6. Adams SL, Greene JS. Absence of a tachycardic response to intraperitoneal hemorrhage. *J Emerg Med* 1986;4(5): 383–9.

7. American College of Obstetrics and Gynecology. Noncontraceptive uses of hormonal contraceptives. Practice Bulletin No. 110. *Obstet Gynecol* 2010;115(1):206–18.

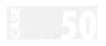

A 36-year-old woman with fever and pelvic pain at 14 weeks' gestation

Frances Casey and Katie P. Friday

History of present illness

A 36-year-old gravida 1, para 0 woman at 14 weeks' gestation by in-vitro fertilization presented complaining of 1 day of fever, abdominal pain, and vaginal bleeding. She described having an intermittent watery vaginal discharge for the past two weeks, which she thought was normal. Several hours prior to presentation, the patient experienced bright red vaginal spotting with passage of small clots. She also had nausea with several episodes of vomiting. She described her pain as cramping across her lower abdomen, rated at a level of 9 on a scale of 0–10.

Gynecologic history was significant for infertility and endometriosis. She has no other significant medical or surgical history. She takes no medications other than a prenatal vitamin.

Physical examination

General appearance: Woman who is tearful and in moderate discomfort

Vital signs:

Temperature: 38.9°C
Pulse: 110 beats/min
Blood pressure: 95/65 mmHg
Respiratory rate: 20 breaths/min
Oxygen saturation: 98% on room air

HEENT: Unremarkable

Cardiovascular: Tachycardic, regular rhythm without murmurs, rubs, or gallops

Lungs: Clear to auscultation bilaterally

Abdomen: Soft, nondistended, diffusely tender to palpation with significant fundal tenderness, fundus consistent with 14 weeks' gestation

Pelvic: Blood-tinged, foul-smelling fluid pooling in vagina on speculum exam, active bleeding visualized at external os. Internal os 1 cm dilated. Cervical motion tenderness present. Fourteen-week-sized diffusely tender uterus. Adnexa not palpable

Laboratory studies:

CBC: Leukocytosis of 13 100/μL (normal 3500–12 500/μL) with 89% neutrophils (normal 50–70%)
Hb: 9.7 g/dL (normal second-trimester pregnancy 9.7–14.8 g/dL)
Ht: 29.2% (normal second-trimester pregnancy 30–39%)
Platelets: 139 × 10³/μL (normal second-trimester pregnancy 155–409 × 10³/μL)

Urinalysis: Clear color, negative for nitrites, glucose, protein, and small leukocytes
Serum electrolytes, renal, and liver functions: Normal
Blood cultures: Sent

Imaging: Transabdominal sonogram (Fig. 50.1) showed a singleton gestation with anhydramnios, located in the lower uterine segment, crown–rump length measuring 8.01 cm consistent with 14 weeks, fetal heart rate 193 beats/min, placenta posterior

How would you manage this patient?

This patient has a septic abortion. The two-week history of clear fluid leaking combined with absence of fluid on sonogram indicates ruptured membranes. This patient is clearly infected as evidenced by tachycardia, temperature to 38.9°C, and a white blood cell count of 13 100/μL. Intrauterine infection is clear from the diffusely tender uterus and foul-smelling fluid leaking from the cervix. Pyelonephritis, another common source of fever in pregnancy, is ruled out with a normal urinalysis.

Blood and urine cultures were obtained, as were cervical nucleic acid amplification tests (NAATs) for gonorrhea and chlamydia. An IV was started and she was rehydrated. She received doses of ampicillin, gentamicin, and clindamycin. She underwent an immediate uncomplicated dilation and evacuation under intravenous sedation in the operating room. She was hospitalized postoperatively and broad-spectrum antibiotics were continued until all signs of infection had

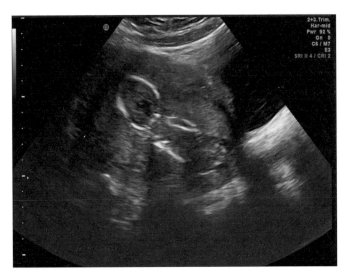

Fig. 50.1 Singleton intrauterine pregnancy 14 weeks with oligohydramnios.

Acute Care and Emergency Gynecology, ed. David Chelmow, Christine R. Isaacs and Ashley Carroll. Published by Cambridge University Press. © Cambridge University Press 2015.

resolved for 48 hours. Blood cultures were positive for *Escherichia coli*.

Septic abortion

A septic abortion is a spontaneous or induced abortion complicated by infection of the products of conception. Septic abortion has most commonly been described in cases of illegal or incomplete induced abortions. In the United States, cases of septic abortion and other abortion-related morbidity and mortality decreased dramatically following legalization of abortion services [1]. Nevertheless, as recently as 2009, a case report described a self-attempted abortion with a coat hanger resulting in sepsis, acute respiratory distress syndrome, and a total abdominal hysterectomy with bilateral salpingo-oophorectomy [2]. Septic abortion is less common during a spontaneous abortion but can occur with retained products or in the setting of prolonged rupture of membranes, as in this case. Other risk factors for septic abortion include concomitant infection with *Chlamydia trachomatis*, immune compromise, and an intrauterine device left in-situ during a pregnancy.

Septic abortions remain one of the leading causes of maternal mortality worldwide. Countries with safe, legal access to abortion services have mortality rates of 1/100 000 as compared to mortality rates as high as 460/100 000 in regions with poor access [3]. Disparities between countries in abortion-related mortality can be attributed to a number of factors including: abortion legislation, stigma, socioeconomic status [4], contraceptive coverage, and the availability of safe, accessible, comprehensive abortion services [5,6].

A septic abortion may present with fever, tachycardia, uterine tenderness, foul-smelling discharge or vaginal bleeding, and lower abdominal pain. Other signs and symptoms may include chills, oliguria, jaundice, and malaise. Presentations may range from mild illness characterized by low-grade fever, mild abdominal pain, and vaginal bleeding to multiorgan failure characterized by tachycardia, tachypnea, hypotension, and an inability to regulate body temperature. A strong suspicion and early recognition of sepsis is important to decrease morbidity and mortality. This patient presented with mild symptoms, but with blood cultures positive for *Escherichia coli*, a delay in diagnosis and treatment could have resulted in multiorgan failure within hours.

Immediate treatment includes aggressive hydration, broad-spectrum antibiotics, and evacuation of uterine contents. A delay in treatment can result in bacteremia, pelvic abscess, septic pelvic thrombophlebitis, disseminated intravascular coagulopathy, septic shock, organ failure, and death [7].

Infections may be polymicrobial and involve gram-negative or gram-positive aerobes, facultative or obligate anaerobes, and sexually transmitted pathogens [7]. The most common organisms include *Escherichia coli*, enterococci, and beta-hemolytic streptococci. Because of the variety of possible agents, no single antibiotic is ideal [8]. Broad-spectrum antibiotics must be started as soon as the diagnosis is suspected after obtaining blood and urine cultures and cervical NAATs. Antibiotic regimens typically include ampicillin (2–3 g IV every 6 h), clindamycin (900 mg IV every 8 h), and gentamicin (loading dose of 2 mg/kg body weight given IV followed by 1.5 mg/kg every 8 h, depending on renal status). Alternative antibiotics with broad-spectrum coverage may also be appropriate. Antibiotics may be tailored once cultures and sensitivities have been reported. For milder infections, single agents may be appropriate. Following 48 hours of clinical improvement, antibiotics may be discontinued.

Evacuation can be performed efficiently in the first trimester with electric or manual vacuum aspiration under local anesthesia or with minimal intravenous sedation. This can be performed at the bedside if a patient is too ill for movement to the operating room. In the case illustrated, the patient had early sepsis, was stable for transfer to the operating room, and dilation and evacuation was accomplished using deep sedation. In the second trimester, a trained provider can perform evacuation of fetal tissue or retained products using forceps under ultrasound guidance. Rapid surgical evacuation is mandatory to achieve clinical improvement and every attempt should be made to facilitate surgical evacuation. Clearly, dilation and time required for uterine evacuation will increase with gestational age. The operating room team must be prepared to manage disseminated intravascular coagulation and hemorrhage, with conversion to hysterectomy if necessary, as these risks are increased in cases of sepsis.

Medication abortion prolongs induction-to-delivery interval and still may require surgical evacuation for retained products of conception. However, if a trained provider is not available, alternative methods of uterine evacuation must be employed according to availability. First- and second-trimester cases could be managed using Hemabate® (carboprost tromethamine), Cytotec® (misoprostol), or Cervidil® (dinoprostone). No studies of misoprostol in the setting of septic abortion have been published, but given its widespread availability, efficacy, and few adverse side effects outside of temperature increase, nausea, and vomiting, misoprostol could facilitate uterine evacuation if surgical methods are not available. While oxytocin has been employed for early induction, it has prolonged induction-to-delivery interval and concern for water intoxication compared to misoprostol. In the second-trimester mechanical dilation can be achieved with a 30 mL Foley catheter balloon placed in the lower uterus and taped to maternal leg for traction [7,9].

Key teaching points

- Immediate treatment includes aggressive hydration, broad-spectrum antibiotics, and evacuation of uterine contents.
- Rapid surgical evacuation is mandatory to achieve clinical improvement. If surgery is not available, alternative means of uterine evacuation must be employed, although surgery is preferred.
- The availability of safe, legal abortion services decreases maternal mortality and morbidity due to septic abortion.

References

1. American Medical Association. Council on Scientific Affairs. Induced termination of pregnancy before and after Roe vs. Wade. Trends in the mortality and morbidity of women. *JAMA* 1992;268(22): 3231–9.

2. Saultes TA, Devita D, Heiner JD. The back alley revisited: Sepsis after attempted self-induced abortion. *West J Emerg Med* 2009;10(4): 278–80.

3. Åhman E, Shah IH. New estimates and trends regarding unsafe abortion mortality. *Int J Gynaecol. Obstet* 2011;115(2):121–6.

4. Dehlendorf C, Weitz T. Access to abortion services: A neglected health disparity. *J Health Care Poor Underserved* 2011;22(2): 415–21.

5. Sedgh G, Singh S, Shah IH, et al. Induced abortion: incidence and trends worldwide from 1995 to 2008. *Lancet* 2012;379(9816):625–32.

6. Fawcus SR. Maternal mortality and unsafe abortion. *Best Pract Res* 2008; 22(3):533–48.

7. Stubblefield PG, Grimes DA. Septic abortion. *N Engl J Med* 1994;331(5): 310–14.

8. Neligan PJ, Laffey JG. Clinical review: Special populations – critical illness and pregnancy. *Crit Care* 2011;15(4):227.

9. Lee VC, Ng EH, Ho PC. Issues in second trimester induced abortion (medical/surgical methods). *Best Pract Res* 2010;24(4):517–27.

Acute fever and tachycardia in a 21-year-old woman during laparoscopy

Thomas C. Peng

History of present illness

A 21-year-old gravida 1, para 1 woman presented to the emergency department with acute onset of lower abdominal pain which started 2 hours prior. She also noted vaginal bleeding with red blood similar to the onset of her menstrual cycle. She uses no contraception and is sexually active. Her last menstrual period was approximately seven weeks ago. She has a history of hyperthyroidism and is intermittently compliant with her methimazole treatment. She thinks it has been at least a year since her thyroid status was checked. She has never had surgery and denies alcohol or tobacco use. She works as a waitress and takes part-time classes so she can become an administrative assistant. Review of systems is negative other than in her presenting complaints.

Physical examination

Vital signs:

Temperature: 37.0°C
Pulse: 110 beats/min
Blood pressure: 150/88 mmHg
Respiratory rate: 20 breaths/min
BMI: 28 kg/m²

HEENT: No neurologic deficit, cranial nerves II–XII are normal
Neck: Supple, no goiter

Cardiovascular: S1 and S2, with pulse of 110 beats/min, without murmur, gallop, or rub
Lungs: Clear to auscultation without rales, rhonchi, nor wheezing
Abdomen: The upper abdomen is soft to palpation and not tender, with normal bowel sounds. Guarding noted in the lower abdomen
Pelvic: On speculum examination, a small amount of vaginal bleeding from the external cervical os identified. The uterus is anteverted and the size is normal for a nonpregnant state. Uterine contour and shape is smooth without irregularity. Abdominal pain is most acute on palpation in the left adnexal area. There is no palpable mass but the examination is limited due to patient discomfort
Extremities: Normal strength with no edema
Neurologic: No focal deficit
Laboratory studies:

Hb: 10 g/dL (normal 11.6–13.9 g/dL)
WBCs: 12 000/μL with 77% neutrophils (normal 5.7–13 600 /μL)
Platelets: 160 000/μL (normal 174 000–391 000/μL)
Creatinine: 0.7 mg/dL (normal 0.4–0.7 mg/dL)
BUN: 10 mg/dL (normal 7–12 mg/dL)
Urine hCG: Positive

Imaging: A pelvic ultrasound was performed (Fig. 51.1)

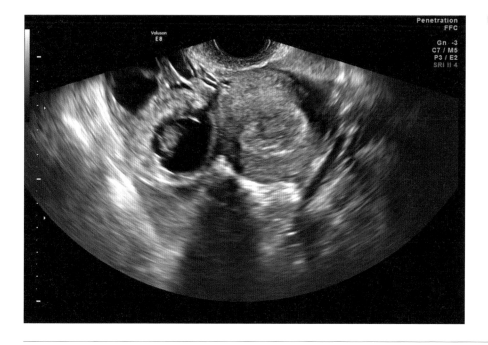

Fig. 51.1 Pelvic ultrasound.

Acute Care and Emergency Gynecology, ed. David Chelmow, Christine R. Isaacs and Ashley Carroll. Published by Cambridge University Press.
© Cambridge University Press 2015.

How would you manage this patient?

The ultrasound image is compatible with the diagnosis of an ectopic pregnancy. The diagnosis was based on identification of a fetal cardiac flicker in the left adnexa, a normal endometrium, and supported with the clinical context of an acute abdomen. The patient was counseled and a laparoscopy was performed under general anesthesia. Upon entry into the abdomen, a mass was noted in the mid-left fallopian tube consistent with an unruptured ectopic gestation and a left partial salpingectomy was performed without complications. During the surgery, the anesthesiologist noted that the patient's heart rate had rapidly increased to 139 beats/min and that her temperature had also rapidly increased to 39.4°C. Estimated surgical blood loss was only 100 mL. There were no surgical complications and total operative time was 30 minutes. The patient was transferred to the intensive care unit postoperatively.

Why did the patient develop a high fever and tachycardia intraoperatively?

The clinical scenario is consistent with thyroid storm.

Thyroid storm

The association of thyroid storm with an ectopic pregnancy has been reported in one case report [1]. Thyroid storm is an uncommon entity, estimated to occur in 1–2% of all hospital admissions, although the actual incidence is not clear due to the absence of laboratory findings that are specific to the diagnosis. It occurs more often in women, and in patients with Graves' disease or multinodular goiter. Typically, a superimposed insult (such as surgery in this case), precipitates the thyroid storm, but other catalysts have been described (Table 51.1).

The mortality rate associated with thyroid storm is estimated at 10–30%, predominantly secondary to the associated multiple organ dysfunction and congestive heart failure and/or cardiac arrhythmias, which include atrial fibrillation, supraventricular tachyarrhythmias, and, rarely, ventricular tachyarrhythmias. These complications, as well as other organ dysfunction including respiratory failure, disseminated intravascular coagulation, hypoxic brain damage, and sepsis, account for the majority of fatal thyroid storm cases [2]. The diagnosis of thyroid storm should be considered and treatment empirically initiated due to the associated morbidity/mortality of the disease. Clinical suspicion should be high in patients with a prior diagnosis of hyperthyroidism (typically Graves' disease), in the context of a precipitating factor or superimposed insult, who then develop fever and tachycardia out of proportion to their illness.

The diagnosis of thyroid storm remains a clinical diagnosis as there are no laboratory or imaging modalities for its confirmation. Laboratory evaluations of serum thyroxine (T4) and/or triiodothyronine (T3) are not significantly different from levels seen in clinical hyperthyroidism. Attempts to

Table 51.1 Reported precipitants of thyroid storm

Thyroid and/or nonthyroidal surgery

Trauma

Vigorous manipulation of thyroid gland

Parturition, including complicated pregnancies

Burns

Myocardial infarction

Pulmonary embolism

Cerebral stroke

Medications, e.g. aspirin overdose

Radio-iodine therapy

Withdrawal of antithyroid medications

Infections

Diabetic ketoacidosis

Acute ingestion of high dose of thyroid hormone

Metastatic thyroid cancer

Struma ovarii

Molar pregnancy

Emotional stress

create scoring systems have been proposed to aid in the diagnosis [3]. The typical symptoms scored would be categorized into organ functions: thermoregulatory dysfunction (fever); cardiovascular dysfunction (tachyarrhythmias and heart failure); central nervous system dysfunction (agitation, delirium, psychosis, extreme lethargy, seizures, and coma); gastrointestinal and hepatic dysfunction (diarrhea, nausea, vomiting, abdominal pain, and unexplained jaundice) [4].

In the absence of definitive laboratory or imaging tests, the utility of a scoring system defines the likelihood of the true presence of thyroid storm. Patients scoring greater than 45 points very likely have thyroid storm present. Using this scoring system, a temperature of greater or equal to 39.4°C (25 points) and a heart rate greater than 139 beats/min (20 points) scores 45 points, as was the case in this patient.

A recent analysis of signs and symptoms of thyroid storm in those patients reported in the literature and in 356 hospitalized Japanese patients confirmed that the most common signs and symptoms include fever (>38°C), noted in 42–55% of patients, and tachycardia greater than or equal to 120 beats/min, noted in 80–82% of patients, or tachycardia greater than 130 beats/min, noted in 68–76% of patients [2]. Clinically, high fever and/or tachycardia is almost universal in all presentations. Less frequent symptoms included central nervous sytem and gastrointestinal symptoms.

Patients with a suspected diagnosis of thyroid storm should be managed in an intensive care unit. The medical management of thyroid storm is the same regimen as for hyperthyroidism, except with higher dosing algorithms. The initial step in treatment is to prevent new thyroid hormone production with thionamides (propylthiouracil, methimazole, or carbimazole). These medications inhibit thyroid peroxidase, a key enzyme involved in the synthesis of T3 and T4. Propylthiouracil (PTU) is the preferred drug of choice due to its additional benefit of inhibition of peripheral conversion of T4 to T3 [5]. T4 is a prohormone for T3. T3 exhibits greater biologic activity as compared to T4, such that inhibition of the peripheral conversion of T4 to T3 decreases the overall thyroid hormone activity. The American Association of Clinical Endocrinologists/American Thyroid Association recommends a 500–1000 mg loading dose of PTU, followed by 250 mg every 4 hours. If methimazole is used for therapy, 60–80 mg per day in divided doses should be administered every 4–6 hours [6]. Beta-blockers, specifically propranolol, may also be added to decrease the risk of tachyarrhythmia. In high doses, propranolol also inhibits the conversion of T4 to T3.

The next step in management is to add iodine to further decrease new thyroid hormone synthesis. The mechanism of how iodine decreases thyroid hormone synthesis is unknown. The addition of iodine should be delayed for at least 1 hour after the administration of PTU or methimazole because administering iodine before the PTU has been effective may result in a paradoxical increase in thyroid hormone synthesis, the "Jod–Basedow effect." Iodide may be administered as a saturated solution of potassium iodide (SSKI) or as Lugol's solution. SSKI can be given as 5 drops (0.25 mL or 250 mg) PO every 6 hours [5]. In patients allergic to iodine, lithium carbonate is an alternative agent to inhibit hormonal release. Lithium also inhibits thyroid hormone synthesis. Another strategy to decrease the level of circulating T4 and T3 is to add cholestyramine, which interrupts the enterohepatic circulation of thyroid hormones. Normally, thyroid hormones are metabolized in the liver and then bound to glucuronides and sulfates, so that this conjugated hormone is excreted into bile. When the conjugated hormone is ultimately released, the free hormone is reabsorbed. By adding cholestyramine, the conjugated hormone remains bound and, thus, is excreted.

Finally, hydrocortisone should be administered to guard against adrenal insufficiency. In hyperthyroid states, there is a subnormal response of the adrenal glands to adrenocortical-stimulating hormone. The American Association of Clinical Endocrinologists/American Thyroid Association recommends a 300 mg IV load of hydrocortisone followed by 100 mg IV dose every 8 hours. An alternative steroid is dexamethasone [6].

Carroll and Matfin [7] have recommended the following mnemonic to guide clinical treatment:

Inhibit synthesis (thioamides)
Inhibit release (iodine)
Inhibit peripheral conversion of T4 to T3 (PTU)
Beta-blockers (typically propranolol)
Inhibit enterohepatic circulation (cholestyramine)

In general, patients with thyroid storm are better managed in an intensive care setting with consultants, which may include endocrinologists and other specialties depending on the organ system complications encountered.

Symptomatic management to decrease fever with acetaminophen and peripheral cooling are appropriate, as is administration of intravenous fluids to address the fluid loss from fever, diarrhea, and/or vomiting.

For this particular patient, her symptoms gradually resolved after three days in the intensive care unit. She was then transferred to a general hospital ward with maintenance methimazole to control her hyperthyroidism. Patients that are compliant with therapy with thionamides will generally have full recovery.

Key teaching points

- In a patient with history of hyperthyroidism subject to a stressful or precipitating event, such as surgery, fever, and tachycardia out of proportion to their diagnosis should raise the suspicion of thyroid storm and prompt early treatment.
- Thyroid storm is entirely a clinical diagnosis and, though uncommon, is associated with a significant risk of mortality.
- The most common signs and symptoms of thyroid storm include fever and tachycardia out of proportion to the existing diagnosis. Other frequently encountered signs and symptoms may include congestive heart failure, gastrointestinal dysfunction, and central nervous system dysfunction.
- Patients with thyroid storm should be managed in an intensive care unit setting.
- Therapy to ameliorate the thyroid storm involves:

  Inhibiting thyroid hormone synthesis with thioamides.
  Inhibiting release of hormones by administering iodine.
  Inhibiting peripheral conversion of thyroxine (T4) to triiodothyronine (T3) with propylthiouracil (PTU).
  Beta-blockers (typically propranolol) to decrease tachyarrhythmia and inhibit T4 to T3 conversion.
  Inhibiting enterohepatic circulation of thyroid hormones (cholestyramine).

References

1. Bahtharia S, Goyal V, Chakrabarti R, Utting H. Ruptured ectopic pregnancy concealing thyroid storm. *J Obstet Gynaecol* 2007;27(2):213–24.

2. Akamizu T, Satoh T, Isozaki O, et al. Diagnostic criteria, clinical features, and incidence of thyroid storm based on nationwide surveys. *Thyroid* 2012;22:661–79.

3. Burch HB, Wartofsky L. Life-threatening thyrotoxicosis. Thyroid storm. *Endocrinol Metab North Am* 1993;22(2): 263–77.

4. Klubo-Gwiezdzinska J, Wartofsky L. Thyroid emergencies. *Med Clin North Am* 2012;96:385–403.

5. Chiha M, Samarasinghe S, Kabaker AS. Thyroid storm: An updated review. *J Intensive Care Med* 2013, Aug 5 [Epub ahead of print].

6. Bahn RS, Burch HB, Cooper DS, et al. Hyperthyroidism and other causes of thyrotoxicosis: Management guidelines of the American Thyroid Association and American Association of Clinical Endocrinologists. *Endocr Pract* 2011;17(3):456–520.

7. Carroll R, Matfin G. Endocrine and metabolic emergencies: Thyroid storm. *Ther Adv Endocrinol Metab* 2010;1:139–45.

A 40-year-old woman with hypertension and first-trimester bleeding

Fidelma B. Rigby and Angela M. Tran

History of present illness

A 40-year-old gravida 2, para 0 woman at 14 weeks' gestation by last menstrual period presents to the emergency department with painless vaginal bleeding. The bleeding began this morning. She is changing a pad every two hours. She has had persistent nausea and vomiting for the past two days. She has not previously sought prenatal care. The pregnancy was unplanned.

Her one prior pregnancy was a hydatidiform mole treated by dilation and curettage (D&C). She has had no other surgeries. She has no medical problems. She takes no medications. She does not desire future pregnancy.

Physical examination

General appearance: Ill-appearing woman in moderate discomfort

Vital signs:

Temperature: 37.1°C

Pulse: 110 beats/min

Blood pressure: 160/110 mmHg

Respiratory rate: 14 breaths/min

Oxygen saturation: 99% on room air

HEENT: Dry mucous membranes, no exophthalmos, no thyromegaly

Cardiovascular: Tachycardic, regular rhythm, no murmurs, rubs, or gallops

Lungs: Clear to auscultation bilaterally

Abdomen: Bowel sounds normoactive; soft, nondistended, and nontender to palpation; fundus palpable 2 cm under the umbilicus; no fetal heart tones audible with Doppler

Pelvic: External genitalia unremarkable; moderate amount of blood from closed cervical os; no cervical motion or adnexal tenderness; no masses; uterus consistent with 18 weeks' size; ovaries not palpable

Extremities: No edema

Neurologic: No focal deficits

Laboratory studies:

Serum beta-hCG: 500 000 mIU/mL

Hb: 11 g/dL

Clean catch urinalysis: 3+ protein, no blood, ketones, nitrites, or leukocyte esterase

Imaging: Ultrasound was obtained of the uterus (Fig. 52.1). Bilateral ovarian cysts were also present, each measuring 6 cm in diameter

How would you manage this patient?

This patient has a complete molar pregnancy, also known as a hydatidiform mole. Her combination of hypertension and

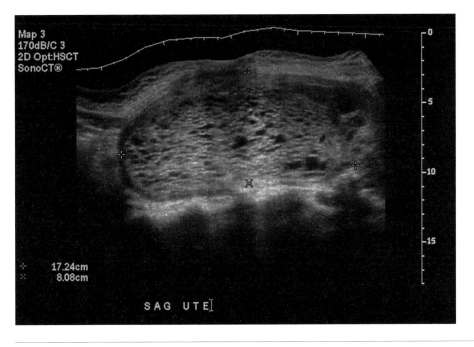

Fig. 52.1 Sagittal ultrasound image of the uterus. Note the vesicular pattern, characteristic of hydatidiform mole. (Image provided by Steven Cohen, MD.)

Acute Care and Emergency Gynecology, ed. David Chelmow, Christine R. Isaacs and Ashley Carroll. Published by Cambridge University Press.
© Cambridge University Press 2015.

Table 52.1 Comparison of partial and complete moles*

Feature	Complete mole	Partial mole
Karyotype	46,XX (90% of cases) or 46,XY	69,XXX or 69, XXY
Fetal tissue	Absent	Present
Chorionic villi	Diffusely hydropic	Focal with variable edema
Trophoblastic hyperplasia	Diffuse, severe	Focal, minimal
Uterine size	28–50% of cases are larger for gestational age	Small for gestational age
Medical complications (hyperemesis, hyperthyroidism, and preeclampsia)	Rare but may occur	Much less common than in complete moles
Risk for gestational trophoblastic neoplasia (GTN)	20%	<5%

* Dighe et al. [1], Berkowitz and Goldstein [4], Zhao et al. [6].

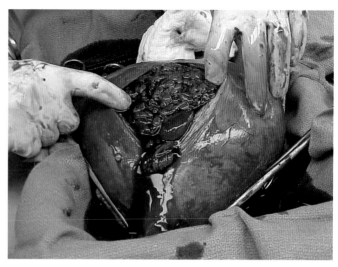

Fig. 52.2 Uterus at time of hysterectomy. The uterus is enlarged greater than expected by dates. The specimen has been opened. Hydropic villi are visible. (Image provided by Steven Cohen, MD.)

proteinuria was indicative of preeclampsia. Platelets, creatinine, and liver function tests were normal. She was admitted to the hospital and her elevated blood pressure was controlled with hydralazine. Her nausea and vomiting were treated with ondansetron. She was typed and cross-matched for two units of packed red blood cells. Chest x-ray was unremarkable. Given her preeclampsia, recurrent mole, and adamant desire not to get pregnant again, she was treated by total abdominal hysterectomy (Fig. 52.2). Her blood pressure had normalized by postoperative day 1. She had an unremarkable postoperative course. The tissue was sent to pathology, and confirmed the diagnosis of complete mole. Her theca lutein cysts resolved after 12 weeks. She was followed with serial serum quantitative beta-human chorionic gonadotropin (beta-hCG) testing, which confirmed resolution of the mole.

Molar pregnancy

Hypertension is common in the emergency care setting, and can be transient and related to patient fear and nervousness and underlying hypertensive disorders. In the setting of early pregnancy bleeding, these two causes likely explain nearly all hypertension present at the time of initial evaluation. It can also be a rare presentation of preeclampsia, which can occur prior to 20 weeks in the setting of molar pregnancy. Preeclampsia is typically defined as systolic pressure greater than or equal to 40 mmHg or diastolic pressure greater than or equal to 90 mmHg on two measurements 6 hours apart, or elevated proteinuria on urine dip or 24-hour collection. It nearly always occurs in the third trimester.

Complete moles are part of a larger spectrum of diseases of the placenta called gestational trophoblastic disease (GTD),

which consists of partial and complete hydatidiform mole and gestational trophoblastic neoplasia (GTN). GTN includes placental site trophoblastic tumor, invasive mole, and choriocarcinoma. A hydatidiform mole is an abnormal pregnancy that results from proliferation of cytotrophoblasts and syncytiotrophoblasts of the placenta. It is characterized by swelling of chorionic villi [1]. Differences between complete and partial moles are summarized in Table 52.1 [1,2,3]. Complete moles are most commonly 46,XX and result from fertilization of an empty ovum by a sperm that duplicates. Most partial moles result from fertilization of a normal ovum by two sperm or fertilization of a normal ovum by one sperm that duplicates. This usually results in a karyotype of 69,XXY [2,4,5]. Partial moles have some component of fetal tissue, varying from nucleated red blood cells to a full fetus. The karyotype of this fetus is usually 69,XXY and early second-trimester fetal growth restriction is typically present. Elevated levels of vascular endothelial growth factor (VEGF) have been implicated in preeclampsia, and increased placental expression of VEGF has been noted in pregnancies with hydatidiform mole [6]

This patient has the two most common risk factors for the development of a complete mole: extremes of maternal age and prior molar pregnancy. Women older than 40 years have a 7.5 times increased risk compared to women aged 21–35, and 1 in 3 pregnancies in women older than 50 years result in a molar pregnancy [4,5]. Partial molar pregnancies do not seem to be associated with increased maternal age [4]. There is a 1% risk for a subsequent molar pregnancy in patients who have had a previous one [1]. Other less well-defined risk factors include oral contraceptive pill use, tobacco use, and vitamin deficiencies.

The most frequent presenting symptoms for hydatidiform moles are painless vaginal bleeding and hyperemesis, which are found in 87% and 8% of cases respectively [5]. The patient in this case has both of these classic findings. Painless vaginal bleeding is a common symptom, and mole is a rare cause of the bleeding. Threatened and spontaneous abortion or ectopic pregnancy are far more common causes of first-trimester bleeding, and are generally the focus of first-trimester bleeding evaluations. Hydatidiform mole should also be included in the differential, although much less frequent than the other causes. In this instance, where preeclampsia was diagnosed so early in pregnancy, molar pregnancy should be specifically investigated. Vaginal bleeding is also common in partial moles, but they may also present as an incomplete or missed abortion where the diagnosis is not made until the specimen undergoes pathologic analysis [5].

This patient has several common physical findings including uterine size greater than expected for gestational age, which is found in 28% of patients. She also had significant hypertension, which should prompt evaluation for preeclampsia as this currently occurs in approximately 1% of patients with moles. This low incidence reflects the current ability to diagnose molar pregnancy early through ultrasound. Older studies from when molar pregnancy was frequently not diagnosed until the second trimester had incidences of preeclampsia as high as 27%. The patient in this case has been diagnosed at 14 weeks, and has a significantly elevated risk. All patients with preeclampsia presenting prior to 20 weeks' gestation should be assessed for molar pregnancy. Rarely, respiratory failure may occur. Unilateral or bilateral theca lutein ovarian cysts occur in about 50% of patients and are caused by hyperstimulation by high levels of hCG [6]. They may be palpable on physical exam. This patient had moderate-sized theca lutein cysts, which were not palpable, likely because the enlarged uterus had caused the ovaries to be located above the level of the pelvis.

Patients with undiagnosed vaginal bleeding should have ultrasonography. Ultrasonography is the diagnostic imaging of choice for hydatidiform moles, and is effective in ruling out the more common causes of first-trimester bleeding. Earlier diagnosis in the first trimester, instead of second or third trimester, coupled with improved ultrasound resolution has led to a notable change in the ultrasound findings of a complete hydatidiform mole. The textbook "snowstorm" description has been replaced by a vesicular pattern, as seen in this patient (Fig. 52.1) [1]. While definitive diagnosis typically requires a pathologic specimen, presence of these ultrasound findings are adequate to guide management. Partial moles may also show similar cystic spaces within the placenta, though the appearance will be more focal in distribution and the transverse diameter of the gestational sac may be increased [4]. Ultrasound may also visualize theca lutein cysts.

Patients with hydatidiform mole can have other medical problems, particularly hyperthyroidism and preeclampsia. Advances in ultrasound resolution and the availability of beta-hCG testing have allowed earlier diagnosis, making preeclampsia and hypertension much less frequent than in the past. Patients with hypertension should be assessed for preeclampsia and patients with hyperthyroid symptoms should have thyroid studies ordered. Anemia is present in 5% of

patients. The hyperemesis and preeclampsia found in complete molar pregnancies are very rare in partial moles [5]. All resolve rapidly after evacuation of the mole.

Typical laboratory findings include a markedly elevated serum hCG level. Complete molar pregnancies may present with normal levels of serum hCG, but about half of patients with complete moles have hCG levels greater than 100 000 mIU/mL. Less than 10% of patients with partial moles have an hCG this high [1]. Because hCG levels peak in the late first trimester, a time when a molar pregnancy is often being considered, a single hCG value is not as useful and a complete mole must be differentiated from a normal intrauterine pregnancy, multiple gestation, and pregnancies characterized by large placentas such as ones with intrauterine infections [5].

Hydatidiform mole is primarily managed by surgical evacuation by suction D&C. Patients being taken to the operating room should have a complete blood count with platelets, clotting functions, metabolic panel, and blood type and screen. For those who do not desire fertility, hysterectomy is an option. Patients are still at risk for metastatic GTN after hysterectomy [4,5]. This patient, who was 40 years old, no longer desired fertility, was having her second molar pregnancy, and had developed preeclampsia, chose to have a hysterectomy as it decreased her risk of a future mole and metastatic GTN with this mole, and might allow her preeclampsia to resolve more quickly. Prior to surgery, chest x-ray is typically done to rule out pulmonary edema or metastases [2]. Any associated complications, such as preeclampsia or hyperthyroidism, should be addressed [4,5]. Special considerations include patients with respiratory compromise by physical examination, or when concern is raised by abnormal chest x-ray findings. Respiratory distress syndrome can occur due to high output congestive heart failure, anemia, hyperthyroidism, or preeclampsia. Central venous catheter monitoring and prolonged intubation can be considered in these patients. The patient must also be monitored intraoperatively for respiratory distress, which can occur from trophoblastic embolization, high-output congestive heart failure, and iatrogenic fluid overload [5]. This patient had her blood pressure controlled. In late pregnancy, magnesium is typically administered to patients with preeclampsia to prophylax against seizures. No recommendations exist for seizure prophylaxis in the first half of pregnancy. As this patient was having her procedure under general and was having a procedure that should resolve her preeclampsia quickly, magnesium was not administered.

Patients with theca lutein cysts are at risk for ovarian torsion because of their ovarian enlargement and should be counseled regarding symptoms [1]. This risk should be low after hysterectomy. These cysts should be managed expectantly as they usually resolve within 8–12 weeks after the molar pregnancy is evacuated. They should not be removed at time of hysterectomy [3]. An ultrasound can be done to document resolution.

While risk of persistent GTN is low after hysterectomy, the patient's hCG levels should still be monitored on a weekly basis until they normalize for three weeks, followed by monthly monitoring for six months, as they would be if she had the usual evacuation by D&C. After evacuation, effective contraception is extremely important to ensure a new pregnancy does not start until it is certain that there is no persistent GTN. This is not an issue after hysterectomy.

With early diagnosis and appropriate treatment, prognosis is generally excellent. Availability of hCG assays and ready access to ultrasound has generally allowed earlier diagnosis, and outcomes are better than in the past. With current chemotherapy regimens, most women with GTN are cured, and even those with widespread metastatic disease have greater than 90% cure rates [2,5].

Key teaching points

- Patients with preeclampsia prior to 20 weeks' gestation need evaluation for a hydatidiform mole.
- Most hydatidiform moles are diagnosed early, where medical complications such as hyperthyroidism and preeclampsia are rare. In moles that are diagnosed later, medical complications are more frequent.

- Vaginal bleeding is the most common presentation. Most patients with bleeding have other more common diagnoses which must be ruled out.
- An extremely elevated human chorionic gonadotropin (hCG) level (>100 000 mIU/mL) should raise suspicion for a complete hydatidiform mole.
- Ultrasonography is the diagnostic imaging procedure of choice. With earlier diagnosis, classic findings such as uterine size greater than expected for gestational age and the "snowstorm" appearance of the mole on ultrasonography are much less common.
- Suction dilation and curettage is the treatment of choice for molar pregnancies. In unusual circumstances in women no longer desiring fertility, hysterectomy may be appropriate.
- Human chorionic gonadotropin levels should be followed after treatment of a molar pregnancy. Levels of hCG that plateau or are persistently elevated should prompt an immediate evaluation for gestational trophoblastic neoplasia.

References

1. Dighe M, Cuevas C, Moshiri M, Dubinsky T, Dogra VS. Sonography in first trimester bleeding. *J Clin Ultrasound* 2008;36(6):352–66.

2. Soper JT, Mutch DG, Schink JC. Diagnosis and treatment of gestational trophoblastic disease. Practice Bulletin No. 53. *Gynecol Oncol* 2004;93:575–85.

3. Berkowitz RS, Goldstein DP. Molar pregnancy. *N Engl J Med* 2009;360: 1639–45.

4. Berkowitz RS, Goldstein DP. Current management of gestational trophoblastic diseases. *Gynecol Oncol* 2009;105:3–4.

5. Lurain JR. Gestational trophoblastic disease I: Epidemiology, pathology, clinical presentation and diagnosis of gestational trophoblastic disease, and management of hydatidiform mole. *Amer J Obstet Gynecol* 2010;6:531–9.

6. Zhao M, Yin Y, Guo F, et al. Placental expression of VEGF is increased in pregnancies with hydatidiform mole: Possible association with developing very early onset preeclampsia. *Early Hum Dev* 2013;89:583–8.

Nausea and vomiting at eight weeks' gestation

Brian Bond and Ashley Peterson

History of present illness

A 25-year-old gravida 1, para 0 woman at 8 weeks' gestation presents with 2 weeks of daily nausea. The nausea persists for several hours each day and is associated with vomiting once or twice a day with temporary relief. She has been able to tolerate some small meals and has been drinking plenty of fluids. She denies dizziness, lightheadedness, fevers, chills, abdominal pain, back pain, changes in bowel habits, or urinary symptoms. She denies weight loss, sick contacts, or recent antibiotic use. Prior to this pregnancy, she was healthy with no significant medical or surgical history. She has a full-time job and has been arriving late to work and feeling less productive than usual.

Physical examination

Vital signs:

Temperature: 37.0°C
Pulse: 80 beats/min
Blood pressure: 110/70 mmHg
Respiratory rate: 18 breaths/min
Oxygen saturation: 99% on room air
BMI: 21 kg/m^2

Neck: Supple, thyroid not enlarged
Cardiovascular: Regular rate and rhythm without rubs, murmurs, or gallops
Lungs: Clear to auscultation bilaterally
Abdomen: Soft, nondistended, nontender, normoactive bowel sounds
Pelvic: Eight-week-sized nontender uterus, no adnexal masses, no vaginal bleeding
Extremities: No clubbing, cyanosis, edema, normal skin turgor, no skin tenting
Laboratory studies: Urinalysis is negative for ketones, protein, WBCs, leukocyte esterase, nitrites, and specific gravity was 1.005 (normal 1.002–1.030)
Imaging: Pelvic ultrasound shows a single viable intrauterine pregnancy with a crown–rump length measuring 1.6 cm consistent with 8 weeks' 0 days gestational age

How would you manage this patient?

The patient described is exhibiting findings consistent with nausea and vomiting of pregnancy. Given the absence of signs or symptoms of dehydration, the patient should be managed as an outpatient with dietary modification, avoidance of triggers, and pharmacologic therapy. The patient should be started on scheduled doses of first-line agents such as pyridoxine (vitamin B6) 10 mg PO TID and doxylamine 12.5 mg PO TID. If her symptoms do not improve, promethazine 12.5 mg PO every 6 hours and metoclopramide 5 mg PO every 8 hours as needed, can be added to the regimen. In this scenario, her symptoms improved within a week and completely resolved by 18 weeks of gestation and medications were discontinued.

Nausea and vomiting of pregnancy

Nausea and vomiting of pregnancy is a common complaint during early pregnancy affecting approximately three quarters of the nearly four-million pregnant women in the United States annually. Although often referred to as "Morning Sickness," the symptoms of nausea and vomiting of pregnancy can occur at any time of the day and range in severity from mild (minimal effect on daily life) to severe (significant effects on daily life, resulting in dehydration often requiring hospitalization) [1].

Nausea and vomiting of pregnancy tends to be more common in younger women, primigravidas, women with less than 12 years of education, nonsmokers, and obese women. Risk factors that have been reported in the literature include women who have a past medical history of motion sickness, nausea and vomiting with oral contraceptive use, migraines, or a prior pregnancy complicated by nausea and vomiting. A higher incidence of nausea and vomiting is reported with multiple gestations as compared with women with singleton pregnancies (87% vs. 73%) [2]. Patients taking a prenatal vitamin prior to conception as well as smokers have a decreased risk of nausea and vomiting of pregnancy [3].

There are no set criteria for the diagnosis of nausea and vomiting of pregnancy; however, symptoms typically manifest after 4 and before 9 weeks of gestation and resolve by 16–20 weeks of gestation [4]. In cases where nausea and vomiting present for the first time after nine weeks of gestation or in the presence of abdominal pain, fever, and headache, other causes must be evaluated such as appendicitis, peptic ulcer disease, and pyelonephritis. There is a wide range in the severity of nausea and vomiting associated with early pregnancy and it is difficult to evaluate objectively. The patient's perception of the severity of her symptoms and desire for treatment often directs clinical decision-making.

Acute Care and Emergency Gynecology, ed. David Chelmow, Christine R. Isaacs and Ashley Carroll. Published by Cambridge University Press.
© Cambridge University Press 2015.

Table 53.1 Pharmacologic therapy options for management of nausea and vomiting of pregnancy

Medication (Name)	Class	Dose	Route	Frequency
Vitamin B6 (Pyridoxine)	Vitamin	10–25 mg	PO	TID or QID
Doxylamine (Unisom SleepTabs®)	Antihistamines, 1st generation	12.5 mg	PO	TID or QID
Promethazine (Phenergan®)	Antihistamines, 1st generation	12.5–25.0 mg	PO or PR or IM	Every 4 hours
Dimenhydrinate (Dramamine®)	Antihistamines, 1st generation	50–100 mg*	PO or PR	Every 4–6 hours
Metoclopramide (Reglan®)	Prokinetic	5–10 mg	PO or IM	Every 8 hours
Trimethobenzamide (Tigan®)	Anti-emetic	200 mg	PR	Every 6–8 hours

* Maximum daily dose 400 mg or 200 mg if used in combination with doxylamine.
IM, intramuscularly; PO, *per* os (orally); PR, by rectum; TID, three times daily; QID, four times daily.

Appropriate initial evaluation includes a history and physical examination. Orthostatic vital signs, serum electrolytes, and a urinalysis may assist in evaluation of dehydration but is often not necessary in the initial management in cases of mild or moderate nausea and vomiting. Laboratory evaluation becomes necessary in women with persistent nausea and vomiting that is not responding to medical management and demonstrating signs of dehydration. An obstetric ultrasound can confirm an intrauterine pregnancy, gestational age, and evaluate for multiple gestations or gestational trophoblastic disease, but is often not necessary in the initial diagnosis and management of nausea and vomiting of pregnancy.

Treatment of nausea and vomiting of pregnancy incorporates both nonpharmacologic and pharmacologic therapies. Despite a lack of strong supporting evidence, providers often recommend dietary modification [5]. Recommendations include frequent small meals of bland or dry foods, protein rich snacks, avoiding an empty stomach, eliminating spicy and fatty foods, discontinuing iron supplements, and using ginger supplements. Heartburn and acid reflux should be treated as they are associated with increased severity of nausea and vomiting of pregnancy [6]. P6 acupressure wristbands and nerve stimulation therapy are commercially available products, although evidence has suggested limited benefit with a large placebo effect.

If symptoms do not improve with lifestyle modifications, it is reasonable to start oral or rectal medications to alleviate mild-to-moderate nausea and vomiting of pregnancy. Pyridoxine (vitamin B6) 10–25 mg PO 3–4 times a day taken with or without doxylamine succinate 12.5 mg (contained in over-the-counter sleep aids) is a first-line agent that helps to alleviate mild nausea [7]. This combination was previously marketed in the United States under the trade name Bendectin®, but was voluntarily withdrawn due to safety concerns. Since that time additional studies have confirmed its safety, and in 2013 it was reintroduced in the United States under the trade name Diclegis®. Other oral medications should be added

in a step-wise fashion to alleviate symptoms and changed if no effect is seen within a week or side effects of current medications are intolerable. Antihistamines such as dimenhydrinate or promethazine should be added if first-line therapies have failed. The medication regimen can be expanded to include metoclopramide, promethazine, or trimethobenzamide if nausea and vomiting continue to persist and there are no signs of dehydration (Table 53.1).

Nausea and vomiting of pregnancy is a time-limited condition and is likely related to the peaking of human chorionic gonadotropin concentration. Symptoms, however, can persist for several weeks if not adequately addressed and can lead to lost wages, require hospitalization for intravenous rehydration and medications, and exacerbate psychosocial stressors. Prevention and adequate treatment of symptoms once they arise can improve quality of life during early pregnancy. There is no association with adverse pregnancy outcomes such as miscarriage, perinatal mortality or fetal anomalies in patients with nausea and vomiting of pregnancy [8].

Key teaching points

- Nausea and vomiting of pregnancy is a common complaint during early pregnancy affecting approximately three quarters of the nearly four-million pregnant women in the United States annually.
- Nausea and vomiting of pregnancy is typically self-limiting and usually arises between 4 and 9 weeks and completely resolves by 18–20 weeks' gestation.
- Early recognition of symptoms and prompt treatment with lifestyle modifications and medications is key to improving quality of life in pregnancy.
- Pyridoxine with or without doxylamine succinate is the first-line treatment for nausea and vomiting of pregnancy.
- If first-line treatments fail, step-wise addition of other medications may be necessary to control symptoms.

References

1. American College of Obstetricians and Gynecologists. Nausea and vomiting of pregnancy. Practice Bulletin No 52. *Obstet Gynecol* 2004;103:803–15.

2. Lee NM, Saha S. Nausea and vomiting of pregnancy. *Gastroenterol Clin North Am* 2011;40:309–34.

3. Czeizel AE, Dudas I, Fritz G, et al. The effect of periconceptional multivitamin-mineral supplementation on vertigo, nausea and vomiting in the first trimester of pregnancy. *Arch Gynecol Obstet* 1992;251(4):181–5.

4. Whitehead SA, Andrews PL, Chamberlain GV. Characterisation of nausea and vomiting in early pregnancy: a survery of 1000 women. *J Obstet Gynaecol* 1992;12:364–9.

5. Matthews A, Dowsell T, Haas DM, Doyle M, O'Mathuna DP. Interventions for nausea and vomiting in early pregnancy. *Cochrane Database Syst Rev* 2010, Issue 9. Art. No.:CD007575. DOI: 10.1002/14651858.CD007575.pub2.

6. Gill SK, Maltepe C, Mastali K, Koren G. The effect of acid-reducing pharmacotherapy on the severity of nausea and vomiting of pregnancy. *Obstet Gynecol Int* 2009;2009:585269.

7. Sahakian V, Rouse D, Sipes S, Rose N, Niebyl J. Vitamin B6 is effective therapy for nausea and vomiting of pregnancy: A randomized, double-blind placebo-controlled study. *Obstet Gynecol* 1991; 78:33–6.

8. Weigel MM, Weigel RM. Nausea and vomiting of early pregnancy and pregnancy outcome. A meta-analytical review. *Br J Obstet Gynaecol* 1989; 96(11):1304–11.

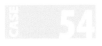

A 27-year-old woman with severe nausea and vomiting in pregnancy

Sarah Peterson

History of present illness

A 27-year-old gravida 3, para 1 woman with a dichorionic diamniotic twin gestation at 9 weeks' gestational age presented to the emergency department for 5 days of severe nausea and vomiting. The patient had been struggling with persistent nausea and vomiting for several weeks, and had been evaluated in another emergency department on two prior occasions for similar symptoms. Symptoms acutely worsened on the day prior to presentation, with an increased frequency of emesis and an inability to tolerate oral liquids or solids. The patient denied abdominal pain, fevers, chills, vaginal bleeding, or vaginal discharge. She complained of mild constipation and symptoms of acid reflux unrelieved by antacids. The patient reported that her symptoms were so distressing that she was considering termination of the pregnancy.

Review of systems was otherwise negative. The patient had no other medical problems and no prior surgeries. She was not on any medications other than prenatal vitamins, which she had been unable to take. Her prior pregnancy had mild nausea that resolved on its own without treatment, and was otherwise uncomplicated.

Physical examination

General appearance: Alert-and-oriented, thin woman in moderate distress with emesis but otherwise well appearing

Vital signs:

Temperature: 36.8°C
Blood pressure: 106/70 mmHg
Pulse: 116 beats/min
Respiratory rate: 22 breaths/min
Oxygen saturation: 98% on room air

HEENT: Dry mucus membranes

Neck: Supple, no lymphadenopathy, no thyromegaly

Cardiovascular: Tachycardic, regular rhythm, normal S1/ S2, no murmurs, rubs, or gallops, no edema

Lungs: Clear to auscultation bilaterally, nonlabored respirations, no wheezes or rales

Abdomen: Soft, mildly tender to palpation in epigastrium, nondistended, hypoactive bowel sounds, no rebound or guarding

Pelvic:

Speculum examination: No blood, discharge, or lesions
Cervix examination: Normal appearing, no cervical motion or adnexal tenderness, cervix closed and long

Uterus: 9-weeks' size

Laboratory studies:

Potassium: 2.9 mmol/L (normal 3.5–5.5 mmol/L)
Leukocyte count: 16 400/μL (normal 3500–12 500/μL) with 77% neutrophils (normal 50–70%)
Urinalysis: 30 mg/dL protein, trace leukocytes, moderate ketones, and a specific gravity of 1.034
Serum lactate concentration: 0.7 mmol/L (normal 0.5–1.6 mmol/L)

Initial treatment in the emergency department consisted of intravenous hydration with two 1 L normal saline fluid boluses and intravenous promethazine. She continued to have emesis.

How would you manage this patient?

The patient has hyperemesis gravidarum. She was admitted for supportive care. Intravenous hydration was continued and her electrolytes were closely monitored. Her hypokalemia was corrected with intravenous potassium. Despite treatment with promethazine 12.5 mg IV every 4 hours and ondansetron 8 mg IV every 12 hours, the patient's nausea and emesis persisted. She continued to lose weight, which prompted initiation of enteral tube feedings. She was continued on a proton pump inhibitor for her gastroesophageal reflux symptoms. Tube feedings were eventually able to be discontinued and her diet was slowly advanced. She was discharged home on hospital day 12 with prescriptions for pyridoxine (vitamin B6), doxylamine, ondansetron, and promethazine. She was advised to eat small frequent meals and was scheduled to return to clinic in one week.

Hyperemesis gravidarum

Pregnancy is often complicated by nausea and vomiting, with up to 80% of women experiencing these symptoms at some point during their pregnancy [1]. While hyperemesis gravidarum is imprecisely defined, it is generally felt to represent the more severe end of the pregnancy-associated nausea and vomiting continuum. Less severe symptoms are very common and are generally called nausea and vomiting of pregnancy. Hyperemesis is second only to preterm labor as an indication for hospital admission during pregnancy, and affects approximately 0.5–2.0% of pregnant women [2]. The symptoms can have significant physical and psychological impacts and can be so distressing that they may lead women to terminate their pregnancies [2].

While definitions for this condition vary, key components include intractable vomiting, weight loss of greater than 5% of prepregnancy weight, dehydration, ketosis, and electrolyte abnormalities [1]. Thyroid and liver abnormalities may also be present. Risk factors include increased placental mass (often due to multiple or molar gestations), female fetus, a personal or family history of hyperemesis, and a history of migraines or motion sickness [2]. Meta-analyses have demonstrated that infection with *Helicobacter pylori* is also associated with an increased risk of hyperemesis [3].

The exact mechanism of hyperemesis gravidarum is not well understood, but human chorionic gonadotropin (hCG) is thought to play a role because of the synchronous temporal relationship between peak hCG concentrations and symptoms of nausea and vomiting in the late first trimester [2]. Conditions causing higher levels of hCG such as multiple gestations and molar pregnancies have been associated with increased nausea and vomiting [1]. This patient's twin pregnancy is a likely explanation for why she has hyperemesis in this pregnancy despite not having it in her prior pregnancy. Estrogen is also thought to contribute, as symptoms are more common with higher estradiol levels. Estrogen stimulates the production of nitric oxide, which relaxes smooth muscle, and it is postulated that this leads to nausea and vomiting by slowing gastrointestinal motility [4]. Cigarette smokers are less likely to have hyperemesis gravidarum, possibly because smoking decreases levels of both hCG and estradiol [2]. Progesterone has also been implicated, as it causes relaxation of the lower esophageal sphincter [4]. Theories of psychogenic causes have fallen out of favor.

Mothers are often concerned about the effects of protracted nausea and vomiting on their developing fetus, and they can generally be reassured that hyperemesis gravidarum is associated with normal pregnancy outcomes. While hyperemesis has been associated with a slightly higher incidence of low-birth-weight infants, there has been no demonstrated increased risk of malformations [2]. Patients with hyperemesis gravidarum actually have a lower incidence of spontaneous abortion, which is hypothesized to result from the abundant synthesis of hCG [2]. Fetal death associated with hyperemesis is rare.

The psychosocial impact on the mother is significant, and may lead to depression, anxiety, somatization, or other psychiatric conditions [2]. While mortality rates are low, a number of severe complications can occur. There have been several reported cases of Wernicke's encephalopathy from severe vitamin B1 deficiency caused by intractable vomiting. Other rare but related complications include splenic avulsion, Mallory–Weiss tears, esophageal rupture, pneumothorax, and acute tubular necrosis [2].

Symptoms are typically worst in the first trimester, peaking around weeks 6–12. Nausea and vomiting can persist beyond 20 weeks' gestational age in up to 20% of women [1]. Timing is an important consideration, as hyperemesis gravidarum typically manifests prior to nine weeks' gestational age. If symptoms begin after nine weeks or are associated with additional symptoms such as abdominal pain, fever, or headaches, alternative

Table 54.1 Differential diagnosis of nausea and vomiting in pregnant women*

Gastrointestinal	Peptic ulcers Cholecystitis Gastroenteritis Appendicitis Hepatitis Pancreatitis Achalasia Bowel obstruction
Genitourinary	Pyelonephritis Nephrolithiasis Ovarian torsion Degenerating fibroids Uremia
Metabolic	Diabetic ketoacidosis Hyperthyroidism Addison disease Porphyria
Neurologic	Migraines Pseudotumor cerebri Vestibular lesions Central nervous system tumors
Pregnancy-related	Acute fatty liver of pregnancy Preeclampsia Mild nausea and vomiting of pregnancy
Iatrogenic	Medication intolerance
Other	Drug or alcohol toxicity Psychological factors

* Modified from the American College of Obstetricians and Gynecologists [2].

diagnoses should be considered [2]. Hyperemesis gravidarum is a diagnosis of exclusion. Other possible causes must be ruled out (Table 54.1 [2]).

Evaluation should include ultrasonography to assess for possible multiple gestation or molar pregnancy [2]. Laboratory testing is warranted when nausea and vomiting is severe and prolonged. Patients with hyperemesis will often have mild elevations in their liver function tests (with AST [aspartate aminotransferase] and ALT [alanine transaminase] typically <300 U/L) [2]. Bilirubin and serum amylase or lipase may also be slightly elevated. A hypochloremic metabolic alkalosis can develop with intractable vomiting and urinalysis often shows increased specific gravity and ketonuria consistent with dehydration [2]. As many as two-thirds of patients with hyperemesis gravidarum will have abnormal thyroid function tests, likely due to cross-reactivity between hCG and thyroid-stimulating hormone (TSH) receptors [4]. Typical findings include increased free thyroxine and suppressed TSH. Patients are typically euthyroid, and the degree of thyroid dysfunction has not been correlated with the severity of symptoms [4]. Therefore, thyroid function studies should not be routinely obtained in patients without clinical features of thyroid dysfunction.

Patients should be admitted to the hospital if they have failed outpatient management or cannot tolerate oral nutritional intake or oral anti-emetics. Subsequent management depends on the degree of the patient's dehydration. If the patient is not significantly dehydrated, dopamine antagonists such as intramuscular or oral metoclopramide or rectal trimethobenzamide should be initiated. Patients with intractable nausea and vomiting accompanied by significant dehydration should be intravenously hydrated with crystalloid solutions to correct dehydration, ketosis, electrolyte and acid-base abnormalities. They should also be administered parenteral anti-emetics. Patients with preexisting psychiatric illnesses should have the management of these problems optimized with counseling, psychotherapy, and medications.

Many options exist for intravenous anti-emetics. Antihistamines such as dimenhydrinate have been widely used and have not been shown to increase the risk of birth defects [5]. Large prospective studies have also demonstrated that metoclopramide and other dopamine antagonists are safe; however, there are no trials demonstrating efficacy. Dopamine antagonists can be helpful in women suffering with reflux esophagitis and dyspepsia because they enhance motility [5]. Phenothiazines such as prochlorperazine, promethazine, and chlorpromazine are also commonly used, and do not appear to be associated with fetal malformations. Neonatal withdrawal and extra-pyramidal effects have been reported in neonates born to mothers using phenothiazines continuously in the third trimester [5]. Ondansetron, a serotonin receptor antagonist often used to control chemotherapy-induced nausea and vomiting, has also been used in patients with hyperemesis despite its cost. One trial demonstrated equal effectiveness to promethazine [2,5]. Lastly, butyrophenones including droperidol have been used to treat hyperemesis gravidarum. A single study with limited power did not demonstrate a statistically significant increase in fetal malformations. Maternal QT interval prolongation has been documented with this medication [2,5] It would be reasonable to commence therapy with either intravenous promethazine, metoclopramide, or dimenhydrinate, depending on provider preference and familiarity. Should these regimens fail, as in our patient, addition of ondansetron may prove helpful.

The use of corticosteroids is controversial. While some studies have shown a decreased rate of hospital readmission with use of methylprednisolone, others have failed to confirm these findings. Methylprednisolone has been associated with a small risk of oral clefting, so corticosteroids should only be used when all alternative regimens have failed [2,5]. One suggested regimen is methylprednisolone 16 mg every 8 hours PO or IV for 3 days, and then tapered over 2 weeks to the lowest effective dose. Six weeks is the maximum recommended duration of use [2].

If patients experience persistent weight loss despite anti-emetics and hydration, enteral or parenteral nutrition options may be necessary. Dextrose and vitamins including intravenous thiamine are recommended when patients have been vomiting for longer than three weeks. Enteral tube feedings should usually be attempted prior to initiation of total parenteral nutrition (TPN), as the latter is associated with potentially life-threatening complications such as infection, thrombosis, and hepatobiliary dysfunction [2,5]. TPN is appropriate for patients who require long-term nutritional support who cannot tolerate enteral feeds.

After initial stabilization, patients may be slowly transitioned to a general diet and oral or rectal anti-emetics. Rectal suppositories including promethazine or trimethobenzamide can be used in patients who are poorly tolerating oral medications. Intravenous fluid resuscitation should be gradually tapered once patients are tolerating oral fluids. If nausea and vomiting persist, laboratory studies for electrolyte abnormalities and ketonemia should be repeated as necessary. Once electrolyte abnormalities have been corrected and patients are tolerating a general diet and oral medications, they may be discharged home with close outpatient follow-up. The Pregnancy-Unique Quantification of Emesis (PUQE) scoring system can be employed to help patients monitor the severity of their symptoms [4].

Patients will usually require continued anti-emetics at after discharge. Vitamin B6 (pyridoxine) and doxylamine (an H1-receptor blocker) in combination has been associated with decreased hospitalization [2]. Randomized, placebo-controlled trials have shown up to a 70% reduction in nausea and vomiting, and this combination has been demonstrated to be safe for the developing fetus [2,5]. Other agents that can be used orally or rectally to control nausea and vomiting in the outpatient setting include promethazine, prochlorperazine, or antihistamines such as dimenhydrate. This patient was sent home on pyridoxine, doxylamine, ondansetron, and promethazine because of the severity of her hyperemesis and the difficulty with which it was controlled. Even with optimal outpatient management, studies have shown a readmission rate of approximately 30% [6].

Key teaching points

- Hyperemesis typically presents prior to nine weeks' gestational age.
- If hyperemesis starts after nine weeks' gestational age, other causes are likely.
- Hyperemesis is a diagnosis of exclusion. Other possible causes of nausea and vomiting in pregnancy must be ruled out.
- Management of patients with hyperemesis gravidarum includes aggressive intravenous fluid replacement, correction of electrolyte abnormalities, thiamine repletion, and pharmacologic therapy with parenteral agents such as dimenhydrinate, metoclopramide, promethazine, and ondansetron.
- Patients should be admitted to the hospital if they have failed outpatient management or cannot tolerate oral nutritional intake or oral anti-emetics.
- Patients should be discharged on a regimen of promethazine and/or ondansetron, pyridoxine, and doxylamine.

References

1. Matthews A, Dowswell T, Haas DM, Doyle M, O'Mathuna DP. Interventions for nausea and vomiting in early pregnancy. *Cochrane Database Syst Rev* 2010, Issue 9. Art. No.: CD007575. DOI: 10.1002/14651858.CD007575. pub2.

2. American College of Obstetricians and Gynecologists. Nausea and vomiting of pregnancy. Practice Bulletin No. 52. *Obstet Gynecol* 2004;103:803–15.

3. Sandven I, Abdelnoor M, Nesheim Bl, et al. *Helicobacter pylori* infection and hyperemesis gravidarum: A systematic review and meta-analysis of case control studies. *Acta Obstet Gynecol Scand* 2009;88:1190–200.

4. Lee NM, Saha S. Nausea and vomiting of pregnancy. *Gastroenterol Clin North Am* 2011;40(2):309–34, vii. DOI 10.1016/j.gtc.2011.03.009.

5. Maltepe C, Koren G. The management of nausea and vomiting of pregnancy and hyperemesis gravidarum – a 2013 update. Canadian Society of Pharmacology and Therapeutics. *J Popul Ther Clin Pharmacol* 2013; 20(2):e184–92.

6. Lacasse A, Laqoutte A, Ferreira E, Bérard A. Metoclopramide and diphenhydramine in the treatment of hyperemesis gravidarum: Effectiveness and predictors of rehospitalisation. *Eur J Obstet Gynecol Reprod Biol* 2009; 143(1):43–9.

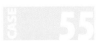

Early pregnancy with vaginal spotting

Kathryn A. Houston and Sarah B. Wilson

History of present illness

A 28-year-old gravida 2, para 0 woman presents to the emergency room with a history of vaginal spotting for 2 days and some mild bilateral pelvic cramping. She has regular 28-day menstrual cycles and the first day of her last menstrual period was approximately 5 weeks ago. She was not using birth control and took a pregnancy test three days ago, which was positive. This pregnancy was not planned but is desired. She has a history of one prior first-trimester miscarriage. The remainder of her review of systems is negative. She has no significant past medical or surgical history. She has no known drug allergies. She does not smoke or drink. She works part time as a preschool teacher.

Physical examination

General appearance: Well-appearing woman in no acute distress

Vital signs:

Temperature: 37.4°C
Blood pressure: 125/70 mmHg
Pulse: 80 beats/min
Respiratory rate: 19 breaths/min
Oxygen saturation: 100% on room air

Cardiovascular: Regular rate and rhythm

Lungs: Clear to auscultation bilaterally

Abdomen: Soft, nontender, no rebound or guarding, no masses

Pelvic:

External genitalia: Normal in appearance
Vagina: Scant dark red blood present
Cervix: No lesions, nulliparous appearing os, no active bleeding
Bimanual exam: Normal size anteverted uterus; no cervical motion, adnexal, or uterine tenderness

Laboratory studies:

hCG: 943 mIU/mL
Urinalysis: Negative
Blood type: O positive

Imaging: A pelvic ultrasound was obtained (Fig. 55.1). The ultrasound showed a normal appearing uterus with an intrauterine echolucency suggestive of a gestational sac. The mean sac diameter measures 5 mm, which would be consistent with an estimated gestational age of approximately 5 weeks. No yolk sac or embryo (fetal pole) is identified. Normal appearing ovaries, no adnexal masses or free fluid

How would you manage this patient?

The patient was counseled regarding her clinical findings of an early pregnancy with uncertain viability given the context of her bleeding. It is also a pregnancy of undetermined location

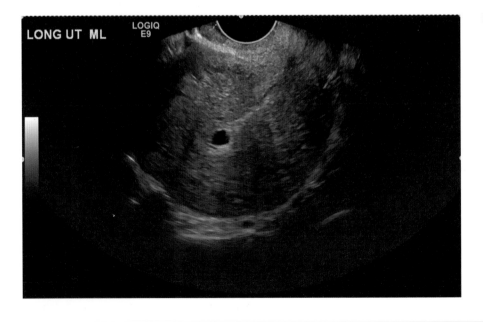

Fig. 55.1 Pelvic ultrasound.

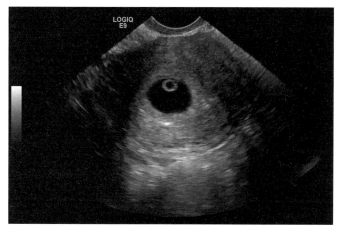

Fig. 55.2 Transvaginal ultrasound.

given the nondiagnostic (although not unexpected) ultrasound findings. An ectopic gestation has not been ruled out given the absence of any defining embryonic growth, and as such the ultrasound echolucency may represent a pseudogestational or "pseudosac" only. The patient's early gestational age limits the ability to have a certain diagnosis and, thus, requires close follow-up and surveillance.

The patient was given precautions to return for any heavy vaginal bleeding or severe abdominal pain and was scheduled for a follow-up assessment in 48 hours, with a repeat human chorionic gonadotropin (hCG) level and ultrasound. Forty-eight hours later she continues to have light vaginal spotting.

hCG: 1926 mIU/mL

Transvaginal ultrasound: See Fig. 55.2. A normal appearing uterus with a gestational sac measuring 8 mm consistent with an estimated gestational age of 5.5 weeks. A yolk sac is visualized within the gestational sac. A fetal pole is not seen. Normal appearing ovaries, no adnexal masses or free fluid

The patient was counseled that she has a confirmed intrauterine pregnancy. Ectopic pregnancy has been ruled out with the presence of a yolk sac appearing within the intrauterine gestational sac. While she still has a risk of miscarriage in the context of the vaginal bleeding, the hCG level continues to rise as would be expected with a viable pregnancy. A follow-up office appointment was scheduled in a week with plans for a repeat ultrasound. Bleeding and pain precautions were reviewed with the patient.

Early pregnancy with vaginal spotting

Women often present in early pregnancy with symptoms of pelvic cramping, pain, or vaginal bleeding. While many of these pregnancies will progress normally, it is important to be able to diagnose both ectopic and nonviable pregnancies in the acute care setting. Evaluation of patients with early pregnancy bleeding or pain can be challenging. Patients are understandably eager to have a diagnosis and are often anxious

regarding their prognosis. A step-wise approach to evaluate the patient's history, serum hCG levels, and transvaginal ultrasounds is necessary to determine the correct diagnosis in early pregnancy. In addition, counseling and clinical follow-up are often an essential part of patient management.

The first step in evaluating any condition of early pregnancy is taking a patient history and trying to identify/calculate the gestational age from the patient's last menstrual period (LMP). This history may unfortunately be limited as menstrual cycles may vary in length and regularity, and patients are not always certain as to when their LMP occurred. To further help determine the best estimated gestational age, any recent history of birth control use or timing of coitus may provide additional clues.

The clinical history should also reference the presence and duration of vaginal bleeding and abdominal/pelvic pain. Ectopic pregnancies commonly present with either bleeding or pain and account for 1–2% of all pregnancies and 6% of maternal deaths in the United States. Intra-abdominal hemorrhage from rupture of the ectopic pregnancy is the cause of death in over 90% of these cases [1]. The goal is to diagnose ectopic pregnancies before tubal rupture in order to prevent morbidity/mortality. Half of women in whom ectopic pregnancy is diagnosed however, have no identifiable risk factors or initial physical findings. Risk factors include a history of pelvic inflammatory disease, prior tubal sterilization, prior ectopic pregnancy, pelvic surgery, assisted reproductive technologies, and smoking [2]. If ectopic pregnancy cannot be ruled out during the initial evaluation by demonstrating embryonic growth within the uterus (as in the case of our patient's first ultrasound), the patient must have close follow-up and an understanding of her circumstances until the diagnosis of an ectopic pregnancy can be excluded.

Finally, the clinical history often includes a discussion regarding the patient's intentions and/or desire for the pregnancy as many patients will have strong feelings that help guide in counseling and further management.

Laboratory assessments with hCG levels are also important in guiding the practitioner as they indicate what developmental milestones should be seen on transvaginal ultrasound. hCG levels, however, are not especially useful in determining actual gestational age as they can vary widely during the first trimester and with multiple gestations. When the hCG measures greater than or equal to 1500–2000 mIU/mL (called the "discriminatory zone"), a fetal pole should be seen on transvaginal ultrasound of a singleton gestation. Failure to visualize a fetal pole on transvaginal ultrasound with an hCG of greater than 2000 mIU/mL should arise suspicion of an ectopic or other nonviable pregnancy. hCG levels should increase by a minimum of 53% over a 48-hour interval in a viable singleton pregnancy [3]. Failure to accomplish this increase is also highly suspicious of a nonviable or ectopic pregnancy. Unfortunately, hCG levels are highly variable in ectopic pregnancies and should not be used alone to confirm the diagnosis. Repeated hCG assessments over time to follow trends, in conjunction with repeated ultrasound evaluations are required to make a confident diagnosis.

In addition to hCG assessments, a patient's blood type, specifically the Rh D antigen status, should be confirmed by a type and screen. Whether to administer anti-D immune globulin to prevent Rh alloimmunization to a patient with threatened abortion and a live embryo or fetus at or before 12 weeks of gestation is controversial, and no evidence-based recommendation can be made. Rh D alloimmunization attributable to threatened abortion prior to 12 weeks' gestation is exceedingly rare. The decision to administer anti-D immune globulin when comparing the overall benefit with the cost of its widespread use has caused many physicians to not routinely administer this in these circumstances [4].

Transvaginal ultrasound is the best imaging modality to diagnose early pregnancy location and confirm viability. Prior to eight weeks' gestation, transvaginal ultrasound is usually necessary to visualize uterine contents as opposed to an abdominal ultrasound. At four to five weeks' gestational age, a gestational sac can usually be seen on a transvaginal ultrasound and its location should be documented. The presence of an intrauterine fluid collection **without** a yolk sac or fetal pole cannot be assumed to be a gestational sac, as it could represent a "pseudosac" [5]. A pseudosac is a small fluid collection located within the uterine cavity appearing in the context of and ectopic pregnancy.

Between five and six weeks' gestation, a yolk sac should typically be seen within the gestational sac. The presence of an intrauterine gestational sac with a yolk sac confirms an intrauterine pregnancy, as was the case in the second ultrasound of this patient. Except in the very rare instance of heterotopic pregnancy, an ectopic has been ruled out.

Between 6 and 7 weeks' gestation, or with a mean gestational sac diameter of 20 mm or greater, a fetal pole (embryo)

should become visible. Visualization of a gestational sac, yolk sac, and embryo with cardiac motion verifies a viable intrauterine pregnancy. If a fetal pole is present, it must be at least 5–7 mm without cardiac motion to diagnose a nonviable pregnancy [5,6]. If the embryo measures less than 5 mm in length, a subsequent scan at a later date will be necessary to assess the presence or absence of cardiac activity.

In this particular case the patient has a confirmed intrauterine pregnancy only after the second ultrasound revealed an intrauterine gestational sac with a yolk sac. The appropriate rise in hCG levels over 48 hours is an encouraging clinical sign and viability will be confirmed when a future scan demonstrates an embryo with cardiac motion.

Key teaching points

- Clinical history to assess last menstrual period/calculate estimated gestational age, human chorionic gonadotropin (hCG) levels, and pelvic ultrasound are the critical components for evaluation of an early pregnancy.
- When the hCG level is greater than 1500–2000 mIU/mL (the "discriminatory zone") an intrauterine gestation should be visible on transvaginal ultrasound. Ultrasound evaluation done prior to this may be nondiagnostic.
- The presence of an intrauterine gestational sac with a yolk sac on ultrasound confirms an intrauterine pregnancy and rules out the possibility of an ectopic pregnancy. A yolk sac should been seen between five and six weeks' gestation.
- hCG levels should increase by greater than 53% over 48-hour period in a normal, viable, singleton pregnancy.
- Serial hCG monitoring and ultrasound evaluation may be necessary to assess early pregnancies presenting with bleeding and uncertain viability or location.

References

1. Chang J, Elan-Evans LD, Berg CJ, et al. Pregnancy-related mortality surveillance – United Sates, 1991–1999. *MMWR* 2003;52(SS02):1–8.

2. American College of Obstetricians and Gynecologists. Medical management of ectopic pregnancy. Practice Bulletin No. 94. *Obstet Gynecol* 2008;111: 1479–85.

3. Barnhart KT, Sammel MD, Rinaudo PF, et al. Symptomatic patients with an early viable intrauterine pregnancy: hCG curves redefined. *Obstet Gynecol* 2004;104:50–5.

4. American College of Obstetricians and Gynecologists. Prevention of Rh D alloimmunization. Practice Bulletin No. 4. *Int J Gynaecol Obstet* 1999; 66(1):63–70.

5. American College of Obstetricians and Gynecologists. Ultrasound in pregnancy. Practice Bulletin No. 101. *Obstet Gynecol* 2009;113: 451–61.

6. Doubilet PM, Benson CB, Bourne T. Diagnostic criteria for nonviable pregnancy early in the first trimester. *N Engl J Med* 2013;369(15): 1443–51.

Positive RPR on initial prenatal labs

Ronald M. Ramus

History of present illness

A 20-year-old gravida 1 woman presents for urgent follow-up after initiation of prenatal care. She is now 12 weeks' pregnant. Her medical history is unremarkable. She has never had surgery and her only medication is a prenatal vitamin. She has had four sexual partners in her lifetime but has never received any gynecologic care or sexually transmitted infection screening prior to her pregnancy. A panel of routine prenatal laboratory studies were performed five days prior, including a rapid plasma reagin (RPR) test. Her test returns with a positive result, at a titer of 1 : 32. A confirmatory test for treponemal specific antibodies was also positive.

Physical examination

General appearance: Well-nourished woman with no discomfort

Vital signs:

Temperature: 37.0°C
Pulse: 80 beats/min
Blood pressure: 120/70 mmHg
Respiratory rate: 16 breaths/min

HEENT: Unremarkable

Neck: Supple

Cardiovascular: Regular rate and rhythm without rubs, murmurs, or gallops

Lungs: Clear to auscultation bilaterally

Abdomen: Soft, nontender

Extremities: No obvious lymphadenopathy. A faint erythematous rash is noted on her palms and soles

Neurologic: Nonfocal

External genitalia: Multiple smooth, moist, flat lesions on the vulva and in the perianal region (Fig. 56.1)

Vagina: Unremarkable, scant discharge

Cervix: Nulliparous, no mucopurulent discharge

Uterus: Approximately 12 weeks' size

Adnexa: Nontender, no masses

Laboratory studies:

CBC: Normal
Negative for chlamydia, gonorrhea, hepatitis B, and HIV

How would you manage this patient?

The patient's laboratory testing confirms a true syphilis infection. The erythematous rash on her palms and soles, as well as the perianal condyloma lata lesions seen are consistent with a diagnosis of secondary syphilis.

The patient was given benzathine penicillin G (Bicillin®) 2.4 million units IM as a one-time dose, and will undergo retesting several weeks later to confirm adequate treatment (her RPR titer should drop at least fourfold). In addition, the RPR will be repeated monthly thereafter throughout the pregnancy to look for evidence of reinfection.

Syphilis

Syphilis is a sexually transmitted disease caused by the spirochete *Treponema pallidum*. The Centers for Disease Control and Prevention (CDC) recommends screening for syphilis in pregnancy. This is typically done at the first prenatal visit, and is repeated in the third trimester in women at high risk for syphilis. High-risk women include sex workers, users of illicit drugs, individuals with HIV, infection with other sexually transmitted diseases, women living in an area with a high incidence of syphilis, a lack of regular prenatal care, uninsured women, poverty, or sexual promiscuity. The RPR test is the most common laboratory study used to screen for syphilis. It is ideally suited for this role due to its simplicity and low cost. An alternative nontreponemal specific screening assay is the VDRL (venereal disease research laboratory) test. The VDRL

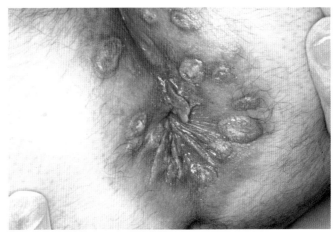

Fig. 56.1 Perianal condyloma lata. This is a common finding with secondary syphilis. The lesions are flat, raised, and moist. (Photograph courtesy of Nick Fiumara, MD.)

Acute Care and Emergency Gynecology, ed. David Chelmow, Christine R. Isaacs and Ashley Carroll. Published by Cambridge University Press. © Cambridge University Press 2015.

Table 56.1 The stages of syphilis seen in pregnancy, with characteristic findings and treatment recommendations

Stage	Clinical findings	RPR titer	Treatment
Primary	Genital chancre, regional lymphadenopathy	High	Bicillin® 2.4 million units × 1
Secondary	Condyloma lata, palmar erythema, generalized lymphadenopathy	High	Bicillin® 2.4 million units × 1
Early latent	None	Usually low	Bicillin® 2.4 million units × 1
Late latent	None	Usually low	Bicillin® 2.4 million units × 3 doses weekly

RPR, rapid plasma reagin.

test was developed before World War 1 and has now largely been replaced by the RPR assay, as both tests use the same antigen but in the RPR test the antigen is bound to a carbon particle to allow visualization of the flocculation reaction (foaming in a test tube) that does not require a microscope. Because the spirochete responsible for syphilis cannot be cultured in the laboratory, serologic testing is essential in making the diagnosis. It is important to remember, however, that the RPR test is not *specific* to syphilis and there are many known false positive RPR associations. This includes connective tissue diseases such as lupus, Lyme disease, malaria, tuberculosis, certain types of pneumonia, intravenous drug use, HIV, and even pregnancy itself. It is estimated that 1–2% of the United States population has false positive nontreponemal specific test results [1]. Therefore, a positive RPR should always be followed by a *treponemal specific* test, most commonly either FTA-ABS (fluorescent treponemal antibody absorption test), MHA-TP (microhemagglutination assay for *T. pallidum*), or TP-PA (*T. pallidum* particle agglutination assay) based on one's local laboratory availability.

Once the treponemal specific test confirms the diagnosis of syphilis, as in the case of this patient, the next step is to perform a physical examination to look for any clinical symptoms of infection. Clinical findings will vary based on the stage of syphilis present (Table 56.1). Primary syphilis is associated with a painless chancre and regional lymphadenopathy. The chancre can be on the vulva, vagina, or cervix and typically spontaneously resolves in three to six weeks. Secondary syphilis is typically apparent anywhere from six weeks to six months after the initial infection. It is associated with a diffuse erythematous rash known to occur all over the body, and notably appears at times on the palms and soles. There may also be evidence of condyloma lata, (flat, moist, nontender lesions on the perineum or perianal regions) and diffuse lymphadenopathy. The rash of secondary syphilis is usually apparent for two to six weeks, but may be subtle and not obvious to the patient or healthcare provider. If there are no clinical findings of syphilis the patient likely has latent disease. Patients with latent disease are typically divided into two groups: early versus late latent disease. Early latent disease is diagnosed when a negative RPR test was noted less than a year prior in the patient's personal history. If there is no evidence to support a

duration of infection of less than a year, the patient is presumed to have late latent syphilis.

Prior to making a diagnosis of latent syphilis one must determine if there is a history of syphilis treatment in the past. A recent study found that 34% of patients appropriately treated for syphilis will have persistent serologic evidence of the disease one year after treatment [2] even though their syphilis has been cured; a condition called "serofast syphilis." Ideally confirmation of this diagnosis requires documentation of appropriate treatment in the past, typically tracked by ones local Health Department. If confirmation of prior treatment is obtained and the RPR titer remains low (typically 1 : 4 or less) then retreatment is not necessary and the patient is considered serofast. If proof of prior treatment is not available, or the titer is 1 : 8 or higher, it is appropriate to presume latent disease or reinfection and to treat accordingly. Untreated infection after many years of latency can lead to tertiary disease, or neurosyphilis. Fortunately, this is extremely rare in pregnancy as gravid women are typically too young to present with signs and symptoms suggestive of a longstanding syphilis infection.

As Table 56.1 indicates, the treatment for syphilis in pregnancy is penicillin. A long-acting penicillin is required, so the typical formulation is benzathine penicillin G (Bicillin), given as a 2.4 million unit dose IM. Penicillin is the clear preferred agent in pregnancy, as none of the alternative antibiotics used to treat syphilis (such as azithromycin, ceftriaxone, or erythromycin) have been shown to be effective in crossing the placenta and treating fetal infection. The CDC currently recommends a single dose of Bicillin for the treatment of primary, secondary, and early latent syphilis in pregnancy [3]; however, many authorities in the field recommend a second dose of Bicillin one week later to provide better treatment for the fetus [4]. Late latent disease requires three doses of Bicillin given at weekly intervals.

Many patients claim to have a penicillin allergy. Since penicillin is the only safe and effective agent to treat syphilis in pregnancy, it is mandatory to perform skin testing to determine if a true allergy exists. If an allergic reaction is documented then one must proceed with a desensitization algorithm prior to penicillin treatment. There are both oral and intravenous regimens to perform desensitization [5], and this is typically done in an inpatient setting in consultation with an Allergy/Immunology specialist.

If syphilis is diagnosed in the second half of pregnancy, fetal ultrasound evaluation should be performed prior to treatment. Congenital infection leads to hydrops fetalis (ascites, pleural effusions, pericardial effusions, subcutaneous edema with placentomegaly, and polyhydramnios), which is seen with ultrasound and is associated with stillbirth, preterm birth, and neonatal death. The risk of congenital infection is related to the stage of disease; perinatal transmission occurs in about 50% of cases of primary or secondary syphilis, but is reduced to 40% with early latent disease and 10% with late latent disease [6]. If there is ultrasound evidence of fetal infection there is a higher risk of the Jarisch–Herxheimer reaction with treatment. The lysis of spirochetes associated with the treatment of syphilis leads to the release of large amounts of lipopolysaccharide (LPS) and endotoxins. These substances elevate circulating cytokine levels, and can cause fever, chills, hypotension, headache, tachycardia, vasodilation, tachypnea, myalgias, and contractions in the mother. In addition, a fetus undergoing the Jarisch–Herxheimer reaction is more likely to have fetal heart rate decelerations or even fetal death. Because of these potential complications with treatment, pregnancies undergoing penicillin therapy for syphilis with evidence of congenital infection in the third trimester are often treated in a Labor and Delivery unit to facilitate monitoring the fetus and delivery if there are any signs of fetal compromise.

Once treatment has been completed, the CDC recommends that repeat serologic titers be obtained at 28–32 weeks' gestation and again at delivery on women treated earlier in pregnancy. If there is a fourfold or higher rise in titers during surveillance following treatment, then one must presume reinfection and retreat the patient. For women at high risk of reinfection or in geographic areas in which the prevalence of syphilis is high, monthly serologic titers may be appropriate. Given the rarity and potential severity of congenital syphilis, many experts consider any pregnant woman diagnosed with syphilis during pregnancy at high risk for re-infection [3].

Key teaching points

- Treponemal specific testing for syphilis is required when a positive screening test (RPR) is obtained. A positive treponemal specific test confirms a true syphilis infection.
- If syphilis testing is positive, one must review the patient's history and any documentation of prior syphilis treatment to confirm if the diagnosis is "serofast syphilis."
- With no history of prior treatment, penicillin is the antibiotic necessary to achieve bacteriocidal levels in the fetus. If the patient has a suspected penicillin allergy, proceed with skin testing for confirmation of such an allergy. If the patient is truly allergic to penicillin, a desensitization protocol is necessary.
- The stage of syphilis determines the risk to the fetus and the appropriate antibiotic treatment regimen.
- Fetal infections may become apparent on ultrasound as evidenced by hydropic fetal changes. Treatment of an infected fetus may lead to a Jarisch–Herxheimer reaction, and because of such, requires appropriate fetal monitoring during treatment.

References

1. Larsen SA. Syphilis. *Clin Lab Med* 1989: 9:545–57.
2. Tong ML, Lin LR, Liu GL, et al. Factors associated with serological cure and the serofast state of HIV-negative patients with primary, secondary, latent, and tertiary syphilis. *PLoS One* 2013;8(7): e70102.
3. Centers for Disease Control and Prevention. Sexually transmitted diseases treatment guidelines, 2010. *MMWR* 2010;59(RR-12):26–40.
4. Kingston M, French P, Goh B, et al. UK national guidelines on the management of syphilis 2008. *Intl J STD & AIDS* 2008:19:729–40.
5. Wendel GD, Stark BJ, Jamison RB, Molina RD, Sullivan TJ. Penicillin allergy and desensitization in serious infections during pregnancy. *N Engl J Med* 1985;312:1229–32.
6. Sanchez PJ, Wendel GD, Grimprel E, et al. Evaluation of molecular methodologies and rabbit infectivity testing for the diagnosis of congenital syphilis and neonatal central nervous system invasion by *Treponema pallidum*. *J Infect Dis* 1993;167(1):148–57.

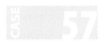

A high-speed motor vehicle accident during pregnancy

Susan M. Lanni

History of present illness

A 25-year-old gravida 2, para 1-0-0-1 woman at 28 weeks' gestation was traveling at posted speed as the unrestrained driver in a car on a major multilane interstate. While driving, her attention waned, and she veered into the adjacent travel lane. She was struck from behind causing her car to spin out of control. Ultimately, her vehicle was hit by two more vehicles traveling in the same direction, and then struck head on by a third car causing her to be ejected from the vehicle. A witness called for emergency medical assistance, which was on scene within five minutes of the crash. There was loss of consciousness. A cervical collar was placed, and her vital signs were rapidly assessed.

Injury assessment/physical examination in the field

General appearance: Suspected head injury based on mechanism of injury, multiple deep and nonhemostatic lacerations and abrasions of the face and arms, legs and chest, a chest contusion extending from T4 level to umbilicus, contusions of the abdomen. Compound fracture of left femur, suspected crush injury of pelvis

Vital signs:

  Pulse: 135 beats/min
  Blood pressure: 167/77 mmHg
  Respiratory rate: 45 breaths/min, shallow, labored
  Oxygen saturation: 96% on 100% FiO_2
  Fetal heart rate: 170 beats/min

Abdomen: Uterine tetany

Ancillary evaluation: Pants soaked and bloody

Course of events

Her respiratory status deteriorated, and she was intubated in the field, as simultaneously intravenous access was obtained. She was transported to a Level 1 trauma facility. Heavy vaginal bleeding was encountered, and blood filled the endotracheal (ET) tube. In the trauma bay, the trauma team and the obstetric team quickly assessed her status, while the neonatal team stood by. The patient was on a backboard tilted to the left, and a FAST (Focused Assessment with Sonography for Trauma) scan revealed significant blood in the abdomen; the fetal heart rate was noted to be 40 beats/min. Maternal asystole was encountered, and chest compressions were initiated, without

regaining a maternal pulse after five minutes. Despite aggressive volume resuscitation with O-negative blood and intravenous fluids, maternal status did not improve. The obstetric team performed emergent Cesarean delivery in the trauma bay via a midline vertical incision; delivery of the cephalic-presenting fetus was 45 seconds after skin incision was made. The neonate was noted to have absent heart rate, poor tone, pale color, and no spontaneous respiratory effort. In addition, the pupils were dilated without reactivity and a depressed parietal bone skull fracture was noted. Resuscitative efforts for the neonate were halted. Meanwhile, the obstetric team repaired the hysterotomy as the trauma team continued resuscitative efforts. Despite an electrical rhythm being obtained, a pulse was never generated. Resuscitative efforts were discontinued at this time.

What is the mechanism of injury?

The mechanism of injury is an unrestrained driver sustaining high speed blunt trauma, causing massive intra-abdominal hemorrhage, acute traumatic membrane rupture and placental abruption, as well as suspected pulmonary hemorrhage from blunt chest trauma. The cephalic-presenting fetus sustained a skull fracture due to the blunt force applied to the maternal pelvis.

Trauma in pregnancy

When all types of trauma are considered, it is suspected that 1 in 12 pregnancies encounter trauma. Certainly, vehicular trauma is but one type, but is the largest contributor to preterm labor and birth, membrane rupture, placental abruption, Cesarean delivery, and intrauterine/neonatal demise resulting from trauma. Pregnancy does not impact severity, mortality, or morbidity of trauma but certainly affects the pattern of injury and the patient's care. Vehicular crashes account for the highest degree of both maternal and fetal/neonatal mortality among all causes of trauma. Outcome of vehicular trauma is affected by seatbelt use; in 2008, 85% of adults surveyed used seatbelts. Seat belt use reduced the likelihood of serious injury in a crash by approximately 45–50% [1]. This is, however, countered by fewer pregnant women at advanced gestational ages wearing seatbelts than by pregnant women below 20 weeks' gestation.

It is estimated that less than 50% of patients are counseled about proper seatbelt use in pregnancy [2]. Seatbelts, both the lap belt and shoulder strap should be used. The lap belt

---

Acute Care and Emergency Gynecology, ed. David Chelmow, Christine R. Isaacs and Ashley Carroll. Published by Cambridge University Press. © Cambridge University Press 2015.

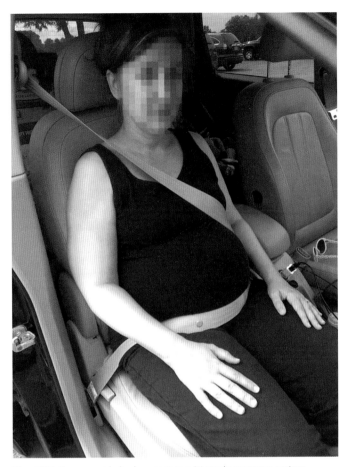

Fig. 57.1 Proper seat belt placement in a 36-weeks pregnant patient. (Photograph courtesy of Susan Lanni, MD; by permission of patient.)

portion should be placed below the pregnant belly and the shoulder strap between the breasts but then lateral to the fundus of the uterus (Fig. 57.1). Airbags and supplemental restraint systems should also be used during pregnancy. Although originally airbags were designed to protect 185-lb male drivers of at least 68 inches at high speeds, as of 2012, all supplemental restraints have been modified to provide safety to women, and in crashes of all speeds [3]. The National Highway Traffic Safety Administration (NHTSA) recommends that the sternum of a pregnant woman be at least 10 inches from the steering wheel or dashboard, and the seat should be adjusted as the abdomen grows.

The evaluation of a pregnant trauma patient is similar to any nonpregnant patient, and begins with the field technicians and paramedics. The ABCs of trauma management apply, as the maternal condition is considered primarily above the fetal condition in all situations and irrespective of gestational age. Physiologic changes associated with pregnancy need to be taken into account to ensure proper care. The increased vascular volume makes the diagnosis of hypovolemia less evident. Lateral displacement of the gravid uterus off the vena cava will ensure adequate venous return and promote maintenance of cardiac output, which is critical where significant intra-abdominal hemorrhage is suspected. Lateral displacement of

the uterus can be accomplished by manually pushing the uterus to the side, or by the use of a wedge under the backboard. In a conscious, stable patient, maintaining the left lateral tilt or decubitus position is sufficient.

Maternal oxygen saturation should be maintained greater than 90% at minimum. At this saturation, the maternal PO_2 is approximately 60 mmHg, which is sufficient to maintain a gradient favoring the delivery of oxygen to the fetus. If saturations fall below 90%, use of supplemental oxygen by nasal cannula, and nonrebreather masks, or ET intubation may be warranted. Intubation is often required for airway protection in the unconscious patient. Aspiration risk is greater when ET intubation is used for the pregnant patient compared to the nonpregnant patient, due to relaxation of the lower esophageal sphincter and altered gastrointestinal motility associated with normal pregnancy physiology. Airway edema may be present in normal pregnancy.

Intravenous access should be obtained in the field, with two 14–18 gauge intravenous catheters. Volume resuscitation using isotonic solutions (normal saline or lactated Ringer's solution) is given in a ratio of 3 : 1 to blood loss. Estimation of blood loss is difficult in a pregnant trauma patient; a 25% loss of blood volume is generally needed to cause a change in maternal vital signs. It is prudent, therefore, to aggressively resuscitate the pregnant trauma patient when hemorrhage is observed or expected. lactated Ringer's solution may have pro-inflammatory effects, and may contribute to multiorgan failure and acute respiratory distress syndrome (ARDS).

Initial hospital care includes injury assessment, maternal vital signs, and evaluation of gestational age and fetal status, which becomes the role of the obstetrician. These factors may affect decisions regarding the care of the mother. Survey of injuries in the pregnant patient should employ all modalities required for adequate assessment, including radiologic studies. CT imaging of the abdomen and pelvis expose the fetus to approximately 3.5 rads; 20–50 rads is required before damage to the fetus should be suspected [4]. Focused Abdominal Sonography for Trauma (FAST) has largely replaced diagnostic peritoneal lavage (DPL) for diagnosis of intra-abdominal bleeding. DPL is disadvantageous in pregnancies of approximately 20 weeks and beyond due to the location of the fundus under the site of entry of the lavage catheter. FAST has the advantage of the immediate ability to "pass the transducer" to the obstetric team for evaluation of the fetus. FAST has high sensitivity (90%) in the first trimester, but low specificity (89%) compared to other trimesters. Negative predictive values approach 100% across trimesters [5].

Placental abruption is not easily diagnosed by ultrasound, but abnormal fetal heart rate patterns especially tachycardia, loss of variability, and late decelerations are observed in the setting of abruption. Uterine contractions greater than 1 every 10 minutes are associated with nearly a 20% rate of placental abruption [6]. Fetomaternal hemorrhage occurs in 10–30% of pregnant trauma patients [7]. In the case of an Rh-negative unsensitized mother, Rh immune globulin should be administered in the standard dose, as 90% of fetomaternal hemorrhages are less than 30 mL in volume [8].

In the above case, the gestational age favors the need to monitor the fetus; however, in light of maternal asystole, monitoring is obviated. Additionally, suspicion of a crush injury to the pelvis predicts poor fetal outcome. Decision to perform perimortem Cesarean delivery should be based on potential survival for the neonate, but may improve survival for the mother also. It is generally performed in the setting of imminent maternal death, or after four minutes of properly performed CPR, as seen in the case above. Neonatal outcomes for fetuses of a viable gestational age (typically 23–24 weeks and above, but are dependent on resources available at the individual hospital) are best when perimortem Cesarean is performed within 5 minutes of maternal asystole [9].

It is estimated that intrauterine death from trauma affects 2.3 per 100 000 live births. Fetal head trauma is almost universally fatal, and when the fetus is in cephalic presentation, the fetal head is cushioned by proportionally less myometrium, allowing the maternal pelvis to contribute to this type of injury. Third trimester is the most common trimester for trauma-related injuries to affect the fetus. Factors that independently portend poor fetal outcomes include maternal loss of consciousness and pelvic injury [10].

Key teaching points

- All pregnant women should be instructed on proper seatbelt use.
- Evaluation of the pregnant trauma patient should always start with the ABCs of life support.
- Lateral displacement of the gravid uterus off of the vena cava will promote maximal venous return and facilitate maintenance of maternal cardiac output.
- All members of the teams caring for the pregnant trauma patient should be apprised of normal pregnancy physiologic changes.
- The mother's status always takes precedence over the fetal status in the situation of resuscitation. If efforts to resuscitate the mother can be improved by uterine evacuation, then delivery should be considered.
- Imaging studies should not be deferred due to risk of radiation exposure to the fetus.
- Perimortem Cesarean delivery for gestations above 24 weeks is ideally performed within 5 minutes of initiation of CPR for maternal cardiac arrest.

References

1. National Highway Traffic Safety Administration. *Final Regulatory Impact Analysis. Amendment to Federal Motor Vehicle Safety Standard 208. Passenger Car Front Seat Occupant Protection.* Washington, DC, US Department of Transportation, National Highway Traffic Safety Administration, 1984. Publication # DOT-HS-806-572. Available at http://www-nrd.nhtsa.dot.gov/pubs/806572.pdf.

2. Sirin H, Weiss HB, Sauber-Schatz EK, et al. Seat belt use, counseling and motor-vehicle injury during pregnancy: results from a multi-state population-based survey. *Matern Child Health J* 2007;11(5):505–10.

3. Segui-Gomez M, Levy J, Graham J. The airbag safety and distance of the driver from the steering wheel [letter]. *N Engl J Med* 1998;339:132–3.

4. American College of Obstetricians and Gynecologists. Guidelines for diagnostic imaging during pregnancy. Committee Opinion No. 299. *Obstet Gynecol* 2004;10(3):647–51.

5. Richards JR, Ormsby EL, Romo MV et al. Blunt abdominal injury in the pregnant patient: detection with ultrasound. *Radiology* 2004;233:463–70.

6. Perlman MD, Tintinnalli JE, Lorenz RP. Blunt trauma during pregnancy. *N Engl J Med* 1990;323:1609–13.

7. Hill C, Pichingpaugh J. Trauma and surgical emergencies in the obstetric patient. *Surg Clin N Amer* 2008;88:421–40.

8. Goodwin TM, Breen MT. Pregnancy outcome and feto-maternal hemorrhage after non catastrophic trauma. *Am J Obstet Gynecol* 1990;162:665–71.

9. Katz VL, Balderston K, Defreest M. Perimortem Cesarean delivery: Were our assumptions correct? *Am J Obstet Gynecol* 2005;192:1916–20.

10. Aboutanos MB, Aboutanos, SZ, Dompkowski D, et al. Significance of Motor vehicle crashes and pelvic injury on fetal mortality: A five-year institutional review. *J Trauma* 2008;65(3):616–20.

A 32-year-old woman with fever and unilateral breast pain

Meghann E. Batten

History of present illness

A 32-year-old gravida 2, para 2 woman presents to an urgent care clinic with complaints of left breast pain, flu-like symptoms, and fever. She is breast-feeding and five weeks postpartum from an uncomplicated spontaneous vaginal delivery. She reports the pain and fatigue began one day prior. Overnight, she developed fever up to 39.8°C, chills, malaise, and worsening breast pain. She took acetaminophen (Tylenol®) and ibuprofen for comfort, but these did not resolve her symptoms. She states that when she nurses on the left side, the breast is exquisitely painful, the baby is fussy, and her milk production seems decreased. She denies nausea, vomiting, diarrhea, or abdominal pain. She has no other medical problems and is not taking any other medications.

Physical examination

General appearance: Healthy woman who appears uncomfortable and tired

Vital signs:

Temperature: 38.5°C
Pulse: 98 beats/min
Blood pressure: 118/76 mmHg
Respiratory rate: 18 breaths/min

Chest: Respirations are nonlabored, lung fields are clear

Cardiac: Regular rate and rhythm

Breast: Right breast is soft, moderately engorged, with no masses noted. Left breast is tender to palpation, erythematous and warm to touch in the left outer quadrant. No masses or fluctuance palpated. Nipples intact bilaterally without lesions or skin break down (Fig. 58.1)

Abdomen: Soft, nontender

Extremities: Nontender, no edema

How would you manage this patient?

The patient has lactational mastitis, a breast infection that occurs during the postpartum period with breast-feeding. She had classic symptoms and high fever, but no evidence of an abscess, so she was treated as an outpatient. She was prescribed a 14-day course of dicloxacillin (500 mg PO QID). She was also educated on adjuvant therapy, including nonsteroidal anti-inflammatory drugs for pain and fever, rest, hydration, massage and warm compresses of the affected breast, and

frequent nursing or pumping to drain the breast. She was afebrile within 24 hours of initiation of antibiotic therapy and pain free within 72 hours. She continued to breast-feed without disruption or difficulty.

Mastitis

Mastitis (also called lactational mastitis or puerperal mastitis) has been defined by the World Health Organization as an inflammatory condition of the breast, which may or may not be accompanied by infection [1]. It is an acute inflammation of the interlobular connective tissue within the breast and ranges from local inflammation with minimal systemic symptoms to abscess and septicemia [2]. It can occur anytime during lactation, but it is most common during the second and third weeks postpartum, with 75–95% of cases occurring within the first 12 weeks postpartum [3]. The reported incidence of mastitis varies widely from 1 to 33% of breast-feeding women. This variance is due to the broad spectrum of methodology for case ascertainment ranging from self-diagnosis to a positive milk culture [1].

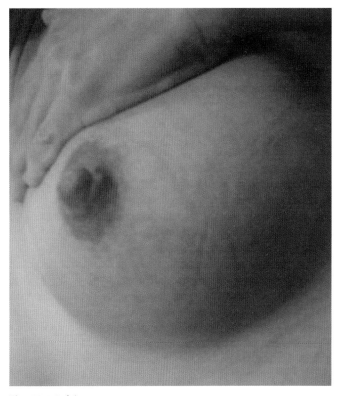

Fig. 58.1 Left breast.

Acute Care and Emergency Gynecology, ed. David Chelmow, Christine R. Isaacs and Ashley Carroll. Published by Cambridge University Press. © Cambridge University Press 2015.

Table 58.1 Differential diagnosis for common lactational problems

	Engorgement	Blocked duct	Mastitis	Abscess
Occurrence during lactation	First-week postpartum	Any time	Any time	Any time
Onset	Gradual	Gradual	Sudden	Sudden
Usual location	Bilateral	Unilateral	Unilateral	Unilateral
Erythema	Bilateral	None	Unilateral	Localized
Heat	Generalized warmth	Little to none	Warm to hot	Hot
Pain	Generalized	Local, mild	Unilateral, moderate–severe	Localized, severe
Appearance/palpation	Firm, enlarged, shiny	Localized lumpy area	Wedge-shaped area of firmness	Swollen discrete lump
Systemic symptoms	Feels well	Feels well	Feels ill	May or may not feel well
Fever	Afebrile	Afebrile	Fever >37.5°C	May or may not have fever

Mastitis is thought to be caused by two primary conditions: milk stasis and infection. Milk stasis can occur as a result of poor breast-feeding latch, incomplete emptying of the breast, over-abundant milk supply, extended periods between feeds, missed feeds, and tight or incorrectly fitting clothing on the breasts. The stagnant milk provides an excellent culture medium for bacterial growth. Infection generally occurs as the result of skin bacteria, though it is not known how the bacteria enters the breast. Because sore nipples are a common finding with mastitis, one theory is that the bacteria enters through a crack or fissure in the nipple [1]. The most common organism involved in mastitis is *Staphylococcus aureus*. Other organisms such as *Streptococcus, Escherichia coli, Haemophilus influenzae, Haemophilus parainfluenzae, Klebsiella pneumoniae, Enterobacter cloacae, Serratia marcescens*, and *Pseudomonas pickettii* have been implicated as well [4].

The differential diagnosis for mastitis includes a range of conditions from normal physiologic processes such as lactational fullness, engorgement, galactoceles, and blocked ducts, to infectious processes such as ductal candidiasis and breast abscess, to more chronic pathology such as Raynaud's phenomenon of the nipple, and inflammatory breast cancer [5]. Table 58.1 includes a comparison of findings for commonly occurring lactational conditions. Diagnosis is based on clinical symptoms including fever, chills, myalgia, flu-like symptoms, breast tenderness and pain, unilateral edema, and erythema in a wedge-shaped area [2]. Milk culture is rarely used because positive cultures can result from normal bacterial colonization and negative cultures do not rule out mastitis. A milk culture may be useful if the infection is severe, unusual, recurrent, or fails to respond to traditional antibiotic therapy [3].

Careful history and physical is crucial to the diagnosis and treatment of mastitis. A detailed breast-feeding history helps identify associated factors including missed feedings, widely spaced feedings, increased stress fatigue, incomplete drainage of the breast, over-abundant milk supply, tight-fitting clothing, and breast pumping [3]. A breast assessment helps to rule out abscess and evaluate for contributing factors such as a crack or

fissure in the nipple. This is especially critical in a patient who has recurrent episodes of mastitis. Breast abscess generally presents as a discrete painful lump with localized heat and erythema and may or may not be associated with fever. If abscess is suspected or mastitis is recurrent, a breast ultrasound may be beneficial [5]. If nipple tenderness is reported or damage such as cracking or bruising is noted, observation of a breast-feeding session by a healthcare professional or lactation consultant may assist with evaluation of the infant's latch. Poor attachment to the breast can occur as a result of flat nipples, obesity, poor positioning, tight frenulum, and prematurity. In this patient, no issues with latch or emptying of the breast were identified. High levels of fatigue and stress, as well as a nursing bra with an underwire were identified as potential contributing factors.

Prompt diagnosis and treatment of mastitis are important in preventing early weaning from breast-feeding. Mastitis has been reported as the third most common reason for weaning with 25% of women citing mastitis as the reason they weaned [6]. Because of the vast benefits of breast-feeding to both mother and infant, the Department of Health and Human Services "Healthy People 2020" and the Surgeon General's Call to Action have emphasized a critical need to increase breast-feeding initiation and continuation rates, particularly to 6 months of age [7]. Swift symptom resolution and correction of predisposing factors may help to reduce premature cessation of breast-feeding due to mastitis.

The primary goals of treatment are facilitating recovery and preventing complications. There is overwhelming consensus that breast-feeding should continue throughout treatment of mastitis. Women should be encouraged to nurse their babies frequently, ideally feeding on the affected side first, with the infant's chin pointing in the direction of the affected area [5]. If nursing is too painful, pumping with an electric or manual pump may be substituted. If over-supply or incomplete emptying is identified, pumping after feeds should be instituted to assist in complete drainage of the breast. Hot compresses and massage during feeds may also help to promote drainage [5]. Supportive therapy to alleviate systemic symptoms includes bed rest, increased fluids, pain medication, and use of anti-inflammatory agents. If systemic symptoms are mild or noninfective mastitis is suspected, these interventions may be sufficient treatment for mastitis [8].

Antibiotic therapy, a mainstay component of mastitis treatment, is controversial. To date, there has been little consensus on which patients require antibiotics, which antibiotic is most appropriate, the timing of treatment, and how long treatment should continue [8]. A Cochrane review of antibiotics in the treatment of mastitis concluded that there is, "Insufficient evidence to confirm or refute the effectiveness of antibiotic therapy for the treatment of lactational mastitis" [8], citing a lack of well-designed, scientific studies such as randomized control trials (RCTs). However, in one study it was found that women who received antibiotic therapy achieved the fastest symptom resolution (2.1 days), as opposed to supportive therapy only (4.2 days), or no therapy (6.7 days). Faster resolution of symptoms is likely to avoid disruption or discontinuation of breast-feeding. In addition, 11% of cases with no intervention developed an abscess while there were no cases of abscess in those women who received antibiotic therapy [8]. When prescribing antibiotics, there must be careful consideration of antibiotic compatibility with breast-feeding. Dicloxacillin (250–500 mg QID) and cephalexin (500 mg QID) are commonly used. Generally a 10–14-day course is recommended [3]. Despite the high fever and rapid onset of systemic symptoms associated with mastitis, patients who undergo appropriate treatment have swift resolution as well. Cessation of fever and systemic symptoms generally occurs within one to three days of antibiotic initiation. Breast pain typically resolves within a week.

Complications arising from mastitis include recurrence, breast abscess and sepsis, which can be fatal. Recurrence may result from incomplete treatment, maternal immunoglobulin A (IgA) deficiency, increased stress/fatigue, or undiagnosed abscess. Daily low-dose antibiotic therapy for prevention of recurrence may be required [5]. Abscess has been reported in 5–11% of mastitis cases [2]. Abscess may be diagnosed on physical examination or with ultrasound. It is generally treated with incision and drainage along with antibiotics (potentially parenteral). Needle aspiration of the abscess, repeated every other day until there is no further purulent accumulation has also been suggested [2]. Sepsis, though rare, can result from delayed or inadequate treatment and requires hospital admission and parenteral antibiotics.

Key teaching points

- Mastitis is characterized by unilateral breast pain and erythema, accompanied by flu-like symptoms including fever, and myalgia. It is caused by milk stasis and infection.
- Treatment requires evaluation and correction of associated factors such as poor infant latch or incomplete emptying of the breast.
- Treatment with antibiotics has been demonstrated to reduce the length of symptoms and the likelihood of abscess. A 10–14 day course is recommended, along with supportive therapy.
- Milk culture should be reserved for recurrence or infection that fails standard therapy.
- Breast abscess and sepsis can occur if treatment is delayed or inadequate.

References

1. Inch, S, von Xylander, S. *Mastitis: Causes and Management.* Geneva, World Health Organization, 2000.

2. Barbosa-Cesnik C, Schwartz K, Foxman B. Lactation mastitis. *JAMA* 2003; 289(13):1609–12.

3. Spencer JP. Management of mastitis in breastfeeding women. *Am Fam Physician* 2008;78(6):727–32.

4. American College of Obstetricians and Gynecologists. *ACOG Practice Bulletin, 2006: Compendium of Selected Publications.* Washington, DC, ACOG, 2006, pp. 284–5.

5. Betzold, CM. An update on the recognition and management of lactational breast inflammation. *J Midwifery Womens Health* 2007; 52(6):595–605.

6. Crepinsek MA, Crowe L, Michener K, Smart NA. Interventions for preventing mastitis after childbirth. *Cochrane Database Syst Rev* 2012, Issue 10. Art. No.: CD007239. DOI: 10.1002/14651858.

7. HealthyPeople.gov. 2020 Topics and objectives: maternal, infant, and child health. Goal 21. Available at http://www.healthypeople.gov/2020/topicsobjectives2020/objectiveslist.aspx?topicId=26.

8. Jahanfar S, Ng CJ, Teng CL. Antibiotics for mastitis in breastfeeding women (review). *Cochrane Database Syst Rev* 2013, Issue 2. Art. No. CD005458. DOI: 10.1002/14651858.

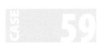

A 36-year-old woman with nipple pain postpartum

Julie Zemaitis DeCesare and Karen Shelton

History of present illness

A 36-year-old gravida 3, para 3 woman presents 2 days postpartum following an uncomplicated vaginal delivery complaining of severe breast soreness and nipple pain with lactation. The pain started with the first feeding, became more intense over the past 12 hours, and has gotten worse with each subsequent feeding. She described the pain as a "searing, burning pain" that gets worse as the feeding progresses. She is anxious and crying. She states she is really committed to breast-feeding this child, and is worried she will not be able to continue. She has successfully breast fed her two previous infants, although she had problems with chronic yeast infections in her breasts with her second child. She is taking no medications other than prenatal vitamins and has no other medical problems. Depression screening was negative.

Physical examination

General appearance: Thin, white woman who is slightly anxious

Vital signs:

Temperature: 37.0°C
Pulse: 70 beats/min
Blood pressure: 100/70 mmHg
Respiratory rate: 14 breaths/min

Abdomen: Soft, nontender uterus palpated 1 cm below the umbilicus

Breast: Bilateral symmetric tenderness, no fluctuance, slight erythema at the nipples, nipples everted (Fig. 59.1)

How would you manage this patient?

The patient has cracked, irritated nipples likely secondary to an improper infant latch. An observational assessment of the feeding session was performed by a lactation consultant. It was observed that the infant's lips were noted to be curled under forming an incomplete seal, and the nipple was not centered in the infant's mouth creating an improper areolar grasp. Instruction on proper latch techniques were provided and recommendations for breast-feeding pillows and other comfort measures were reviewed including pure lanolin solution, rubbing expressed milk into the nipple, and hydrogel pads.

She was advised to feed on the side with the least amount of discomfort first and was fitted with a 24 mm nipple shield.

The patient noted gradual improvement with the next feeding sessions, and went on to breast-feed successfully for 12 months.

Cracked nipples

The Department of Health and Human Services "Healthy People 2020" goal for breast-feeding are 81.9%, 60.6%, and 34.1% in the early postpartum period, 6 months, and 12 months, respectively. In 2010, these breast-feeding rates are 76.5%, 49.0%, and 27.0%, respectively [1] As reviewed in the American College of Obstetricians and Gynecologists "Breast feeding: maternal and infant aspects" [2], breast pain is the second most common reason for early discontinuation of breast-feeding. As a clinician, an understanding of the

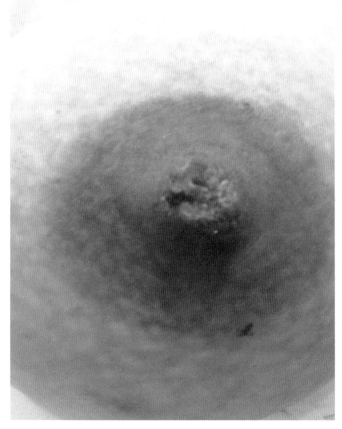

Fig. 59.1 Breast.

Acute Care and Emergency Gynecology, ed. David Chelmow, Christine R. Isaacs and Ashley Carroll. Published by Cambridge University Press. © Cambridge University Press 2015.

causes and treatments of common breast problems resulting in cracked nipples is important to improve current breast-feeding rates.

When a patient presents with cracked nipples, she will often report pain on lactation that is described as burning or searing. The pain gets worse as the feeding session continues, and often starts with one of the first few feeding sessions. Common physical examination findings for nipple pain include bilateral and symmetrical tenderness, slight redness, and dry and flakey skin on the nipple. Small fissures or cracks can be noted upon close inspection of the nipples and areola.

Breast causes of cracked nipples include engorgement, mastitis, plugged milk ducts, yeast, and skin disorders. Almost all women experience some form of breast engorgement in the postpartum period, and most commonly present within the first two weeks. Engorged breasts can promote nipple cracking, as well as act as an entry point for bacteria. Infant causes of nipple cracking include poor latch, improper position, and infant teething, while maternal causes of sore and cracked nipples are improper pumping techniques with mechanical pumps and harsh cleansing agents on the breast. Skin conditions of the breast such as psoriasis, thrush, and contact dermatitis can cause also cause nipple soreness and cracking while breast-feeding [3].

If a woman develops cracked nipples, the treatment is multifactorial. Supportive care is first line, and it is important to encourage the mom to continue to breast-feed despite the discomfort. Feeding from the less painful side first is important, as the infant suck is less vigorous after they are somewhat satiated. Additionally, frequent small feedings can help facilitate a less vigorous suck. Expressing some milk and gently rubbing into the nipples can sooth the tender area. Pure lanolin rubbed into the nipples before and after feeding can prevent chafing and cracking. It is important to change wet nursing bras/undergarments to keep the breast clean, dry and to prevent chaffing. Use of a commercial available nursing nipple pad can facilitate this. Hydrogel pads are used to sooth chaffed and cracked nipples. These dressings are designed to keep the breast moist to facilitate healing, provide immediate pain relief and adsorb drainage. Finally, it is key to promote proper hand washing, as cracked breasts are very prone to infectious complications.

If supportive care does not quickly improve, a nipple shield is recommended. This is a nipple-shaped sheath worn over the areola and nipple during breast-feeding. Shields vary in size and are made of soft, thin silicone with holes at the end of the nipple section to allow breast milk to pass through (Fig. 59.2). Nipple shields are used to allow mothers to continue breast-feeding until her cracked or sore nipples heal. Nipple shields should be of temporary use and aim is always to return to regular breast-feeding.

Thrush or yeast will need to be treated in both the mother and infant, and should be suspected as a cause of cracked nipples if the mother complains of persistent redness, itchy

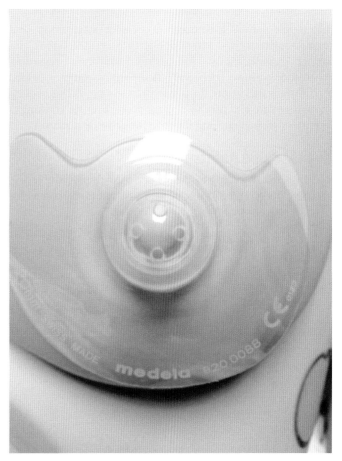

Fig. 59.2 Nipple shield.

or burning nipple pain, shooting pains in the breast after feeding, or intense pain that is not improved with better latch and positioning. The nipples and areola may appear pink or red, shiny, or flaky. This condition should be suspected when the infant has thrush, or the mother has persistent erythema. Treatment of the mother with oral fluconazole (Diflucan®) for 10–14 days, as well as treating the infant with nystatin is appropriate. Mastitis should also be considered as a cause of nipple soreness and erythema; however, it can be differentiated from other causes by fever and fluctuance.

Prevention of cracked nipples in the breast-feeding experience is crucial for long-term success. Keys to prevention include the correct latch and position early on. Education and observation of the feeding experience can correct the latch before any breast problem occurs. Prevention of engorgement will also preclude cracked nipples. Feeding on demand, as much as every two hours in the newborn period, helps to prevent this condition. Additionally, manually expressing milk prior to feeding can help the infant more effectively latch. Taking the baby off the breast, by gently breaking suction with the tip of a clean maternal finger will prevent trauma from occurring at the nipple. Proper hygiene to the breast decreases contamination with skin flora; however, harsh/heavily scented cleansers can themselves be a source of breast trauma.

In summary, it is important to address and acknowledge that nipple pain is a common occurrence in lactation, and present solutions and interventions to prevent cracking and further complications. Antepartum education regarding expectations, proper latch, and infant position can be provided by clinicians well before the first feeding session. Techniques on supportive care and how to manage/prevent nipple cracking is important to facilitate and improve breast-feeding rates.

Key teaching points

- Most breast-feeding women experience nipple pain at some point, and it is one of the most common reasons for early discontinuation of breast-feeding.

- Improper latch is one of the most common causes of nipple pain and cracked nipples.
- Prevention of cracked nipples by education regarding proper latch and proper infant position for feeding can be provided in the antepartum period.
- Use of lanolin, hydrogel dressings, and nipple shields are interventions that can be employed once the cracking has occurred.

References

1. Centers for Disease Control and Prevention. Breastfeeding. Available at http://www.cdc.gov/breastfeeding/data/nis_data/

2. American College of Obstetricians and Gynecologists. Breast feeding: maternal and infant aspects. Committee Opinion No. 361. *Obstet Gynecol* 2007; 109(2 Pt 1):479–80. Reaffirmed 2013.

3. Lawrence R, Lawrence R. *Breastfeeding: A Guide for the Medical Professional*, 7th edn. Maryland Heights, MO, Elsevier Health Sciences, 2010.

A woman in first-trimester pregnancy with fever, malaise, nausea, and vomiting

Saweda A. Bright and Susan M. Lanni

History of present illness

A 25-year-old gravida 3, para 1 woman with dichorionic twin pregnancy at approximately 8 weeks' gestational age by last menstrual period presented with complaints of intractable nausea and vomiting. She had been seen at an outside facility 4 times within the last 10 days for similar complaints without improvement. Two days prior to presentation, she noticed a productive cough with green sputum, nasal congestion, a sore throat, and a headache. She noted body aches, malaise, and fatigue for a couple of days. She noted a temperature of 39.4°C on the day prior to admission. She also had some loose stools for about three days prior to presentation. She denied sick contacts or changes in eating habits.

She had no medical problems. Prior surgeries included a dilation and curettage for a missed abortion and a Cesarean delivery. Her second pregnancy was complicated by hyperemesis gravidarum for which she was admitted several times. She had a three pack-year history of tobacco use prior to pregnancy. She quit smoking when she learned she was pregnant. Her only medication was prenatal vitamins.

Physical examination

General appearance: Ill-appearing woman with no acute distress

Vital signs:

Temperature: 38.3°C
Pulse: 109 beats/min
Blood pressure: 134/81 mmHg
Respiratory rate: 22 breaths/min
Oxygen saturation: 96% on room air

HEENT: Nontender sinuses, erythematous oral pharynx, no exudate, neck soft, mildly tender, no thyromegaly, mild cervical lymphadenopathy

Cardiovascular: Tachycardic, regular rhythm, no peripheral edema

Pulmonary: Clear to auscultation bilaterally, no crackles or wheezes

Abdomen: Normoactive bowel sounds, soft, nontender

Extremities: No calf tenderness bilaterally

Laboratory studies:

WBCs: 10 500/μL with 92% neutrophils
Platelet count: 351 000/μL
Hb: 12.2 g/dL

Electrolytes, liver function tests, and lipase: Within normal limits
Urinalysis: Significant for large ketones and trace protein
Rapid influenza immunofluorescence amplification assay: Positive for the presence of influenza A. No influenza B virus was detected by the amplification test

Imaging:

Transvaginal ultrasound: Confirmed viability of intrauterine dichorionic twin gestation through the presence of cardiac activity

Chest x-ray: Showed opacity in lingual segment adjacent to the left-heart border consistent with a region of bronchopneumonia. The right lung appeared clear without evidence of focal airspace disease. There was no evidence of pulmonary edema or pleural effusion (Fig. 60.1)

How would you manage this patient?

The patient has influenza and was given oseltamivir orally for treatment. Her productive cough and radiographic findings were concerning for superimposed pneumonia, so she was also started on ceftriaxone and azithromycin to cover community-acquired pathogens. By hospital day 3, her symptoms had improved significantly. She was transitioned to oral antibiotics. She was discharged home with prescriptions to complete a 10-day course of oseltamivir and a 5-day course of azithromycin. She was given follow-up with her primary obstetrician in one week and was doing well at that visit. She went on to have an

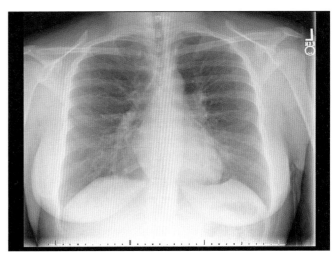

Fig. 60.1 Chest radiograph.

Acute Care and Emergency Gynecology, ed. David Chelmow, Christine R. Isaacs and Ashley Carroll. Published by Cambridge University Press.
© Cambridge University Press 2015.

otherwise uncomplicated pregnancy and delivered her twins at 38 weeks' gestational age.

Pregnant women with influenza

Early diagnosis and initiation of therapy is important when caring for pregnant women with influenza. The decision to perform a rapid influenza test in this patient was made based on her clinical symptoms, namely her fever, cough, and sore throat. Because of the risks of complications associated with delay in initiating treatment, any pregnant woman who is suspected to have influenza should receive rapid testing. Patients with fever and sore throat may also be evaluated for streptococcal pharyngitis. In patients who present with a productive cough, such as this case, clinicians should consider a chest radiograph to evaluate for focal consolidation or other signs suggestive of superimposed bacterial pneumonia.

The influenza virus is a RNA virus in the family, Orthomyxoviridae. There are three types of influenza viruses, A, B, and C, which are responsible for respiratory illnesses in humans. Types A and B cause seasonal epidemics in the United States in the winter, whereas type C causes a mild respiratory illness. Influenza A is further divided into subtypes based on surface antigenic proteins hemagglutinin (H) and neuraminidase (N). There are 17 different hemagglutinin and 10 different neuraminidase subtypes. Both influenza A and B types can be further divided into different strains. Currently, influenza A H1N1 and H3N2 are the viruses that cause infections in the United States [1] and are the targets for prevention strategies.

Of all clinical signs and symptoms, fever and cough are the two best predictors of a positive influenza antigen test. In a retrospective pooled analysis of 3744 subjects, Monto and colleagues [2] found that the combination of development fever and cough within 48 hours of onset of the initial symptom had a positive predictive value of 79% for influenza infections. Other typical clinical findings include myalgia, headache, nasal congestion, weakness, decreased appetite, and sore throat. Without treatment, the natural course is an average incubation of approximately two days, with recovery for most patients within a few days to a week.

According to the World Health Organization, populations of patients who are at increased risk for severe illness as the results of infection with influenza include pregnant women, children younger than five years of age, the elderly, and individuals with underlying health conditions such as HIV/AIDS, asthma, and chronic heart or lung disease [3]. Additional high-risk groups include patients with diabetes and cancer or other immunosuppressive conditions. Influenza is more likely to cause severe infection in women who are pregnant compared to women who are not pregnant. Pregnant women are also more likely to have serious side effects, such as pneumonia or even death, as a result of influenza infection. Infection may lead to serious complications such as stillbirth, decreased birth weight, preterm delivery, or neonatal death. Pregnant patients experienced greater mortality during influenza pandemics of 1918–1919, 1957–1958, and 2009 [4].

Cardiac, respiratory, and immunologic changes that occur during pregnancy contribute to the increased susceptibility of pregnant women to more severe illness and complications. In addition to increased blood volume and decreased functional residual capacity, pregnancy is associated with suppression of humoral and cell-mediated immunologic functions. During pregnancy, there is suppression of T-helper and T-cytotoxic cells, which decrease interferon, interleukin, and tumor necrosis factor-alpha. Interferons are a key component of the antiviral response of the immune system.

Because pregnant women can have more serious complications when infected with influenza virus, early treatment is recommended. Antiviral drugs can shorten the duration of illness by 1–2 days, especially if started within 48 hours of symptom onset. Treatment consists of antiviral drugs and supportive care. For pregnant women, treatment with antiviral medications should begin as early as possible, even if it is later than two days since the onset of symptoms. Oseltamivir and zanamivir are neuraminidase inhibitors that are both active against influenza A and B strains. Both are acceptable treatment options in pregnancy, but oseltamivir is preferred in pregnant women due to better oral bioavailability. Zanamivir is administered by inhalation, so it should be avoided in patients with respiratory diseases, such as asthma.

Updated recommended treatment regimens can be located on the Centers for Disease Control and Prevention (CDC) website for seasonal influenza (www.cdc.gov/flu). The current treatment regimen for oseltamivir is 75 mg PO BID for 5 days. The treatment dose for zanamivir is 2 inhalations, 10 mg total, BID for 5 days.

Oseltamivir and zanamivir should be used for post-exposure prophylaxis in pregnant women who have had close contact with a confirmed or suspected case of influenza during the period of time that individual would have been infectious. The infectious period lasts from 1 day before the onset of symptoms until 24 hours after defervescence. The post-exposure chemophophylaxis regimen consists of oseltamivir 75 mg PO once daily for 10 days or zanamivir 2 inhalations, 10 mg total, once daily for 10 days. This patient was given oseltamivir for her influenza, as well as azithromycin to cover probable superimposed community-acquired pneumonia.

The American College of Obstetricians and Gynecologists recommends that all pregnant women who are pregnant during the influenza season receive the inactivated influenza vaccine as an integral part of their routine prenatal care [4]. Patients with known contraindications to the inactivated influenza vaccine should not receive the vaccine, despite the increased risks associated with the disease during pregnancy. Vaccination can occur in any trimester and should be strongly encouraged for pregnant women. To protect the newborn, it is also recommended that household contacts and caregivers of infants less than six months of age receive the influenza vaccine. The effectiveness of the influenza vaccine changes from year to year. Overall, the CDC reports the vaccine effectiveness point estimate as 60% with a confidence interval of between 50 and 70% [5].

Many pregnant women may refuse vaccination due to fear associated with potential harmful effects of thimerosal. Thimerosal is a mercury-based preservative that is used in multidose vials of the inactivated influenza vaccine. The CDC, the National Institutes of Health, the Food and Drug Administration, and the American Academy of Pediatrics, along with other agencies, have reviewed several studies conducted on the safety of thimerosal and concluded that the small amounts of thimerosal in the vials are not harmful [6]. Furthermore, there is no association between thimerosal exposure and autism [6].

Pregnant women who receive the inactivated influenza vaccine transfer immunity to their unborn babies through antibodies to the influenza virus. Thus, babies are protected from influenza virus before they are mature enough to receive the influenza vaccine.

Key teaching points

- Influenza should be suspected in any pregnant patient with fever and cough who presents during the influenza season.
- Early treatment is crucial in pregnant patients with influenza and oseltamivir is the preferred treatment.
- All pregnant women should be vaccinated with the inactivated influenza vaccine as a part of routine prenatal care.

References

1. Centers for Disease Control and Prevention. Seasonal influenza. Types of influenza viruses. Available at http://www.cdc.gov/flu/about/viruses/types.htm.

2. Monto A, Gravenstein S, Elliott M, et al. Clinical signs and symptoms predicting influenza infection. *Arch Intern Med* 2000;160:3243–7.

3. World Health Organization. Vaccines against influenza WHO position paper – November 2012. *Wkly Epidemiol Rec* 2012;87(47):461–76. Available at http://www.who.int/wer/2012/wer8747.pdf.

4. The American College of Obstetricians and Gynecologists. Influenza vaccination during pregnancy. Committee Opinion No. 468. *Obstet Gynecol* 2010;116:1006–7.

5. Centers for Disease Control and Prevention. Seasonal influenza. Vaccine effectiveness: How well does the flu vaccine work? Available at http://www.cdc.gov/flu/about/qa/vaccineeffect.htm.

6. Centers for Disease Control and Prevention. Seasonal influenza. Thimerosal and 2013–2014 seasonal flu vaccines. Available at http://www.cdc.gov/flu/protect/vaccine/thimerosal.htm.

First-trimester flu-like symptoms in a 31-year-old woman

Lilja Stefansson and Susan M. Lanni

History of present illness

A 31-year-old healthy gravida 2, para 1-0-0-1 woman at 10 weeks' gestation presents to the emergency department complaining of a one-week history of flu-like symptoms. She works as a nurse in a pediatrics clinic and states that she is only concerned about this illness because she is pregnant and wants to "make sure everything is ok." She reports that she received the flu vaccine and waited this long to present as she thought the illness would be short-lived, but is now interested in obtaining a workup because a coworker told her to ask about cytomegalovirus (CMV) testing. She states that her first pregnancy was uncomplicated and she delivered vaginally at term. This pregnancy has been uncomplicated to date and she has had a first-trimester dating ultrasound confirming a singleton gestation with no abnormal findings.

Physical examination

General appearance: Woman appears ill and fatigued, but awake, alert, and oriented × 3

Vital signs:

Temperature: 38.0°C
Pulse: 102 beats/min
Blood pressure: 118/76 mmHg
Respiratory rate: 16 breaths/min
Oxygen saturation: 99% on room air

HEENT: Cervical lymphadenopathy

Cardiovascular: Mild tachycardia, no murmurs, rubs, or gallops

Respiratory: Clear to auscultation bilaterally all fields

Abdomen: Soft, nontender, nondistended

Laboratory studies:

WBCs: 11 000/μL
Hb: 11.0 g/dL
AST: 60 U/L
ALT: 80 U/L
Other tests were all within normal range

Imaging: Bedside transabdominal ultrasound showed single living intrauterine pregnancy, consistent with 10 weeks' gestation, fetal heart tones 150 beats/min. Normal appearing placenta

You discuss the findings with the patient and counsel her regarding the various diagnoses in the differential. She agrees to viral testing. You perform influenza, Epstein–Barr virus,

and CMV immunoglobulin M/immunoglobulin G (IgM/IgG) studies, which are all negative. She is diagnosed with a likely viral-illness and prior to sending her home, you counsel her to notify her obstetrician regarding this presentation to the emergency department. You inform her that she could potentially still have a diagnosis of CMV despite negative results, as antibody testing is variable and a negative IgM result does not rule out CMV. You explain to her that CMV can result in neurologic deficits in the fetus, most commonly sensorineural hearing loss.

The patient informs her obstetrician about her illness and reports that her condition has improved. She has opted for close monitoring with serial ultrasounds. One month later she had a normal scan, and two months later she presented for her anatomy ultrasound scan (Fig. 61.1) with the following findings:

Gestational age:

Composite gestational age: 19 weeks 1 day
Clinical gestational age: 19 weeks 1 day

Estimated weight: Normal (276 g ± 40 g)

Amniotic fluid: Maximum vertical pocket 52 mm

Morphology evaluation: Hyperechogenic bowel noted. Otherwise, unremarkable fetal anatomic survey, nasal bone present, normal humerus length

Summary: A single living intrauterine pregnancy with normal fetal growth and fluid for given gestational age; normal placenta; normal cervix. No additional aneuploidy

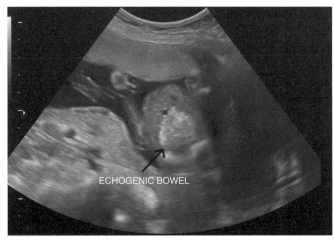

ECHOGENIC BOWEL

Fig. 61.1 Transabdominal ultrasound.

Acute Care and Emergency Gynecology, ed. David Chelmow, Christine R. Isaacs and Ashley Carroll. Published by Cambridge University Press. © Cambridge University Press 2015.

markers were noted on the scan. Differential includes: CMV aneuploidy versus cystic fibrosis versus bleeding in early pregnancy

The patient underwent genetic counseling. She reports that she has not had any bleeding during this pregnancy. She was offered and accepted the recommended testing: maternal serum CMV antibody and avidity testing, cystic fibrosis screening, and amniocentesis. The results of the tests were:

Routine prenatal serum studies:

Cystic fibrosis 32 mutation panel screen: Negative
Maternal serum analyte screen: Negative

Additional studies after echogenic bowel diagnosed:

CMV IgG: Positive
CMV IgM: Positive
Avidity testing: 0.47
(Reference values for avidity testing: Low avidity index, ≤0.50; intermediate avidity index, 0.51–0.59; high avidity index, ≥0.60)

Amniocentesis results:

CMV PCR of amniotic fluid: Positive
Karyotype: 46XY, normal male karyotype

How will you now manage this patient and how will you answer her questions regarding fetal effects of CMV exposure?

This patient had exposure to CMV early in her pregnancy, which can have lasting neurologic fetal effects. Exposure in the first trimester can have more serious health implications for the pregnancy and serial ultrasounds are indicated to monitor growth and progression of findings. Currently there is no approved therapy for CMV, but there is a developing body of evidence for the use of CMV-specific hyperimmune gamma-globulin infusion therapy to mitigate fetal damage.

Cytomegalovirus exposure in the first trimester

Cytomegalovirus (CMV) is the most common congenital infection, affecting 0.2 –2.0% of neonates. It is a double-stranded DNA herpes virus that is transmitted by contact with bodily fluids such as saliva, urine, blood, or sexual contact [1]. Children in daycare centers commonly acquire this infection and can transmit it to family members. One feature common to the herpesviridae family is that they cause a primary infection that becomes quiescent, but can reactivate in the future. Primary infections may have only minor flu-like symptoms or reactive adenopathy as their only manifestations. Reactivated CMV is typically asymptomatic, but is hallmarked by active viral shedding. Acute primary infection has an incubation period of 28–60 days and results in an IgM response usually 2–3 weeks following exposure. However, the IgM response is variable and resolves in approximately 30–60 days, followed by an IgG response, which persists. Due to the inconsistency of the IgM response, serologic testing may be unreliable. When infection occurs, adults are generally asymptomatic, but approximately 15% may present with flu-like symptoms including fever, chills, and malaise, and abnormal laboratory findings such as leukocytosis and abnormal liver function tests. Primary maternal infection prevalence ranges between 0.7 and 4.0%, with the risk of transmission to the fetus as high as 40% [1]. The rate of vertical transmission increases proportional to the gestational age at time of infection; however, transmission that occurs earlier in the pregnancy is associated with worse outcomes [2]. If infection occurs in the first trimester, approximately 25% of fetuses will be infected [3]. The prevalence of recurrent infection can be as high as 13.5%, but the risk of vertical transmission to the fetus with maternal CMV recurrence decreases to 0.15–2.00%. Vertical transmission to the fetus occurs transplacentally and is more likely to occur in the first half of pregnancy; fetal infection can also occur during delivery or postpartum through breast-feeding [1]. Most infants are asymptomatic at birth; however, 10% will have symptoms, and of these, approximately one-third will die and a majority of the remainder will develop sequelae, the most common being sensorineural hearing loss [1,2,4]. Manifestations of infection vary, including jaundice, thrombocytopenia, hepatosplenomegaly, and nonimmune hydrops. Infection via intrapartum exposure from cervical fluids or postpartum from breast-feeding tends to be asymptomatic at birth and remains so, reiterating the clinical significance of exposure earlier in the pregnancy and via transplacental passage to the fetus.

There are several ways to diagnose a primary infection in the pregnant patient if clinical suspicion of CMV infection arises. In several European countries, CMV testing is done as part of routine prenatal care. Of the 4 million babies born in the United States every year, only 5–6% of the approximately 40 000 infected will exhibit signs of infection. Antenatal testing is not routine here and is generally only performed when concern for infection is raised. Maternal CMV can be detected via serologic testing for IgG antibodies approximately four weeks apart if exposure is known. Evidence of a primary CMV infection is confirmed when an initial negative IgG seroconverts to positive over the intervening four weeks, or if titers increase greater than fourfold [1]. IgM titers are not as reliable to use as an indicator for primary infection as these may not be positive in an acute infection or they can persist for several months afterwards. Avidity testing is only performed if the IgG antibody is positive but can provide information regarding the timing of the infection. Avidity testing is an index of the specificity of the IgG antibody for its antigen. A low avidity (values are lab. dependent) is indicative of a primary infection, and likely occurred in the past six months. Higher avidity index values, greater than 0.7–0.8, generally occurs with more long-standing infections [5]. The fetal compartment can be tested directly for CMV infection using

Table 61.1 Manifestations of CMV in the fetus and the neonate

Ultrasonographic findings associated with CMV	Clinical sequelae of CMV in neonate
Fetal growth restriction	Asymptomatic
Cerebral calcifications	Microcephaly
Ventriculomegaly	Sensorineural loss
Microcephaly	Neurologic deficits
Hepatomegaly	Chorioretinitis
Splenomegaly	Learning disabilities
Hyperechogenic bowel	Psychomotor retardation
Oligohydramnios	Hepatomegaly
Polyhydramnios	Splenomegaly
Pleural effusion	Jaundice
Hydrops	Hemolytic anemia
Placental enlargement (placental thickness >35 mm)	Thrombocytopenic purpura
	Death
CMV, cytomegalovirus.	

amniotic fluid via PCR (sensitivity 77–100%) or culture (sensitivity 50–69%). In the first half of pregnancy, the utility of diagnosing CMV infection via fetal serologies is questionable, as the fetal immune system has not matured enough to develop antibodies, therefore minimizing the effective diagnosis of CMV infection. In addition, it requires Percutaneous Umbilical Cord Blood Sampling (PUBS), a procedure that has a higher rate of fetal loss than amniocentesis. In the newborn, urine can be PCR tested as the primary organ of replication in the fetus is the kidney; testing can also be performed on infected bodily fluids including saliva and blood [1].

Most infections are diagnosed based on fetal ultrasound findings, which may include calcifications of the lateral border of the ventricles, echogenic bowel, hydrops, ascites, hepatosplenomegaly, and ventriculomegaly (Table 61.1). The severity of the disease is not correlated with the amount of CMV virus detected in amniotic fluid; rather, it can be determined by clinical findings such as sonographic evidence of central nervous system infection [1].

Currently, there are no approved therapies for CMV infection. There is a developing body of literature regarding the antenatal intravenous administration of hyperimmune globulin to the mother, and neonatal ganciclovir for reducing the occurrence of central nervous system damage and hearing loss in newborns [1,2].

It is important to counsel pregnant patients on appropriate prevention strategies, particularly in those patients at high risk for contracting CMV. Patients at high risk are those that work around or live with children or immunocompromised people, women from lower socioeconomic backgrounds, those born outside the United States, those with other sexually transmitted diseases, and women whose first pregnancy occurred below the age of 15. Prevention strategies include basic hygiene measures such as frequent hand washing, use of personal protective equipment such as gloves, gowns and goggles, caution when handling physiologic fluids from children including diapers, using condoms, and avoiding needle-sharing for intravenous drug abusers.

Key teaching points

- Cytomegalovirus (CMV) is the most common congenital infection, affecting 0.2–2.0% of all neonates.
- CMV is transmitted through body fluids.
- Fetal infection has a poorer prognosis when it occurs earlier in the pregnancy.
- The most common clinical sequelae from CMV infection in the neonate is sensorineural hearing loss.
- Diagnosis is usually made after clinical suspicion arises from ultrasonographic findings concerning for CMV infection. Testing can be performed through maternal serologies (IgM, IgG, avidity testing, PCR, and culture); on fetus through amniotic fluid (PCR, culture).
- Prevention of CMV occurs primarily through methods such as hand washing and hygiene. There is no vaccine for CMV, but there is some developing evidence regarding CMV hyperimmune gamma-globulin given to the mother during pregnancy and ganciclovir administered to the neonate.

References

1. American College of Obstetricians and Gynecologists. Perinatal and parasitic infections. Practice Bulletin No. 20. *Int J Gynaecol Obstet* 2002;76(1):95–107. Reaffirmed 2011.

2. Visentin S, Manara R, Milanese L, et al. Early primary cytomegalovirus infection in pregnancy: maternal hyperimmunoglobulin therapy improves outcomes among infants at 1 year of age. *Clin Infect Dis* 2012;55:497–503.

3. Nigro G, Adler SP, Parruti G, et al. Immunoglobulin therapy of fetal cytomegalovirus infection occurring in the first half of pregnancy – a case control study of the outcome in children. *J Infect Dis* 2012;205:215–27.

4. Lipitz S, Yinon Y, Malinger G, et al. Risk of cytomegalovirus-associated sequelae in relation to time of infection and findings on prenatal imaging. *Ultrasound Obstet Gyneol* 2013;41:508–14.

5. Leruez-Ville M, Sellier Y, Salomon LJ. et al. Prediction of fetal infection in cases with cytomegalovirus immunoglobulin M in the first trimester of pregnancy: a retrospective cohort. *Clin Infect Dis* 2013;56:1428–35.

Abdominal pain and distension seven days after egg retrieval for planned IVF

Richard Scott Lucidi

History of present illness

A 28-year-old gravida 0 woman is brought into the emergency department by her husband with complaints of abdominal pain, abdominal distension, nausea, and difficulty breathing. Her symptoms began that afternoon and have become progressively worse. She states that her pain is on both sides of her lower abdomen and that it is difficult to breathe, especially when lying down. She has mild nausea but denies vomiting, diarrhea, or fever. She cannot remember the last time she urinated.

Her history is significant for anovulatory infertility due to polycystic ovary syndrome. She has been undergoing in-vitro fertilization (IVF) treatment. A phone call to her reproductive endocrinologist reveals that her egg retrieval was 7 days prior and 32 oocytes were obtained. Her peak estradiol level was 4231 pg/mL. She had a single embryo transferred to her uterus two days ago.

Her only medications are prenatal vitamins and vaginal progesterone. She has no other medical problems, and has never had surgery.

Physical examination

General appearance: Well-developed, well-nourished woman in mild discomfort and mild respiratory distress

Vital signs:

Temperature: 37.0°C
Pulse: 115 beats/min
Blood pressure: 102/62 mmHg
Respiratory rate: 24 breaths/min
Oxygen saturation: 99% on room air
Height: 66 inches
Weight: 124 lb

Cardiovascular: Tachycardic, regular rhythm, no murmur, no jugular venous distention

Pulmonary: Tachypneic, breaths are shallow, lungs are clear

Abdomen: Distended, fluid wave is present, diffusely tender

Extremities: No edema is seen

Laboratory studies:

WBCs: 16 100/μL (normal 3900–11 700/μL)
Hb: 15.3 g/dL (normal 12–15 g/dL)
Ht: 46% (normal 34.8–45.0%)
hCG: 22 mIU/mL (normal <5 mIU/mL)
Sodium: 131 mEq/L (normal 135–145 mEq/L)
Potassium: 5.5 mEq/L (normal 3.7–5.2 mEq/L)
Creatinine: 1.1 mg/dL (normal 0.5–1.0 mg/dL)

Imaging: A pelvic ultrasound is obtained (Fig. 62.1)

Intravenous analgesics and anti-emetics were administered.

How would you manage this patient?

This patient has ovarian hyperstimulation syndrome (OHSS). Her history of a recent IVF treatment and her constellation of symptoms support the diagnosis. Although abdominal pain and a positive pregnancy test would usually prompt consideration of ectopic pregnancy in the differential diagnosis, that would not be likely in this case. Her embryo transfer was only two days ago, so it would be too early for her to have symptoms from an ectopic pregnancy. It would also be too early for a pregnancy to have detectible human chorionic gonadotropin (hCG) levels. Her positive pregnancy test is due to the exogenous hCG used in the IVF stimulation.

Her laboratory abnormalities of hyponatremia, hyperkalemia, leucocytosis, and hemoconcentration, as well as her respiratory difficulty, indicate severe disease and the need for inpatient management. She should be admitted for pain management, intravenous volume replacement, venous thrombosis prophylaxis, and correction of her electrolyte abnormalities. Since this patient had nausea but no vomiting, oral opiates, such as oxycodone, are a good first option for pain management. Intravenous opiates may be required if vomiting

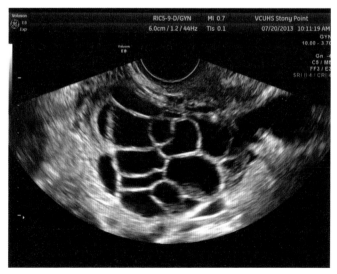

Fig. 62.1 Transvaginal ultrasound of the right ovary.

Acute Care and Emergency Gynecology, ed. David Chelmow, Christine R. Isaacs and Ashley Carroll. Published by Cambridge University Press. © Cambridge University Press 2015.

Table 62.1 Symptoms, signs, and laboratory abnormalities of OHSS

	Symptoms	Signs	Lab. abnormalities
Mild	Abdominal discomfort Nausea/vomiting Abdominal distension	Enlarged ovaries on ultrasound	
Severe	Shortness of breath Rapid weight gain	Tachypnea Tachycardia Hypotension Tense ascites Oliguria	Hyponatremia (<135 mEq/L) Hyperkalemia (>5 mEq/L) Hemoconcentration (Hct >45%) Leukocytosis (WBCs >15 000/μL) Creatinine >1.2 Elevated liver enzymes

OHSS, ovarian hyperstimulation syndrome.

develops. Fluid replacement and correction of the electrolyte abnormalities can be achieved with a 1 L bolus of normal saline followed by continuous infusion at 150 mL/h. Heparin 5000 U SQ BID should be started for venous thrombosis prophylaxis.

Ovarian hyperstimulation syndrome

Ovarian hyperstimulation syndrome (OHSS) is a potential complication of in-vitro fertilization treatment and other ovarian stimulation treatments involving gonadotropins. In its severe form, OHSS affects approximately 1% of women undergoing ovarian hyperstimulation [1]. This patient has a number of risk factors for OHSS, including treatment with exogenous gonadotropins, young age (<35 years), low body weight, polycystic ovary syndrome, high estradiol levels, larger number of follicles stimulated, and use of hCG. Although not present in this patient, prior OHSS is also a risk factor.

Although the pathophysiology of OHSS is not clear, increased capillary permeability and extravasation of fluid into the peritoneal cavity are the hallmarks of the disease [2]. The third-spacing of fluid results in an increase in total-body water, decreased intravascular volume, and the symptoms, signs, and laboratory abnormalities of the disease (Table 62.1). Although the increased capillary permeability begins in the ovaries, it can spread to other tissues resulting in pulmonary and peripheral edema. The risk of thromboembolic disease is also increased in women with severe OHSS. This may be due to the hemoconcentration and inactivity associated with abdominal discomfort [2], or it may be that underlying thrombophilias are predisposing factors for the development of severe OHSS [3]. In addition to thromboembolism, other life-threatening complications of OHSS include adult respiratory distress syndrome (ARDS), renal failure, and hemorrhage from ovarian rupture [2].

OHSS typically presents in patients following gonadotropin treatment for infertility and is rare in patients not treated with gonadotropins or in patients treated with other medications such as clomiphene. It typically presents 3–7 days following hCG treatment but can present as late as 17 days after hCG [4]. Most patients initially develop abdominal discomfort (99%) and other symptoms and signs are often present (Table 62.1).

Ultrasound will often show enlarged ovaries that are typically 5–12 cm but may measure up to 25 cm. Ovarian rupture can occur with aggressive abdominal or pelvic examination so these should be avoided in favor of ultrasound examination. The initial laboratory evaluation should include a complete blood count and metabolic panel to assess sodium, potassium, creatinine, aspartate aminotransferase (AST) and alanine aminotransferase (ALT). Abnormal results of these tests are shown in Table 62.1 and inpatient management should be considered for patients with abnormal results.

OHSS is a common complication of ovarian stimulation and is usually a self-limiting disorder that resolves spontaneously within a few days. The duration and severity can worsen, especially in patients who conceive. This worsening is likely from continued hCG exposure.

The American Society for Reproductive Medicine Practice Committee [2] points out that, while OHSS has traditionally been classified as mild, moderate, or severe, the signs and symptoms of the disease represent a continuum not amenable to a specific classification system. However, management is dictated by the severity. Mild OHSS can usually be managed in the outpatient setting with oral hydration using at least 1 L of sports drinks or other electrolyte-supplemented beverages, oral analgesics, and daily weights with instructions to monitor for signs of progressive disease (weight gain of >2 lb daily, increasing abdominal girth or discomfort, urine output <1 L/day). Acetaminophen or opiates should be used for analgesia. Nonsteroidal anti-inflammatory drugs should be avoided while pregnancy is a possibility. Patients should continue monitoring for two weeks or until menses occurs.

Hospitalization should be considered if the diagnosis is unsure, vomiting prevents oral hydration, or pain is severe enough to require intravenous analgesics. Hospitalization should also be considered if any sign or laboratory abnormality of severe disease is present. In this case, the patient's tachypnea, tachycardia, oliguria, electrolyte abnormalities, and hemoconcentration merit inpatient management.

Inpatient management of OHSS is primarily supportive and consists of intravascular volume replacement and correction of electrolyte abnormalities. Normal saline is recommended instead of lactated Ringer's due to the hyponatremia that is often present. Plasma expanders such as 25% albumin (50–100 g over 4 hours) may be used when normal saline infusion fails to maintain normal hemodynamic status and urine output. Thromboembolic prophylaxis with heparin (5000 U SQ every 12 hours) or low-molecular-weight heparin (Lovenox® 40 mg SQ daily) is also recommended for patients with intravascular hemoconcentration until the hematocrit normalizes (Ht <38%). Diuretics such as furosemide can be used, but their use should be avoided until after the intravascular volume has normalized. Inpatient monitoring should continue until pain improves, electrolytes are within the normal range and the hemoconcentration has resolved. A falling hematocrit indicates mobilization of fluid into the intravascular space and is usually not an indication of hemorrhage. If hyperkalemia is present, an ECG should be obtained. If peaked T waves, ST segment depression, or prolonged PR or QRS intervals are present, prompt treatment with calcium gluconate is indicated. If no ECG abnormalities are present, the hyperkalemia can be corrected more slowly with sodium polystyrene sulfonate USP (Kayexelate®).

Paracentesis may be required to alleviate abdominal pain or respiratory symptoms. This can be accomplished under ultrasound guidance using either a transabdominal or transvaginal approach. In otherwise healthy women with OHSS, large volumes can usually be safely removed.

Prevention of OHSS involves careful monitoring during ovarian stimulation and the recognition of risk factors. Since prior OHSS is a risk factor, this patient will be at high risk should she undergo similar treatment in the future. "Coasting"

for up to three days has been shown to decrease the risk of OHSS without lowering pregnancy rates. Coasting involves delaying hCG and withholding gonadotropin stimulation until estradiol levels fall below 2500 pg/mL. Gonadotropin-releasing hormone (GnRH) agonists (leuprolide) can be used to induce an endogenous luteinizing hormone (LH) surge instead of hCG to reduce the risk. Using a lower dose of hCG (5000 mIU instead of 10 000 mIU) will also reduce the risk of OHSS [4].

Key teaching points

- Mild ovarian hyperstimulation syndrome (OHSS) is a common complication of ovarian stimulation with gonadotropins.
- Severe OHSS is an uncommon but potentially life-threatening complication.
- OHSS is self-limited and treatment is primarily supportive to alleviate symptoms and prevent complications of the disease.
- Risk factors for OHSS include gonadotropin ovarian stimulation, prior OHSS, young age, low body weight, polycystic ovary syndrome, high estradiol levels, large follicle counts, and human chorionic gonadotropin (hCG) (during stimulation or from a resulting pregnancy).
- Common symptoms and signs of OHSS include abdominal pain and bloating, shortness of breath, ascites, hyponatremia, hyperkalemia, and hemoconcentration.
- Potential life-threatening complications of OHSS include pulmonary embolism, ovarian rupture and hemorrhage, hypovolemic shock, and electrolyte-induced arrhythmias.

References

1. Schenker JG. Clinical aspects of ovarian hyperstimulation syndrome. *Eur J Obstet Gynecol Reprod Biol* 1999;85:13–20.

2. Practice Committee of the American Society for Reproductive Medicine.

Ovarian hyperstimulation syndrome. *Fertil Steril* 2008;90(Suppl 3): S188–93.

3. Dulitzky M, Cohen SB, Inbal A, et al. Increased prevalence of thrombophilia among women with severe ovarian

hyperstimulation syndrome. *Fertil Steril* 2002;77:463–7.

4. Lucidi RS. *Ovarian Hyperstimulation Syndrome.* Available at http:// emedicine.medscape.com/article/ 1343572-overview.

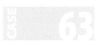

Irregular bleeding in a 39-year-old nulliparous woman desiring fertility

PonJola Coney

History of present illness

A 39-year-old gravida 0 woman is seen who is anxious because her menses have gotten "much heavier" and she is worried. Up until six months ago her cycles were monthly, lasting five to six days and requiring four to five sanitary pad changes per day. However, over the last six months her cycles now last seven to nine days and seem twice as heavy, requiring nine to ten pad changes per day, and often with golf ball-sized clots noted. She also reports several episodes of light bleeding between cycles. She is unmarried, not sexually active, uses no contraception, but is very anxious to maintain fertility and is thinking about "freezing her eggs."

Her medical history is notable for obesity and her only surgical history is a repair of a diaphragmatic hernia as a neonate. She reports menarche at age eight, and denies any sexually transmitted infections, abnormal cervical screens, or vasomotor symptoms. She is on no medications other than a multivitamin. She is employed as a pharmacy technician and does not smoke or drink alcohol. She has no known family history of cancers.

Physical examination

General appearance: A pleasant, anxious-appearing woman
Vital signs:

All within normal limits
BMI: 42 kg/m^2
HEENT: Normal
Neck: Normal thyroid exam
Chest: Clear bilaterally
Cardiac: Regular rate and rhythm
Abdomen: Obese. No masses or tenderness appreciated. Surgical scars noted
Pelvic: Revealed normal external genitalia, normal vagina, and a nulliparous cervix. The bimanual examination was limited due to the patient's habitus. No obvious abnormalities were appreciated
Laboratory studies:

Hb: 10.7 g/dL (normal 14–18 g/dL)
Ht: 31.3% (normal 36–48%)
Urine pregnancy test: Negative
Imaging: Pelvic ultrasound was performed. Endovaginal ultrasound of the pelvis showed an anteverted uterus with normal shape and contour measuring 6.9 × 5.5 cm, and an endometrial stripe measuring 2.2 cm

How would you manage this patient?

Office endometrial sampling was obtained to aid in diagnosing the etiology of the patient's abnormal uterine bleeding with associated anemia. Pathology was consistent with complex hyperplasia with atypia (Figs 63.1 and 63.2).

Due to the patient's strong desire for childbearing, she was started on medroxyprogesterone acetate (MPA) 30 mg daily for the next 6 months. A follow-up dilation and curettage done in the operating room after her six months of treatment revealed benign endometrial tissue only. She is currently considering her fertility options and consulting a Reproductive Endocrine and Infertility specialist.

Endometrial hyperplasia

The most common presenting symptom of endometrial abnormalities is abnormal uterine bleeding and, specifically, endometrial hyperplasia is an entity preceded by abnormal uterine bleeding more than 80% of the time. Bleeding irregularities identified in the clinical history often prompt endometrial assessment with tissue sampling for histology (an endometrial biopsy), as was the case in this patient.

Hyperplasia is a microscopic diagnosis found when endometrial tissue reveals an increased proliferation (or overgrowth) of cells which can then result in a greater

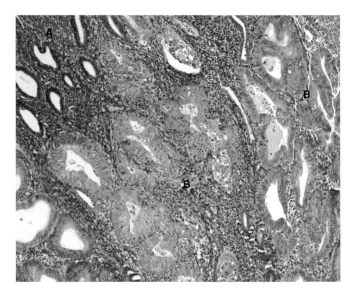

Fig. 63.1 Benign, small endometrial glands [A] adjacent to [B] crowded glands with complex contours. 100× H&E. (Courtesy of Department of Pathology, Medical College of Virginia Hospitals.)

Acute Care and Emergency Gynecology, ed. David Chelmow, Christine R. Isaacs and Ashley Carroll. Published by Cambridge University Press. © Cambridge University Press 2015.

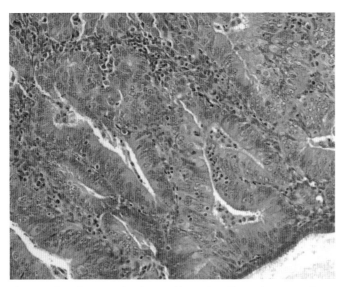

Fig.63.2 Complex atypical endometrial hypoplasia. The endometrium shows significant cytologic atypia (large nuclei, vesicular chromatin, prominent nucleoli) within the crowded glands. 200× H&E. (Courtesy of Department of Pathology, Medical College of Virginia Hospitals.)

gland-to-stroma ratio than what is observed in the normal endometrium (Fig. 63.1). Microscopically, cells may initially resemble normal cells but are increased per unit volume. Nuclear atypia indicates the presence of nuclear enlargement and poses a higher cumulative risk of developing endometrial carcinoma. Women with conditions of prolonged unopposed estrogen stimulation, nulliparity, a BMI greater than 30 kg/m^2, and irregular menstruation are at greater risk for developing hyperplasia [1,2,3].

There are currently two recommended diagnostic classifications for endometrial hyperplasia: (1) The revised 1994 World Health Organization (WHO) hyperplasia system, and (2) the Endometrial Intraepithelial Neoplasia (EIN) Classification System. The WHO hyperplasia system is based on morphologic features of architectural complexity and nuclear atypia. This system recognizes cytological atypia as the defining feature for distinguishing genuine simple and complex endometrial hyperplasias from those that have higher potential to be precancerous – simple and complex atypical endometrial hyperplasias. Simple hyperplasia refers to diffuse and variably sized glands with a normal ratio of glands to stroma. Complex hyperplasia consists of architecturally irregular glands, and an increased gland-to-stroma ratio. When nuclear enlargement with evenly dispersed or clumped chromatin is present, atypical hyperplasia (simple or complex) is diagnosed.

The EIN classification system was proposed in 2000 to develop pathologic criteria for the categories of benign, pre-malignant, and malignant disease in an effort to predict clinical outcomes of endometrial hyperplasia. Benign "endometrial hyperplasia" (EH) replaces simple and complex hyperplasia while "endometrial intraepithelial neoplasia" (EIN) represents the immediate precursor of endometrioid adenocarcinoma with a 45-fold increased cancer risk. The foundation of this system is its reproducibility and its ability to detect precursors

for disease progression to carcinoma more accurately than the WHO system; however, to date, the WHO classification remains more widely used. Both classification systems attempt to capture the differences in severity across the spectrum of endometrial hyperplasia [2,3] and in both, atypia remains the defining feature in differentiating precancerous from purely hyperplastic lesions.

While solid data representing the clinical course of endometrial hyperplasia is lacking, endometrial hyperplasia with atypia poses a real risk of progression to carcinoma. The long-term risk of women developing cancer when diagnosed with hyperplasia (without atypia) is less than 5%, but the risk among women with atypical hyperplasia approaches 30%. The presence of atypical cells is understood to increase the risk of progressing to cancer, but there is generally poor reproducibility in histologic assessments by pathologists and no biomarkers have been identified to aid in this process. The often incomplete sampling of the entire uterine cavity further compromises diagnostic abilities when office techniques of endometrial sampling are incorporated. While the incidence of endometrial hyperplasia is most common in postmenopausal women, the risk for women aged 35–44 is 6.2% and thus, incorporates the reproductive years [1,2,3,4].

Treatment protocols for hyperplasias have not been standardized, but nonsurgical management with progestin therapy (as opposed to hysterectomy) remains appropriate in hyperplasias without atypia given the overall low risk of progression to carcinoma, particularly in the patient who desires fertility preservation. There are no randomized controlled trials and therefore no standard hormonal doses or regimens have been developed. Published results to date have investigated continuous treatment with MPA (10–30 mg/day), megestrol (100–320 mg/day), or cyclic administration with norethisterone (NET) (15 mg/day for 10 days/month). Higher doses (up to 600 mg/day) may be used in cases with atypia present and even in early endometrial carcinoma. The levonorgestrel-releasing intrauterine device (LNG-IUD), (Mirena®) holds great promise as it releases a daily local uterine dose of 20 µg of levonorgestrel, but randomized controlled trials are lacking to determine whether the LNG-IUD is safe and effective for treating atypical endometrial hyperplasia. Side effects of these regimens are generally well tolerated, but may include irregular vaginal bleeding, mood changes, headaches, edema, weight gain, or more concerning thromboembolic events [5,6,7].

Published studies show regression outcomes up to 90% for oral treatment and up to 92% for the LNG-IUD for simple and complex or benign hyperplasia. The progesterone concentrations in the uterine mucosa when delivered through an intra-uterine device placed directly into the uterine cavity are reported to exceed that of the oral treatment and are associated with higher patient satisfaction resulting in greater patient compliance. Treatment regimens are generally continued for a minimum of 3 months up to 24 months, and repeated for failures or recurrences [5,6,7]. Endometrial sampling is generally repeated following medical therapy. The choice of sampling technique (office procedures vs. operative) tends to represent the preference and experience of the physician.

In a large retrospective study, women were followed for a minimum of five years after their initial successful progestin treatment demonstrated regression, to the time of future relapse. Relapse rates for simple/complex hyperplasia versus atypical hyperplasia were 28% and 50% respectively [8]. Relapse rates for women treated with LNG-IUD for simple/complex hyperplasia versus atypical hyperplasia were 13% and 27% respectively. Relapses also occurred sooner with oral therapy than with intrauterine therapy, but the treatment interval is generally shorter for oral therapy [8]. From a practical standpoint, atypical hyperplasia poses a higher chance of relapse versus simple/complex hyperplasia (without atypia), and future clinical surveillance and management options should be mindful of this when caring for the patient who desires fertility preservation.

Infertility treatment, particularly the use of ovulation induction drugs and assisted reproduction following conservative progestin treatment of endometrial hyperplasias, has not been shown to increase the risk of recurrence of the disease. Furthermore, a resulting pregnancy seems to have an advantageous effect on patient outcomes [9,10]. In one retrospective study of 36 patients who received conservative treatment for endometrial cancer or atypical complex endometrial hyperplasia, 26 went on to receive infertility treatment. Eighteen of these patients (69%) conceived and 16 of these patients went on to deliver healthy babies. Three of the 16 women who delivered babies experienced a recurrence, while 7 women who did not accomplish pregnancy experienced a recurrence. In addition, 7 (70%) of the 10 women who did not undergo any infertility treatments experienced recurrence. Overall, while the data is limited by small numbers, 38.5% of women who underwent infertility therapy had a recurrence of their endometrial pathology versus 70% of women who had a recurrence despite not pursuing infertility treatments. The time to recurrence was not significantly different among the groups, averaging 13–23 months [10].

Considering the gap in knowledge that remains regarding the risks of progression for any endometrial hyperplasia diagnosis, the decision to choose conservative hormonal management rests with the physician and patient after a review of both risks and benefits. The objective of conservative hormonal management is to induce endometrial regression and avoid hysterectomy. Endometrial hyperplasia when treated in a timely fashion allows for future fertility options in women who may desire such, as was the case in this patient.

Key teaching points

- Endometrial hyperplasia is preceded by abnormal uterine bleeding in more than 80% of the time.
- Two classification systems (World Health Organization [WHO] and Endometrial Intraepithelial Neoplasia [EIN]) exist for classifying endometrial hyperplasia. The presence of atypia is the defining feature in differentiating lesions more likely to be precancerous.
- Conservative management using progestin for endometrial hyperplasia is a valid management option to preserve fertility, but requires close follow-up surveillance.
- Pregnancy is feasible after medical management of endometrial hyperplasia with good outcomes noted in small studies. Limited existing data suggests that ovarian stimulation or ovulation induction and assisted reproductive techniques do not increase the overall risk of recurrence of hyperplasia.
- Considering our current knowledge gaps regarding predicting the risk of progression to cancer, as well as difficulties with histologic reproducibility for any hyperplasia diagnosis, choosing conservative treatment with hormonal management rests with the physician and patient after appropriate counseling.

References

1. Reed SD, Newton KM, Clinton WL et al. Incidence of endometrial hyperplasia. *Am J Obstet Gynecol* 2009;678:e1–6.

2. Lacey JV, Sherman ME, Rush BB, et al. Absolute risk of endometrial carcinoma during 20-year follow-up among women with endometrial hyperplasia. *J Clin Oncol* 2010;28:788–92.

3. Trimble CL, Method M, Leitao M et al. for the Society of Gynecologic Oncology Clinical Practice Committee. Management of endometrial precancers. *Obstet Gynecol* 2012; 120:1160–75.

4. Haidopoulos D, Simou M, Akrivos N et al. Risk factors in women 40 years of age and younger with endometrial carcinoma. *Acta Obstet Gynecol Scand* 2010;89:1326–30.

5. Ozdegirmenci O, Kayikcioglu F, Bozkurt U et al. Comparison of the efficacy of three progestins in the treatment of simple endometrial hyperplasia without atypia. *Gynecol Obstet Invest* 2011;72:10–14.

6. Gallos ID, Shehmar M, Thangaratinam S et al. Oral progestogens vs. levonorgestrel-releasing intrauterine system for endometrial hyperplasia:a systematic review and metaanalysis. *Am J Obstet Gynecol* 2010;203(547):e1–10.

7. Hubbs JL, Saig R, Abaid LN, et al. Systemic and local hormone therapy for endometrial hyperplasia and early adenocarcinoma. *Obstet Gynecol* 2013;121:1172–80.

8. Gallos ID, Krishan P, Shehmar M et al. Relapse of endometrial hyperplasia after conservative treatment: a cohort study with long-term follow-up. *Hum Reprod* 2013;28:1231–6.

9. Ricciardi E, Maniglio P, Frega A et al. Fertility-sparing treatment of endometrial cancer precursors among young women:a reproductive point of view. *Eur Rev Med Pharmacol Sci* 2012;16:1934–7.

10. Ichinose M, Fujimoto A, Osuga Y, et al. The influence of infertility treatment on the prognosis of endometrial cancer and atypical complex endometrial hyperplasia. *Int J Gynecol Cancer* 2013;23:288–93.

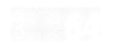

A 24-year-old woman with her third pregnancy loss

Richard Scott Lucidi

History of present illness

A 24-year-old gravida 3, para 0 woman presents to your acute care clinic with complaints of vaginal bleeding that she describes as "like a period." She is currently at 8 weeks' gestational age confirmed by an ultrasound 2 weeks ago that showed a 5 mm fetal pole with cardiac motion. She denies any pain but has symptoms consistent with early pregnancy including breast tenderness and nausea. She is tearful and worried about this pregnancy since she has had two prior pregnancy losses. The first pregnancy passed spontaneously without complications. Her second pregnancy was managed with cervical dilation and uterine curettage; however, the surgical pathology showed no products of conception and a second curettage was successfully performed with products of conception obtained. Her only medication is prenatal vitamins. A prior three-dimensional pelvic ultrasound showed a septate uterus (Fig. 64.1.)

Physical examination

General appearance: Well-developed, well-nourished woman in no discomfort but with mild emotional distress

Vital signs:

Temperature: 37.0°C
Pulse: 90 beats/min
Blood pressure: 102/62 mmHg
Respiratory rate: 16 breaths/min
Oxygen saturation: 99% on room air
BMI: 23 kg/m^2

Pelvic: Blood is on the perineum and in the vagina. Moderate active bleeding is present from the cervical os. The uterus is anteverted, six weeks' size, and nontender. No cervical motion tenderness is present. The cervix is closed. There is no adnexal mass or tenderness

Laboratory studies:

hCG: 9200 mIU/mL (normal <5 mIU/mL)
Hb: 14.3 g/dL (normal 12–15 g/dL)
Ht: 43% (normal 34.8–45%)

Imaging: A pelvic ultrasound is obtained that shows an intrauterine pregnancy with an irregularly shaped gestational sac and a 5-mm fetal pole without cardiac motion

How would you manage this patient?

This patient is hemodynamically stable; however, the lack of interval growth between the ultrasound exams two weeks apart and the absence of previously seen cardiac motion confirms the diagnosis of a missed abortion. Since this is her third miscarriage, the diagnosis of recurrent pregnancy loss (RPL) is also appropriate.

Expectant management, medical management, and surgical management with dilation and curettage are options for the management of a missed abortion in a stable patient. Since she also has the diagnosis of recurrent pregnancy loss, consideration should be given to performing a dilation and curettage in order to obtain tissue for cytogenetic analysis [1]. Karyotype analysis of the products of conception would provide information to assess whether the loss was random or likely due to her structural uterine abnormality. An abnormal karyotype in the products of conception may guide further evaluation toward parental chromosomal abnormalities. A normal karyotype in the products of conception may guide the evaluation toward endocrine abnormalities, antiphospholipid antibodies, or toward the treatment of her uterine septum.

Ultrasound guidance during the dilation and curettage procedure would help to assure that the products of conception are evacuated. With a uterine septum, it is possible to curette the uterine cavity on only one side of the septum and failing to obtain tissue on the opposite side of the septum. This scenario happened in the patient's second miscarriage.

Patients with a septate uterus have a high incidence of first-trimester loss (44%) and surgical correction of the septum decreases the incidence (17%) [2,3]. This patient should be scheduled for hysteroscopic correction of her septum in a nonemergent setting following resolution of this pregnancy.

Although a probable cause of her RPL is evident with the septum, further evaluation of other causes including hormonal abnormalities (thyroid dysfunction, uncontrolled diabetes, hyperprolactinemia), antiphospholipid antibodies (lupus anticoagulant, anti-cardiolipin antibodies, anti-β_2 glycoprotein antibodies) and balanced chromosomal abnormalities (translocations, inversions) should be offered as more than one etiologic factor is often present [4].

Pregnancy loss is an emotional experience and couples with RPL may have heightened grief, depression, or anxiety. Sensitivity to these issues is necessary and psychological counseling should be offered.

Acute Care and Emergency Gynecology, ed. David Chelmow, Christine R. Isaacs and Ashley Carroll. Published by Cambridge University Press.
© Cambridge University Press 2015.

Recurrent pregnancy loss

Recurrent pregnancy loss (RPL) is defined as two or more consecutive first-trimester losses of clinical pregnancies [2,3]. Although 15–25% of pregnancies result in a spontaneous loss, only 5% of women will have two consecutive losses, and only 1% will have three or more losses. The risk of miscarriage in subsequent pregnancies is also influenced by the number of prior losses. After 2 losses the risk is 30% and after 3 losses the risk is 33% [3]. Thus, the definition of RPL is based on both decreased prevalence and increased risk.

The definition also specifies losses of clinical pregnancies. Clinical pregnancies are defined by ultrasonic visualization or histopathologic examination [1]. Ectopic pregnancies result from a different set of possible etiologies and are not included. Also, positive pregnancy tests that resolve spontaneously – chemical pregnancies – are not included since there is no data on associated risks following these pregnancies.

Although the potential etiologies of RPL are controversial, consensus exists for a small number of accepted etiologies (Table 64.1) including uterine structural abnormalities, parental chromosomal abnormalities, maternal endocrine disorders, and antiphospholipid antibody syndrome (APS).

Women with congenital uterine malformations have a higher incidence of pregnancy loss. Although no prospective

Table 64.1 Etiologies of recurrent pregnancy loss

Etiology	Recommended tests	Treatment
Anatomic	Sonohysterogram or Hysterosalpingogram or Hysteroscopy	Hysteroscopic removal of uterine septum, synechia or submucous myomas IVF with gestational surrogate for uncorrectable abnormalities
Parental chromosomal abnormalities	Karyotype	Preimplantation genetic diagnosis Donor sperm or donor oocytes
Endocrine	Thyroid-stimulating hormone Prolactin Fasting blood sugar or HgbA1C if symptomatic	Thyroid replacement Bromocriptine Insulin or insulin-sensitizing agents
Antiphospholipid antibody syndrome	Lupus anticoagulant Anticardiolipin IgG and IgM Anti-β2 glycoprotein IgG and IgM	Aspirin 81 mg Heparin 5000 U SQ BID with pregnancy

BID, twice a day; HgbA1C, hemoglobin A1C; IgG, immunoglobulin G; IgM, immunoglobulin M; IVF, in-vitro fertilization; SQ, subcutaneous.

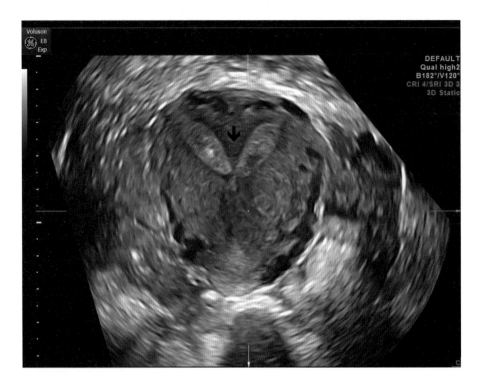

Fig. 64.1 Three-dimensional pelvic ultrasound.

trials exist on which to base firm conclusions, the general consensus is that women with RPL be evaluated with hysterosalpingogram, sonohysterogram, or hysteroscopy and that identified abnormalities can be more fully evaluated by MRI or three-dimensional ultrasound. Consensus also exists that those women with a significant uterine abnormality undergo surgical correction [2]. This patient has a clearly visible septum on three-dimensional ultrasound and hysteroscopic resection should be offered.

Balanced structural chromosome abnormalities are present in 2–5% of couples with RPL. Balanced translocations, either reciprocal or Robertsonian, are the most common type of structural abnormality in patients with RPL. When germ cells with these balanced translocations undergo meiosis they result in unbalanced oocytes or sperm with high frequency. These abnormalities are thought to be more commonly inherited from the mother since unbalanced sperm are less likely to result in fertilization; however, karyotype testing of both partners is indicated. Couples found to have a chromosomal abnormality should be referred for genetic counseling. Treatment options include donor eggs or sperm, and preimplantation genetic diagnosis (PGD) of embryos created via in-vitro fertilization.

The American Society of Reproductive Medicine (ASRM) recommends screening patients with RPL for thyroid and prolactin abnormalities with TSH and prolactin levels [2]. Poorly controlled diabetes is also a risk factor for miscarriage and women with symptoms of diabetes should be screened with a fasting blood glucose or HbA1C.

Antiphospholipid antibody syndrome (APS) is associated with RPL and treatment with aspirin and heparin improves pregnancy outcomes. Patients with RPL should be screened for the lupus anticoagulant, anticardiolipin immunoglobulin G and immunoglobulin M (IgG and IgM), and anti-β2 glycoprotein IgG and IgM. Positive tests should be confirmed 12 or more weeks after the initial test, and patients with persistent titers should be treated with aspirin 81 mg daily and 5000 U of unfractionated heparin SQ BID.

For more than 50% of couples with RPL, no etiology will be identified following evaluation. However, live birth rates of 35–85%, depending on age and parity, are typically achieved in the subsequent pregnancy without treatment.

Key teaching points

- Recurrent pregnancy loss (RPL) is defined as two or more consecutive losses of clinical pregnancies.
- Structural uterine abnormalities, parental chromosome abnormalities, maternal endocrine abnormalities, and antiphospholipid antibodies are potential causes of RPL.
- No cause is identified in more than 50% of couples with RPL.
- The prognosis in subsequent pregnancies for live-birth is good.

References

1. Royal College of Obstetricians and Gynaecologists. *The Investigation And Treatment Of Couples With Recurrent First-Trimester And Second Trimester Miscarriage.* Green-top Guideline 17, April 2011. Available at http://www. rcog.org.uk/files/rcog-corp/GTG17recurrentmiscarriage.pdf.

2. Practice Committee of the American Society for Reproductive Medicine. Evaluation and treatment of recurrent pregnancy loss: a committee opinion. *Fertil Steril* 2012;98:1103–11.

3. American College of Obstetricians and Gynecologists. Management of recurrent pregnancy loss. Practice Bulletin No. 24. *Int J Gynecol Obstet* 2002;78:179–90.

4. Petrozza JC. *Recurrent Early Pregnancy Loss.* Available at http://emedicine. medscape.com/article/260495-overview.

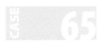

A 38-year-old woman with worsening postpartum fatigue

Amanda H. Ritter

History of present illness

A 38-year-old gravida 1, para 1 woman presented 3 months postpartum with worsening fatigue, lethargy, and depression. She had a term spontaneous vaginal delivery of an 8-lb boy, but her delivery was complicated by a retained placenta and postpartum hemorrhage of approximately 2000 cc. She required a manual placental extraction and uterine curettage, and was transfused four units of packed red blood cells postpartum. Afterwards, the patient had an otherwise uneventful course but was unable to breast-feed her infant due to a failure to lactate. She still has not had return of menses. The patient initially attributed her fatigue and lethargy to being a new mother. However, these symptoms have progressively worsened. She also reports cold intolerance, inability to lose weight, and decreased libido.

She denies any other medical problems and has had no surgeries. She uses condoms for birth control. She takes no medications.

Physical examination

General appearance: Obese, white woman in no acute distress
Vital signs:

Temperature: 37.0°C
Pulse: 54 beats/min
Blood pressure: 100/70 mmHg
Respiratory rate: 12 breaths/min
Oxygen saturation: 99% on room air

HEENT: Mild alopecia present; unremarkable otherwise
Neck: Supple, no thyromegaly
Cardiovascular: Bradycardic rate; regular rhythm without murmurs, rubs, or gallops
Lungs: Clear to auscultation bilaterally
Breast: Normal appearing breasts bilaterally, no masses palpated, no nipple discharge expressed
Abdomen: Soft, obese, nondistended, active bowel sounds present. No tenderness to palpation in upper or lower quadrants bilaterally
Pelvic: Normal appearing external genitalia. Vaginal mucosa within normal limits, scant discharge. Parous cervix without lesions. Bimanual examination with small, anteverted, mobile, nontender uterus. No cervical motion tenderness. No adnexal masses or tenderness to palpation bilaterally

Extremities: Patches of erythematous, scaly skin on hands and anterior lower extremities
Neurologic: Delayed 2+ deep tendon reflexes, bilaterally; nonfocal otherwise
Initial laboratory studies:

Urine pregnancy test: Negative
Hb: 11.5 g/dL
MCV: 83 fL

How would you further evaluate this patient?

This patient presents with amenorrhea, absence of lactation, fatigue, cold intolerance, and decreased libido. From her workup thus far, subsequent pregnancy and pelvic anatomic abnormalities have been excluded as a cause for her amenorrhea. Additionally, her remaining symptoms and clinical findings are suggestive of possible depression, hypothyroidism, or malfunctioning of the hypothalamic–pituitary–ovarian axis. A thyroid-stimulating hormone (TSH) level should be ordered to evaluate thyroid function as the next most likely cause of her symptoms. This patient's TSH was 0.06 µIU/mL (0.35–5.5 µIU/mL). Her free thyroxine (T4) was 0.4 ng/dL (0.8–1.8 ng/dL). The low TSH and free T4 indicate a problem with the pituitary itself. At this time, further investigation of the hypothalamic–pituitary–ovarian axis is necessary with testing of cortisol, adrenocorticotropic hormone (ACTH), follicle-stimulating hormone (FSH), luteinizing hormone (LH), and prolactin. All of these values were low: cortisol 5 µg/dL (5–23 µg/dL), ACTH 10 pg/mL (9–52 pg/mL), FSH less than 0.3 mIU/mL, LH less than 0.1 mIU/mL, and prolactin 1.5 ng/mL (2–39 ng/mL). This patient shows evidence of panhypopituitarism, so imaging of the pituitary itself was ordered to further delineate a cause for this patient's symptoms. MRI of the brain revealed an empty sella with minimal pituitary tissue.

How would you manage this patient?

This patient has Sheehan syndrome. She presents with the typical history of postpartum hemorrhage, failure to lactate, and amenorrhea. She also displays symptoms of other pituitary deficiencies, including hypothyroidism. Her laboratory findings are significant for pan-hypopituitarism, and her imaging shows an empty sella turcica. Once the diagnosis was made, treatment was initiated with both steroids and levothyroxine under the guidance of an endocrinologist. Her symptoms

Acute Care and Emergency Gynecology, ed. David Chelmow, Christine R. Isaacs and Ashley Carroll. Published by Cambridge University Press.
© Cambridge University Press 2015.

gradually begin to improve after initiation of hormone replacement therapy, and she is followed at regular intervals by both her gynecologist and endocrinologist.

Sheehan syndrome

Sheehan syndrome is a process that was first described by Harold L. Sheehan in the 1930s. Sheehan syndrome involves persistent hypopituitarism after pituitary ischemia caused by obstetrical blood loss and hypotension or shock. This syndrome has become much rarer because of advances in the prevention and management of postpartum hemorrhage and the availability of blood products for transfusion. However, cases of Sheehan syndrome still happen, most frequently in developing countries with limited obstetrical resources or in areas where home births are still common [1].

Sheehan syndrome involves a wide range of clinical presentations, ranging from immediate postpartum circulatory failure to mild symptoms manifesting many years after the sentinel event [2]. The average time between the inciting incident and clinical manifestations varies from 1 to 40 years, and the timing of onset of presenting symptoms does not often correlate with the severity of symptoms [3]. The speed and onset of symptoms is determined by the extent of pituitary damage. Because the pituitary gland has significant reserve capacity, more than 75% of the gland must be destroyed before symptoms become evident [2]. In less severe cases of Sheehan syndrome, the absence of lactation after pregnancy due to low levels of prolactin is often the first evidence of postpartum pituitary necrosis. Affected women typically have failure of return of menses and scant regrowth of shaved pubic hair, both as a result of gonadotropin failure. Secondary hypothyroidism, adrenal insufficiency, and growth hormone deficiency, manifested as low levels of TSH, free T4, cortisol, ACTH, and growth hormone often appear later [1,2]. Growth hormone deficiency has been found in all reported cases of Sheehan syndrome, whereas other hormones typically thought to be routinely involved, like TSH and prolactin, are actually variably present [4]. When Sheehan syndrome presents acutely, women may be confused, stuporous, or comatose. These findings are all indications of severe hyponatremia, which can be another manifestation of Sheehan syndrome. In these cases, immediate cortisol and thyroxine replacement should be administered to enable the correction of the hyponatremia [2].

While radiologic imaging is not necessary for the diagnosis of Sheehan syndrome, evidence of partial or complete pituitary necrosis, or empty sella, on imaging further supports the diagnosis [1]. An empty sella may be visualized on MRI or CT (arrow, Fig. 65.1) [2]. Pituitary MRI is the most sensitive imaging for detecting Sheehan syndrome [3]. However, an empty sella is not specific for Sheehan syndrome. According to Sert and colleagues, an empty sella is visualized in approximately 28.5% of MRI images and 20% of high-resolution CT images in women with Sheehan syndrome [2]. Given that an

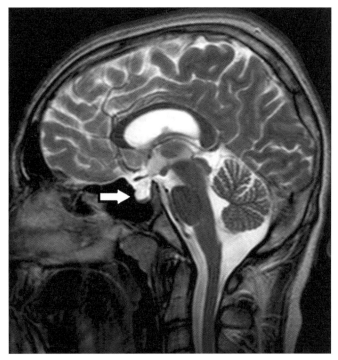

Fig. 65.1 Empty sella (arrow) on MRI. Image from: Empty sella syndrome. http://en.wikipedia.org/wiki/Empty_sella (Accessed November 21, 2013).

empty sella is not diagnostic of Sheehan syndrome, other diagnoses presenting with this radiograph finding must also be ruled out, including postpartum necrosis of a pituitary adenoma and lymphocytic hypophysitis [3].

The management of Sheehan syndrome should begin with the replacement of the target hormones that have been found to be deficient. Adrenal function should be corrected first as adrenal insufficiency can be life-threatening [1]. The minimum glucocorticoid dose required to correct clinical symptoms should be administered and must be tailored to each individual case [3]. The administration of thyroid hormone replacement alone in a patient with unrecognized adrenal insufficiency can be extremely dangerous, as thyroid hormone replacement can increase the metabolic clearance of cortisol and exacerbate an adrenal crisis [1]. Once adrenal replacement is adequate, thyroid hormone replacement should be initiated and titrated to maintenance levels based on periodic serum TSH testing and clinical symptoms. Premenopausal women with gonadotropin deficiency should be administered estrogen and progesterone. If a woman with Sheehan syndrome desires to become pregnant, ovulation induction may be necessary. Growth hormone replacement improves waist circumference, lipid profiles, visceral fat, and importantly, quality of life [3].

Key teaching points

- The classic presentation of Sheehan syndrome involves a history of significant postpartum hemorrhage requiring blood transfusions or volume repletion followed by failure of lactation and amenorrhea or other evidence of anterior pituitary malfunction.

- The differential diagnosis of Sheehan syndrome includes pregnancy, depression, hypothyroidism, pituitary adenoma, and lymphocytic hypophysitis.

- Radiographic imaging may display an empty sella, but this is not diagnostic of Sheehan syndrome. Pituitary MRI is the most sensitive imaging modality for Sheehan syndrome.

- The onset and severity of symptoms can be extremely variable. Symptoms may be acute and so extreme as to cause hemodynamic instability and altered mentation. Conversely, hypopituitarism may gradually begin as long as 40 years postpartum.

- Treatment involves stabilization of the patient if symptoms are acute and severe. Deficient hormones need replacement. Steroids must be initiated prior to thyroid hormone replacement to prevent adrenal crisis.

References

1. Tessnow AH, Wilson JD. The changing face of Sheehan's syndrome. *Am J Med Sci* 2010;340:402–6.

2. Sert M, Tetiker T, Kirim S, Kocak M. Clinical report of 28 patients with Sheehan's syndrome. *Endocr J* 2003; 50:297–301.

3. Karaca Z, Tanriverdi F, Unluhizarci K, Kelestimur F. Pregnancy and pituitary disorders. *Eur J Endocrinol* 2010; 162:453–75.

4. Dejager S, Gerber S, Foubert L, Turpin G. Sheehan's syndrome: Differential diagnosis in the acute phase. *J Int Med* 1998;244: 261–6.

A 19-year-old woman with primary amenorrhea

Amy Brown and Nicole W. Karjane

History of present illness

A 19-year-old woman presents to the emergency department with lower abdominal pain. The pain started gradually 12 hours earlier and has progressively worsened in intensity. It is sharp in nature and localized to her left lower quadrant. She recalls that she has mild cramping pains in her lower abdomen every few weeks for years, but they have never been this intense. She denies any vaginal bleeding or discharge. She has never had a menstrual cycle and has never had vaginal intercourse.

Review of systems is negative for nausea, vomiting, diarrhea, constipation, fever, or chills. Her only medical history consists of mild scoliosis that has never required intervention. She takes no medications and has no known allergies. She was hospitalized at age eight for pyelonephritis, but is otherwise healthy and has never had surgery.

Physical examination

General appearance: Well-groomed, well-nourished woman in mild distress

Vital signs:

Temperature: 36.9°C
Pulse: 95 beats/min
Blood pressure: 133/76 mmHg
Respiratory rate: 18 breaths/min
Oxygen saturation: 99% on room air
BMI: 21 kg/m^2

HEENT: Normal

Cardiovascular: Regular rate and rhythm, normal S1 and S2, no murmurs, no edema

Lungs: Clear bilaterally without wheezes, good respiratory effort

Breasts: Tanner stage V breast development

Abdomen: Soft, moderately tender in left lower quadrant, minimal suprapubic or right lower quadrant tenderness. No distension, rebound or guarding. No masses palpable

Genitourinary: Tanner stage V pubic hair development, external genitalia (Fig. 66.1); unable to pass speculum or perform bimanual examination

Laboratory studies:

CBC and basic metabolic panel: Normal
Urinalysis: No blood, leukocytes, nitrites, or protein. Trace ketones present
Urine beta-hCG: Negative

Imaging: Trans-abdominal ultrasound reveals no definite uterus but approximate 2 × 2 × 1 cm mass of tissue posterior to the normal bladder. No evidence of an endometrial stripe or cervical anatomy. Right ovary normal. Left ovary contains a 3 cm cyst with fluid layering consistent with hemorrhage. Normal blood flow visualized to the ovaries bilaterally without evidence of torsion

The patient was given 30 mg IV ketorolac (Toradol®) in the emergency department and reported great improvement of her pain.

How would you manage this patient?

The patient's normal vital signs, laboratory evaluation, non-acute physical examination findings, and ovarian imaging suggest symptoms due to a hemorrhagic corpus luteal cyst. More concerning, however, is the patient's amenorrhea and findings on genital examination, which are suggestive of Mullerian agenesis.

The patient was referred for an outpatient gynecologic evaluation scheduled within 48 hours. A repeat ultrasound showed normal ovaries and a small, rudimentary uterus without endometrium. A karyotype was obtained confirming a 46,XX chromosome pattern. All endocrine laboratory studies were normal. The patient was diagnosed with complete Mullerian agenesis, also known as Mayer–Rokitansky–Küster–Hauser syndrome. She was ultimately started on vaginal dilator

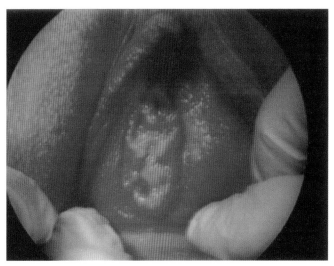

Fig. 66.1 External genitalia.

Acute Care and Emergency Gynecology, ed. David Chelmow, Christine R. Isaacs and Ashley Carroll. Published by Cambridge University Press.
© Cambridge University Press 2015.

therapy, received extensive counseling, and plans to consult with a fertility specialist in the future.

Primary amenorrhea and Mullerian agenesis

Primary amenorrhea is defined as either a lack of menses by age 14 without evidence of pubertal development (axillary or pubic hair growth, breast development), or a lack of menses by age 16 if other evidence of puberty is present [1]. Potential etiologies are multiple and can be classified as either **anatomic** or **endocrine** abnormalities. A flow-diagram of the initial workup is shown in Fig. 66.2.

Anatomic causes of primary amenorrhea can be divided into abnormalities of the Mullerian organs (uterus, fallopian tubes, cervix, and superior 2/3 of the vagina) or of the distal outflow tract (inferior 1/3 of the vagina or labia). Mullerian agenesis is the most prevalent of these anatomic disorders and is second only to gonadal dysgenesis (an endocrine abnormality) as the leading cause of primary amenorrhea [1]. It encompasses a large number of potential anatomical variants depending on the degree of fusion of the Mullerian ducts in utero [2]. The patient in this scenario has Mayer–Rokitansky–Küster–Hauser syndrome, a form of Mullerian agenesis defined by congenital aplasia of the uterus and superior 2/3 of the vagina [3]. Approximately 50% of these

patients have other congenital anomalies, the most common being renal (horseshoe kidney, unilateral renal agenesis, or ectopic kidneys) and skeletal (scoliosis or other vertebral anomalies) [2]. Multiple genes have been implicated as a potential cause for these malformations, but there is no clear consensus as to whether this is a unifactorial or multifactorial condition [3].

Patients with complete Mullerian agenesis usually present in the outpatient setting due to concerns of amenorrhea. They may, however, present earlier if any of the associated anatomical abnormalities are discovered as incidental finding on imaging, or if they are seeking medical attention for symptoms unrelated to the Mullerian agenesis, as in this case with the patient presenting for pain due to a functional ovarian cyst. Additionally, 2–7% of patients with Mullerian agenesis will have rudimentary uterine horns that contain active endometrium. These patients will often present with symptoms of menstrual obstruction or pelvic pain due to retrograde menstruation and endometriosis formation [2]. Removal of the noncommunicating horn may be indicated for symptom relief in these cases.

Disorders of the distal outflow tract encompass any abnormality of the inferior 1/3 of the vagina or labia. The most common of these are an imperforate hymen (1 in 1000 women) and a transverse vaginal septum (1 in 80 000 women)

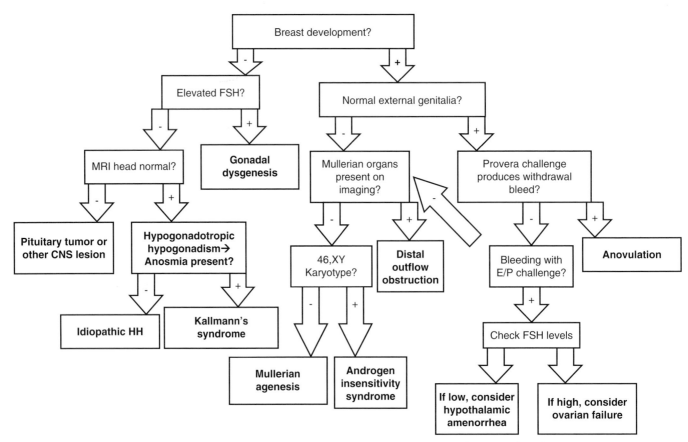

Fig. 66.2 Evaluation of primary amenorrhea. CNS, central nervous system; E/P, estrogen/progesterone; FSH, follicle-stimulating hormone; HH, hypogonadotropic hypogonadism.

[1]. Patients with these disorders often present with cyclic pelvic pain in the absence of menstrual bleeding due to the outflow obstruction. Because these pain symptoms most commonly prompt medical evaluation prior to concerns for primary amenorrhea, these conditions will likely be diagnosed and managed (prior to age 16) and, thus, remain less common than gonadal dysgenesis and Mullerian agenesis as an etiology of true primary amenorrhea. Surgical correction of the outflow obstruction is curative.

When primary amenorrhea is associated with an endocrine etiology, it can be divided into disorders of the hypothalamus, pituitary, or gonads. The initial laboratory evaluation is guided by the physical examination findings, particularly the presence or absence of pubertal development. In patients without breast development, a follicle-stimulating hormone (FSH) should be measured. Patients with absent pubertal development and low FSH levels should undergo an MRI of the brain to rule out a CNS lesion as the cause. Most of these patients will be diagnosed with hypogonadotropic hypogonadism, a hypothalamic disorder characterized by congenital gonadotropin-releasing hormone (GnRH) deficiency. Kallmann syndrome is the most common of these disorders and is associated with anosmia, or lack of smell [1]. Rare cases of idiopathic hypogonadotropic hypogonadism without anosmia have also been reported. Though functional hypothalamic disorders (typically due to stressors, eating disorders, or intensive exercise) are common causes of *secondary* amenorrhea, they rarely present as primary amenorrhea except in severe cases [1].

The pituitary is responsible for approximately 5% of primary amenorrhea cases, which are typically discovered by abnormalities in pituitary hormone levels, most often prolactin. Patients presenting with primary amenorrhea and new-onset headaches or vision changes, particularly bilateral hemianopsia (temporal visual field defects), should undergo an evaluation for a pituitary tumor, as the mass effect of a growth can produce these associated clinical symptoms.

Gonadal dysgenesis, also referred to as "primary ovarian insufficiency," is the most frequent cause of primary amenorrhea [1]. Just over half of these patients have Turner syndrome, which is typically characterized by the absence of all or part of one X chromosome (45,X karyotype) and streak ovaries (the ovaries are replaced by functionless fibrous tissue). Clinically, Turner's stigmata include short stature, neck-webbing, and primary amenorrhea. Turner's patients may also have concurrent congenital heart and renal defects. Up to 40% of patients with gonadal dysgenesis may have a 46,XX or XY karyotype. Those who are XY or have the sex-determining region of the Y chromosome are recommended to undergo gonadectomy due to the risk of developing a gonadal malignancy [1].

Evaluation of primary amenorrhea should always start with a thorough history and physical examination to determine the stage of pubertal development. In patients with breast development, functional gonads can generally be assumed and, thus, the next step is to determine whether normal external genitalia, vagina, and cervical anatomy are present.

Imaging via ultrasonography may be required in patients who cannot tolerate a pelvic examination. Patients with ultrasonographic evidence of menstrual obstruction may need to be further evaluated by MRI to clarify their pelvic anatomy and to define the specific anomaly. In patients without a patent vagina or uterus, karyotyping should be performed to determine whether the diagnosis is Mullerian agenesis or androgen insensitivity syndrome (AIS). AIS results in an apparently female phenotype at birth in a 46,XY patient due to lack of testosterone activity at the external genitalia. Unlike patients with Mullerian agenesis, however, those with AIS generally have scant pubic hair due to the insensitivity of peripheral androgen receptors to circulating testosterone. Since the karyotype is 46,XY, testicles are present (instead of ovaries) and, hence, produce anti-Mullerian hormone in utero, resulting in an absence of Mullerian organs. There is a 25% risk of developing testicular malignancy with AIS, thought to be due to the presence of intra-abdominal testes. As such, surgical removal of the testes should be prophylactically performed once puberty is complete [4].

In patients with primary amenorrhea, normal pubertal development, and normal pelvic anatomy, a progestin challenge is helpful diagnostically once pregnancy has been ruled out. If bleeding occurs in response to the progestin challenge, the etiology of the amenorrhea is anovulation, and the patient should be evaluated for etiologies of this such as thyroid dysfunction, prolactinomas, and polycystic ovary syndrome. If no withdrawal bleeding follows the progestin challenge, an estrogen plus progestin challenge should be prescribed. Bleeding in response to an estrogen/progesterone challenge confirms a patent outflow tract, but leaves concern for gonadal failure. Patients with gonadal failure after puberty should be evaluated for Turner syndrome as well as the Fragile X premutation.

Long-term management of primary amenorrhea is dictated by the etiology of the disorder. Patients with an imperforate hymen or transverse vaginal septum (anatomic distal outflow obstructions) should undergo surgical correction, which will result in resolution of amenorrhea and cure [1]. In the case of the patient described with Mullerian agenesis, as well as those with AIS, a number of surgical techniques have been described for the creation of a neovagina. Despite surgical procedures that can create a functional vagina, vaginal dilator therapy is still considered the first-line intervention and in motivated patients and has a success rate of over 90% [3]. Patients with Mullerian agenesis should also be offered counseling regarding their diagnosis and reproductive options. While they will be unable to carry a fetus due to the absence of the uterus, they are able to have their own biological children via in-vitro fertilization (IVF) technology using a gestational carrier [2]. Those with AIS do not have this ability since they have neither a uterus nor ovaries; thus, adoption and surrogacy are the only options.

Patients with primary amenorrhea from endocrine dysfunction typically require hormone treatments. Patients with gonadal dysgenesis should be treated initially with low-dose estrogen therapy to initiate normal pubertal maturation and bone growth. Once adequate breast development is present and/or the patient has breakthrough bleeding, the patient should be transitioned to estrogen/progesterone therapy for prevention of early bone loss and other estrogen deficiency symptoms while protecting against endometrial hyperplasia. These patients may conceive using IVF with donor eggs and should likewise be offered counseling regarding fertility options. The management of pituitary lesions depends on the etiology. Prolactinomas are generally treated with dopamine agonists as first-line therapy, whereas more significant lesions may require referral to a neurosurgeon for management. Hypogonadotropic hypogonadism can be treated by hormone replacement therapy (similar to those with gonadal dysgenesis) once CNS lesions have been ruled out. These patients will need treatment with gonadotropins or pulsatile GnRH if pregnancy is desired [1]. Special consideration should be given to emotional and social factors for patients with primary amenorrhea and support groups may be highly beneficial.

Key teaching points

- Primary amenorrhea is defined as either a lack of menses by age 14 without evidence of pubertal development, or a lack of menses by age 16 if other evidence of puberty exists.
- Patients with primary amenorrhea should be evaluated to determine the etiology which can be classified as either anatomic or endocrine in origin.
- Anatomic causes of primary amenorrhea include abnormalities of Mullerian organs (uterus, fallopian tubes, cervix, superior 2/3 of the vagina), or of the distal outflow tract (inferior 1/3 of the vagina or labia).
- Endocrine causes of primary amenorrhea include disorders of the hypothalamus, pituitary, or gonads.
- Women with primary amenorrhea should receive comprehensive therapy which, depending on the diagnosis, may include hormone therapy, vaginal dilator use, surgical interventions, emotional counseling, and consultation with fertility specialists.

References

1. Practice Committee of the American Society for Reproductive Medicine. Current evaluation of amenorrhea. *Fertil Steril* 2008;90:S219–25.

2. American College of Obstetricians and Gynecologists. Mullerian agenesis: Diagnosis, management, and treatment. Committee Opinion No. 562. *Obstet Gynecol* 2013;121: 1134–7.

3. Pizzo A, Lagana AS, Sturlese E, et al. Mayer–Rokitansky–Kuster–Hauser syndrome: Embryology, genetics, and clinical and surgical treatment. *Obstet Gynecol* 2013;2013:628717. DOI: 10.1155/2013/628717.

4. Hughes IA, Werner R, Bunch T, Hiort O. Androgen insensitivity syndrome. *Semin Reprod Med* 2012; 30:432–42.

A 26-year-old woman with secondary amenorrhea

Mary T. Sale and Nancy A. Sokkary

History of present illness

A 26-year-old gravida 0 woman presents with complaint of 6 months of amenorrhea. She reports menarche at age 13 and describes her periods as having always been irregular. Over the last two years they have become increasingly less frequent. She has also experienced weight gain and increasingly troublesome facial hair growth. She denies any vaginal dryness, hot flashes, nipple discharge, or new headache.

She is sexually active with her long-term boyfriend. They use condoms for contraception. Her only prior surgery was a laparoscopic appendectomy. She has no other significant medical or family history. She takes no medications.

Physical examination

General appearance: Well-nourished woman in no acute distress

Vital signs:

Temperature: 37.0°C
Pulse: 64 beats/min
Blood pressure: 142/88 mmHg
Respiratory rate: 14 breaths/min
Oxygen saturation: 98% on room air
Weight: 224 lb
Height: 66 inches
BMI: 36 kg/m^2

Neck: Supple, no thyromegaly

Cardiovascular: Regular rate and rhythm

Lungs: Clear to auscultation bilaterally

Breast: Symmetric, no nipple discharge, no lumps

Abdomen: Soft, nondistended, nontender in all quadrants

Pelvic:

Normal appearing external female genitalia with excessive pubic hair extending to the inner thighs
Speculum exam: Well rugated, moist vaginal walls. No cervical discharge. Normal appearing nulliparous cervix without lesions
Bimanual exam: Small, anteverted uterus. No cervical motion tenderness. No adnexal masses

Extremities: No clubbing, cyanosis, or edema

Neurologic: Nonfocal

Skin: Increased hair growth on chin, upper lip, abdomen, and chest. Moderate acne is present

Laboratory studies:

Urine pregnancy test: Negative
TSH: 3.2 μIU/mL (normal 0.50–4.70 μIU/mL)
Serum prolactin: 16 ng/mL (normal for nonlactating women: 2–29 ng/mL)

Imaging: Endovaginal ultrasound was obtained (Figs 67.1 and 67.2)

How would you manage this patient?

This patient has secondary amenorrhea due to polycystic ovarian syndrome (PCOS). She was counseled on lifestyle modifications and prescribed cyclical oral contraceptive pills. She began a vigorous exercise program and lost 35 lb. Her acne improved. Nine months later, she discontinued her oral contraceptive pills and had spontaneous regular monthly cycles.

Secondary amenorrhea is defined as greater than three months without a period in a woman who has undergone menarche. In the acute setting it is sufficient to rule out common causes of amenorrhea: pregnancy, thyroid dysfunction, and hyperprolactinemia. However, the evaluation (Table 67.1) may need to be more extensive depending on the symptoms associated with amenorrhea. If other symptoms such as hot flashes or vaginal dryness are present, estradiol, luteinizing hormone (LH), and follicle-stimulating hormone (FSH) should be tested to evaluate for primary ovarian insufficiency (POI). If women are underweight or have other systemic illnesses, gonadotropin (FSH and LH) levels should also be evaluated to assess for hypogonadotropic hypogonadism. Alternatively, a progestin challenge can be given to evaluate for endogenous estrogen production. If androgenic symptoms are present, like this case, PCOS should be considered. This patient has secondary amenorrhea with clinical symptoms of androgen excess including acne and increased hair growth. Her initial laboratory evaluation was unremarkable, excluding other causes. Her endovaginal ultrasound demonstrated multiple peripheral cysts (Fig. 67.1) and ovarian volume greater than 10 cm^3 (Fig. 67.2). She meets criteria for the diagnosis of PCOS.

Polycystic ovarian syndrome

Polycystic ovarian syndrome (PCOS) is a common endocrine disorder that can present at any time during a woman's reproductive years, and affects from 6 to 15% of women [1,2,3]. Woman with PCOS typically have a combination of irregular

---

Acute Care and Emergency Gynecology, ed. David Chelmow, Christine R. Isaacs and Ashley Carroll. Published by Cambridge University Press.

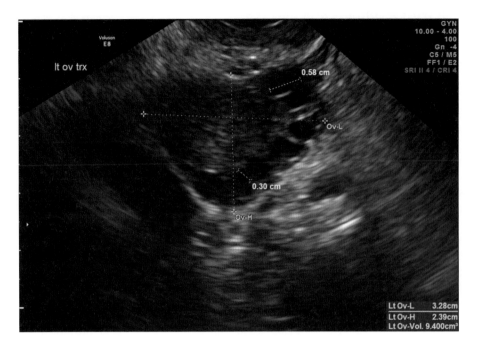

Fig. 67.1 Endovaginal ultrasound demonstrating left ovary in 26-year-old woman with amenorrhea.

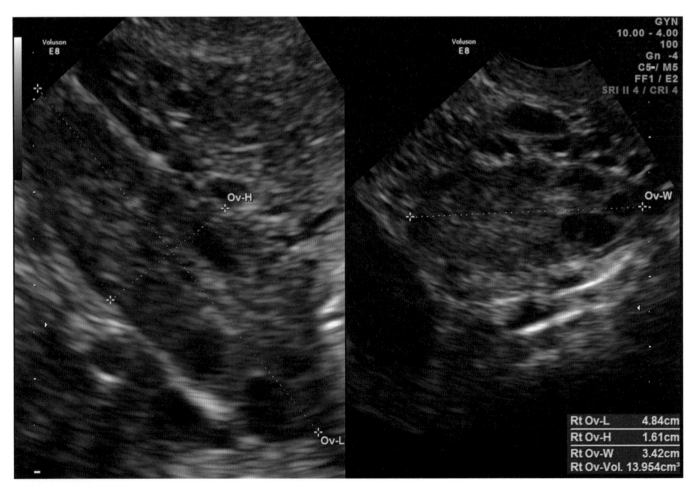

Fig. 67.2 Endovaginal ultrasound demonstrating right ovary in 26-year-old woman with amenorrhea.

cycles or secondary amenorrhea, hyperandrogenism, and abnormal ovarian morphology [1]. Three different diagnostic criteria exist. They all require at least two of the following: anovulation, clinical or laboratory evidence of hyperandrogenism, and polycystic ovaries on ultrasound. They also require exclusion of other diagnosis (Table 67.1) [2].

The pathophysiology of PCOS is complex and not entirely understood. Hyperandrogenism may be due to increased ovarian sensitivity to LH or abnormal gonadotropin-releasing hormone (GnRH) pulsatility resulting in increased circulating LH. Insulin resistance also plays a key role in increased androgen levels [2,4]. While the syndrome likely starts *in utero* and has a heritable component, environmental factors such as obesity also contribute [4].

Evaluation of secondary amenorrhea includes a full history and physical examination to evaluate for symptoms of hypothyroidism, pregnancy, primary ovarian insufficiency, and hyperprolactinemia. When PCOS is considered as part of the differential, pelvic ultrasound should be considered. Polycystic ovaries on ultrasound are defined as the presence of 12 or more antral follicles measuring 2–9 mm in diameter (Fig. 67.1), or total ovarian volume greater than 10 mL (Fig. 67.2) [3]. Sonographic findings of polycystic ovaries are observed in 20–30% of the general population and by themselves are not diagnostic for PCOS [2]. Laboratory tests should be performed to rule out other etiologies of secondary amenorrhea or oligomenorrhea. If androgen symptoms are severe, the differential diagnosis should be expanded to include an androgen-secreting tumor and if the patient is an adolescent, testing should be performed for late-onset congenital adrenal hyperplasia (Table 67.1).

Patients with PCOS can experience secondary amenorrhea due to anovulation. The consequent unopposed estrogen can lead to endometrial hyperplasia which, if left untreated, can progress to uterine cancer [1,4]. In a patient with anovulation,

Table 67.1 Laboratory evaluation of oligoovulation/secondary amenorrhea

Differential diagnosis	Laboratory test
Pregnancy	Urine pregnancy test or serum beta-hCG
Hypothyroidism	TSH
Hyperprolactinemia	Prolactin
Hypogonadotropic-hypogonadism/ primary ovarian insufficiency	LH/FSH, estradiol
Androgen-secreting tumor*	Testosterone, DHEA-S
Late-onset congenital adrenal hyperplasia†	17-Hydroxyprogesterone

* Significant signs of androgenization
† Adolescents
DHEA-S, dehydroepiandrosterone sulfate; FSH, follicle-stimulating hormone; hCG, human chorionic gonadotropin (hCG); LH, luteinizing hormone; TSH, thyroid-stimulating hormone.

one goal of therapy is to prevent endometrial hyperplasia either through resumption of spontaneous cycles or administering progestin. In a woman presenting with history of prolonged anovulation due to PCOS, endometrial biopsy should be performed to evaluate for endometrial hyperplasia or cancer. Biopsy should be performed in women over age 45 who have bleeding from suspected ovulatory dysfunction. The American College of Obstetricians and Gynecologists guidelines [5] recommend endometrial sampling in younger women if they have had "prolonged" periods of unopposed estrogen or have failed medical treatment. The guidelines do not define "prolonged" but a determination should be made based on length of unopposed estrogen in conjunction with other risk factors such as degree of obesity [5]. If abnormalities are diagnosed, they should be treated. If the biopsy shows no evidence of hyperplasia or cancer, multiple hormonal therapies exist for prevention of hyperplasia. Hormonal therapy requires the delivery of progestin, which can be administered through combined hormonal contraceptives (pills, patch, or ring), or cyclic or continuous progestin alone. Frequently used progestins include oral medroxyprogesterone (10 mg PO for 10–14 days each month) or depot medroxyprogesterone acetate (150 mg IM every 3 months). The levonorgestrel intrauterine device is another convenient way of delivering continuous progestin. Combined hormonal contraceptives have the added benefit of improving androgenic symptoms. While nearly all patients can be managed with medical therapy, hysterectomy is a potential option in women who have completed childbearing and do not tolerate or cannot comply with medical therapy [5].

Other treatment options can be used in combination. Therapy for PCOS includes lifestyle modification, particularly weight reduction, metformin, and anti-androgens. Lifestyle modification including diet and cardiovascular exercise is first-line therapy for this patient because she is obese. A 5% reduction in body mass index leads to resumption of spontaneous menses in 60% of women with PCOS [6]. Weight loss can also decrease the risk of hyperplasia by decreasing peripheral estrogen production. Metformin improves metabolic parameters and is also effective in decreasing serum androgens and promoting the return of spontaneous menstrual cycles. Some studies have found a resumption of regular cycles in 50% of women within 6 months of initiation of metformin [6]. Anti-androgens, including spironolactone, flutamide, and finasteride have not been found to have an additional treatment benefit when used in combination with oral contraceptive pills [1]. Clomiphene citrate is effective for ovulation induction in women with PCOS-related infertility [6].

Key teaching points

- Polycystic ovarian syndrome (PCOS) is a diagnosis of exclusion. Other causes of amenorrhea and excessive androgen syndromes must be excluded to make the diagnosis.

- Diagnostic criteria for PCOS include anovulation, clinical, or laboratory evidence of hyperandrogenism, and sonographic evidence of abnormal ovaries (>12 follicles measuring 2–9 mm or total ovarian volume >10 mL).
- Women with secondary amenorrhea from PCOS are at increased risk of endometrial hyperplasia and malignancy.

- Cyclic or continuous progestin is effective for protecting the endometrium in women with anovulation or oligoovulation from PCOS. Progestin can be delivered through combined hormonal contraceptives, oral progestin, depot medroxyprogesterone, or the levonorgestrel intrauterine device.

References

1. Fauser BC, Tarlatzis BC, Rebar RW, et al. Consensus on women's health aspects of polycystic ovary syndrome (PCOS): The Amsterdam ESHRE/ASRM-Sponsored 3rd PCOS Consensus Workshop Group. *Fertil Steril* 2012;97(1):28–38.

2. Azziz R, Carmina E, Dewailly D, et al. The Androgen Excess and PCOS Society criteria for the polycystic ovary syndrome: The complete task force report. *Fertil Steril* 2009;91(2):456–88.

3. Hart R, Hickey M, Franks S.Definitions, prevalence and symptoms of polycystic ovaries and polycystic ovary syndrome. *Best Pract Res Clin Obstet Gynaecol* 2004;18(5):671–83.

4. American College of Obstetricians and Gynecologists. Polycystic ovary syndrome. Practice Bulletin No. 108. *Obstet Gynecol* 2009;114:936–49.

5. American College of Obstetricians and Gynecologists. Management of abnormal uterine bleeding associated with ovulatory dysfunction. Practice Bulletin No. 136. *Obstet Gynecol* 2013;122:176–85.

6. Bates GW Jr., Propst AM. Polycystic ovarian syndrome management options. *Obstet Gynecol Clin North Am* 2012;39(4):495–506.

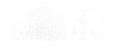

Irregular bleeding in a 25-year-old woman

Anita K. Blanchard

History of present illness

A 25-year-old gravida 0, para 0 woman presents to the emergency department complaining of heavy vaginal bleeding. Her current menses began eight days ago preceded by a three-month absence of menses. She reports menarche at age 16 with irregular cycle intervals. She notes an alternating pattern of absent menses for 6–12 weeks followed by heavy bleeding lasting up to 10 days. Currently she notes passage of quarter-sized clots and soaked pads every four hours. She complains of fatigue but denies any dizziness. She denies abdominal pain, nausea, vomiting, or diarrhea. She denies any history of blood dyscrasia, epistaxis, or bruising. She is sexually active with one male partner. They intermittently use male condoms for contraception. No vulvar, vaginal, or abdominal trauma is reported. She is otherwise healthy and takes no other medications.

Physical examination

General appearance: A well-hydrated woman in no distress
Vital signs:

  Temperature: 37.1°C
  Pulse: 88 beats/min
  Blood pressure: 102/64 mmHg
  Respiratory rate: 12 breaths/min
  BMI: 36 kg/m^2

HEENT: No goiter or thyroid prominence
Cardiovascular: Regular rate and rhythm without murmur or gallop
Lungs: Clear to auscultation bilaterally
Breasts: No discharge, no masses bilaterally
Abdomen: Soft, nondistended and nontender to palpation, bowel sounds present
Pelvic: Normal external genitalia, no clitoromegaly. Blood noted at the introitus. Approximately 7 cc of dark blood is seen in the vagina. Normal appearing cervix; no vaginal or cervical lacerations or lesions are noted. Normal-sized, anteverted uterus with no adnexal masses palpated
Neurologic: Alert and oriented, nonfocal findings on exam
Skin: No frontal balding, mild acne, mild hirsuitism with skin findings notable for hair growth on upper lip, chin, mid-sternum, periaerolar region, and thighs
Laboratory studies:

  Urine hCG test: Negative
  A CBC is ordered: Hb was 9.4 mg/dL

Imaging: Transvaginal ultrasound images reveal a normal-sized anteverted uterus. Ovaries are normal size with 12–14 follicles noted on the periphery of each ovary (Fig. 68.1)

How would you manage this patient?

This patient has chronic anovulation as a result of polycystic ovary syndrome. She was treated with a combined oral contraceptive pills to regulate her cycle and was scheduled to return to the outpatient clinic for further evaluation of her androgen excess.

Anovulation and the differential diagnosis

Pregnancy and malignancy should be excluded in any reproductive-aged woman who presents with abnormal vaginal bleeding. The source of the bleeding should also be confirmed. Abnormal uterine bleeding associated with ovulatory dysfunction is characterized by irregular uterine bleeding in which uterine structural abnormalities have been ruled out by imaging, typically transvaginal ultrasonography. Irregular uterine bleeding can be ovulatory or anovulatory. Causes of anovulation include physiologic etiologies associated with adolescence, perimenopause, pregnancy, or lactation. With the onset of menstruation, anovulation is frequent. It is estimated that 85% of menstrual cycles are anovulatory in the 1st year after menarche. This percentage decreases to about 59% by year 3 of menstruation [1]. Pathologic causes of anovulation include endocrine abnormalities such as hyperandrogenic disorders, hypothalamic dysfunction, pituitary and thyroid disorders, and premature ovarian failure. Iatrogenic causes include radiation and medications, particularly chemotherapy and exogenous hormones.

Chronic anovulation is common in reproductive-aged women and is often characterized by oligomenorrhea followed by heavy and or prolonged menses. In the absence of ovulation, the corpus luteum does not form and the ovary does not secrete progestin to stabilize and differentiate the endometrial lining. Unopposed estrogen promotes stimulation and proliferation of the endometrium, which continues without the progesterone withdrawal-induced menstrual shedding. The thickened endometrium is vascular and lacks stromal support [2]. When bleeding occurs there is irregular, unsynchronized shedding of the lining producing noncyclic, unpredictably heavy, and prolonged menses. Patterns of irregular bleeding from chronic anovulation may be reported as early as menarche and can continue until menopause. In patients who

Acute Care and Emergency Gynecology, ed. David Chelmow, Christine R. Isaacs and Ashley Carroll. Published by Cambridge University Press. © Cambridge University Press 2015.

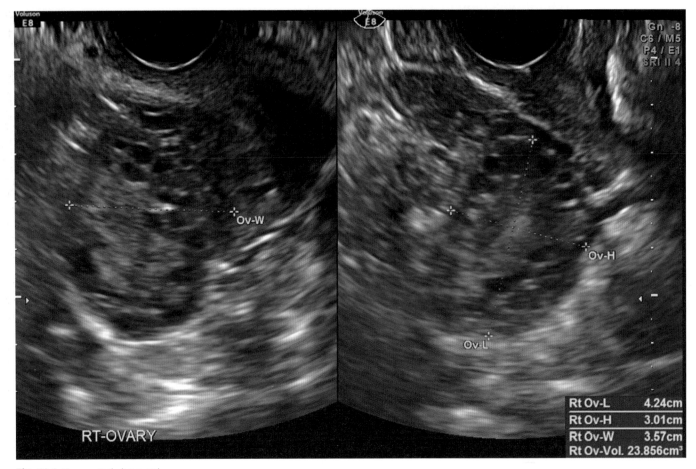

Fig. 68.1 Transvaginal ultrasound.

present with vaginal bleeding with chronic anovulation, urgent or long-term intervention strategies depend on the acuity of the bleeding episode including quantifying the amount of blood loss, assessing active bleeding and identifying symptomatic anemia. A subset of patients with chronic anovulation have polycystic ovary syndrome.

Polycystic ovary syndrome

Polycystic ovary syndrome (PCOS) was first described by Irving Stein and Michael Leventhal in 1935 [3]. PCOS is a clinical diagnosis that may present with a spectrum of symptoms. There are several classification systems that have been used to define PCOS (Table 68.1) [4,5,6,7]. The Rotterdam criteria revised in 2003 provide the most commonly used definition [5]. Menstrual irregularity, androgen excess and ovarian morphologic changes are defining characteristics of PCOS. The prevalence of PCOS is estimated at 5–8% in women [8]. It is the most common endocrine disorder in reproductive-aged women. The pathophysiology of the disorder is not completely understood but the familial associations imply a genetic component. The clinical presentation of PCOS including the symptoms and comorbidities can vary with a heterogeneous phenotypic expression.

Management of PCOS is based on symptoms. In the current clinical scenario, the patient presents with an eight-day history of menorrhagia. Acute management focuses on assessment of hemodynamic state and blood loss. She is not actively bleeding and her anemia is relatively asymptomatic. Chronic anovulatory bleeding in a nonacute setting can be managed on an outpatient basis with hormonal regulation of the cycle. Treatment options include combined oral contraceptive pills and progestins, including medroxyprogesterone acetate or the levonorgestrel intrauterine device. If active hemorrhage is noted resulting in severe anemia, blood transfusion may be indicated with a short course of intravenous estrogen therapy until the bleeding subsides. Supplemental iron therapy should be initiated to replace depleted iron stores. Long-term hormonal interventions depend on patient history, contraceptive needs, and fertility planning.

After an acute assessment and plan, long-term follow-up addressing health implications of PCOS is imperative. In addition to menstrual irregularity, other potential sequelae of PCOS including androgen excess, obesity, insulin resistance, and infertility should be properly managed in an outpatient setting.

Patients with features of androgen excess should complete an endocrine evaluation to rule out alternative causes of

Table 68.1 Diagnostic criteria for PCOS

NIH 1990 [4]	Chronic anovulation Clinical and/or biochemical signs of hyperandrogenism (with exclusion of other etiologies; e.g., congenital adrenal hyperplasia) *(Both criteria needed)*
Rotterdam criteria 2003 [4,5]	Oligomenorrhea and/ or anovulation Clinical and/or biochemical signs of hyperandrogenism Polycystic ovaries *(Two of three criteria needed)*
AE-PCOS Society 2006 [4]	Clinical and or biochemical signs of hyperandrogenism Ovarian dysfunction (oligo-anovulation and/or polycystic ovarian morphology) *(Both criteria needed)*
NIH Methodology Workshop on PCOS 2012 [6]	Recommend maintaining the broad inclusionary diagnostic criteria of Rotterdam while specifically identifying the phenotype: • Androgen excess + ovulatory dysfunction • Androgen excess + polycystic ovarian morphology • Ovulatory dysfunction + polycystic ovarian morphology Androgen excess + ovulatory dysfunction + polycystic ovarian morphology

AE, Androgen excess; NIH, National Institutes of Health; PCOS, polycystic ovary syndrome.

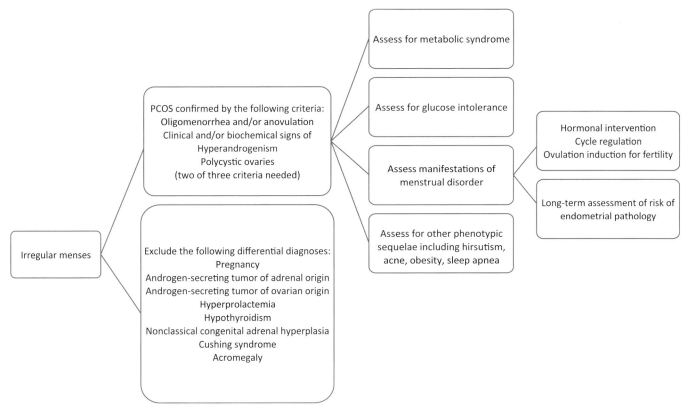

Fig.68.2 Algorithm for evaluation of irregular menses. (Adapted from [9].)

hirsuitism. A biochemical assessment of hyperandrogenism identifies other endocrinopathies, including late-onset congenital adrenal hyperplasia and Cushing syndrome. Androgen-secreting tumors of the ovary or adrenal are also excluded (Fig. 68.2). The clinical assessment of androgen excess is subjective, both age and ethnicity may contribute to body hair distribution. The Ferriman Gallwey score is sometimes used by clinicians as a standard method of documenting hirsutism. Approximately 5% of reproductive-aged women are hirsute as defined by a Ferriman Gallwey score above 8. PCOS is the most common endocrine disorder associated with hirsutism. Oral contraceptive pills are the first line of treatment in a patient without contraindications. Oral contraceptive pills increase the hepatic production of steroid hormone-binding globulin, which binds free circulating testosterone. Spironolactone, an aldosterone antagonist that inhibits dihydrotestosterone binding and inhibits 5-α reductase, is a second-line therapy that decreases androgen production. Other oral antiandrogen medical therapies include flutamide and finasteride. Cosmetic hair removal and topical eflornithine cream can also retard hair growth.

In addition to irregular bleeding, PCOS has other gynecologic impacts, including an increased risk of infertility and endometrial disorders. In evaluating a woman with PCOS who desires pregnancy, other health risks should be excluded. Counseling and lifestyle modification with an improved diet and exercise regimen may be helpful in an overweight or obese patient. Ovulation induction can be achieved with clomiphene citrate. Successful therapy is noted with a reported cumulative singleton live-birth rate of 72% [10]. Second- and third-line therapy for clomiphene citrate-resistant anovulatory patients may include exogenous gonadotropins, laparoscopic ovarian surgery, or in-vitro fertilization [10]. Long-term anovulation and oligomenorrhea without hormonal regulation also increases the risk of endometrial hyperplasia and endometrial adenocarcinoma. An endometrial biopsy can exclude endometrial pathology and in chronic anovulation disordered proliferative endometrium is often found. Other assessment modalities include hysteroscopy with dilatation and curettage for individuals at risk.

Patients with PCOS are also at risk for chronic medical disorders including obesity, metabolic syndrome, and insulin insensitivity. These medical disorders can predispose affected patients with PCOS to dyslipidemia, cardiovascular disease, type 2 diabetes mellitus, and sleep apnea. Patients should be adequately screened and counseled about the potential sequelae of PCOS. Individual risk assessments should be based on the phenotypic presentation.

Key teaching points

- Anovulation is a common cause of abnormal uterine bleeding in patients who do not have structural uterine abnormalities.
- Patients presenting with anovulation should be evaluated for physiologic and pathologic etiologies. Physiologic causes include adolescence, pregnancy, lactation, and perimenopause. Pathologic causes include hyperandrogenic anovulation, hypothalamic dysfunction, hyperprolactinemia, thyroid disorder, primary pituitary disease, premature ovarian failure, and iatrogenic sources.
- Polycystic ovary syndrome (PCOS) is a common cause of chronic anovulation and androgen excess.
- Management of PCOS is based on presenting symptoms. Minimizing long-time sequelae and comorbidities are optimal treatment strategies.

References

1. Apter D. Endocrine and metabolic abnormalities in adolescents with a PCOS-like condition: Consequences for adult reproduction. *Trends Endocrinol Metab* 1998;9:58–61.

2. American College of Obstetricians and Gynecologists. Management of abnormal uterine bleeding associated with ovulatory dysfunction. Practice Bulletin No. 136. *Obstet Gynecol* 2013;122:176–85.

3. Ferriman D, Gallwey JD. Clinical assessment of body hair growth in women. *J Clin Endocrinol Metab* 1961;21:1440–7.

4. National Institutes of Health. *Evidence-based Methodology Workshop on Polycystic Ovary Syndrome, December 3–5, 2012. Executive Summary.* Available at https://prevention.nih.gov/docs/programs/pcos/FinalReport.pdf.

5. Rotterdam ESHRE/ASRM-Sponsored PCOS Consensus Workshop Group. Revised 2003 consensus on diagnostic criteria and long-term health risks related to polycystic ovary syndrome. *Fertil Steril* 2004;81:19–25.

6. Amsterdam ESHRE/ASRM-Sponsored Third PCOS Consensus Workshop Group. Consensus on women's health aspects of polycystic ovary syndrome (PCOS). *Fertil Steril* 2012;97:28–38.

7. Azziz R, Carmina E. Dewailly D, et al. The Androgen Excess and PCOS Society criteria for the polycystic ovary syndrome: The complete task force report. *Fertil Steril* 2009;91:456–88.

8. Azziz R, Woods KS, Reyna R, et al. The prevalence and features of the polycystic ovary syndrome in an unselected population. *J Clin Endocrinol Metab* 2004;89:2745–9.

9. Ehrmann DA. Polycystic ovary syndrome. *N Engl J Med* 2005; 353:1223–36.

10. Tarlatzis BC, Fauser BC, Legro RS, et al. Thessaloniki ESHRE/ASRM-Sponsored PCOS Consensus Workshop Group: Consensus on infertility treatment related to polycystic ovary syndrome. *Fertil Steril* 2008;89:505–22.

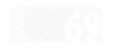

A 28-year-old woman with irregular bleeding requiring transfusion

Ronan A. Bakker

History of present illness

A 28-year-old obese gravida 0 woman presents to the emergency department complaining of general malaise, weakness, lightheadedness, and heavy vaginal bleeding. She had a single episode of "blacking out" earlier in the day, which led her to seek medical care. The bleeding has been "as much as a regular period" if not heavier for the last eight days. She has been passing golf-ball-size clots and has been changing pads every one to two hours. She reports the pads are completely "soaked through." For the last seven days, the patient has felt worsening weakness, lightheadedness and shortness of breath culminating in a syncopal episode earlier today. She has cramping abdominal pain which is tolerable and not severe in nature (3 out of 10 on the pain scale).

Her "periods" have been irregular since graduating from college, occurring every two to three months. In the last two years she has begun to have worsening intermenstrual bleeding and the bleeding episodes have become heavier and longer in duration. They usually last for five to eight days.

She has had scant medical care. She denies a history of sexually transmitted infections. She has never been transfused, but has been on iron supplementation in the past for anemia. She takes no prescription medications and does not take the iron on a consistent basis. She denies a history of nose bleeds, easy bruising, or bleeding gums. She has not had any prior surgery and has no other known medical problems.

Physical examination

General appearance: Woman appearing tired and pale
Vital signs:

Temperature 37.3°C
Heart rate: 125 beats/min
Blood pressure: 95/45 mmHg
Respiratory rate: 24 breaths/min
Oxygen saturation: 97% on room air
BMI: 38 m/kg^2

HEENT: Hirsutism and acne noted on face
Cardiovascular: Tachycardia; no murmurs, rubs, or gallops
Respiratory: Clear to auscultation bilaterally
Abdominal: Mild bilateral lower abdominal discomfort, normal bowel sounds, no distention

Pelvic:

Speculum exam: Three scopettes of blood removed from vaginal vault and several quarter-size clots noted. Moderate amount of blood noted to be coming from cervical os. Cervix appears normal
Bimanual exam: No cervical motion tenderness; normal uterus; mild generalized pelvic tenderness. Examination of adnexa limited by habitus

Laboratory studies:

Urine pregnancy test: Negative
Hb: 5.4 g/dL

How would you manage this patient?

The patient had a presumed heavy anovulatory bleed leading to significant anemia. The patient was admitted to the hospital and transfused 2 units of packed red blood cells and administered a 1-L fluid bolus of normal saline. An endometrial biopsy was performed. After the transfusion, she felt much improved and her tachycardia resolved. Repeat hemoglobin drawn 4 hours after the transfusion was 7.8 g/dL. Because of the heaviness of the bleeding and significant anemia, the patient was started on high-dose intravenous estrogen for 24 hours. The bleeding decreased substantially and the patient was then switched to 3 times a day dosing of a combined monophasic oral contraceptive containing 35 μg of ethinyl estradiol for a 7-day period, followed by once daily dosing. Her bleeding resolved. Her endometrial biopsy showed proliferative endometrium with stromal breakdown. She was seen in follow-up, and continued on cyclic oral contraceptive pills for long-term management of her bleeding. Her acne and hirsutism in combination with her abnormal bleeding were strongly indicative of polycystic ovarian syndrome (PCOS), which was addressed separately at her follow-up visit.

Treatment of heavy bleeding

Effective treatment of heavy bleeding requires determining the cause. A urine pregnancy test should be performed in all reproductive-aged patients with unexplained bleeding as pregnancy-related bleeding is managed completely differently from other causes, and undiagnosed ectopic pregnancy is life threatening. The timing of the bleeding episodes must be determined, as it can help differentiate bleeding from the different causes. The PALM-COEIN system classifies uterine bleeding abnormalities by their pattern and etiology [1]. In this

Acute Care and Emergency Gynecology, ed. David Chelmow, Christine R. Isaacs and Ashley Carroll. Published by Cambridge University Press. © Cambridge University Press 2015.

instance, a clinical picture of irregular, unpredictable bleeding episodes is present. Based on the history and clinical findings obtained during examination of the patient, a picture of abnormal uterine bleeding with ovulatory dysfunction (AUB-O) is most likely. The patient is obese and has clinical signs of androgen excess with hirsutism and acne, making PCOS the probable cause of her chronic anovulation. Her history suggests that the problem is longstanding, which is typical for PCOS. Given her uterus was felt to be normal on palpation, a structural problem such as a large myoma is less likely. However, her anovulatory bleeding could be compounded by a small submucosal myoma or endometrial polyp.

Patients with anovulation can have significant bleeding leading to life-threatening volume loss and hemodynamic instability. Patients with heavy bleeding and hypovolemia should have intravenous access for fluid administration and if need be, transfusion. Assessment of blood loss and hemodynamic status of the patient will dictate the need for surgical or medical management. Hemoglobin and hematocrit status should be obtained. Blood products should be cross-matched for patients who have symptomatic hypovolemia or life-threatening acute bleeding. Patients with lesser bleeding but where transfusion may be necessary should have a type and screen sent. The patient should be hemodynamically stabilized while completing the evaluation and initiating therapy.

Thyroid-stimulating hormone (TSH) and prolactin levels can be drawn to rule out other possible etiologies of heavy AUB, such as significant thyroid abnormalities and hyperprolactinemia, which are common causes of lighter bleeding or amenorrhea, but less frequent causes of heavy bleeding. Ultrasound is warranted to rule out an anatomic abnormality leading to excessive bleeding, particularly if the pelvic examination suggests a uterine abnormality. Screening for possible underlying clotting disorder should be done by way of thorough patient history, especially in younger patients. Coagulation studies should be drawn if the patient has a history of heavy bleeding associated with procedures, recurrent epistaxis, easy bruising, frequent gum bleeding, or family history of bleeding symptoms. Coagulation disorders are more common than previously thought, with up to 20% of women with heavy menstrual bleeding potentially having an underlying coagulation disorder [2]. To assess for coagulation disorder, complete blood count with platelets, prothrombin time, and partial thromboplastin time should be drawn, with further testing depending on the results.

Patients with AUB-O continuously produce normal levels of estrogen. They have absent or infrequent ovulation, and consequently absent or infrequent endogenous progesterone to counteract estrogen-stimulated endometrial proliferation. Without progesterone withdrawal to help stabilize and control this growth, a fragile, unstable, thickened vascular endometrial layer forms that is prone to intermittent sloughing. As in this patient, the bleeding can be very heavy and prolonged [3]. Progestin is the treatment of choice in women with light and moderate bleeding. Progestin requires an adequately thick proliferative endometrium on which to work. With heavy bleeding, the endometrial lining becomes denuded. Estrogen becomes the treatment of choice to help stimulate the growth of the endometrium. Once bleeding has decreased, the estrogen-stimulated endometrial growth is sufficient to respond to progestin [4]. The need to restore an adequate endometrial lining in women with heavy anovulatory bleeding explains their potential poor response to progestin alone, and the preference for high-dose estrogen. High-dose estrogen also serves to stimulate clotting of vessels within the endometrial lining, which in turn decreases the vaginal bleeding [5]. The recurrent heavy bleeding episodes are caused by the instability of the endometrial layer and its irregularity [4].

Prolonged unopposed estrogen is the predominant risk factor for endometrial hyperplasia and cancer. The risk of endometrial cancer in women aged 20–34 with anovulatory bleeding is 1.6% and for women aged 35–44 it is 6.2% [3]. Given the chronicity of her anovulation and unopposed estrogen exposure, her risk of developing endometrial hyperplasia or cancer is increased and her endometrium should be evaluated. Per the American College of Obstetricians and Gynecologists, any patient younger than 45 years of age with AUB and unopposed estrogen exposure, failed medical management, or persistent vaginal bleeding, requires endometrial sampling [1]. This patient had evidence of prolonged unopposed estrogen and appropriately underwent endometrial sampling. Her biopsy showed proliferative endometrium with stromal breakdown, a typical finding in anovulatory bleeding, and effectively confirmed the absence of hyperplasia or cancer.

Given her acute blood loss and hypovolemia, conjugated estrogen was administered. She was administered 25 mg IV conjugated estrogen every 4 hours for a total of 24 hours. As an alternative, high-dose oral contraceptives (Table 69.1 [2]) can be administered. High doses of estrogen can cause nausea and vomiting, so anti-emetics can be administered prophylactically. Most patients will have resolution or marked decrease in vaginal bleeding, allowing for transition to combined oral contraceptive pills. This regimen should be for seven days, three times daily, and then decreased to daily dosing [2]. Some providers use more complicated tapers, but these are often difficult for patients to follow. When initiating estrogen-based contraception, patients are carefully screened for potential contraindications. These contraindications do not necessarily apply in situations of acute, potentially life-threatening vaginal bleeding. In this situation the risks of the bleeding are much higher, and the estrogen can be used very short term, limiting the risks of the medication. Minor contraindications to estrogen-based contraception like smoking and older age or hypertension should not preclude short-course high-dose estrogen. Surgery should be reserved for treatment failure or situations where bleeding is profuse and there is insufficient time for medical management. Dilation and curettage is usually attempted first, although curettage of an already denuded

Table 69.1 Treatment options for acute abnormal uterine bleeding from AUB-O

Drug	Dose	Frequency
Conjugated equine estrogen	25 mg IV	Every 4–6 hours for total of 24 h
Combined oral contraceptives	Monophasic pill with minimum of 35 µg ethinyl estradiol PO	3 times a day for 7 days
Medroxyprogesterone acetate	20 mg PO	3 times a day for 7 days
Tranexamic acid	1.3 g PO or 10 mg/kg IV	3 times a day for 5 days

Adapted from American College of Obstetricians and Gynecologists [2].
AUB-O, abnormal uterine bleeding with ovulatory dysfunction; IV, intravenous; PO, *per os* (orally).

endometrium may not be effective. Endometrial ablation, uterine artery embolization, or hysterectomy may be required if curettage fails. Curettage will treat only the acute bleeding and not prevent future episodes [2].

The patient requires long-term progestin administration to prevent recurrent episodes. Oral contraceptives are an easy formulation, and give other benefits in terms of contraception and improvement in PCOS-related hair growth and acne. This patient had no contraindications, and should plan on staying on her oral contraceptives long term. Unless she corrects her underlying PCOS through weight loss or other means, she should expect her abnormal bleeding will recur if she stops.

Other therapies can be used for patients who present with minimal-to-moderate acute vaginal bleeding (Table 69.1). Use of progestin alone or combined oral contraceptives are effective. One study found that bleeding stopped in 88% of participants who took combined oral contraceptives and in 76% of women who took medroxyprogesterone acetate [6]. Alternate progestin or combined oral contraceptive formulations are also likely effective. Another option is the use of tranexamic acid; however, its use has only been studied in patients with chronic AUB [2].

Key teaching points

- Establishing the etiology of abnormal uterine bleeding (AUB) will help in determining appropriate management. The PALM-COEIN system was intended to help clarify the diagnosis of AUB.
- Patients with heavy bleeding need assessment of hemodynamic parameters, and may need blood replacement.
- Pharmacological management is first-line therapy for treatment of acute abnormal uterine bleeding with ovulatory dysfunction (AUB-O). Alternatives include intravenous conjugated estrogen, combined oral contraceptive pills, oral progestin, or tranexamic acid. Progestin alone is typically adequate for moderate-to-light bleeding. For patients with heavy bleeding, estrogen is typically required.
- Surgical treatment should be reserved for patients failing medical management.
- Patients with life-threatening AUB-O are at risk for recurrence, as well as hyperplasia or cancer, unless the underlying problem is corrected or progestin is administered long term.

References

1. American College of Obstetricians and Gynecologists. Diagnosis of abnormal uterine bleeding in reproductive-aged women. Practice Bulletin No. 128. *Obstet Gynecol* 2012;120:197–206.

2. American College of Obstetricians and Gynecologists. Management of acute abnormal bleeding in nonpregnant reproductive-aged women. Committee Opinion No. 557. *Obstet Gynecol* 2013;121:891–6.

3. American College of Obstetricians and Gynecologists. Management of abnormal uterine bleeding associated with ovulatory dysfunction. Practice Bulletin No. 136. *Obstet Gynecol* 2013;122:179–85.

4. Bayer SR, DeCherney AH, Clinical manifestations and treatment of dysfunctional uterine bleeding, *JAMA* 1993;269:1823–8.

5. Heistinger M, Stockenhuber F, Schneider B, et al. Effect of conjugated estrogens on platelet function and prostacyclin generation in CRF. *Kidney Int* 1990;38:1181–6.

6. Munro MG, Mainor N, Basu R, Brisinger M, Barreda L. Oral medroxyprogesterone acetate and combination oral contraceptives for acute uterine bleeding: a randomized controlled trial. *Obstet Gynecol* 2006;108:924–9.

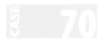
A 29-year-old woman with secondary amenorrhea after a septic abortion

Nancy D. Gaba and Gaby Moawad

History of present illness

A 29-year-old gravida 3, para 1-0-2-1 woman presents to your office reporting no menses since her second spontaneous abortion, which she experienced 6 months prior. She has a history of regular menstrual cycles preceding her two recent spontaneous abortions, and one uneventful normal spontaneous vaginal delivery four years ago. Her first spontaneous abortion was diagnosed at 11 weeks' gestation, and was treated with dilation and curettage. The most recent spontaneous abortion was diagnosed at nine weeks' gestation, when she presented to the emergency department with five days of heavy bleeding per vagina. A dilation and sharp curettage was performed; however, the patient returned 3 days later with a fever to 39.4°C, a tender uterus, leucocytosis, and retained products of conception identified on ultrasound. Another dilation and sharp curettage was performed and the patient received postoperative antibiotics as an outpatient for seven days. The remainder of her postoperative course was unremarkable thereafter but she continues to report cyclic pelvic pain since that event. Her medical history is otherwise unremarkable. She is sexually active with one partner, with whom she desires another pregnancy. She has not been using any contraception. She smokes socially and works as a sales associate.

Physical examination

General appearance: Well-developed, well-nourished young woman
Vital signs:

Temperature: 37.1°C
Pulse: 80 beats/min
Blood pressure: 110/70 mmHg
Respiratory rate: 16 breaths/min
BMI: 24 kg/m^2

Breasts: No masses, adenopathy, or nipple discharge
Abdomen: Soft, nontender, no masses
External genitalia: Normal
Vagina: Normal mucosa, no lesions, scant discharge
Cervix: Parous, no lesions
Uterus: Normal size, minimally tender, retroflexed, mobile
Adnexa: Nontender, no masses
Laboratory studies: Urine pregnancy test: Negative

How would you manage this patient?

This patient has secondary amenorrhea, and given the context of her recent obstetrical history, the differential diagnosis places Asherman syndrome (also known as intrauterine adhesions [IUAs]), which developed as a result of her septic abortion in combination with the repeated instrumentation of her uterus, high on the list of concerns.

Once pregnancy had been excluded, an attempt to pass a small dilator and uterine sound in the office was performed to determine if any cervical or uterine obstruction was present. The uterus sounded to 8 cm and was easily measured. In this case, where the suspicion for IUAs was high, a hysteroscopy was performed (Fig. 70.1).

Intraoperative findings were consistent with dense IUAs and a hysteroscopic resection of the adhesions was performed with the resectoscope. There were no complications at the time of surgery.

At the completion of the procedure, a normal uterine cavity was visualized (Fig. 70.2).

Six weeks after the hysteroscopic procedure, the patient resumed a light menses. Since then her menses have become

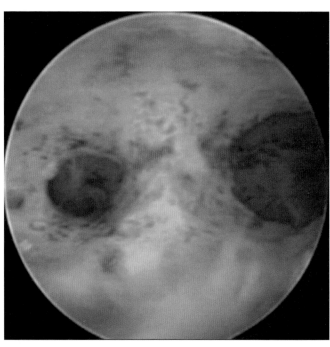

Fig. 70.1 Before hysteroscopic resection of the adhesions.

Acute Care and Emergency Gynecology, ed. David Chelmow, Christine R. Isaacs and Ashley Carroll. Published by Cambridge University Press.
© Cambridge University Press 2015.

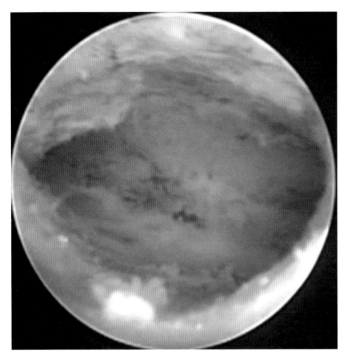

Fig. 70.2 After hysteroscopic resection of the adhesions.

more normal, lasting three to four days every month. She continues to attempt conception.

Asherman syndrome

The initial description of intrauterine adhesions (IUAs) was first published by Heinrich Frisch in 1894, but the problem was not studied in detail until Joseph Asherman published his work on the topic in 1949. Asherman syndrome is typically manifested by the formation of fibrous adhesions involving the uterine cavity, and sometimes, the internal cervical os and the cervical canal. These adhesions can lead to amenorrhea. It was later recognized that IUAs may result from any trauma to the endometrium, and can also have a significant impact on future fertility. IUAs occur most commonly after surgical management of incomplete abortion (50%), as in the patient described here, postpartum hemorrhage (24%), and surgically performed elective abortion (17.5%) [1]. Other etiologic factors that can lead to IUAs include myomectomy (especially hysteroscopic removal of opposing fibroids, or when the endometrial cavity is breached via laparoscopy/laparotomy), hysterotomy, Cesarean delivery, tuberculosis, caustic abortifacients, and post-pregnancy instrumentation of the endometrium including uterine packing or balloon tamponade.

The presumed mechanism by which the adhesions are formed is trauma to the basalis layer of the endometrium. Although a Cochrane review [2] concluded that medical and surgical abortion have equal pregnancy rates after five years, the specific complication of IUAs was not addressed. It is commonly assumed that IUAs are more prevalent following instrumentation of the uterus, particularly if there are retained products or repeat instrumentation. Several investigators have attempted to address the question of the likelihood of developing IUAs after a secondary procedure becomes necessary for the removal of placental remnants, as in the patient in this case. Westendorp and colleagues reported on a prospective analysis of 50 women undergoing surgical management for retained placental tissue [3]. Among these women, 40% were found to have IUAs on hysteroscopy conducted 3 months after the instrumentation, and of these, 75% had moderate to severe IUAs [3]. Other studies, which examined only women having one primary surgical evacuation in the case of a spontaneous abortion, have found the rate of IUAs to be as low as 8% in comparative prospective trials [4]. The patient described here desires future fertility and, given her concerning obstetric history, all efforts should be made to accurately determine if her secondary amenorrhea is due to Asherman syndrome and, if so, to restore normal anatomy.

The gold standard for diagnosis of IUAs is hysteroscopy. Although traditional ultrasound, three-dimensional ultrasound, saline infusion ultrasound, and hysterosalpingography (HSG) have all been utilized for evaluation of the uterine cavity, hysteroscopy provides an accurate "real-time" opportunity to examine the extent of the IUAs. Hysteroscopy also enables the physician to not only accurately diagnose and classify the uterine adhesions, but provides the opportunity for simultaneous therapeutic intervention. There can be some benefit to performing a preoperative ultrasound, as the thickness of the endometrium can be used to evaluate improvement after treatment. Conversely, MRI has not been found to be useful, and is considerably more expensive than other diagnostic modalities [5]. Several authors have tried to create classification systems for IUAs, although none of these have received unanimous endorsement. All of these systems rely on hysteroscopy, although in some cases other diagnostic tests such as HSG are used. The goal of these efforts are to help advise the patients regarding the severity of their adhesive disease and the prognosis or likelihood of pregnancy following treatment [6].

The management of severe IUAs and the resulting amenorrhea has been well studied, although there is currently no single approach that has been shown to create significantly superior outcomes. In a small retrospective review of 12 cases, Myers and Hurst found that a comprehensive approach, including preoperative oral estradiol, intraoperative hysteroscopic synechiolysis, placement of a triangular balloon catheter, and subsequent placement of a copper intrauterine device (IUD), resulted in resumption of menses in all patients and a 67% pregnancy rate [7]. Robinson and colleagues reported that serial postoperative blunt adhesiolysis of recurrent synechiae resulted in an improvement in menstrual flow in 95% of women and pregnancy in 46% of women over their 2-year study period [8]. Other studies have evaluated expectant management, cervical probing, and dilation and curettage; however, these are all associated with higher rates of failure and/or complications and, thus, should not be used [5].

Ancillary treatments to hysteroscopic adhesiolysis including physical barriers; (IUDs, Foley catheters, Cook balloons, amnion grafts, hyaluronic acid); hormone therapy (estrogen, estrogen plus progesterone); vascular flow modifiers (nitroglycerin, sildenafil); and antibiotic therapy have all been studied. Although they all have shown some benefit in preventing the reformation of adhesions, no single therapy stands out as significantly better than the others [5,6,9]. Several recommendations to prevent Asherman syndrome and IUAs are typically recommended. The general principle is to avoid any trauma to the basalis layer, especially in patients who are pregnant or immediately postpartum. Post-abortal curettage should be avoided whenever possible. Medical management of elective and spontaneous abortion should be offered whenever feasible. Consideration to treat retained products of conception with agents such as misoprostol should be considered in an effort to avoid unnecessary uterine instrumentation. Finally, hysteroscopic evacuation of retained products, using a resecting loop under direct visualization instead of blind curettage, can also be considered depending on the surgical skill of the clinician [10].

The patient described here might have avoided the initial curettage if alternative management of her incomplete abortion, such as misoprostol, had been provided. Short-interval office hysteroscopy, given the clinical suspicion of IUAs, could have also been helpful, with early interventions such as blunt lysis of adhesions possibly preventing the development of the dense IUAs pictured above.

Key teaching points

- Asherman syndrome is manifested by the formation of fibrous adhesions involving the uterine cavity, and possibly the internal cervical os and/or cervical canal, which may lead to amenorrhea and infertility.
- Intrauterine adhesions (IUAs) occur most commonly after surgical management of an incomplete abortion, postpartum hemorrhage, elective abortion, or other surgical procedure that involves the endometrial cavity and disrupts the endometrial basalis layer.
- The gold standard for the diagnosis of IUAs is hysteroscopy.
- Hysteroscopic adhesiolysis is the preferred treatment for IUAs.

References

1. Valle RF, Sciarra JJ. Intrauterine adhesions: Hysteroscopic diagnosis, classification, treatment, and reproductive outcome. *Obstet Gynecol* 1988;158(6):1459–70.

2. Nanda K, Peloggia A, Grimes D, Lopez L, Nanda G. Expectant care versus surgical treatment for miscarriage. *Cochrane Database Syst Rev* 2006, Issue 2. Art. No. CD003518.

3. Westendorp IC, Ankum WM, Moi BW, Vonk J. Prevalence of Asherman's syndrome after secondary removal of placental remnants or a repeat curettage for incomplete abortion. *Hum Reprod* 1998;13(12):3347–50.

4. Tam WH, Lau WC, Cheung LP, Yuen PM, Chung TK. Intrauterine adhesions after conservative and surgical management of spontaneous abortion. *J Am Assoc Gynecol Laparosc* 2002; 9(2):182–5.

5. Deans R, Abbott J. Review of intrauterine adhesions. *J Minim Invasive Gynecol* 2010;17(5):555–69.

6. Yu D, Wong Y, Cheong Y, Xia E, Li T. Asherman syndrome – one century later. *Fertil Steril* 2008;89(4): 759–79.

7. Myers EM, Hurst BS. Comprehensive management of severe Asherman syndrome and amenorrhea. *Fertil Steril* 2012;97(1):160–4.

8. Robinson JK, Colimon LM, Isaacson KB. Postoperative adhesiolysis therapy for intrauterine adhesions (Asherman's syndrome). *Fertil Steril* 2008;90(2): 409–14.

9. March CM. Management of Asherman's syndrome. *Reprod Biomed Online* 2011;23(1):63–76.

10. Golan A, Dishi M, Shalev A, et al. Operative hysteroscopy to remove retained products of conception: Novel treatment of an old problem. *J Minim Invasive Gynecol* 2011;18(1): 100–3.

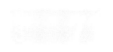

Worsening dysmenorrhea in a 14-year-old girl

Nicole W. Karjane

History of present illness

A 14-year-old girl presents to the emergency department with a 5-day history of severe pelvic pain. This episode began on the first day of her menstrual period and has been progressively worsening. She reports crampy pain with menses since menarche approximately six months ago. The pain is located slightly to the right of midline and occasionally radiates to her back. Initially, her cramping was mild and improved with ibuprofen; however, with each menstrual period, her pain has gotten worse and more resistant to treatment with nonsteroidal anti-inflammatory drugs (NSAIDs). Her pediatrician started her on oral contraceptive pills (OCPs) after her third menstrual period, but her pain has continued to intensify with each cycle, such that she has missed multiple days of school. Her menses have been regular, lasting about 4–5 days, with an interval of 28–29 days. Although her pain was originally just with the duration of her menses, for the past three months it has been lingering for several days after her bleeding stops. She reports that she has no difficulty using tampons, but she must always use a pad in addition to the tampon to avoid soiling her underwear. She denies fevers, chills, nausea, vomiting, diarrhea, or constipation. She has never been sexually active. Her medical history is significant for right renal agenesis that was incidentally diagnosed at age five during the workup of abdominal pain, and she has had no prior medical illnesses or surgeries.

Physical examination

General appearance: Nontoxic appearing girl who is apprehensive and in moderate distress

Vital signs:

Temperature: 37.0°C
Pulse: 92 beats/min
Blood pressure: 115/62
Respiratory rate: 18 breaths/min
Oxygen saturation: 100% on room air

HEENT: Normal

Cardiovascular: Regular rate and rhythm without murmurs, rubs, or gallops

Lungs: Clear to auscultation bilaterally

Breasts: Tanner stage IV breast development

Abdomen: Soft, tender throughout lower abdomen, right greater than left, nondistended, no guarding or rebound tenderness, palpable mass to right of midline just above pubic symphysis at area of maximal tenderness

Genitalia: Normal external genitalia, normal, well-estrogenized hymen. Bimanual examination reveals a tense bulge in the right vagina that begins 2 cm cephalad to the introitus and extends to the cervix. No cervical motion tenderness, but unable to delineate uterine size due to patient discomfort

Laboratory studies: Urine pregnancy test: Negative

Imaging: A transabdominal pelvic ultrasound showed a large cystic mass filling the pelvis, normal appearing uterus above the mass, unable to identify ovaries. The patient was admitted, given intravenous narcotics, and MRI of the pelvis was ordered (Figs 71.1, 71.2, and 71.3)

How would you manage this patient?

The patient's diagnosis is dysmenorrhea due to menstrual outflow obstruction in a patient with uterine didelphys, obstructed hemivagina and ipsilateral renal agenesis. This diagnosis was made based on history and examination and confirmed on MRI. The patient was taken to the operating room where her physicians performed an examination under anesthesia and excision of the obstructive vaginal septum. The

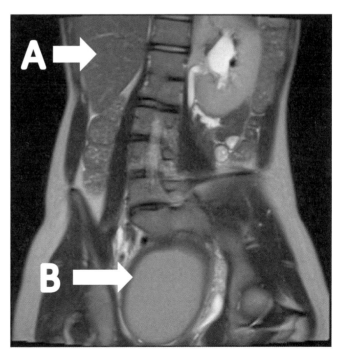

Fig. 71.1 Right-sided renal agenesis (A) as well as the obstructed hemivagina (B).

Acute Care and Emergency Gynecology, ed. David Chelmow, Christine R. Isaacs and Ashley Carroll. Published by Cambridge University Press.
© Cambridge University Press 2015.

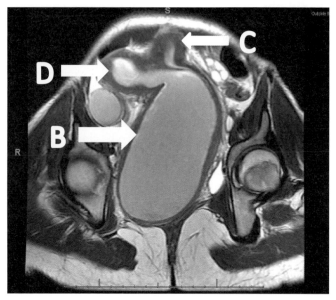

Fig. 71.2 Coronal view of the obstructed hemivagina (B), the normal left uterus in the midline (C), and the obstructed right uterus that is deviated to the right (D).

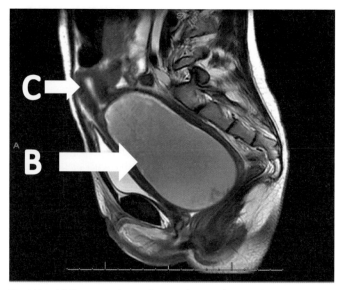

Fig. 71.3 Midline, sagittal view showing the nonobstructed uterus (C) overlying the obstructed hemivagina (B).

patient's pain resolved following surgery, and her dysmenorrhea gradually improved over the next several months.

Obstructive hemivagina

Dysmenorrhea, or painful menses, is the most common presenting menstrual disorder in adolescent females. Most of these young patients are ultimately diagnosed with primary dysmenorrhea, or cyclic menstrual pain without an identifiable cause; however, there are many potential causes of dysmenorrhea that must be considered. These include endometriosis, pelvic inflammatory disease, leiomyomas, and menstrual obstruction.

The initial assessment of an adolescent with dysmenorrhea includes a thorough history, with particular attention to menstrual history and sexual history. Physical examination should include an adequate abdominal examination and visualization of the external genitalia. In virginal patients with regular menses and normal external genitalia, pelvic examination can generally be avoided during the preliminary evaluation, particularly if they are able to use tampons. Patients with a history of sexual activity should undergo speculum examination and bimanual pelvic examination to evaluate for sexually transmitted infections, and those with infections should be treated appropriately. In addition, a urine pregnancy test should be obtained to rule out pregnancy associated bleeding and pain.

The release of prostaglandins that occurs during sloughing of the endometrium is thought to be the cause of primary dysmenorrhea; therefore, NSAIDs are a reasonable first-line treatment in young women with dysmenorrhea once the initial evaluation is complete. OCPs are also effective in the treatment of dysmenorrhea as they decrease the production of uterine prostaglandins. Oral contraceptive use has been shown to improve dysmenorrhea in over 70% of women [1] and may be used as first- or second-line treatment depending on patient preference and the need for contraception. Patients who fail to respond to combination therapy with both NSAIDS and OCPs require further workup to determine the etiology of their menstrual pain. This workup should be guided by the history and examination. In patients with a normal, adequate pelvic examination and no evidence of infection, endometriosis must be considered as an etiology. If the initial history and examination are concerning for an obstructive anomaly, as in the patient described in this case, imaging is indicated to confirm the diagnosis and clarify the anatomy.

It is well-established that women with Mullerian anomalies are at higher risk for concomitant renal anomalies, and vice versa. Therefore, when patients with known renal anomalies present with dysmenorrhea, as did this patient, the practitioner should have a high index of suspicion for a Mullerian anomaly. Initial imaging of the pelvis with ultrasound is a reasonable first step, however, MRI is often required to make a definitive diagnosis [2,3]. Once an anomaly is identified, prompt surgical intervention should be undertaken to relieve any obstruction and to prevent the possible long-term consequences of menstrual obstructions such as endometriosis and adhesive disease.

Uterine didelphys with obstructed hemivagina and ipsilateral renal agenesis, also referred to as obstructed hemivagina and ipsilateral renal anomaly (OHVIRA) syndrome or Herlyn–Werner–Wunderlich syndrome, has been well-described in the medical literature dating back to as early as 1922. Embryologically, it appears to be caused by an abnormal development of both the Wolffian duct and the ipsilateral Mullerian duct, resulting in renal agenesis (or other anomaly) as well as incomplete fusion of the Mullerian duct with its contralateral side and with the more distal urogenital sinus [4,5]. As with many unilateral birth defects, this anomaly is significantly more likely to occur on the right side of the body than the left side, for reasons that remain unclear [4]. Although the most common findings in this syndrome are uterine dildelphys, obstructed hemivagina, and ipsilateral renal agenesis, numerous anatomic variants have been reported. These variants may occur in up to 27% of cases and include a septate uterus with an obstructed hemivagina, a bicornuate bicollis uterus with an obstructed hemivagina, a bicornuate uterus with a septate cervix and obstructed hemivagina, and a uterine didelphys with unilateral cervical atresia [5]. The possibility of alternate anatomic variants makes MRI in these patients essential to define the anomaly and treat the circumstances appropriately.

Definitive treatment of uterine didelphys with obstructed hemivagina involves excision of the obstructive vaginal septum. This is generally performed in the operating room by incising the bulging longitudinal vaginal septum, excising it up to the level of the cervix, and marsupializing the vaginal epithelium with absorbable suture. Attempts to perform needle drainage of the hematocolpos without excising the septum should be avoided, as this may seed the obstructed hematocolpos with bacteria and lead to an ascending pelvic infection with subsequent abscess formation, adhesive disease, and/or sepsis.

Concomitant laparoscopy was previously advocated in patients with OHVIRA to aide in the diagnosis. More recently, however, it appears that the correct diagnosis can generally be made on the basis of history, examination and imaging, and therefore laparoscopy may be avoided in most cases [6]. Because menstrual obstruction and the resultant retrograde menstruation may cause endometriosis, considering concomitant laparoscopy to evaluate and treat endometriosis implants

may be reasonable. The natural history of endometriosis in patients with obstructive anomalies, however, is unclear, and spontaneous resolution often occurs following correction of the causative obstruction. It seems prudent, therefore, to reserve laparoscopy to patients with persistent symptoms following correction of their menstrual obstruction, or to patients in whom the diagnosis remains unclear after the initial workup.

Key teaching points

- Dysmenorrhea that is refractory to conservative management with nonsteroidal anti-inflammatory drugs and oral contraceptive pills should be further evaluated for potential anatomic causes.
- Although most patients with menstrual obstructions present with cyclic pain without menses, patients with a partial obstruction will present with worsening dysmenorrhea refractory to medical management.
- Young women with known renal anomalies are at higher risk for concomitant Mullerian anomalies. Therefore, practitioners should have a high index of suspicion when these patients have persistent menstrual complaints in order to avoid delays in diagnosis.
- Patient with suspected menstrual obstructions should undergo MRI to accurately define the anomaly and aid in surgical planning.
- Uterine didelphys with obstructed hemivagina and ipsilateral renal anomaly (OHVIRA) is an uncommon yet well-defined entity that is treated with excision of the obstructive vaginal septum.

References

1. American College of Obstetricians and Gynecologists. Noncontraceptive uses of hormonal contraceptives. Practice Bulletin No. 110. *Obstet Gynecol* 2010;115:206–18.

2. Church DG, Vancil JM, Vasanawala SS. Magnetic resonance imaging for uterine and vaginal anomalies. *Curr Opin Obstet Gynecol* 2009;21(5):379–89.

3. Behr SC, Courtier JL, Qayyum A. Imaging of Müllerian duct anomalies. *Radiographics* 2012;32(6):E233–50. DOI: 10.1148/rg.326125515.

4. Vercellini P, Daguati R, Somigliana E, et al. Asymmetric lateral distribution of obstructed hemivagina and renal agenesis in women with uterus didelphys: Institutional case series and a systematic literature review. *Fertil Steril* 2007;87(4):719–24.

5. Fedele L, Motta F, Frontino G, Restelli E, Bianchi S. Double uterus with obstruced hemivagina and ipsilateral renal agenesis: pelvic anatomic variants in 87 cases. *Hum Reprod* 2013;28(6):1580–3.

6. Smith NA, Laufer MR. Obstructed hemivagina and inpsilateral renal anomaly (OHVIRA) syndrome: Management and follow-up. *Fertil Steril* 2007;87(4):918–22.

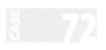

A seven-year-old girl with vaginal bleeding

Nicole W. Karjane

History of present illness

A seven-year-old girl is brought to the emergency department by her mother because of persistent vaginal bleeding. Her mother reports that she has had blood-stained underwear for the past three weeks. The bleeding is minimal but has been persistent despite efforts to improve hygiene by front to back wiping, sitz baths, and using a bland topical emollient, as recommended by her pediatrician. Her mother notes only slight improvement despite these efforts. There are no other associated symptoms that her mother has noticed. Specifically, the child and mother report no fevers, vomiting, bowel changes, abdominal or genital pain, and no vaginal itching or foul-smelling discharge. Both the patient and her mother deny a history or concern for trauma or abuse. She has no significant past medical or surgical history, takes no medications, and reports no recent illnesses. The patient gets routine well-child checks by her pediatrician that have been uneventful.

Physical examination

General appearance: Well-appearing girl who is apprehensive but in no distress

Vital signs:

Temperature: 37.0°C
Pulse: 92 beats/min
Blood pressure: 95/50 mmHg
Respiratory rate: 16 breaths/min
Oxygen saturation: 100% on room air

HEENT: Normal

Neck: supple, without thyromegaly or lymphadenopathy

Cardiovascular: Regular rate and rhythm

Lungs: Clear to auscultation bilaterally

Breasts: Tanner stage I breast development

Abdomen: Soft, nontender, nondistended, no palpable masses

Genitalia: Tanner stage I pubic hair development with fair hygiene and normal prepubertal external genitalia. There were no vulvar or perineal lesions, lacerations, excoriations, or erythema. In frog-leg positioning with labial traction, a normal annular hymen without notches or lacerations is noted. Visualization above the hymen was limited due to patient's inability to cooperate with further examination, but there was a small greyish mass noted and no active bleeding visualized

How would you manage this patient?

The patient was taken to the operating room for examination under anesthesia. Vaginoscopy was performed (Fig. 72.1).

How would you manage this patient?

The diagnosis is prepubertal vaginal bleeding due to a retained foreign body, in this case, toilet paper. The examination under anesthesia was significant for normal prepubertal external genitalia, a normal hymen, and a foreign body within the vagina. Saline vaginoscopy revealed several pea-size wads of toilet paper, which were irrigated out of the vagina during the procedure. The remainder of the vagina was normal appearing. The patient did well postoperatively and was instructed on proper wiping and continued good hygiene measures. She had no further bleeding.

Prepubescent vaginal bleeding

Vaginal bleeding prior to puberty is a medical problem that requires thorough investigation. Neonates may experience physiologic vaginal bleeding in the first weeks of life due to withdrawal of maternal estrogen; however, beyond that,

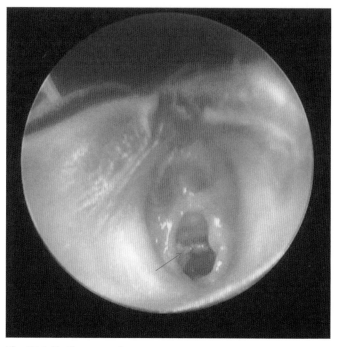

Fig. 72.1 Findings on vaginoscopy.

Acute Care and Emergency Gynecology, ed. David Chelmow, Christine R. Isaacs and Ashley Carroll. Published by Cambridge University Press. © Cambridge University Press 2015.

vaginal bleeding before puberty must be considered pathologic until proven otherwise. The differential diagnosis of prepubertal vaginal bleeding includes: trauma, abuse, vulvovaginitis, condyloma, urethral prolapse, cervical, vaginal, or urethral masses, estrogen-producing ovarian tumors, vaginal foreign bodies, excoriations, or bleeding from the gastrointestinal or genitourinary tract.

To evaluate girls with vaginal bleeding, it is essential to take a thorough history to exclude trauma or abuse as an etiology. Girls who report abuse or who have perineal trauma should be evaluated by a specialized child sexual assault team that includes trained forensic nurses. Once abuse or trauma has been ruled out, the possibility of exogenous estrogen exposure should be explored, as well as history of recent illnesses that could predispose the patient to vulvovaginitis caused by a specific bacterial pathogen. A recent history of group A streptococcal pharyngitis may lead to streptococcal vaginitis, while a history of recent diarrheal illness may suggest a *Shigella* vaginitis as the etiology of vaginal bleeding. Other associated symptoms may also guide the differential diagnosis. Nighttime peri-anal itching, for example, may signify pinworms, whereas, persistent vulvar itching may be caused by a vulvar dermatitis or lichen sclerosis.

On examination, careful attention should be paid to Tanner staging, as evidence of estrogen exposure would be concerning for precocious puberty (central or peripheral), estrogen-secreting ovarian tumors, or exogenous estrogen exposure due to use of hormone creams or tablets (either intentional or accidental). On abdominal examination, a pelvic mass would be concerning for an ovarian tumor and should be followed-up with imaging of the pelvis and evaluation of tumor markers. Thorough examination of the external genitalia, including the urethral orifice and peri-anal region, should be performed, with careful attention to hygiene and estrogen status of the genitalia. Survey of the genitalia should note any discharge, lesions or lacerations that may be present. Generally, the hymen and distal vagina can be easily visualized without discomfort to the patient by using labial traction, which involves gently grabbing the labia majora and pulling away from the patient, or by examining the patient in knee–chest position. Labial separation, which is performed by gently pulling the labia majora laterally, is generally less effective at providing adequate visualization. If discharge is present, specimens should be obtained for culture.

In cases where a foreign body is visualized, as in this patient, removal of the foreign body may be accomplished in the outpatient setting. Options for removing soft foreign bodies from the vagina include using a cotton-tipped applicator and twirling it within the vagina or, more commonly, vaginal lavage [1]. Vaginal lavage can be performed by passing a small urethral catheter beyond the hymen and flushing the vagina with warm saline. With either procedure, care should be taken to avoid the hymen, as it is particularly sensitive to the touch in most prepubertal girls. This may be facilitated by having an assistant use gentle labial traction to open the introitus while the catheter or swab is passed into the vagina. Most patients tolerate the procedure very well and without significant discomfort; however, if the patient is reluctant or unwilling to cooperate, examination under anesthesia may be necessary, as was the case in this patient.

Examination under anesthesia can usually be accomplished in the frog-leg position using labial traction. Using this technique, the hymen can be visualized in its entirety, and air enters the vagina to allow for visualization of the distal vagina as well. Vaginoscopy is then performed using normal saline as the distention medium with either a 3 mm pediatric cystoscope or a 4–5 mm diagnostic hysteroscope [2,3]. The surgeon advances the scope above the hymen to examine the vagina and cervix while gently pressing the labia majora together to maintain distention of the vagina and improve visualization. Any foreign bodies are generally flushed out with the saline. If the foreign body is solid, it may require removal with endoscopic graspers, forceps, or by gently milking it out via rectal examination. Placing a speculum into the vagina in a prepubertal girl is rarely necessary and should be avoided if possible, as it can cause unnecessary lacerations, abrasions, and discomfort.

Vaginal foreign bodies are a common cause of vaginal bleeding in prepubertal girls [4,5]. Though foul-smelling discharge makes one consider foreign body as a potential etiology, most girls with a vaginal foreign body do not, in fact, have a foul-smelling discharge [4,6]. Toilet paper appears to be the most common foreign body; however, other items such as coins, paper clips, safety pins, dice, beads, crayons, and even batteries have been reported. Removal of the foreign body, followed by proper perineal hygiene, should promptly resolve the associated vaginal bleeding. If bleeding persists, investigation for other sources (or for another foreign body) must be undertaken. This is particularly true of cases that are treated in the outpatient setting. For example, if vaginal lavage was performed in the office with apparent successful removal of the foreign body, the next step would be an examination under anesthesia with vaginoscopy to evaluate for a persistent foreign body or for a secondary diagnosis.

Key teaching points

- A vaginal foreign body is the most common cause of vaginal bleeding in prepubertal girls.
- Toilet paper is the most common vaginal foreign body, but other items have been reported.
- In cooperative patients, vaginal foreign bodies may be removed in the office setting using vaginal lavage with warm saline.
- Patients who are uncooperative with examination in the office may need to be evaluated under anesthesia, in which case, saline vaginoscopy will likely be both diagnostic and therapeutic.
- Vaginal bleeding that persists following removal of the foreign body should be further evaluated for other potential etiologies.

References

1. Emans SJ, Laufer MR. *Pediatric and Adolescent Gynecology*, 6th edn. Philadelphia, PA, Lippincott Williams & Wilkins, 2012.

2. Golan A, Lurie S, Sagiv R, Glezerman M. Continuous-flow vaginoscopy in children and adolescents. *J Am Assoc Gynecol Laparosc* 2000;7(4):526–8.

3. Nakhal RS, Wood D, Creighton SM. The role of examination under anesthesia (EUA) and vaginoscopy in pediatric and adolescent gynecology: A retrospective review. *J Pediatr Adolesc Gynecol* 2012;25: 64–6.

4. Paradise JE, Willis ED. Probability of vaginal foreign body in girls with genital complaints. *Am J Dis Child* 1985;139:472–6.

5. Fishman A, Paldi E. Vaginal bleeding in premenarchal girls: A review. *Obstet Gynecol Surv* 1991;46: 457–60.

6. Stricker T, Navratil F, Sennhause FH. Vaginal foreign bodies. *J Paediatr Child Health* 2004;40:205–7.

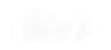

A four-year-old girl falls while exiting the bathtub

Sarah H. Milton and Elisabeth McGaw

History of present illness

A four-year-old girl presented to the emergency department after slipping while getting out of the bathtub. She was accompanied by her mother who witnessed the fall. Both reported that she fell in a manner that she straddled the edge of the bathtub. After the fall she immediately began to cry and complain of pain. Her mother then noted bleeding from "between her legs" and was able to see what she thought looked like a "cut." The patient's mother was able to apply pressure to the area which slowed the bleeding, and then brought her immediately to the emergency department for evaluation. Upon questioning, the patient is tearful and nods that she is in pain. She points to her genitals when asked where she hurts. She denies any other source of pain. She is unable to answer any further questions. The mother adds that she and her daughter were the only two people home at the time of the accident, that her daughter does not have any known medical problems, has never had surgery, and has never been hospitalized. When questioned separately, both the patient and her mother deny any history of physical or sexual abuse directed toward the patient.

Physical examination

General appearance: Tearful child, clinging to her mother
Vital signs:

  Temperature: 37.0°C
  Pulse: 85 beats/min
  Blood pressure: 107/68 mmHg
  Respiratory rate: 18 breaths/min
  Oxygen saturation: 100% on room air
Neurologic: Nonfocal
HEENT: Normocephalic, atraumatic
Cardiovascular: Regular, rate, and rhythm
Respiratory: Chest clear to auscultation bilaterally
Abdomen: Soft, nontender, nondistended, normal bowel sounds
Extremities: No other bruises or injuries noted
Genitourinary: The examination is limited by patient discomfort (Fig. 73.1). Dried blood is noted on the medial thighs and external genitalia. There is Tanner stage I pubic hair development. There is a laceration of the left labia majora extending from just below the level of the clitoris down to the perineal body, approximately 3 cm in length with minimal active bleeding. There is minimal ecchymosis on left labia majora, minora and perineal body adjacent to laceration. The depth of laceration is difficult to discern due to patient cooperation
Laboratory studies: CBC was normal

What is your diagnosis?

The patient has an accidental straddle injury with a perineal laceration. The recognition of active bleeding and the size of the laceration warrant surgical intervention.

How would you manage this patient?

The inability to adequately perform a genitourinary examination further substantiates the need for examination under anesthesia. The patient was taken to the operating room where an examination revealed a 3 cm laceration that was 1 cm in depth and extended from the left labia majora down the perineal body to 1 cm anterior to the anus. The laceration was repaired with a 3–0 synthetic absorbable suture with excellent anatomic reapproximation and hemostasis. The patient was able to be discharged from the hospital the next day at which time she was able to void and ambulate comfortably while taking only oral pain medications. At a two-week follow-up visit, the area was well healed with only a faint visible scar.

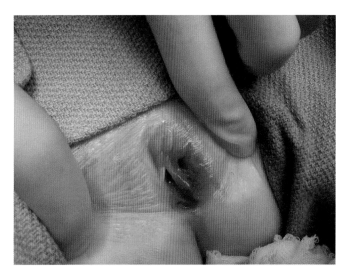

Fig. 73.1 A four-year-old girl after falling while exiting the bath tub. (Photograph courtesy of Shalon Nienow, MD.)

Acute Care and Emergency Gynecology, ed. David Chelmow, Christine R. Isaacs and Ashley Carroll. Published by Cambridge University Press. © Cambridge University Press 2015.

Straddle injuries

Pediatric patients presenting with genital trauma pose a particular challenge to the provider. While these injuries are relatively rare, their evaluation and management can provoke significant anxiety in the patient and their caregivers. Genital trauma may be accidental or may be the result of sexual abuse. A careful history and physical examination to rule out abuse is warranted in any patient who has sustained genital trauma. Providers should place particular emphasis on creating a safe environment for the interview and physical examination as children who have sustained perineal trauma are often particularly frightened and vulnerable.

Accidental genital trauma can occur as the result of straddle injuries, motor vehicle accidents, animal bites, burns, falls, and penetrating injuries [1]. By far the most common mechanism of accidental injury to the genital tract in pediatric females is straddle injury, accounting for over 80% of cases [2]. Straddle injuries, which can result in lacerations or hematoma formation, occur as a result of blunt trauma to the genital region incurred during an accidental fall where the patient straddles an object, railing or other obstacle. Although less common, vaginal insufflation injury is also reported in which rapid distension of the vagina results in tearing of the vaginal walls with resultant bleeding. This mechanism of injury has been reported in association with falls while water or jet skiing and in association with water slides [3]. While the majority of accidental trauma occurs in the home, outdoor and sports-related activities are also commonly implicated [4]. The average age of patients sustaining an accidental genital tract injury is 5.5–6.5 years of age [3,4,5].

The presentation of traumatic injury to the genital tract is variable. Accidental injury may result in ecchymoses, abrasions, hematomas, or lacerations [1]. Penetrating trauma is more likely to result in laceration of the hymen or vagina [3]. Conversely, blunt trauma commonly results in vulvar damage including ecchymoses, abrasions, hematomas, and lacerations [3]. In straddle injuries specifically, the most common injury sustained is a laceration and the most commonly involved area is the posterior vulva as was the case in this patient [2]. While most patients with a history of sexual abuse will have normal or nonspecific physical examination findings, these patients may also present with any combination of the aforementioned findings [6]. Because of the significant variability in physical examination following sexual abuse, providers must be vigilant in their assessment of history and risk factors to aid in identification of patients who have been the victims of assault [6,7].

Evaluating a child who has sustained a traumatic genital injury is particularly challenging. Careful attention to the history is necessary to assess the severity of injury as well as to screen for abuse. History should be obtained from the patient alone whenever possible with collateral information obtained from the caregiver and/or witnesses to the injury [1,7]. As in any trauma patient, initial evaluation should focus on vital signs and a primary survey to identify any hemodynamic instability that would warrant emergent intervention. Laboratory evaluation varies based on severity of injury. A complete blood count should be ordered if bleeding has been significant or is persistent. Once the primary survey is performed, it is followed by a complete physical examination, including a targeted genitourinary examination [3]. Positioning the child for examination of the genitalia can be accomplished with the patient frog-legged or supine, or with the child in knee-chest position. If examination reveals active bleeding, a laceration, or a hematoma, it is critical to fully assess the extent of the injury. If assessment is limited by patient cooperation, pain or bleeding, force, or coercion should never be used. Sedation can be used in the emergency department to obtain better visualization or the patient may require an examination under anesthesia to evaluate the extent of the injury [3]. Speculum examination is usually not necessary and is reserved for evaluation of significant vaginal lacerations or unidentified bleeding. If the use of a speculum is needed in a prepubertal patient, sedation or anesthesia should be used [1]. In addition, depending on the extent of injury and the age of the patient, the pediatric gynecologist can consider utilizing cystoscopy or vaginoscopy to better visualize genital injuries [3].

Genital trauma is commonly managed conservatively [2]. Abrasions that are bleeding can be treated with cold compresses and pressure. In most cases, vulvar hematomas also respond favorably to conservative management [3]. The mass effect of a large hematoma can compress the urethra and render the patient incapable of voiding. Therefore, if any urinary retention is noted, a Foley catheter should be placed until the hematoma decreases in size. A nonexpanding hematoma in a hemodynamically stable patient should be managed with cold compresses, analgesia, and rest [1,3]. These conservative measures commonly result in resolution of the hematoma over several weeks without surgical intervention [8]. Rapid expansion of a hematoma or hemodynamic instability warrant surgical evacuation [3].

Small, hemostatic genital lacerations, particularly in prepubertal girls, generally respond favorably to conservative management [3], commonly healing in a matter of days [8]. Application of nightly topical estrogen cream to lacerations in prepubertal girls facilitates healing [3]. Moderately sized lacerations or those with bleeding may be amenable to repair in the emergency department with local anesthesia in appropriately selected patients. Lacerations that are bleeding persistently, are large, or potentially involve the urethra, vagina, or anal region require surgical exploration and management. Intraoperatively the extent of the injury should be carefully delineated and the laceration should be repaired in layers (when of significant depth) with a synthetic absorbable suture [3]. Any patient who has sustained genital trauma should have an appropriate plan for analgesia, should be voiding (spontaneously or in the case of large vulvar hematomas via indwelling catheter), and should have close pediatric or gynecologic follow-up [1,3].

Key teaching points

- In pediatric patients who have sustained genital trauma, providers must screen for sexual assault with a careful history and physical examination.
- Initial evaluation of a patient with genital trauma involves assessment of vital signs and hemodynamic stability, followed by a complete physical examination including a targeted genitourinary examination.
- If examination of the genitalia in a pediatric patient is limited by patient cooperation, pain or bleeding, an examination with sedation or under anesthesia in the operating room should be performed. Care should be taken to avoid using force or coercion to facilitate examination.
- Vulvar lacerations are the most common injury resulting from accidental genital trauma in pediatric patients. If hemostatic, lacerations may be managed conservatively with a plan for analgesia and close follow-up.
- Vulvar hematomas should be managed conservatively unless they are expanding rapidly or the patient is hemodynamically unstable.

References

1. Benjamins LJ. Genital trauma in pediatric and adolescent females. *J Pediatr Adolesc Gynecol* 2009;22: 129–33.

2. Spitzer RF, Kives S, Caccia N, et al. Retrospective review of unintentional female genital trauma at a pediatric referral center. *Pediatr Emerg Care* 2008;24:831–5.

3. Emans SJ, Laufer MR. *Pediatric and Adolescent Gynecology*, 6th edn. Philadelphia, PA, Lippincott Williams & Wilkins, 2012.

4. Saxena AK, Steiner M, Hollwarth ME. Straddle injuries in female children and adolescents: 10-year accident and management analysis. *Indian J Pediatr* 2013; Jul 4 [Epub ahead of print].

5. Bond GR, Dowd MD, Landsman I, Rimza M. Unintentional perineal injury in prepubescent girls: a multicenter prospective report of 56 girls. *Pediatrics* 1995;95:628–31.

6. Adams JA, Harper K, Knudson S, et al. Examination findings in legally confirmed child sexual abuse: It's normal to be normal. *Pediatrics* 1994;94:310–17.

7. Kellog N. The evaluation of sexual abuse in children. *Pediatrics* 2005;116:506–12.

8. Mcann J, Miyamoto S, Boyle C, et al. Healing of non-hymenyl genital injuries in prepubertal and adolescent girls: a descriptive study. *Pediatrics* 2007;120:1000–11.

Worsening cyclic pain and amenorrhea in a 13-year-old girl

Sarah H. Milton

History of present illness

A 13-year-old adolescent girl presented to the emergency department with a complaint of cramping and lower abdominal pain that was increasing in severity. Her pain was constant, located in the midline, did not radiate, and was not relieved by acetaminophen. Further questioning revealed a history of similar type pain that had been occurring cyclically for the last three months. She reported mild constipation and lower back pain, but denied nausea, vomiting, fever, chills, or urinary symptoms. She had no prior medical or surgical history, was premenarchal and denied prior sexual activity. She is accompanied by her mother who reports no other changes in her daughter's school performance or social interactions.

Physical examination

General appearance: Thin adolescent woman in moderate distress

Vital signs:

Temperature: 37.1°C
Pulse: 120 beats/min
Blood pressure: 92/46 mmHg
Respiratory rate: 22 breaths/min
Oxygen saturation: 100% on room air

Cardiovascular: Tachycardia, with regular rhythm

Breast: Tanner stage IV breast development

Respiratory: Chest clear to auscultation bilaterally

Abdomen: Soft, nondistended, normal bowel sounds, with tenderness to palpation suprapubically. There is a midline mass palpable which was smooth, mobile and tender. The mass extended approximately 4 cm above pubic symphysis. No rebound or guarding

Genitourinary: Normal labia with tense, bulging, bluish translucent membrane just cephlad to the vaginal introitus. Tanner stage IV pubic hair development

Laboratory studies:

WBCs: Normal
Hb: Normal

How would you manage this patient?

This 13-year-old adolescent has an imperforate hymen with resultant hematocolpos and hematometria. The diagnosis was suspected based on the classic presentation of an adolescent patient with cyclic abdominal pain and amenorrhea. This suspicion was confirmed by the genitourinary examination which revealed the classic tense bluish, translucent membrane (indicative of an imperforate hymen) with proximal hematocolpos. The patient was given narcotic pain medications, and the gynecology team was consulted. She was taken to surgery the following day where she underwent successful excision of the imperforate hymen with evacuation of the hematocolpos and hematometria. She recovered well and was discharged the day of her surgery without incident.

Imperforate hymen

Pathologic conditions of the hymen largely result from failed canalization of the lumen of the vaginal canal and the vaginal vestibule during embryonic life [1]. The hymen is usually patent at birth; however, several pathologic variations in the development of the hymen can occur including septation, microperforation or complete occlusion termed "imperforate." Imperforate hymen is the rarest of these variations and is found in 0.05–0.10% of newborn girls [1]. Although the majority of cases are sporadic, genetic transmission has also been reported with both dominant and recessive inheritance patterns [2].

An imperforate hymen most commonly comes to clinical attention in adolescence when menarche occurs and the distal vaginal occlusion results in painful hematocolpos (menstrual blood accumulated in the vagina) [3]. These young girls give a history of several months of cyclic pelvic pain. They may also experience back pain, nausea, vomiting, urinary frequency, and constipation as a result of the mass effect of the hematocolpos and hematometria [4]. Although less common, these patients may present with peritoneal signs as a result of retrograde flow of menstrual blood through fallopian tubes and into the peritoneal cavity [1]. A microperforate hymen or a septate hymen will not obstruct menstruation. These conditions commonly come to clinical attention when patients encounter difficulty with insertion of a tampon or with vaginal intercourse [4].

A careful examination of the external genitalia is recommended by the American Academy of Pediatrics [5]. Despite this recommendation, the incidental diagnosis of imperforate hymen in the newborn period is uncommon [3]. In this circumstance, there is not proximal distension of the vagina by blood or fluid which makes visualization and diagnosis more difficult. Very infrequently, a newborn examination may reveal a thin, white bulging membrane at the vaginal introitus. This pathologic finding is the result of accumulation of genital tract

Acute Care and Emergency Gynecology, ed. David Chelmow, Christine R. Isaacs and Ashley Carroll. Published by Cambridge University Press.
© Cambridge University Press 2015.

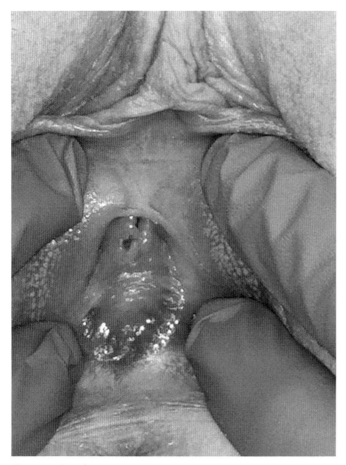

Fig. 74.1 Genital examination.

secretions produced secondary to in-utero exposure to maternal estrogen [4]. The result of these secretions in a newborn with an imperforate hymen is the development of a mucocolpos, which is generally asymptomatic, but more readily identified on routine newborn examination.

An imperforate hymen is a clinical diagnosis. A characteristic history of cyclic pelvic pain in an adolescent patient, in conjunction with a genital examination revealing a tense bulging membrane at the vaginal introitus is sufficient for diagnosis as was the case in this patient. On occasion, the diagnosis may be more difficult if the thickness of the obstructing membrane cannot be readily determined by physical examination (Fig. 74.1). In these circumstances, the differential diagnosis includes Mullerian anomalies, including a transverse or longitudinal vaginal septum, labial adhesions, androgen insensitivity syndrome, or complete Mullerian agenesis. Correct diagnosis is essential prior to operative intervention as the management of the aforementioned conditions varies widely and is not universally surgical. If the diagnosis of imperforate hymen is in question, a MRI is the best test to evaluate the pelvic anatomy prior to intervention [6,7]. Particularly in newborn girls, ultrasound may also be of use to determine the thickness of the obstructing tissue and identify pelvic structures [8].

If diagnosis of an imperforate hymen is suspected in an adolescent patient, gynecologic consultation should be obtained prior to any attempt to alleviate obstruction. While management of an imperforate hymen is surgical, it is not a surgical emergency. Initial emphasis should be placed on analgesia with a plan for surgical decompression in the operating room by a trained gynecologic surgeon. Once adequate anesthesia is obtained in the operating room, the distended hymenal tissue can be injected with a local anesthetic, and a cruciate incision is made in the hymen to evacuate the hematocolpos. The excess hymenal tissue is then excised, and the mucosal margins are reapproximated to prevent scarring and provide hemostasis [1].

In a newborn girl with an imperforate hymen (with or without a mucocolpos present), surgical excision of the hymen is encouraged. This can be accomplished in the operating room and is identical to the procedure described above. If the hymenectomy is deferred in the newborn period and performed at puberty, one must be mindful of the risk of a painful hematocolpos forming with initiation of menses. Because hymenectomy is facilitated by well-estrogenized tissue, it should be deferred until after puberty if the diagnosis is made outside of the newborn period [4].

Microperforate and septate hymens should only be surgically managed if they are symptomatic [4]. The most common complaints in patients with these conditions are inability to insert a tampon and difficulty with sexual intercourse. Surgical procedures are individualized and should be performed by a gynecologic surgeon with experience in hymenal pathology.

Complications of hymenectomy are rare. Most patients recover well and do not have any long-term reproductive consequences from the surgery [9]. Because familial associations have been described, any offspring of a woman with a history of an imperforate hymen should be carefully examined in the newborn period for evidence of the condition [2].

Key teaching points

- Imperforate hymen is a relatively rare condition that should be considered in all adolescent patients presenting with cyclic abdominal pain and amenorrhea.

- All newborn girls should have a thorough pediatric examination of their external genitalia shortly after birth, which can facilitate early diagnosis and repair of an imperforate hymen.

- In most cases, a thorough history and examination should be sufficient for diagnosis of an imperforate hymen and for surgical planning. If, however, the diagnosis is uncertain, the best imaging study to clarify and identify pelvic structures is an MRI.

- Obstruction of menstruation resulting from an imperforate hymen is not a surgical emergency. Emphasis should be placed on analgesia while obtaining timely consultation by a gynecologist trained to confirm the diagnosis and plan a nonemergent surgical intervention.

- Surgical repair of an imperforate hymen by hymenectomy is best performed when tissue is well estrogenized, either in the immediate newborn period or after puberty.

References

1. Rock JA, Jones HW. *TeLinde's Operative Gynecology*, 10th edn. Philadelphia, PA, Lippincott Williams & Wilkins, 2008.

2. Sakalkale R, Samarakkody U. Familial occurrence of imperforate hymen. *J Pediatr Adolesc Gynecol* 2005;18(6): 427–9.

3. Posner JC, Spandorfer PR. Early detection of imperforate hymen prevents morbidity from delays in diagnosis. *Pediatrics* 2005;115(4): 1008–12.

4. Emans SJ, Laufer MR. *Pediatric and Adolescent Gynecology*, 6th edn. Philadelphia, PA, Lippincott Williams & Wilkins; 2012.

5. McInerny TK. *American Academy of Pediatrics Textbook of Pediatric Care*. Washington, DC, American Academy of Pediatrics, 2009.

6. Church DG, Vancil JM, Vasanawala SS. Magnetic resonance imaging for uterine and vaginal anomalies. *Curr Opin Obstet Gynecol* 2009;21(5):379–89.

7. American College of Obstetricians and Gynecologists. Müllerian agenesis: diagnosis, management, and treatment. Committee Opinion No. 562. *Obstet Gynecol* 2013;121:1134–7.

8. Blask AR, Sanders RC, Rock JA. Obstructed uterovaginal anomalies: demonstration with sonography. Part II. Teenagers. *Radiology* 1991;179(1): 84–8.

9. Rock JA, Zacur HA, Dlugi AM, et al. Pregnancy success following the surgical correction of imperforate hymen as compared to the complete transverse vaginal septum. *Obstet Gynecol* 1982;59:448–51.

Worsening cyclic pain and amenorrhea in a 13-year-old girl with a normal appearing but short vagina

Nicole W. Karjane

History of present illness

A 13-year-old adolescent girl presents to the emergency department with severe pelvic pain. She reports the pain began several months ago, was cramping in nature, and lasted approximately seven days. Since the initial episode, she has had worsening cyclic pelvic pain every 4–5 weeks that lasts 7–10 days. Initially, the pain was moderate and had improved with ibuprofen; however, each episode has been increasingly resistant to nonsteroidal anti-inflammatory drugs, and her pain is now intolerable. She reports thelarche at age 10 and pubarche shortly thereafter, but she has not yet had her first menstrual period. On review of systems, she has no fevers, chills, nausea, vomiting, diarrhea, or urinary complaints. She does report mild constipation and low back discomfort. She is otherwise healthy, reports no history of sexual activity or abuse, and has never had surgery.

Physical examination

General appearance: Nontoxic-appearing woman who is apprehensive and in moderate distress
Vital signs:

Temperature: 37.0°C
Pulse: 96 beats/min
Blood pressure: 115/62 mmHg
Respiratory rate: 18 breaths/min
Oxygen saturation: 100% on room air

Cardiovascular: Regular rate and rhythm without murmurs, rubs, or gallops
Lungs: Clear to auscultation bilaterally
Breasts: Tanner stage IV breast development
Abdomen: Soft, tender throughout lower abdomen, nondistended, with no guarding or rebound tenderness; however, examination is limited by the patient's discomfort. On palpation, there is fullness in the lower abdomen to approximately 2 cm above the pubic symphysis at the area of maximal tenderness
Genitalia: Normal external genitalia, normal, well-estrogenized hymen, vagina normal caliber, with length of 4 cm, unable to visualize or palpate cervix
Imaging: MRI is performed (Fig. 75.1)

How would you manage this patient?

The diagnosis is transverse vaginal septum with resultant hematocolpos and hematometra. The patient's history of progressively worsening cyclic pelvic pain around the time of expected menarche is typical of obstructed menstruation. MRI revealed a normal cervix (arrow A in Fig. 75.1), mild hematometra, and a dilated upper vagina (arrow B in Fig. 75.1) with an approximately 5 mm transverse vaginal septum. Her pain was controlled with intravenous narcotics, and she was posted for surgery. In the operating room, she underwent successful resection of the transverse vaginal septum with the z-plasty technique and was advised to use vaginal dilators postoperatively in order to prevent scar formation at the anastomosis line. Her pain resolved immediately, she was discharged home, and she was doing well at her follow-up visits.

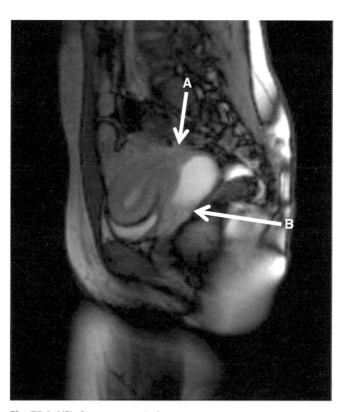

Fig. 75.1 MRI of transverse vaginal septum.

Acute Care and Emergency Gynecology, ed. David Chelmow, Christine R. Isaacs and Ashley Carroll. Published by Cambridge University Press.
© Cambridge University Press 2015.

Menstrual obstruction can be caused by a number of etiologies, the most common of which is imperforate hymen, with an estimated incidence of 1 in 2000 women [1]. In this patient, the initial examination was not consistent with an imperforate hymen, which has the classic appearance of a bluish, tense bulge at the introitus; therefore, an MRI was performed to further delineate the anatomy. It is essential to delay surgical intervention until the exact obstructive anomaly is identified in order to facilitate surgical planning and avoid inappropriate procedures. Though imperforate hymen is the most common cause of obstructed menstruation, other potential etiologies must be considered and include a transverse vaginal septum, with an incidence of approximately 1 in 70 000 women [2], and other rare anomalies like distal vaginal atresia or agenesis, and cervical agenesis. In addition, approximately 2–7% of patients with Mullerian agenesis (congenital absence or underdevelopment of the uterus, vagina, or both) will have rudimentary uterine horns that contain active endometrium and thus may present with symptoms of menstrual obstruction [3]. All of these anomalies require more significant surgical resection and postoperative care than imperforate hymen; therefore, proceeding to the operating room prior to adequate diagnostic testing is ill-advised.

Imaging modalities that may be helpful in making the diagnosis in cases of menstrual obstruction include ultrasound and MRI; however, MRI is most helpful in characterizing anomalies of the reproductive tract, particularly in distinguishing the location and thickness of a vaginal septum and identifying the presence or absence of a uterine cervix [4]. Cases of cervical agenesis are particularly important to identify, as creating a fistula between the vagina and uterus in the absence of a cervix may place the patient at significant risk for ascending infection, sepsis and even death [5]. Traditional treatment of cervical agenesis has been hysterectomy; however, fertility preserving procedures have been reported with varying success rates. Patients with cervical agenesis and desire for fertility preservation are best managed at institutions with experience dealing with these procedures.

The etiology of the transverse vaginal septum is thought to be failure of canalization and/or fusion of the Mullerian ducts and urogenital sinus during embryogenesis. The location of the septum may be in the upper vagina (46%), middle vagina (35%), or lower vagina (19%) [6]. Treatment of the transverse vaginal septum involves excision of the septum with re-anastamosis of the vaginal epithelium above and below the excised septum. Drainage of the hematocolpos from below without excision of the septum may place the patient at risk for persistent obstruction and ascending infection and should not be performed. In cases of a thick septum, surgical excision may be delayed, and the patient may opt to perform preoperative dilator therapy to help thin out the septum and facilitate excision. Alternatively, the z-plasty technique is thought to increase the circumference of the anastamosis line and thus reduce the risk of stenosis [7]. In rare cases, a skin graft may be required when the septum is so thick that the vaginal epithelium from the upper vagina does not reach that of the lower vagina. This can generally be avoided, however, by performing the procedure when significant hematocolops is present or by using preoperative dilators as described above, both of which can serve to increase the amount of vaginal epithelium to be mobilized and reduce the thickness of the vaginal septum.

Pregnancy is possible following surgical excision of the transverse vaginal septum; however, pregnancy rates are reported to be significantly lower in these women compared to those with a history of an imperforate hymen [6]. The reason for this discrepancy is unclear, but it is speculated that an imperforate hymen is more likely to be diagnosed and corrected promptly, thus decreasing the likelihood of resultant endometriosis.

Key teaching points

- Cyclic pelvic pain in a normally developed adolescent at the age of anticipated menarche is suspicious for obstructed menstruation.
- Though imperforate hymen is the most common cause of menstrual obstruction, other etiologies must be considered prior to surgical intervention, particularly if the initial examination is not consistent with the classic "bluish bulge" appearance of imperforate hymen.
- MRI is the imaging modality of choice to evaluate for anomalies of the female reproductive tract and to aid in surgical planning.
- Transverse vaginal septum is treated with surgical excision of the septum and reanastamosis of the upper and lower vagina.

References

1. Parazzini F, Cecchetti G. The frequency of imperforate hymen in northern Italy. *Int J Epidemiol* 1990;19(3):763–4.

2. Banerjee R, Laufer MR. Reproductive disorders associated with pelvic pain. *Semin Pediatr Surg* 1998;7(1):52–61.

3. American College of Obstetricians and Gynecologists. Müllerian agenesis: diagnosis, management, and treatment. Committee Opinion No. 562. *Obstet Gynecol* 2013;121:1134–7.

4. Church DG, Vancil JM, Vasanawala SS. Magnetic resonance imaging for uterine and vaginal anomalies. *Curr Opin Obstet Gynecol* 2009;21(5):379–89.

5. Emans SJ, Laufer MR, *Pediatric and Adolescent Gynecology*, 6th edn. Philadelphia, PA, Lippincott Williams & Wilkins, 2012.

6. Rock JA, Zacur HA, Dlugi AM, et al. Pregnancy success following the surgical correction of imperforate hymen as compared to the complete transverse vaginal septum. *Obstet Gynecol* 1982;59:448–51.

7. Garcia RE. Z-plasty correction for the congenital transverse vaginal septum. *Am J Obstet Gynecol* 1967;99: 1164–5.

A 19-month-old girl with labial adhesions and acute urinary retention

Hong-Thao Thieu and Meredith S. Thomas

History of present illness

The patient is a 19-month-old girl who presents to a tertiary care pediatric and adolescent gynecology clinic with acute dysuria and voiding difficulty. She has been followed by her pediatrician for labial agglutination for approximately one year. At the time of diagnosis she was noted to have thin labial adhesions that were transparent and affected only the posterior portion of the fold. As prescribed, her mother had been applying topical estrogen (Premarin®) cream to the labial adhesions twice daily for the past year but never achieved complete separation. Over the last week prior to presentation she has been fussy, crying with urination, and her mother notes a foul smell in her diaper. Review of systems is negative for fevers, back pain, nausea, vomiting, and diarrhea.

Physical examination

General appearance: Well-developed, well-grown 19-month-old girl who appears fussy, crying, and resistant to examiner

Vital signs:

Temperature: 37.0°C
Pulse: 120 beats/min
Blood pressure: 95/60 mmHg
Respiratory rate: 22 breaths/min
Oxygen saturation: 100% on room air
Height: 32.67 inches
Weight: 26 lb
BMI: 17 kg/m²

Cardiovascular: Normal S1, S2 without murmurs, rubs, or gallops

Respiratory: Clear to auscultation bilaterally

Abdomen: Soft and nontender without masses or hernias; no distention was appreciated

Gynecologic: Tanner stage I breast and pubic hair development. There is nearly 100% agglutination of the labia except for a small urethral outlet (Fig. 76.1)

Laboratory studies:

Urine: Appears cloudy
Urinalysis: 1+ Leukocyte esterase, 1 RBC, 1 WBC, few bacteria, specific gravity 1.021
Urine culture: 10–50 000 cfu mixed bacterial flora

How would you manage this patient?

This 19-month-old girl with known labial adhesions presents after a year of treatment failure following conservative management with topical estrogen. Given her voiding complaints, suspicion for urinary tract infection and treatment failure in the setting of high degree of agglutination, this patient qualifies for surgical management.

The patient was taken to the operating room where the labia were grasped bilaterally and extended to allow visualization of the thin line of adhesion and a small incision into the thin adhesion was made with electrocautery. The labia were then completely separated with gentle manual traction and blunt dissection. The line of adhesion remained hemostatic (Fig. 76.2).

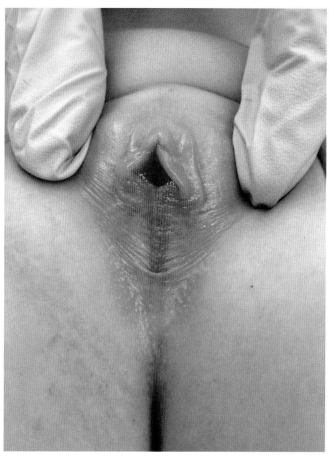

Fig. 76.1 Labial adhesion in 19-month-old girl with one year of treatment failure, presenting with urinary difficulty.

Acute Care and Emergency Gynecology, ed. David Chelmow, Christine R. Isaacs and Ashley Carroll. Published by Cambridge University Press.

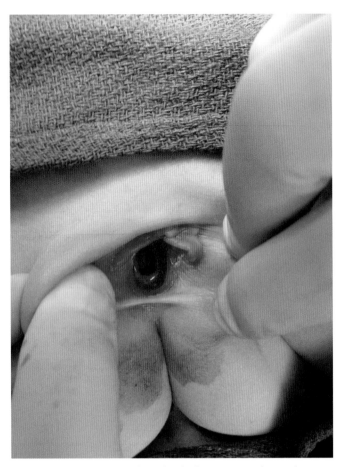

Fig. 76.2 Labial separation achieved with electocautery and manual separation under general anesthesia.

Labial adhesions

Labial adhesions are a relatively common pediatric gynecologic complaint and prevalence has been cited as up to 20% of pediatric populations presenting for routine primary care [1]. The prevalence differs largely among different studies, and this is likely secondary to the wide clinical presentation with a large percentage of cases being asymptomatic. The true prevalence is difficult to accurately calculate given the wide range of clinical presentations.

The above clinical scenario illustrates several of the common presentations of labial adhesions. Clinical presentation varies from asymptomatic, thus an incidental finding of adhesions on routine exam, to acute urinary retention necessitating emergent surgical intervention. Common complaints include vulvovaginitis, positional pain, bleeding, urinary incontinence, and urinary tract infections. It is important to recognize the range of symptoms associated with labial adhesions in order to appropriately triage treatment goals. Practice Bulletin No. 93 by the American College of Obstetricians and Gynecologists (ACOG) recommends that treatment is reserved for those patients presenting with symptoms [2]. As above, the first-line treatment recommendation is topical estrogen cream.

As with any thorough evaluation, it is important to establish a differential diagnosis prior to proceeding with treatment and to rule out alternative etiologies of the presenting complaint or clinical finding. The differential diagnosis for labial adhesions includes congenital anomalies such as vaginal agenesis and vaginal septum, hymenal abnormalities such as an imperforate hymen, and clitoromegaly. Typically the pathophysiology of labial adhesions is thought to be secondary to a physiologic nadir in systemic estrogen and an inciting factor of vulvar irritation. This nadir corresponds with the peak incidence of agglutination presentation, which is 2.5 years of age [1]. A rare but important historical element that must be considered with labial adhesions is potential for abuse. Typical diaper rash is thought to be enough of an insult to initiate adhesions, but one would not want to miss abuse in the outpatient setting.

Approach to treatment depends on severity of symptoms. ACOG recommends topical estrogen for symptomatic patients followed by one month of emollient cream to prevent reagglutiation of raw labial edges after separation [2]. Topical estrogen such as Premarin (0.625 mg/g) should be applied twice daily to the midline of the adherent labia [3]. If the twice-daily application is not successful, the application can be increased to three or four times per day. One alternative to estrogen cream that has been recently studied is topical steroids [2]. A study by Myers and colleagues looked retrospectively at a cohort of patients with labial adhesions who were treated with betamethasone and found the treatment to be as effective as estrogen [4]. However, a retrospective comparison by Eroglu and colleagues, published a few years later, looked at the use of betamethasone, estrogen, and a combination of the two and found essentially no difference [5]. Estrogen cream remains the first-line treatment but betamethasone may be a safe second-line treatment for those who fail estrogen therapy.

Some common pitfalls of treatment are not concentrating the application to the midline. Signs of too-wide application are treatment failure and hyperpigmentation. The patient in our case was treated conservatively for one year but never achieved complete separation. When she presented, her symptoms had worsened. Presentation with urinary retention and suspected urinary tract infection is an indication for surgical intervention. Additional characteristics that may be an indication for surgical intervention are thick adhesions, greater than 90% of the vestibule affected, and small uretheral opening [6].

Reagglutination is a preventable complication of any labial separation, whether manual or passive with topical cream. The parents in this case were instructed to keep the raw edges of the adhesion moist with a topical agent such as Aquaphor® cream or A&D® ointment. When this patient presented for her 6-week postoperative visit she was doing well but was found to have a small 5 mm area of re-agglutination near the posterior forchette. At this time the parents were instructed to reintroduce Premarin topical cream until complete separation was achieved. By her second follow-up visit one month later, she had achieved complete separation and this was further maintained with A&D ointment.

Key teaching points

- Labial adhesions are a common presenting complaint in the pediatric population and treatment options are decided based on severity of symptoms.

- Topical estrogen cream application is sufficient for most cases of labial adhesions, and manual or surgical separation should be reserved for only the most severe symptoms such as urinary dysfunction or retention.

- Once separation is achieved, continued use of lubricants or moisturizers will help to maintain separation until the labial skin is completely healed.

References

1. Murram D. Treatment of prepubertal girls with labial adhesions. *J Pediatr Adolesc Gynecol* 1999;12: 67–70.

2. American College of Obstetricians and Gynecologists. Diagnosis and management of vulvar skin disorders. Practice Bulletin No. 93. *Obstet Gynecol* 2008;111:1243–53.

3. Tebruegge M, Misra I, Nerminathan V. Is the topical application of oestrogen cream an effective intervention in girls suffering from labial adhesions? *Arch Dis Child* 2007;92: 268–71.

4. Myers J, Sorensen C, Wisner B, et al. Betamethasone cream for the treatment of pre-pubertal labial adhesions. *J Pediatr Adolesc Gynecol* 2006;19: 407–11.

5. Eroglu E, Yip M, Oktar T, Kayiran S, Mocan H. How should we treat prepubertal labial adhesions? Retrospective comparison of topical treatments: estrogen only, betamethasone only, and combination estrogen and betamethasone. *J Pediatr Adolesc Gynecol* 2011;24:389–91.

6. Bacon J. Prepuberal labial adhesions: evaluation of a referral population. *Am J Obstet Gynecol* 2002;187:327–32.

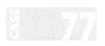
A 13-year-old girl with irregular menses and significant weight gain

Tiffany Tonismae and Eduardo Lara-Torre

History of present illness

A 13-year-old girl presents with her mother to discuss her irregular menses. Her menarche was at age 10 and her periods have been irregular since. Sometimes she bleeds every month and sometimes she skips a month or two. Her menses often last four to six days, or less. She has no dysmenorrhea. She reports that her last menstrual period started four weeks ago and consisted of five days of spotting.

Her mother is also concerned because her daughter has gained almost 15 lb over the past 3 months. Both deny changes in activity level or appetite. She is currently in the seventh grade and is very active with cheerleading. Her mom reports her daughter always watches what she eats, as she wants to be "thin" so she can be a better cheerleader. She also complains of some nausea over the past two to three months but denies loss of appetite, diarrhea, or emesis.

With both the mother and the daughter present, you ask if she could be pregnant and the mother immediately dismisses the possibility. She states her daughter is always under her observation and is a "good girl." Her mother denies that her daughter has a boyfriend.

She is otherwise healthy. She has no other known medical problems and has never had surgery. She takes no medications.

Physical examination

General appearance: No acute distress; healthy-appearing teenage girl

Vital signs:

Temperature: 36.9°C
Pulse: 64 beats/min
Blood pressure: 110/65 mmHg
Respiratory rate: 20 breaths/min
BMI: 23.9 kg/m^2

HEENT: Normal

Cardiovascular: Regular rate and rhythm without murmurs, rubs, or gallops

Lungs: Clear to auscultation bilaterally, no wheezing

Abdomen: Soft, nontender, nondistended. An abdominal mass is palpated half way between umbilicus and pubic symphisis. It is nonmobile and nontender

Pelvic: Deferred at this point in the encounter

How would you manage this patient?

After the initial examination (as you do on all your adolescent patients), you ask the patient's mother to step out of the room for private questions regarding teenage high-risk behaviors. The mother agrees. In private, the patient denies any alcohol, tobacco, or drug use. She admits she has a boyfriend in the eighth grade. When you ask about sexual activity, she becomes very tearful and cannot answer the question. She nods her head in agreement when you ask if she is having sex. You ask her if you can run some tests to see if she could be pregnant. She agrees but does not want you to tell her mom the results.

Laboratory studies:

Urine pregnancy test: Positive
HIV testing and urine NAATs for gonorrhea and chlamydia sent

Imaging: Bedside transabdominal ultrasound shows a 16-week intrauterine pregnancy, fetal heart rate 145 beats/min

How would you manage this patient?

This is a case of a teen pregnancy. Pregnancy is always of concern when a sexually active patient presents with irregular bleeding or increased weight. Although a urine pregnancy test confirms pregnancy, it does not determine dates or location of the pregnancy. Both can be best determined with ultrasound. Abdominal ultrasound is appropriate if the uterine fundus is palpable. Transvaginal ultrasound should be reserved for early gestations and pregnancies of undetermined location to minimize discomfort and distress to the teenage patient. In our case, the confidential discussion with the teen allowed eliciting further information that was not available with the mother present, and to focus our diagnostic interventions towards pregnancy and further counseling and care.

Once the diagnosis of pregnancy was confirmed, the findings were discussed with the patient. She was asked if she desired her mother to be present for further counseling on options. You discussed that you supported her privacy, but were available to assist in the disclosure as needed. She agreed to have her mother in the room and options were discussed as a group.

Once the patient's mother was informed of the pregnancy, options were discussed for the management of pregnancy including obstetrical care and parenthood, adoption, or pregnancy termination. The patient desired to continue the pregnancy and prenatal care was initiated.

Acute Care and Emergency Gynecology, ed. David Chelmow, Christine R. Isaacs and Ashley Carroll. Published by Cambridge University Press.
© Cambridge University Press 2015.

Teen pregnancy

Teen pregnancy refers to pregnancies occurring in girls younger than age 20. Most data regarding teen pregnancy, complications, outcomes, and risk factors in the United States refers to girls aged 15–19, with limited data for pregnancies occurring in girls aged 10–14 [1]. Approximately 750 000 teens in the United States between the ages of 15 and 19 become pregnant each year, with a pregnancy rate of 42 per 1000 in teens between the ages of 15 and 17 years. Though this rate has declined over the past few decades (Fig. 77.1), the teen pregnancy rate in the United States still remains one of the highest among industrialized nations, approximately twice that of Europe and Canada [2].

There are a number of clear risk factors for teen pregnancy (Table 77.1 [1]). Certain racial and socioeconomic groups are

at higher risk of teen pregnancy. In the United States, African-American teens continue to have the highest teen pregnancy rate, followed by Hispanic teens [1]. Pregnancies are more common among those coming from lower levels of income or education. Having an older sibling who was a teen mother is also a risk factor [2]. Patients with these risk factors are more likely to seek prenatal care late, and have less access to reliable contraception services.

Most teen pregnancies are unintended, and teens often have presented to providers requesting information about their options in pregnancy prevention and contraception almost 12 months after initiation of sexual activity. Almost 26% of teens choose to have an elective abortion, with the increased incidence in unintended teen pregnancy in minority groups such as Hispanic and African Americans accounting for a larger amount of abortions performed in the United States [1]. Forty-four states require parental consent or notification to care for girls under the age of 18, and it is important for providers to know the requirements in their state when counseling teens. The Guttmacher Institute (www.guttmacher. org) provides information regarding federal and state specific rules and regulations guiding the provision of reproductive services for teens including pregnancy care, abortion, and contraception [3,4]. Teens are also at risk as they may seek an unsafe abortion performed by someone lacking skills or sanitary conditions. It is estimated that 14% of all unsafe abortions are performed on teens. More than 90% of teens who give birth choose to raise the infants. Adoption is utilized by unmarried teens under age 17 as an option to manage pregnancy about 8% of the time [2].

Table 77.1 Risk factors for adolescent pregnancy*

Lack of support
Living in disadvantaged/impoverished conditions
Minority background
History of abuse
Lack of parental involvement
Single-parent household
Use of alcohol or drugs
Early dating
Little perceived opportunity for success
Child of an adolescent pregnancy
School drop-out

* Modified from Kost and Henshaw [1].

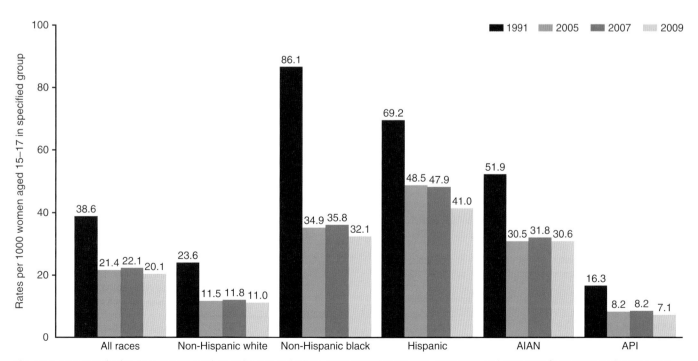

Fig. 77.1 Birth rates for female teenagers aged 15-17 by race and ethnic origin: United States 1991, 2005, 2007, and 2009. Data for 2009 are preliminary. AIAN, American Indian or Alaska Native; API, Asian or Pacific Islander. (Source: CDC/NCHS, National Vital Statistics System.)

Teen pregnancies are often associated with increased pregnancy related complications, in part because adolescents often do not receive early prenatal care, placing them at higher risk for both preterm birth and low birth weight babies [2]. Teens are also at risk for poor nutritional status, low pre-pregnancy weight, poor pregnancy weight gain, poverty, unmarried status, low educational levels, smoking, and drug use, which are additional risk factors for adverse pregnancy outcomes [5]. Teen pregnancies have a higher rate of neonatal death with up to a three times increased risk of infant death in the first year of life compared to children born to older women (women aged 20 or older) [2]. Certain congenital anomalies are also more common including those affecting the central nervous system (anencephaly, spina bifida, hydrocephaly, and microcephaly), gastrointestinal anomalies (gastroschisis, omphalocele) and musculoskeletal anomalies (cleft lip/palate, polydactyly, syndactyly, adactyly) [2]. Infants born to teen mothers are also at increased risk of neonatal infection and abuse.

Teen pregnancy has a large negative impact on the teens after childbirth. Teen mothers are less likely to receive a high school diploma, are more likely to require public assistance or welfare, and are more likely to live in poverty [2]. Teen moms are also at increased risk of having another pregnancy as a teen, with 25% of teen births having a subsequent teen pregnancy [5]. The children of teen mothers have increased rates of substance abuse, depression, and early sexual activity, as well as developmental delay and difficulty with academics. Daughters of teen mothers are also more likely to become teen mothers themselves, thus repeating this unfortunate cycle [2].

It is important to talk with teens about contraception before the first sexual encounter and even more so after the first teen pregnancy. Even with increasing use of contraception by teens at the time of first intercourse, almost 50% of teen pregnancies occur within the first 6 months of their initial sexual encounter [5]. All options for contraception should be discussed starting with long-acting reversible contraception (LARC), such as implants and intrauterine devices, as well as injectables, oral/vaginal contraception, barrier methods or abstinence. The American College of Obstetricians and Gynecologists advocates for the use of LARC and its safety in this age group [6]. Teens should also be made aware of options for emergency contraception and how to access them.

Counseling is key when clinicians take care of pregnant teens. The importance of prenatal care should be reviewed for those deciding to continue with the pregnancy. A discussion of other options including abortion and adoption is necessary to allow for all alternatives to be considered before making a decision. Providers who do not perform abortions should provide information about local clinics and practitioners where this service is available, as well as review time constraints for decision making. In teens who continue with obstetrical care and delivery, counseling during pregnancy should include a discussion and plan for postpartum contraception. LARC methods should be recommended to decrease the risk of subsequent teen pregnancy.

Key teaching points

- Teen pregnancy is a common occurrence and should be always kept at the top of the differential diagnosis in sexually active teens with abnormal bleeding or amenorrhea.
- A confidential discussion with the patient should always be undertaken to discuss issues the patient would be more comfortable discussing in private and to address high-risk behaviors and circumstances.
- Laws about parental disclosure vary from state to state. Providers caring for teens must be aware of the laws in their states including provision of confidential services, emancipation rules, and parental involvement requirements.
- Pregnant teens should be counseled on all options for the pregnancy including abortion, adoption, and pregnancy continuation and parenthood. Practitioners should be able to refer the patient for any desired option that they cannot provide themselves.
- Contraception should be discussed with all teen patients. Ideally this discussion should occur prior to the first sexual encounter. Plans for postpartum contraception should be developed during pregnancy, with a focus on long-acting reversible contraception methods.

References

1. Kost K, Henshaw S. *US Teenage Pregnancies, Births and Abortions, 2008: National Trends by Race and Ethnicity*, 2012. Available at http://www.guttmacher.org/pubs/USTPtrends08.pdf.

2. Black AY, Fleming NA, Rome ES. Pregnancy in adolescents. In Fisher M, Lara-Torre E, eds. *Adolescent Medicine: State of the Art Reviews*. Elk Grove Village, IL, American Academy of Pediatrics, 2012, pp. 123–38.

3. Ventura SJ, Abma JC, Mosher WD, et al. *National Vitals Statistics Reports. Estimated Pregnancy Rates by Outcomes for the United States*, 1990–2004. Available at http://www.cdc.gov/nchs/data/nvsr56/nvsr56_15.pdf.

4. National Abortion Federation. *Threats to Abortion Rights: Parental Involvement Bills*. Available at http://www.prochoice.org/policy/states/parental_involvement.html.

5. Klein JD. Adolescent pregnancy: current trends and issues. *Pediatrics* 2005;116:281–6.

6. American College of Obstetricians and Gynecologists. Adolescents and long-acting reversible contraception: implants and intrauterine devices. Committee Opinion No. 539. *Obstet Gynecol* 2012;120:983–8.

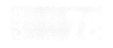

A 14-year-old girl with anemia

Layson L. Denney and Sarah H. Milton

History of present illness

A 14-year-old adolescent girl presented with a 3-day history of fatigue. She denied pain, fever, recent illness, sick contacts, difficulties sleeping, and symptoms of depression. She reported that her menstrual period ended two days ago and that she generally feels fatigued around the time of her menses, but her symptoms were worse this cycle.

Her medical history is significant for menarche at age 12. Her menstrual cycles were initially irregular, but are now regular and 28 days. She generally soaks through a pad every two hours. She was seen by her pediatrician at ages five and eight for epistaxis. She reported frequent bruising, which she attributes to playing soccer. Her mother underwent a hysterectomy at age 37 for heavy bleeding, and her maternal grandmother had a history of "heavy periods." There are no known diagnoses of bleeding disorders in the family.

Physical examination

Vital signs:

Temperature: 36.5°C
Pulse: 110 beats/min
Blood pressure: 123/76 mmHg
Respiratory rate: 20 breaths/min
Oxygen saturation: 100% on room air

HEENT: Normocephalic, atraumatic, conjunctival pallor
Cardiovascular: Tachycardic, regular rhythm with no murmurs, rubs, or gallops
Lungs: Clear to auscultation bilaterally
Abdomen: Soft, nontender, nondistended, normal bowel sounds
Extremities: Multiple bruises on bilateral lower extremities in various stages of healing; no cyanosis, clubbing, or edema; normal capillary refill
Neurologic: Nonfocal
Pelvic: Deferred
Laboratory studies:

Hb: 8.8 g/dL (normal 12.0–15.0 g/dL)
WBCs: 7000/μL (normal 3900–11 700/μL)
Platelet count: 250 000/μL (normal 172 000–440 000/μL)
Pregnancy test: Negative
PPT (partial thromboplastin time): 67 s, corrected with 1 : 1 mixing with normal plasma (normal 25–36 s)

PT (prothrombin time) and INR (international normalized ratio): Both within normal limits
VVWF:Ag (von Willebrand factor antigen): 25 IU/dL (normal 50–160 IU/dL)
VWF:RCoA (ristocetin cofactor activity): 20 IU/dL (normal 50–160 IU/dL)
Factor VIII activity level: 50% of normal

How would you manage this patient?

The patient has von Willebrand disease (VWD), type I. This diagnosis should be suspected based on the history and was confirmed with laboratory results revealing anemia, a prolonged partial thromboplastin time (PTT), normal prothrombin time (PT) and international normalized ratio (INR), and decreased von Willebrand factor antigen (VWF:Ag), ristocetin cofactor activity (VWF:RCoA) and factor VII activity. Low levels of VWF:Ag, VWF:RCoA, and factor VIII suggest a quantitative defect that is consistent with type I VWD [1]. The patient was referred to a hematologist where the diagnosis was confirmed with repeat VWD laboratory testing. The patient was started on iron supplements and oral contraceptive pills, which resulted in return of her hemoglobin to normal levels, resolution of symptoms, and marked improvement in her heavy menstrual bleeding (HMB).

VWD is the most common inherited bleeding disorder. It is caused by mutations that lead to quantitative or qualitative impairment of von Willebrand factor (VWF). After endothelial injury, VWF is released from endothelial cells and activated platelets. It functions in primary hemostasis by forming adhesions between exposed collagen and platelets and between individual platelets, strengthening the platelet plug. In addition, VWF functions in the intrinsic pathway of secondary hemostasis as a carrier protein of factor VIII, aiding in fibrin clot formation [1]. VWD is categorized into three types, which sequentially increase in severity. Type I is a quantitative deficiency and has an autosomal dominant inheritance pattern. Type II is a qualitative deficiency and has autosomal dominant and recessive inheritance patterns. Type III is defined by severely decreased or absent VWF and has an autosomal recessive inheritance pattern [1].

Clinical characteristics of VWD include easy bruising, excessive bleeding from minor wounds, prolonged mucosal bleeding (such as epistaxis or bleeding after a dental procedure) and, in severe cases, soft tissue bleeding and hemarthrosis [2]. Although VWD can affect both sexes, special considerations in

Acute Care and Emergency Gynecology, ed. David Chelmow, Christine R. Isaacs and Ashley Carroll. Published by Cambridge University Press.
© Cambridge University Press 2015.

women with VWD include HMB, postpartum hemorrhage, and other gynecologic conditions involving blood loss.

Identification of patients with a bleeding disorder begins with a thorough history. Emphasis should be placed on any history of excessive bleeding. Because of the inheritance patterns of VWD, a detailed family history of any bleeding abnormalities should be obtained. A careful medication history is important as any antiplatelet medications can exacerbate or instigate bleeding [1]. In women, careful attention to the menstrual history is important as HMB is the most common presenting symptom of VWD, experienced by 32–100% of women with VWD [3]. While the prevalence of VWD in the general population is 1%, the prevalence is 11–16% among women with HMB [4]. Careful attention to the menstrual history is particularly relevant in the adolescent population as HMB at menarche is often the first sign of VWD. The American College of Obstetricians and Gynecologists emphasizes obtaining a thorough menstrual history at the first reproductive health visit between the ages of 13 and 15. This visit should serve as an opportunity to evaluate patients for HMB indicative of a bleeding disorder [5]. A quantitative

approach to obtaining a menstrual history is preferred in which the clinician should inquire about the number of pads used, the frequency with which they are changed, and should consider the use of a menstrual calendar or pictorial bleeding assessments [2]. This patient's combination of HMB as an adolescent and history of epistaxis should raise concern.

If the diagnosis of VWD is suspected based on history and physical examination, an initial laboratory evaluation should be performed including a complete blood count with peripheral smear and coagulation studies [1,2]. An isolated PPT time that corrects on 1:1 mixing study with otherwise normal labs merits testing for VWD [6]. To test for VWD specifically, the provider should obtain a VWF ristocetin cofactor activity, VWF antigen, and clotting factor VIII activity assay (Fig. 78.1 [7]). Generally, a VWF ristocetin cofactor activity level of less than 30 IU/dL is characteristic of VWD. However, these levels may be influenced by diverse characteristics including age, race, timing in the menstrual cycle, pregnancy, or inflammation. Referral to a hematologist for complete workup and definitive diagnosis is warranted. Additionally, classification of VWD into subtypes is complicated and is based on the

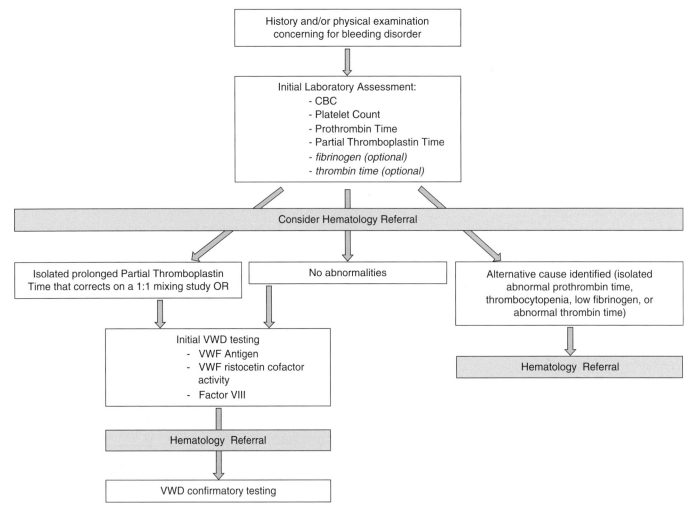

Fig. 78.1 Laboratory workup for patients with a history concerning for a bleeding disorder. (Adapted from [7].)

degree of quantitative and qualitative deficiencies in VWF and is best performed by a trained hematologist [1]. This patient had abnormalities on all of these tests.

It is important to identify women with VWD early due to the impact the disease can have on long-term health [8]. Women with bleeding disorders are more likely to develop any condition involving bleeding, such as hemorrhagic ovarian cysts and "Mittelschmerz" or midcycle pain [3]. Women with VWD are more likely than women without a bleeding disorder to experience exacerbated symptoms of common gynecologic conditions including endometriosis (30% vs. 13%), leiomyomas (32% vs. 17%), endometrial hyperplasia (10% vs. 1%), and polyps (8% vs. 1%), and ultimately are more likely to undergo hysterectomy (26% vs. 9%) [9]. Kirtava and colleagues found an increased incidence of miscarriage among women with VWD (15% vs. 9% of controls), as well as an increased risk of postpartum hemorrhage in women with VWD (59% vs. 21% of controls) [9]. They were also more prone to vulvar or vaginal hematomas, as well as delayed postpartum hemorrhage with a mean time to presentation of 15.7 days [9]. Additionally, women with VWD reported an increased negative effect of menstruation on their lives as compared to their peers [9].

Management of VWD is aimed at preventing bleeding and treating bleeding complications when they arise by increasing the levels of VWF and factor VIII [1]. Bleeding prophylaxis in women primarily focuses on the prevention of HMB. Combined hormonal contraception (oral contraceptive pill, patch, or vaginal ring) is first line for prevention of HMB associated with VWD. Combined hormonal contraception is highly efficacious with 88% of women with VWD reporting improvement in their HMB after initiation of treatment with oral contraceptive pills [1,2]. VWF levels are increased by oral contraceptive pills, and, so laboratory assessment should be obtained prior to initiating them, as was done in this patient. The levonorgestrel intrauterine device is also effective in the treatment of HMB and is a suitable alternative therapy for all age groups [2,10,11]. Transexamic acid and ε-aminocaproic acid, both antifibrinolytics, are other treatment options and are often used in conjunction with oral contraceptive pills to control HMB [5].

Patients with VWD are at significant risk of bleeding with invasive procedures. Preoperative consultation with a hematologist is important so that laboratory studies can be ordered and a pre- and postoperative treatment plan can be developed. For hemostatic control where blood loss occurs, 1-desamino-8-D-arginine vasopressin (DDAVP) can be administered to stimulate release of VWF from endothelial cells. DDAVP is intended for use over short intervals of 48–72 hours [6]. If a longer period of treatment is necessary, recombinant factor VIII and VWF concentrate can be administered to replace inherent deficiencies with exogenous factors [6].

Obstetric complications are common in women with VWD, which further underscores the importance of early diagnosis as these complications are more readily managed if the diagnosis of VWD is known prior to conception [9]. During pregnancy, patients should have VWD laboratory testing prior to any invasive procedure. All patients should have testing in the third trimester with the goal of achieving factor VIII and ristocetin cofactor levels greater than 50 IU/dL prior to delivery through 3–5 days afterward [1]. A patient with type I disease with a factor VIII or ristocetin cofactor levels less than 50 IU/dL, or any patient with type II or type III disease is a candidate for prophylaxis and delivery should be in a facility skilled in hemostasis with specialist help available [1]. For acute replacement at the time of delivery, VWF concentrate should be used instead of desmopressin as desmopressin can cause hyponatremia when administered with oxytocin [1,6]. Given the inheritance patterns of VWD, all women with it should be referred to a genetic counselor to discuss the genetic implications of the disease [6]. Further, their fetuses are at risk and invasive fetal procedures and operative vaginal delivery should be avoided given the potential for fetal hemorrhage.

Key teaching points

- Providers should obtain a menstrual, past medical and family history as part of the initial reproductive health visit to aid in the identification of patients with von Willebrand disease (VWD).
- The most common symptom in women with VWD is heavy menstrual bleeding (HMB). VWD should be high on the differential diagnosis in an adolescent with HMB and anemia.
- Early diagnosis of von Willebrand disease can prevent unnecessary bleeding complications.
- No single test reliably identifies VWD, and laboratory results are affected by various factors; patients should be referred to a hematologist for specific diagnosis, continued monitoring, and any necessary prophylaxis for invasive procedures or management of the peripartum period.
- First-line treatment for HMB in VWD is combined hormonal contraceptives.

References

1. Nichols WL, Hultin MB, James AH, et al. Von Willebrand disease (VWD): Evidence-based diagnosis and management guidelines, the National Heart, Lung, and Blood Institute (NHLBI) expert panel report (USA). *Haemophilia* 2008;14:171–232.

2. American College of Obstetricians and Gynecologists. Von Willebrand Disease in women. ACOG Committee Opinion No. 451. *Obstet Gynecol* 2009;114: 1439–43.

3. James, AH. More than menorrhagia: a review of the obstetric and gynecological manifestations of bleeding disorders. *Haemophilia* 2005;11:295–307.

4. Kouides PA. Current understanding of von Willebrand's disease in women:

Some answers, more questions. *Haemophilia* 2006;12(Suppl 3): 143–51.

5. American College of Obstetricians and Gynecologists. The initial reproductive health visit. Committee Opinion No. 460. *Obstet Gynecol* 2010;116: 240–3.

6. Yawn BP, Nichols WL, Rick ME. Diagnosis and management of von Willebrand disease: Guidelines for primary care. *Am Fam Physician* 2009;80:1261–8.

7. The National Heart, Lung, and Blood Institute. *The Diagnosis, Evaluation, and Management of von Willebrand Disease*. NIH Pub. No. 08–5832, December 2007. Available at http://www.nhlbi.nih.gov/guidelines/vwd/vwd.pdf.

8. Ragni MV, Bontempo FA, Hassett AC. Von Willebrand disease and bleeding in women. *Haemophilia* 1999; 5:313–17.

9. Kirtava A, Drews C, Lally C, Dilley A, Evatt B. Medical, reproductive and psychosocial experiences of women diagnosed with von Willebrand's disease receiving care in haemophilia treatment centres: a case-control study. *Haemophilia* 2003;9:292–7.

10. Kingman CE, Kadir RA, Lee CA, Economides DL. The use of levonorgestrel-releasing intrauterine system for the treatment of menorrhagia in women with inherited bleeding disorders. *BJOG* 2004;111:1425–8.

11. American College of Obstetricians and Gynecologists. Management of abnormal uterine bleeding associated with ovulatory dysfunction. Practice Bulletin No. 136. *Obstet Gynecol* 2013;122:176–85.

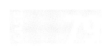

A 13-year-old girl with vulvar irritation and new-onset behavioral problems

Meredith Gray and Eduardo Lara-Torre

History of present illness

A 13-year-old girl is brought to your office by her mother for evaluation of vulvar irritation. The mother reports seeing her daughter constantly touching and scratching her vulva. Her daughter has also been complaining of pain with urination and vaginal itching. The patient denies any vaginal discharge, but has had irregular bleeding and sometimes spotting between periods. She is currently having spotting. She also reports that it feels "raw down there," and will not let her mother look at the area. She denies any local irritants or trauma. She has also been complaining of headaches and stomach aches for the past three months, and has difficulty falling asleep at night. The mother further expresses her concern by recounting recent changes in her daughter's behavior. She describes her as secretive and withdrawn from her friends over the past three to four months. The patient used to enjoy going to her grandfather's house on weekends, but recently has asked her mom if she can just stay at home. You ask her if you can take a look at her vulvar area, and she agrees but wants her mother present during the exam.

When you step out of the room to allow her to change, the mother finds you in the hall and reports that her daughter recently got in trouble at school for showing her genitalia to other children and using sexually explicit language. You ask the mother to please allow you to interview the patient in private. You reenter the room and gently ask the patient, "I understand your mother is worried about you, can you tell me more about that?" The patient does not offer up any further information and becomes tearful.

Physical examination

General appearance: Normally developed teenaged girl in no acute distress, but tearful and nervous

Vital signs:

Temperature: 36.7°C
Pulse: 98 beats/min
Blood pressure: 95/63 mmHg
Respiratory rate: 20 breaths/min
Height: 66 inches
Weight: 100 lb

HEENT: Unremarkable

Neck: Supple

Cardiovascular: Regular rate and rhythm without rubs, murmurs, or gallops

Lungs: Clear to auscultation bilaterally

Abdomen: Soft, nontender, nondistended, active bowel sounds present. No masses palpated. No bruising, cuts, or scars

Extremities: Unremarkable. No bruising

Genital examination (supine frog-leg position): Tanner stage III pubic hair development. Erythema of the labia and perineum is present. No warty lesions, abrasions, or scarring are present. Gentle traction to separate the labia reveals a hymenal laceration with a deep notch at 5 o'clock and evidence of recent bleeding. The full extension of the laceration is visualized. No other hymenal notches, bumps, or lacerations are appreciated. There are no anal lacerations. The urethral meatus and clitoris appear normal

Laboratory studies:

Urine pregnancy test: Negative
Wet mount preparation: No yeast, clue cells or trichomonads
Gonorrhea and chlamydia NAATs obtained on urine specimen

How would you manage this patient?

Child sexual abuse is suspected in this case. The findings of a posterior hymenal transection, deep notches, and perforations raise the suspicion for abuse, but are not diagnostic [1]. The differential diagnosis includes another type of genital injury, such as a straddle injury, which she denies; a congenital variation, which does not present with pain and bleeding; and dermatologic conditions, which do not injure or transect the hymen. A transection of the hymen between 4 and 8 o'clock suggests penetration, but does not confirm sexual abuse [1]. Consensual intercourse between similarly aged adolescents must also be considered. This adolescent's behavioral changes, in particular her sexualized actions and fear to interact with a male relative, are cause for concern and contribute to the suspicion of sexual abuse. Making sure the teen understands that is not her fault, asking her permission to involve her mom for assistance, and making sure she is ready to participate in the examination will allow for a less traumatic experience and facilitate the actual exam. Performing the nongenital examination components first will also allow you to establish a better rapport before performing the genital examination and addressing the affected areas. In this case, a complete description of the history and examination findings was documented including the child's position during the

Acute Care and Emergency Gynecology, ed. David Chelmow, Christine R. Isaacs and Ashley Carroll. Published by Cambridge University Press.

exam. The position used to perform the examination as well as a detailed description of the findings will allow for standardization in case a second examination by a different practitioner is needed. The mother and the teen were informed of the concern for possible abuse in a nonaccusatory manner. The patient was referred to a child forensic nurse examiner, where further documentation and evidence collection took place. She was also enrolled into the local Child Advocacy Center for counseling and follow-up. The suspected abuse was reported to Child Protective Services and the local Police, as required by law.

Child sexual abuse

Child sexual abuse is any sexual activity with someone under the age of 18 years old in which he or she cannot comprehend, give consent, or that violates the laws and norms of society. The US Department of Health and Human Services reports that more than 60 000 children are sexually abused annually, which translates into approximately 1% of children experiencing some form of sexual abuse [2].

Most cases of child abuse are detected when a child discloses that he or she has been abused [3]. The diagnosis of abuse is often based on the child's history alone. Pediatric providers are obligated to screen for abuse (including physical and sexual abuse) at each visit. Screening is generally accomplished by looking for signs of abuse during the general examination such as burns or bruising, as well as by direct questioning to the child or adolescent when suspicion is present. In teens, spending time alone to confidentially address mental health, substance abuse and sexuality is part of the routine visit and is used to directly ask questions regarding abuse. Simple questions such as "Has anyone touched you in a way that made you feel uncomfortable?" should be used, and the use of complex medical language should be avoided as adolescents and children tend to not respond well to its use. In our case, the physical examination findings are highly suggestive of abuse; however, rarely are such clear examination findings such as an acute hymen tear present. Many types of abuse (fondling, exhibitionism, voyeurism, or pornography) are less physically intrusive and leave no physical evidence. For this reason, a careful history and a high index for suspicion from the medical provider are the most important parts of the evaluation.

The history should be obtained with and without the parent or guardian present when possible and without leading questions or strong shows of emotion. The history taken by the medical professional has weight in the legal system and can be used in court as part of the evidence to reach a verdict [4]. Therefore, careful descriptions of the victims' answers, including quotations, should be documented. Expert interviewers often use audiotape or videotape during the interview in accordance with state guidelines.

Victims of abuse struggle with fear, guilt, shame, and embarrassment. These feelings can result in behavioral changes. Most complaints that are possible indicators of sexual abuse are nonspecific. Indirect evidence of sexual abuse can include sleep problems, changes in appetite (increased or decreased), behavioral changes, abdominal pain, anxiety and depression, use of sexual language or behaviors unexpected at the child's chronological age, bladder or bowel control problems, or changes in school performance [5]. Teenagers may turn to substance abuse, running away, or promiscuity.

The physical examination should not result in more emotional trauma to the victim. All actions should be explained to the patient before the examination is performed. It is helpful to have the parent or adult not suspected of abuse present for the exam. A child or adolescent should be examined by a healthcare provider with appropriate training and experience; someone who can interpret normal anatomy, nonspecific findings, and findings associated with healed or new trauma. Special training and certification is required to become a forensic examiner. Although residency programs in Obstetrics and Gynecology as well as Emergency Medicine may train physicians to perform these types of assessments, certified forensic nurse examiners undergo specialized training through postgraduate courses on evidence collection, identification of injuries, documentation guidelines, and post-abuse referrals. Those dealing with children undergo even further training as the approach to children with abuse requires different skills to be able to deal with both patients, and their parents. An immediate evaluation of assault is required if the patient is symptomatic with complaints such as active bleeding from a genital injury, vaginal discharge, vulvar/vaginal pain, or if the abuse has been suspected to have occurred within 72 hours [4]. Otherwise, the examination should be deferred until an experienced clinician or sexual abuse center can be involved. The use of standardized techniques for the interview and exam, as those provided by a pediatric forensic nurse examiner, provides a more reliable source of information to use in court and should be used when available.

A thorough physical examination should be performed looking for signs of physical abuse, neglect, or self-inflicted injuries. The examination should be meticulously documented in writing and with drawings or photography. For children and early adolescents the genital and anal structures can be visualized with the patient in frog-legged or knee-chest prone position. Gentle traction on the labia allows the examiner to inspect the outer vagina and hymen without the need for an internal exam. A bimanual or speculum examination when needed should be targeted to the age of the patient and the clinical presentation. An examination under anesthesia is suggested on those prepubertal children with acute injuries and may include the use of vaginoscopy when the injuries affect the internal genitalia. In adolescents, the use of a speculum smaller than the traditional Graves or Petterson, such as the Huffman speculum (1/2 inches wide × 4 inches long), could facilitate the internal exam, without adding significant discomfort. Table 79.1 lists findings during an examination that are concerning for abuse.

Table 79.1 Findings suspicious for sexual abuse*

Abrasions or bruising of genitalia
Acute or healed tear in the posterior hymen extending to the base of the hymen
Markedly decreased or absent posterior hymenal tissue
Injury to or scarring of the posterior fourchette
Anal bruising or lacerations
Vaginal discharge in the prepubertal patient

* From Adams [3].

Approximately 5% of victims acquire a sexually transmitted disease from their abuser [6,7]. Postpubertal patients should be tested for sexually transmitted diseases (STDs) and pregnancy, as well as offered emergency contraception if applicable. However, more selective criteria can be used for prepubertal children based on the type of abuse, the age of the child, the examination findings, and the prevalence of the diseases in the area. For the most up-to-date recommendations on the screening and treatment of children and adolescents suspected of sexual abuse refer to the Centers for Disease Control and Prevention (CDC) guidelines [7].

All healthcare providers in the United States are required by law to report suspected or confirmed cases of child sexual abuse. Local requirements may vary by state or even by jurisdiction, and providers should check their local agencies such as the Attorney General's office or the local Child Protective Services (CPS) office for details. In most counties a call to the local police department and CPS complies with the requirement. The CPS office is generally staffed by social workers and specialists in child abuse that can guide the provider on the next steps after the initial report. The CPS office will facilitate referrals for the multidisciplinary needs of the patients including medical care, social work, short- and long-term psychological therapy, as well as assist the victims and their caregivers in navigating the legal implications of the abuse. First and foremost our goal is to protect the child and provide healing and safety for our patients.

Key teaching points

- Child sexual abuse should be considered by any practitioner who takes care of a pediatric population when new behavior problems exist and/or physical complaints arise without a clear etiology.
- The evaluation of sexual abuse requires careful questioning and a detailed physical examination with detailed documentation. Such evaluations are best performed by a trained professional, such as a Pediatric Forensic Nurse examiner whenever possible.
- Behavioral changes, abdominal pain, bowel and bladder control problems, sexually advanced language or behavior, substance abuse, or changes in school performance are potential indirect evidence of abuse.
- Posterior hymeneal transections, deep notches, and perforations are findings suspicious for abuse, but are not diagnostic.
- All physicians in the United States are required by law to report suspected as well as known cases of child abuse. Patient history and provider suspicion of abuse are the most important components in the diagnosis.

References

1. Berkoff MC, Zolotor AJ, Makoroff AL, et al. Has this prepubertal girl been sexually abused? *JAMA* 2008;300: 2779–92.
2. Children's Bureau. *Child Maltreatment 2010.* Available at http://www.acf.hhs.gov/programs/cb/pubs/cm10/cm10.pdf.
3. Adams J. Approach to the interpretation of medical and laboratory findings in suspected child sexual abuse: A 2005 revision. *APSAC Advisor* 2005;**Summer**:7–13
4. Adams JA, Kaplan RA, Starling SP, et al. Guidelines for medical care of children who may have been sexually abused. *J Pediatr Adolesc Gynecol* 2007;20:163–72.
5. National Institute for Health and Clinical Excellence. *When to Suspect Child Maltreatment.* Clinical Guidelines CG89, July 2009. Available at http://www.nice.org.uk/CG89.
6. American Academy of Pediatrics. Sexually transmitted diseases in adolescents and children. In Pickering LK, ed. *Red Book: 2012 Report of the Committee on Infectious Diseases*, 29th edn. Elk Grove Village, IL, American Academy of Pediatrics, 2006, p. 166.
7. Centers for Disease Control and Prevention. *Sexually Transmitted Diseases. Treatment Guidelines, 2010.* Available at http://www.cdc.gov/std/treatment/2010/sexual-assault.htm.

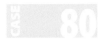

A 10-year-old girl with lower abdominal pain

Lisa Rubinsak and Ellen L. Brock

History of present illness

A 10-year-old girl presents to the emergency room (ER) with a 4-day history of lower abdominal pain that she describes as "constant cramping." She also reports nausea and vomiting associated with the pain a few days ago, but this has resolved. She was seen at another ER when the pain first started, and a CT scan there was reported as "fluid in the endometrium." She was sent home with narcotic analgesics. She was given a follow-up appointment with a gynecologist in the community, but was not able to afford the significant copay. She is again seeking care in the ER as the pain has persisted.

Her past medical history is significant only for obesity. She has not had her first menses but does have breast and pubic hair development. She has never had surgery. She takes no medications.

Physical examination

General appearance: Girl who is in no acute distress
Vital signs:

Temperature: 39.2°C
Pulse: 117 beats/min
Blood pressure: 113/64 mmHg
Respiratory rate: 12 breaths/min

Lungs: Clear to auscultation
Abdomen: Soft, nondistended; mildly tender to palpation in the periumbilical and suprapubic areas with no rebound or guarding
Pelvic (limited to external inspection):

Vulva: Presence of pubic hair, normal appearing virginal hymen, and no bleeding

Laboratory studies:

WBCs: 12 200/μL
Hb: 10.3 g/dL
Ht: 30.8%
Platelet count: 262 000/μL
Sodium: 138 mEq/L
Potassium: 4.3 mEq/L
Chloride: 108 mmol/L
HCO3⁻: 25 mmol/L
Glucose: 122 mg/dL
BUN: 6 mg/dL
Creatinine: 0.46 mg/dL

Imaging: Bedside abdominal ultrasound on admission showed uterus measuring $12.5 \times 10 \times 2$ cm. Right ovary enlarged, measuring $6.7 \times 4.9 \times 4.4$ cm. Fluid collection proximal to uterus measuring 4.2×4.8 cm. MRI is performed (Figs 80.1a,b & 80.2)

How would you manage this patient?

The patient has an ovarian torsion. She was taken to the operating room for diagnostic laparoscopy, where left ovarian torsion and enlarged paratubal cyst were seen (Fig. 80.3). The patient underwent a paratubal cystectomy, and the ovarian torsion was relieved. Figure 80.4 shows the appearance after the torsion was relieved, with improved color in the fallopian tube. The patient's pain was greatly improved postoperatively and she was discharged home the day following surgery.

Pediatric ovarian torsion

Ovarian torsion occurs when adnexal structures twist on their vascular support. Typically, the ovary and fallopian tube rotate together around the broad ligament. As torsion occurs, venous and lymphatic drainage are obstructed. If ovarian torsion goes undiagnosed, arterial blood supply can become compromised. This can ultimately result in infarction, tissue necrosis and loss of ovarian function [1].

Ovarian torsion is uncommon in the pediatric and adolescent population, with estimated incidence of 4.9 per 100 000 females aged 1–20 years [1]. Despite its rarity, it should always be considered in the differential diagnosis of abdominal pain, as ovarian salvage depends on early diagnosis and surgical management. Patients typically present with acute-onset abdominal pain that is localized to one side, more commonly in the right lower quadrant [2,3]. This asymmetry could be due to the presence of the sigmoid colon in the left pelvis lessening the chance for torsion on this side [4]. It has also been proposed that patients with right-sided pain may be more likely to have surgery because of initial concerns for appendicitis [3]. Nausea and vomiting often accompany adnexal torsion. Leukocytosis and fever may indicate necrosis of the ovary, however, normal a white blood cell count does not rule out torsion [3].

Ovarian torsion is a surgical diagnosis, but imaging can often be helpful. Transvaginal ultrasound findings can vary widely in cases of torsion with rates of correct diagnosis ranging from 23 to 74% [5]. The most frequent finding is an

Acute Care and Emergency Gynecology, ed. David Chelmow, Christine R. Isaacs and Ashley Carroll. Published by Cambridge University Press. © Cambridge University Press 2015.

(a)

(b)

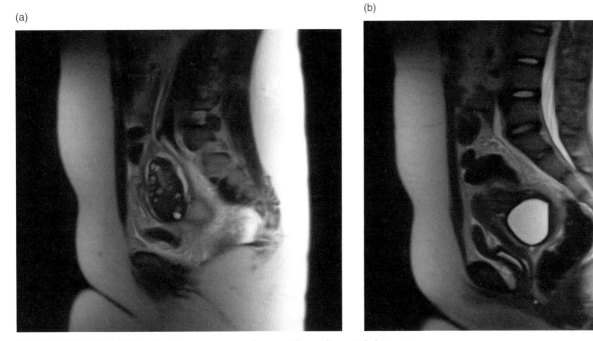

Fig. 80.1 (a,b) Sagittal MRI imaging shows an engorged ovary with an adjacent tubal structure.

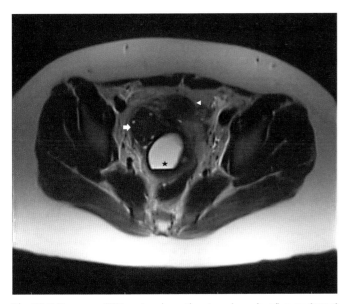

Fig. 80.2 Transverse MRI imaging shows the uterus (arrowhead), ovary (arrow) and paratubal cyst (star).

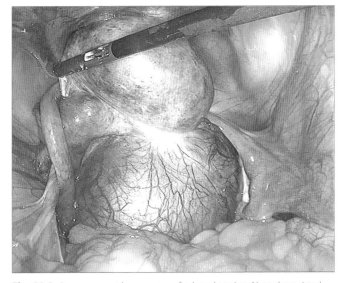

Fig. 80.3 Appearance at laparoscopy of adnexal torsion. Note the twisted infundibulopelvic ligament and the engorged ovary atop the large paratubal cyst.

enlarged ovary or adnexal mass [2]. The absence of adnexal blood flow on Doppler-enhanced imaging is an indicator of torsion, but normal vascular flow does not reliably rule out the diagnosis. If torsion is suspected clinically the patient should undergo laparoscopic evaluation even with normal vascular flow is present. In subacute or chronic cases with less clear clinical presentations, MRI can further assist with the diagnosis. MRI was ordered for this patient because of her prolonged course of pain and her relatively benign exam. The most

specific MRI findings for adnexal torsion are thickening of the tube and an adnexal cystic mass with thickening of the cyst wall [6].

Over the past decade, management of ovarian torsion has moved away from surgical resection. Complete resection of ischemic appearing adnexa was previously performed because it was thought that a blue/black appearing ovary indicated irreversible necrosis. There was also a fear that simple relief of the torsion ("untwisting" the ovary on its pedicle) could

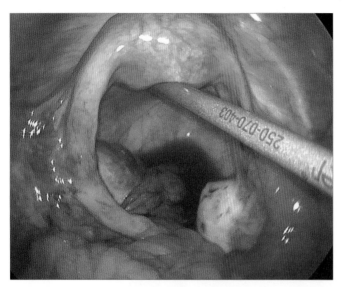

Fig. 80.4 Appearance of the pelvis following relief of the torsion and removal of the paratubal cyst. The ovary is still enlarged but the engorgement and purple color are already resolving.

leave a malignancy in situ or dislodge a thrombus from pelvic veins and cause a thromboembolic complication [2,4]. More recent studies have shown that the intraoperative appearance of the adnexa does not correlate with recovery of ovarian function. In a case series of ovarian torsion patients, all 14 patients who followed up postoperatively were found to have functional ovaries on ultrasound or biopsy despite intra-operative ovarian appearance described as worrisome for moderate to severe ischemia [7]. Similarly, Celik and colleagues found successful return of normal ovarian function in 13 of 14 patients who had relief of torsion despite necrotic appearance on gross examination [8]. Studies have also shown that thrombo-embolic complications are extremely rare. Since 1900, there have been two reported cases of pulmonary embolism associated with ovarian torsion following adnexal resection and no reports of thromboembolism following simple relief of torsion [4]. Malignancy risk in pediatric ovarian torsion cases is also low and data suggest that presence of an ovarian mass should not deter attempted ovarian salvage. Incidence of malignant

neoplasm has been estimated at less than 0.5% of all cases of torsion in the pediatric population [1].

Timely diagnosis and surgical intervention is important in ovarian conservation. The amount of time from torsion to permanent ovarian necrosis is unknown. There are animal studies that demonstrate ovarian reperfusion following relief of torsion if time to intervention was less than 36 hours [3]. In a case series of 22 ovarian torsion patients, those operated on within 8 hours of initial presentation had a salvage rate of 40%, while those operated on within 24 hours had a salvage rate of 33%, and those whose operative intervention was more than 24 hours after initial presentation had no ovaries salvaged [9]. While the differences in ovarian salvage rates were not statistically significant in the study, the trend suggests the importance of early surgical management. The same study also found no correlation between duration of symptoms and ovarian infarction. An ovary can undergo intermittent torsion where adnexal structures twist followed by an uncoiling and reperfusion. This alternating cycle can present as prolonged symptoms prior to diagnosis, but can result in continued viability of ovarian tissue. With no exact time known to cause permanent ovarian necrosis, prolonged pain prior to presentation should not deter prompt evaluation and surgical intervention.

Key teaching points

- Ovarian torsion should be considered in any woman with lower quadrant abdominal pain.
- The most common finding on ultrasound is an enlarged ovary or adnexal mass.
- Normal vascular flow to the ovary on ultrasound does not rule out the diagnosis of ovarian torsion.
- MRI or CT may be useful in an unclear clinical presentation with subacute or chronic symptoms.
- If there is clinical suspicion of torsion, operative intervention should occur in a timely manner.
- Current recommendations for treatment are conservative management with relief of the torsion alone regardless of the gross appearance of the ovary.
- Risks of malignancy and thromboembolic events are very low and should not deter attempted ovarian conservation.

References

1. Guthrie BD, Adler MD, Powell EC. Incidence and trends of pediatric ovarian torsion hospitalizations in the United States, 2000–2006. *Pediatrics* 2010;125:532–8.

2. Poonai N, Poonai C, Lim R, Lynch T. Pediatric ovarian torsion: case series and review of the literature. *Can J Surg* 2013;56:103–8.

3. Rossi BV, Ference EH, Zurakowski D, et al. The clinical presentation and surgical management of adnexal torsion in the pediatric

and adolescent population. *J Pediatr Adolesc Gynecol* 2012;25:109–13.

4. Tsafrir Z, Azem F, Hasson J, et al. Risk factors, symptoms, and treatment of ovarian torsion in children: the twelve-year experience of one center. *J Minim Invasive Gynecol* 2012;19:29–33.

5. Mashiach R, Melamed N, Gilad N, Ben-Shitrit G, Meizner I. Sonographic diagnosis of ovarian torsion: accuracy and predictive factors. *J Ultrasound Med* 2011;30:1205–10.

6. Rha SE, Byun JY, Jung SE, et al. CT and MR imaging features of adnexal torsion. *Radiographics* 2002;22:283–94.

7. Aziz D, Davis V, Allen L, Langer J. Ovarian torsion in children: Is oophorectomy necessary? *J Pediatr Surg* 2004;39(5):750–3.

8. Celik, A. Ergun O, Aldemir H, et al. Long-term results of conservative management of adnexal torsion in children *J Pediatr Surg* 2005;40(4): 704–8.

9. Anders JF, Powell EC. Urgency of evaluation and outcome of acute ovarian torsion in pediatric patients. *Arch Pediatr Adolesc Med* 2005;159: 532–5.

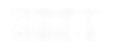

Complete procidentia in a 70-year-old woman

Jordan Hylton and Saweda A. Bright

History of present illness

A 70-year-old gravida 4, para 4 woman presents to the urgent care clinic with complaints of a bulge in her vagina. She reports that she has felt as though her "bottom may fall out" for years and has noticed progressive bulging in her vaginal area for approximately one year. She initially noticed "bulging" during bowel movements or with coughing spells. She now reports a more persistent bulge requiring manual reduction to initiate voids. She has noticed spotting for the last two weeks and increased soreness. She denies urinary or fecal incontinence.

Her past medical history includes well-controlled hypertension for which she takes hydrochlorothiazide and she has had no prior surgical procedures. She had four uncomplicated term vaginal deliveries.

Physical examination

General appearance: Well-appearing woman who is mildly anxious

Vital signs:

Temperature: 37.0°C

Pulse: 78 beats/min

Blood pressure: 124/83 mmHg

Respiratory rate: 16 breaths/min

Oxygen saturation: 98% on room air

Heart: Regular rate and rhythm, no murmurs noted

Lungs: Clear to auscultation bilaterally, no wheezing, rhonchi, or rales

Abdomen: Soft, nontender, thin abdomen, no organomegaly, rebound or guarding

Genitourinary:

External genitalia: Normal appearing, minimal atrophy, no lesions noted

Complete uterine prolapse with the cervix extending 10 cm from the hymen (Fig 81.1). There is moderate cervical erythema and friability with mild ulceration. The uterus is reducible with gentle pressure applied. No adnexal masses

Laboratory studies: Urinalysis within normal limits without evidence of infection

How would you manage this patient?

The patient has symptomatic complete uterine procidentia. She was counseled regarding conservative management with a pessary as well as surgical options. She was not sexually active and elected for a trial of a pessary. She was fitted with a 2.5-inch-long stem gelhorn pessary at her gynecology office, which provided immediate relief in her pressure symptoms. She was also started on estrogen vaginal cream to be used twice weekly to promote healing of the cervical ulcer. She returned to the office in a week to confirm appropriate size of her pessary and she was very pleased with the placement. She was then followed for routine visits every three months to remove and clean the pessary. By six months her cervical ulcer had completely resolved.

Pelvic organ prolapse

The pelvis is a complex system of connective tissue, muscle and ligamentous support which is responsible for many functions including the security of the pelvic organs. With time and considering many factors, this system may fail which can result in pelvic organ prolapse to varying degree. Prolapse occurs in at least one of three vaginal compartments: the apex, the anterior vagina, and the posterior vagina. Apical defects are the most common and involve the cervix or apex of the vaginal vault descending within or out of the vagina. Anterior vaginal wall prolapse often includes the bladder and is referred to as a cystocele whereas posterior wall prolapse often includes the rectum and is called a rectocele. If the prolapse contains small bowel it is referred to as an enterocele. Complete procidentia is the term that is used to describe the phenomena that occurs

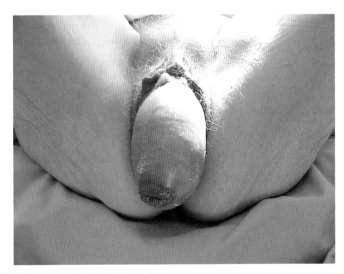

Fig. 81.1 Complete uterine prolapse.

Acute Care and Emergency Gynecology, ed. David Chelmow, Christine R. Isaacs and Ashley Carroll. Published by Cambridge University Press.
© Cambridge University Press 2015.

when the uterus or vagina is entirely prolapsed outside the level of the hymenal ring and is the most advanced stage of pelvic organ prolapse as seen in the patient above.

Risk factors for developing prolapse include advancing age, vaginal births, genetic predisposition, and pelvic surgery.[1] Conditions associated with abnormal collagen fiber, as well as those that lead to increased intra-abdominal pressure, such as chronic airway disease or cough, constipation, and obesity, may also contribute to pelvic organ prolapse. Symptoms of prolapse can widely vary from patient to patient and may or may not correlate with the degree of prolapse. Many patients are asymptomatic and found to have prolapse on a routine pelvic examination. Most other patients complain of varying degrees of pressure or a bulging sensation in the vagina that often is worse with lifting or straining. Women may need to reduce the prolapse manually in order to void or defecate. Some will also complain of concomitant urinary symptoms such as urgency or incontinence. Others have bowel symptoms such as constipation, obstructed defecation, or fecal incontinence.

Obtaining a clear history is important for proper diagnosis and treatment. A survey may be used to assess the extent to which the patient's symptoms have affected her quality of life. The Pelvic Floor Impact Questionnaire as well as Pelvic Floor Distress Inventory surveys are available and commonly used. Associated symptoms such as urinary and fecal incontinence, urgency, retention, and constipation should be discussed and evaluated to survey if patients may need multiple treatment considerations.

Patients are typically examined in dorsal lithotomy position and are asked to valsalva in order to examine the maximum degree of prolapse. The first part of the examination includes assessment of the genital hiatus and perineal body during valsalva. Next, the anterior and posterior compartments of the vagina can be assessed using half of a speculum or a Sims speculum to retract the opposite vaginal wall during a valsalva. Finally, the apex of the vagina is assessed using a speculum to visualize the apex and inspect the maximum degree of descent during a valsalva. If the patient notes that the maximum degree of prolapse is not seen during the supine exam, she may be examined in the standing position.

There are two common staging guidelines for classification of pelvic organ prolapse; the Pelvic Organ Prolapse Quantification system (POP-Q) and the Baden–Walker Staging. The POP-Q is the most recognized system and is consistently used in clinical research. In this system, nine points are measured in centimeters relative to the hymen allowing for a standardized and objective measurement tool to define prolapse, however some have argued that this system is too time consuming or confusing for everyday clinical practice. However one chooses to document prolapse, it is important to assess and document the degree of prolapse in each of the three vaginal compartments as described above. [1]

Treatment of pelvic organ prolapse is dependent upon the degree of symptoms experience by the patient. For those who are asymptomatic, no further treatment is necessary. Patients with minimal to mild symptoms can opt to be managed expectantly, including the use of estrogen cream as well as pelvic floor muscle exercises [2]. For patients who would like to avoid surgery, a pessary can be an acceptable treatment option. Pessary devices are used by some physicians as routine first-line therapy given adequate patient compliance and satisfaction [3]. It is a good solution for patients who are poor surgical candidates. A pessary, usually a plastic or silicone insert, can be fitted in the office after appropriate patient counseling and education. Complications surrounding pessary use are secondary to poor fit and surveillance [4].

For some patients surgery may be a better option or their ultimate choice for management. Decisions regarding approach are based on patient's history, clinical exam, comorbidities, and individual treatment goals. Surgical procedures include sacrocolpoplexy, uterosacral ligament suspension, sacrospinous ligament fixation, and anterior or posterior colporrhaphy. A hysterectomy at the time of repair is a common approach; however, it is not required for those who prefer to preserve their uterus. For patients with complete procidentia who are not sexually active and have no further interest in intercourse, a colpocleisis is a surgical option that can be performed under regional anesthesia and has close to 100% success rate [1].

Key teaching points

- Asymptomatic patients or those with mild symptoms can be offered expectant management with conservative or no treatment.
- For most patients pessary devices are an excellent choice for initial therapy.
- Surgical options may be considered on an individualized basis.

References

1. American College of Obstetricians and Gynecologists. Pelvic organ prolapse. Practice Bulletin No. 85. *Obstet Gynecol* 2007;110:717–29.

2. Ismail SI, Bain C, Hagen S. Oestrogens for treatment or prevention of pelvic organ prolapse in postmenopausal women. *Cochrane Database Syst Rev* 2010, Issue 9. Art. No.: CD007063. DOI: 10.1002/14651858.CD007063. pub2.

3. Bugge C, Adams EJ, Gopinath D, Reid F. Pessaries (mechanical devices) for pelvic organ prolapse in women. *Cochrane Database Syst Rev* 2013, Issue 2. Art. No.: CD004010. DOI: 10.1002/14651858.CD004010.pub3.

4. Royal College of Obstetricians and Gynaecologists. *The Management of Post Hysterectomy Vaginal Vault Prolapse.* Green-top Guideline No. 46, October, 2007. Available at http://www.rcog.org.uk/files/rcog-corp/uploaded-files/GT46Posthysterectomy VaginalProlapse2007.pdf.

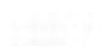

Incontinence in a 50-year-old woman after pessary placement

Tanaz R. Ferzandi

History of present illness

A 50-year-old postmenopausal woman presents to an urgent care clinic due to new-onset urinary incontinence following placement of a pessary for uterine prolapse. She recently went to her primary gynecologist in her hometown for a routine annual visit. At that time she reported a three-year history of a worsening "vaginal bulge" and was found to have grade 3 uterine prolapse per the Baden–Walker assessment scale [1]. A pessary was inserted and the patient noted relief of her pressure symptoms and improvement in constipation, but then shortly thereafter began noticing bothersome symptoms of urinary leakage, which was not an issue prior to the placement of her pessary. She now has complaints of urinary leakage with cough, sneeze and when she tried to attend an exercise class. She has mild overactive bladder symptoms and nocturia, but she is not as bothered by these issues. She has no other medical problems and has had no prior surgeries.

Physical examination

General appearance: Well-developed woman in no acute distress

Vital signs:

Pulse: 67 beats/min
Blood pressure: 130/60 mmHg
Respiratory rate: 16 breaths/min
BMI: 24 kg/m^2

Abdomen: Soft, nontender, nondistended, no palpable masses

Pelvic:

Normal external vulvar and vaginal tissue without any visible lesions
Vulvar atrophy is noted
#5 Ring with support pessary removed (Fig. 82.1)
Negative empty supine stress test
Post-void residual is obtained with a straight catheter for 25 cc
Speculum exam: Atrophy noted, but no erosions or lesions
With maximum valsalva, the genital hiatus is 4 cm and the cervix is distal to the hymen by 2 cm. Both the anterior wall and posterior wall of the vagina protrude to but not beyond the hymenal ring (stage III pelvic organ prolapse or grade 3 uterine prolapse)

Bimanual exam: Uterus is normal sized, midline, and no adnexal masses appreciated
Rectovaginal exam: Fascial defect palpated along the posterior vagina, normal external
Anal sphincter tone and strength: No masses in the rectal vault

Laboratory studies: Urine dipstick is negative for leukesterase, nitrites, and blood

How would you manage this patient?

This patient has new-onset stress urinary incontinence that was unmasked with the reduction of her prolapse with the pessary. Given the type of pessary that the patient had inserted, another # 5 Ring with Support and Knob (Fig. 82.2) was inserted. The patient was offered surgical management of her prolapse, but she opted to continue with the new pessary given her lifestyle and that she was overall content with its use. She was instructed on how to insert, clean and replace her pessary. She was also prescribed vaginal estrogen cream (1 g per vagina, at night, 3 times weekly) to treat the vaginal atrophy. She returned to the clinic in a week to check on her symptoms and to assure

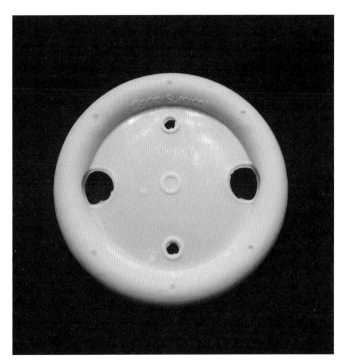

Fig. 82.1 Ring with Support.

Acute Care and Emergency Gynecology, ed. David Chelmow, Christine R. Isaacs and Ashley Carroll. Published by Cambridge University Press.
© Cambridge University Press 2015.

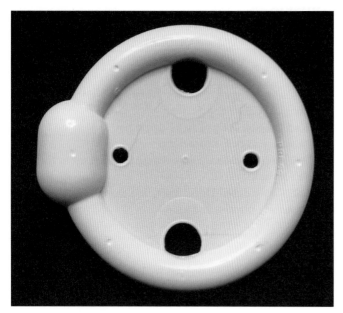

Fig. 82.2 Ring with Knob and Support.

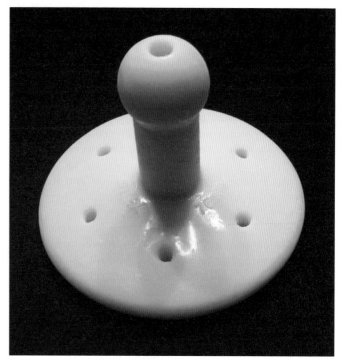

Fig. 82.3 Gellhorn.

that the pessary was comfortable. She reported a 50% improvement in her incontinence symptoms and was pleased with the results as a means for conservative management of her prolapse.

Pelvic organ prolapse

Pelvic organ prolapse is common but the exact prevalence is difficult to ascertain due to many reasons, including the manner in which the studies were conducted, type of classification system used to quantify the prolapse, and the likelihood that many women do not report or seek help for the condition. Pessaries are an excellent method of treatment for many patients, especially in those who desire to avoid surgery, and pessaries have been in use for centuries. In fact, Hippocrates (fifth century BC) commented on the use of a half pomegranate dipped in wine to reduce prolapse. Modern pessaries are made of inert silicone and come in several varieties [2].

To determine the right candidate for a pessary, multiple factors need to be assessed on an individual basis. This includes whether the patient has healthy vaginal epithelium, the ability of the patient to return for routine pessary exams, need for vaginal estrogen, current sexual function, ability to empty the bladder efficiently, and whether a patient might want to remove and insert the pessary herself. It is recommended to have the patient come in for a fitting, and the pelvic organ prolapse quantification assessment can guide selection of a pessary [1]. The most commonly used pessaries are the Ring and Gellhorn (Fig. 82.3). The Gellhorn is usually reserved for those patients with more advanced prolapse and those who are no longer sexually active due to the difficulty associated with removal. After fitting the patient for a pessary, it is recommended she takes some time in the examination room and performs various maneuvers such as bending, squatting,

or jumping to ensure a comfortable fit and appropriate size. If the pessary is the correct size, it should be very comfortable to the patient. The patient is then asked to use the bathroom to assure that she can void, and simulate having a bowel movement (i.e. valsalva) to ascertain if they will expel the pessary. The patient then returns one week later to assess overall function and for a speculum examination to assess the health of the vaginal tissue. In postmenopausal women, we highly recommend concomitant use of a vaginal estrogen cream or ring (the latter serves us very well as we can insert the ring for patients who might have difficulty self-administering the cream, and it will coincide with return visits, as we can replace the ring for them). For patients who use the ring, we place it proximal to the pessary. Patients present every three months to have the pessary removed, cleaned and the vaginal tissue inspected. It is very important to use a speculum and assess not only the lateral walls, but to rotate the speculum and inspect the anterior and posterior walls of the vagina for erosions/abrasions. If such are seen, we then proceed with a "pessary holiday" by having the patient discontinue use of the pessary for a period of time, usually one to three months, depending on extent of damage to the vaginal epithelium, to allow the vaginal epithelium to heal. More liberal use of the vaginal estrogen cream is advised during this time to promote healing. The patient then returns for an examination at the end of this period to ensure proper healing before reinitiating pessary use.

In patients who have concurrent incontinence, or present with such after placement of a pessary, we recommend usage of an incontinence ring pessary or one that has a "knob." The knob is placed anteriorly behind the pubic bone to help with stabilization of the hypermobile urethra. It is difficult to assess to what degree the knob is efficacious, but it's a viable option to help prevent incontinence. In fact, we often warn patients that they might have leakage after the placement of a pessary due to occult incontinence. Symptoms of leakage are often thwarted by the acute angulation of the urethra caused by the prolapse. It is thought that reduction of the prolapse with a pessary unmasks stress urinary incontinence since the angle of the urethra returns to a more normal plane. During the exam, the patient may also be evaluated with an "empty supine stress test." This is a simple and inexpensive method to diagnose for stress urinary incontinence and potential intrinsic sphincter deficiency. With the patient having voided earlier, and while she's in the dorsal lithotomy position, she is asked to cough. If she leaks, it is diagnostic of stress urinary incontinence with 98% positive predictive value [3]. For women who present with incontinence following a pessary placement it is also important to consider other causes of incontinence including urinary tract infections and urinary retention with overflow incontinence. For the patient above, she was evaluated for each of these with a urinalysis and a post-void residual urine assessment, respectively.

Long-term outcomes with pessary use were addressed in a couple of studies. The majority of patients who trial a pessary utilized it for over 5 years, with only minor complications (pain/discomfort 6.9%, excoriation or bleeding 3.2%, disimpaction or constipation 2%) [4]. In another retrospective study, over 14% had continuation of use over 14 years [5]. With regards to counseling for patients who might want to get information regarding progression of prolapse, a recent study monitored 64 women (median follow-up 16 months) who chose expectant management by sequential pelvic organ prolapse quantification system (POP-Q) examinations. They noted that a change in leading edge greater than or equal to 2 cm was significant, and the leading edge ranged from −1.5 to +7 cm. Most of the women were stage II or III prolapse. No change in leading edge was found in 78%, while 19% had progression, and 3% had regression. On multivariate analysis, no variables were associated with change. In this study, 63% of women were satisfied and chose to continue with observation, while 38% chose a pessary or surgery [6].

Key teaching points

- A pessary is an excellent method of treatment for pelvic organ prolapse, especially in those who desire to avoid surgery.
- The most commonly used pessaries are the Ring and Gellhorn.
- In patients who have concurrent incontinence, or present with such after placement of a pessary, the use of an incontinence ring pessary or one that has a "knob" may be beneficial.
- For women who present with incontinence following a pessary placement it is also important to consider other causes of incontinence, including urinary tract infections and urinary retention with overflow incontinence.

References

1. American College of Obstetricians and Gynecologists. Pelvic organ prolapse. Practice Bulletin, No. 85. *Obstet Gynecol* 2007;110:717–29.

2. Oliver R, Thakar R, Sultan AH. The history and usage of the vaginal pessary: a review. *Eur J Obstet Gynecol Reprod Biol* 2011;156:125–30.

3. Lobel RW, Sand PK. The empty supine stress test as a predictor of intrinsic urethral sphincter dysfunction. *Obstet Gynecol* 1996;88(1):128–32.

4. Lone F, Thakar R, Sultan AH, Karamalis G. A 5-year prospective study of vaginal pessary use for pelvic organ prolapse. *Int J Gynecol Obstet* 2011;114:56–9.

5. Sarma S, Ying T, Moore K. Long-term vaginal ring pessary use: discontinuation rates and adverse events. *BJOG* 2009;116:1715–21.

6. Gilchrist AS, Campbell W, Steele H, et al. Outcomes of observation as therapy for pelvic organ prolapse: A study in the natural history of pelvic organ prolapse. *Neurourol Urodyn* 2013;32(4):383–6.

A periurethral mass in a 25-year-old woman

Barbara L. Robinson

History of present illness

A 25-year-old gravida 3, para 1 woman presents to the office complaining of a 1-year history of a vaginal bulge, dyspareunia, and intermittent urinary incontinence. She can feel pressure in the vagina but cannot see a bulge protruding from the introitus. She admits to dyspareunia with both initial insertion and deep penetration. She denies incontinence of urine with coughing, laughing, sneezing, or urgency. However, she experiences post-void dribbling. The feels as if she never completely empties her bladder as she constantly feels the urge to void. She has had three urinary tract infections in the past year, but denies a history of pyelonephritis, nephrolithiasis, hematuria, or urinary hesitancy. She is in a stable relationship with one sexual partner in the past year. She has a remote history of trichomoniasis. Otherwise her medical and surgical histories are negative.

Physical examination

General appearance: Well-nourished woman in no acute distress

Vital signs:

Temperature: 37.2°C
Pulse: 68 beats/min
Blood pressure: 128/70 mmHg
Respiratory rate: 18 breaths/min
Oxygen saturation: 99% on room air

Abdomen: Soft, nontender, nondistended, obese, no organosplenomegaly

External genitalia: Unremarkable

Bladder: Nontender, no palpable masses

Urethra: Meatus midline, suburethral fullness and tenderness. No discharge from the meatus with compression of the midurethra

Vagina: Loss of epithelial rugations in the midurethral area, otherwise no lesions; scant clear discharge; Bartholin's and Skene's glands are unremarkable

Cervix: Parous, no mucopurulent discharge, no lesions

Uterus: Small, anteverted, nontender, mobile

Adnexa: Nontender, no masses

Laboratory studies:

Urine dipstick: Moderate leukocyte estrace, negative nitrites, pH 6.0, trace blood, specific gravity 1.015, negative ketones, negative glucose, negative bilirubin
Urine culture: Negative

Cystourethroscopy was performed in the office with a rigid 30° cystourethroscope after application of 2% lidocaine gel to the urethra

Imaging: MRI was ordered

How would you manage this patient?

The diagnosis is a urethral diverticulum. Pelvic examination revealed an anterior vaginal bulge with loss of epithelial rugations in the midurethral area (Fig. 83.1a,b). On cystourethroscopy the diverticular ostium was identified in the right, posterior aspect of the midurethra (Fig. 83.2). MRI revealed a 3 cm suburethral mass with an ostium at the 7-o'clock position on the urethra. Under general anesthesia in the operating room, a urethral diverticulectomy was performed vaginally. The patient was discharged home on the day of surgery and the Foley catheter remained in place for two weeks. Before discontinuing the Foley catheter, voiding cystourethrography (VCUG) was performed which revealed an intact repair as there was no extravasation of contrast from the urethra. The patient had an uneventful postoperative recovery.

Urethral diverticulum in a female

A urethral diverticulum is a localized protrusion or outpouching of the urethral mucosa into the surrounding nonurothelial tissues [1]. Urethral diverticula are more prevalent among females and most commonly present between the ages of 20 and 60, although they have been reported in adolescents and the elderly [2,3]. Urethral diverticula are uncommon as the prevalence ranges from 0.6 to 6% in adult women, with less than 0.02% of women affected annually [2,4].

The pathogenesis of urethra diverticula remains uncertain; however, the majority of cases are thought to be acquired rather than congenital as they rarely occur in neonates. Congenital diverticula have been proposed to result from a remnant of Gartner's duct, abnormal union of primordial folds or persisting cell rest, especially those of Mullerian origin [1]. Most commonly urethral diverticula are thought to develop as a result of repeated infection of the periurethral glands that become obstructed and enlarged eventually forming a suburethral abscess which eventually ruptures into the urethral lumen [2]. Other possible etiologies include trauma of the lower genital tract from obstetric injury or complication during urethral instrumentation, transurethral bulking procedures, or midurethral sling placement [2]. The majority of urethra diverticula are benign; however, 10% have

Acute Care and Emergency Gynecology, ed. David Chelmow, Christine R. Isaacs and Ashley Carroll. Published by Cambridge University Press. © Cambridge University Press 2015.

(a)

(b)

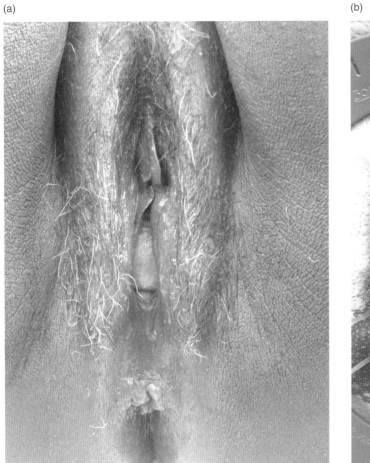

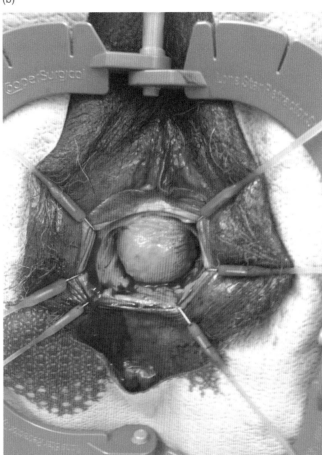

Fig. 83.1 (a,b) Examination of the anterior vaginal wall with a urethral diverticulum.

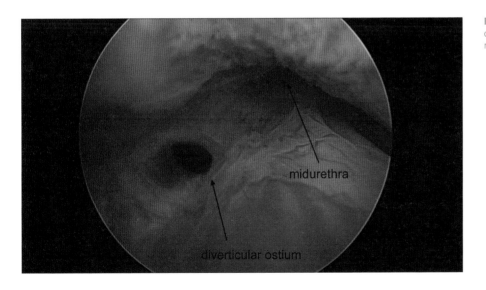

Fig. 83.2 Cystourethroscopy using a 30° cystoscope. A diverticular ostium at 7-o'clock in the midurethral is identified.

midurethra

diverticular ostium

atypical glandular findings, including invasive carcinoma [5]. Thus, careful assessment and follow-up is recommended for all patients with a history and examination concerning for a urethral diverticulum.

Women with urethral diverticula present with a variety of nonspecific symptoms, which may make diagnosis challenging, leading to treatment delays. The classic triad of symptoms includes post-void dribbling, dysuria, and dyspareunia. However, many women present with other complaints including recurrent urinary tract infections, urinary incontinence, urinary frequency and urgency, gross hematuria, urinary retention, pelvic and urethral pain, and purulent urethral discharge [2,5].

Diagnosis of a suspected urethral diverticulum begins with a thorough physical examination with emphasis on the distal genitourinary tract. The external genitalia should be inspected for lesions and anatomic anomalies. The periurethral and Bartholin's glands should be evaluated for tenderness, erythema, and enlargement. The urethral meatus should be carefully inspected for purulent discharge, lateral deviation, or prolapse. The anterior vaginal wall should be visualized noting the presence or absence of epithelial rugations. An identified bulge should be gently palpated to assess tenderness and consistency. In 13–40% of women with urethral diverticulum, urine or purulent material may be expressed from the urethral meatus with gentle compression of the anterior abdominal wall mass [2]. A urinalysis should be performed and, if suspicious for infection, a culture should be sent to exclude infection.

Imaging of the urethra is typically performed to confirm the diagnosis of urethral diverticulum and to assist in surgical planning. VCUG was the initial imaging method used to evaluate the female urethra; however, the accuracy of this technique for suspected urethra diverticula is only 65–85% [6]. Additionally, this modality requires bladder catheterization and patient voiding during the examination, which may be uncomfortable for the patient. Transvaginal ultrasound is an inexpensive and noninvasive method to visualize the urethra but its use is operator dependent and has not been well studied for diagnosis of urethral diverticula. CT voiding urethrography has been shown to have high diagnostic accuracy; however, its disadvantages are similar to that of VCUG [6]. MRI is now considered imaging study of choice for diagnosing urethral diverticula. It provides superb soft-tissue contrast, which allows delineation of the urethral anatomy and its supporting structure with diagnostic sensitivity up to 100% [6]. Urethroscopy may be used as an adjunct to MRI to provide information on the anatomic relationship between the urethra and diverticular ostium. However, urethroscopy is limited in that it does not provide information on the size and complexity of the diverticulum. It has been shown to have a diagnostic accuracy of 15–85% [6].

Expectant management with close observation is acceptable among asymptomatic women with urethral diverticula that do not have malignant characteristics. Similarly, conservative management with prophylactic antibiotics, needle aspiration, or digital compression may be used upon initial presentation. Complete vaginal excision of the diverticulum or vaginal diverticulectomy is the preferred surgical treatment for women with a suburethral diverticulum. For the less common circumferential or dorsal diverticula, a more invasive procedure requiring division of the urethra may be required. Genitourinary tract infections, including infectious cystitis and diverticular abscess, should be treated before proceeding with diverticulectomy. Postoperatively a transurethral Foley catheter should be maintained for one to three weeks to minimize the risk of urethral stricture or formation of urethrovaginal fistula. VCUG may be performed to verify the integrity of the repair before Foley removal, but such imaging is not required. Some providers choose to retrograde fill the bladder with methylene-blue or indigo carmine-dyed solution and look for extravasation of dye during the vaginal speculum examination. If there is extravasation of contrast or dye on either study, the Foley catheter should be replaced for at least one additional week.

Key teaching points

- The classic triad of symptoms of a urethral diverticulum includes post-void dribbling, dysuria, and dyspareunia. However, many women present with other complaints including recurrent urinary tract infections, urinary incontinence, urinary frequency and urgency, gross hematuria, urinary retention, pelvic and urethral pain, and purulent urethral discharge.
- The majority of urethra diverticula are benign; however, 10% have atypical glandular findings, including invasive carcinoma.
- MRI is considered imaging study of choice for diagnosing urethral diverticula with a diagnostic sensitivity up to 100%. Urethroscopy may be used as an adjunct to MRI to provide information on the anatomic relationship between the urethra and diverticular ostium.

References

1. Foley CL, Greenwell TJ, Gardiner RA. Urethral diverticula in females. *BJU Int* 2011;108(Suppl 2):20–3.

2. Antosh DD, Gutman RE. Diagnosis and management of female urethral diverticulum. *Female Pelvic Med Reconstr Surg* 2011;17(6):264–71.

3. Burrows LJ, Howden NL, Meyn L, Weber AM. Surgical procedures for urethral diverticula in women in the United States, 1979–1997. *Int Urogynecol J Pelvic Floor Dysfunct* 2005;16(2):158–61.

4. El-Nashar SA, Bacon MM, Kim-Fine S, et al. Incidence of female urethral diverticulum: A population-based analysis and literature review. *Int Urogynecol J* 2014;25(1):73–9.

5. Thomas AA, Rackley RR, Lee U, et al. Urethral diverticula in 90 female patients: A study with emphasis on neoplastic alterations. *J Urol* 2008; 180(6):2463–7.

6. Singla P, Long SS, Long CM, Genadry RR, Macura KJ. Imaging of the female urethral diverticulum. *Clin Radiol* 2013;68(7):e418–25.

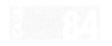

A periurethral mass in a 45-year-old woman

Andrew Galffy and Christopher Morosky

History of present illness

A 45-year-old gravida 3, para 1 woman presents to the office for an annual gynecologic examination and routine screening. She reports that over the past three months she has noticed increasing pressure in the vagina and worsening pain with intercourse. She denies menstrual irregularities, urinary frequency, hesitancy or dribbling, dysuria, dyspareunia, or abnormal vaginal discharge.

Her previous medical history is significant for obesity and hypothyroidism. She takes 100 µg of levothyroxine PO every day. Her previous surgical history includes a postpartum bilateral tubal ligation and two prior dilation and curettage procedures. Her obstetrical history includes a first-trimester termination of pregnancy, a first-trimester spontaneous abortion, and a term normal spontaneous vaginal delivery. All of her previous Pap smears and mammograms have been normal. She denies a history of sexually transmitted infections.

Physical examination

General appearance: Obese woman in no apparent distress
Vital signs:

Temperature: 36.8°C
Pulse: 82 beats/min
Blood pressure: 122/82 mmHg
Respiratory rate: 16 breaths/min
Oxygen saturation: 99% on room air

Cardiovascular: Regular rate and rhythm without murmurs, rubs, or gallops
Lungs: Clear to auscultation bilaterally
Abdomen: Soft, nontender and nondistended, no guarding or rebound, normal active bowel sounds
External genitalia: Normal appearing with no lesions, masses, or discoloration
Vagina: An approximately 4-cm smooth, mobile, nontender mass is palpable in the anterior vaginal wall. The mass is moderately firm, and compression does not produce a discharge from the urethral meatus. There is no distortion of the surrounding structures. On visual inspection, the vaginal epithelium covering the mass is without abnormality (Fig. 84.1)
Cervix: Easily visualized past the anterior vaginal wall mass. Normal in appearance
Uterus: Normal sized and anteverted
Adnexa: Nontender and without masses

Imaging: A T2-weighted contrast MRI of the pelvis reveals a 4.1 × 4.2 cm mass located within the anterior vaginal wall. The mass is clearly separated from the urethra and has homogenous enhancement (Fig. 84.2)

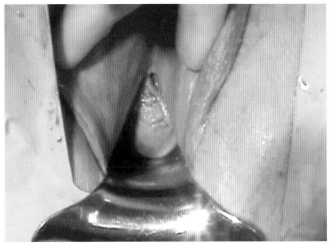

Fig. 84.1 A 4 cm anterior vaginal wall mass that is firm and nontender.

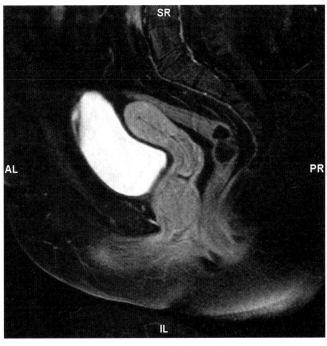

Fig. 84.2 A T2-weighted MRI of the pelvis shows the anterior vaginal wall mass.

Acute Care and Emergency Gynecology, ed. David Chelmow, Christine R. Isaacs and Ashley Carroll. Published by Cambridge University Press.
© Cambridge University Press 2015.

How would you manage this patient?

The patient has an extrauterine leiomyoma located in the anterior vaginal wall. She underwent a transvaginal excision with layered closure. Histologic examination revealed interlacing bundles of benign smooth muscle cells. Due to the proximity of the urethra to the area of excision, the patient wore an indwelling catheter for two weeks to prevent urethrovaginal fistula formation. At her four-week follow-up visit she was completely healed and without complication.

Periurethral masses

Symptomatic periurethral masses are an uncommon occurrence. Description of their workup and management in the literature is mostly limited to case reports or case series [1]. There are a number of pathologic conditions within this anatomic area that may give rise to a periurethral mass and may cause patients to present with a variety of symptoms. Often, however, the clinician may find a mass through palpation of the anterior vaginal wall during the routine physical examination of an asymptomatic patient.

The differential diagnosis of a periurethral mass can be divided into three major categories [2]. The first category is anterior vaginal wall prolapse. Prolapse is a common condition, especially in parous patients. Typically, patients with anterior vaginal wall prolapse present with the complaint of a bulge in the vagina that is worse with increased intra-abdominal pressure or prolonged standing. These patients commonly have some degree of stress urinary incontinence. Physical examination reveals prolapse along the entire anterior vaginal wall that is worsened with Valsalva techniques. A discrete periurethral mass is seldom encountered in the patient with prolapse.

Conditions specific to the urethra and urologic system are the next category and include urethral diverticulum, periurethral fibrosis, ectopic ureterocele and Skene's gland abscesses. These patients will commonly have some degree of urinary symptoms, including dysuria, frequency, hesitancy, incomplete emptying or dribbling of urine. Compression of the periurethral mass often results in expression of urine or purulent material from the urethra. This maneuver has been termed, "milking the urethra."

The final category is benign and malignant neoplasms arising from the vagina and urethra. These include vaginal leiomyoma, vaginal wall inclusion cysts, Gartner's duct cysts, vaginal cancer and urethral cancer. The combination of a periurethral mass and bloody discharge from the urethra should raise the suspicion for a malignant condition. These patients should be worked-up in collaboration with a gynecologic or urologic oncologist. The discovery of any periurethral mass warrants further investigation because although most periurethral masses are of benign etiology, proper diagnosis is essential for management decisions.

When beginning the diagnostic workup, the initial presentation of the patient will often aid in exclusion of many of the pathologies listed above. For instance, in the case of our patient she reported increased vaginal pressure and dyspareunia, however she had no complaints of bleeding, discharge, dysuria or incontinence. Also the mass was firm, smooth, and mobile, which suggests a solid and not cystic mass. The fact that it was smooth and mobile also reduces the chance of it being malignant. While these findings are extremely informative, additional workup is needed due to the diversity of the differential diagnosis and the relatively low incidence of most of the conditions on our list.

The next step is to obtain an imaging study that will most effectively aid in obtaining the diagnosis and therefore planning the appropriate management. The most efficient imaging modality to start with when working up a discrete periurethral mass is generally ultrasound. Even when suspicion for urethral diverticulum, the most common discrete periurethral mass, is high, voiding cystourethrography (VCUG) and retrograde positive pressure urethrography are no longer recommended for routine evaluation due to their low sensitivity, exposure to radiation, and lack of providing additional information [3,4,5]. A study comparing ultrasound to VCUG found that both techniques were able to diagnose 13 of 15 urethral diverticula, however ultrasound was also able to diagnose periurethral cysts and leiomyomas not detected by VCUG [6].

The most effective imaging modality available to diagnose periurethral masses is MRI. Some authors argue that MRI should always be the first-line imaging modality despite its increased expense and limited availability when compared to ultrasound [7]. When the mass is evidently solid, MRI is a reasonable initial choice as it can substantially aid not only in diagnosis but also surgical planning. MRI provides multiplanar resolution lending superior tissue resolution and allows for differentiation between normal anatomic variants, soft tissue masses, and urethral pathology. The MRI findings of our patient showed that the mass was located within the anterior vaginal wall and clearly separated from the urethra with homogenous enhancement. The decision was made to excise the mass so as to obtain a pathologic diagnosis.

The histologic evaluation revealed interlacing bundles of benign smooth muscle cells consistent with a leiomyoma. While the vast majority of leiomyoma are found within the uterine corpus, the rare appearance of extrauterine leiomyomas is occasionally encountered. Extrauterine leiomyomas have been noted to present in various ways: benign metastasizing, parasitic, intravenous leiomyomatosis, leiomyomatosis peritonealis disseminata, and other miscellaneous locations have been reported [8,9]. In general, leiomyomas with rare growth patterns tend to be found in women of reproductive age, often with a history of uterine surgery. It is still unclear if these tumors occur from hematogenous spread of smooth muscle cells from the uterus or if they arise from proliferation of smooth muscle cells in the extrauterine location.

Surgery should be performed by an experienced vaginal surgeon whenever in close proximity to the urethra due to the concern of urethral injury and subsequent urethrovaginal fistula formation following such procedures. The use of a layered closure when repairing the incision is used to reduce the risk of fistula formation and prevent stricture that can cause urethral obstruction. In certain cases where large excisions are required, the use of interpositional flaps or grafts may be required. In addition, the use of a transurethral indwelling catheter for two weeks can prevent urethrovaginal fistula formation and urethral stricture.

Key teaching points

- Periurethral masses can present with a broad range of symptoms including urinary complaints, pain with intercourse, or a bulge or pressure in the vagina. However, many patients may be asymptomatic when they are discovered to have a periurethral mass on routine examination.

- Abnormal variants of the distal urologic tract can present as distinct periurethral masses. These include urethral diverticulum, periurethral fibrosis, ectopic ureterocele, and Skene's gland abscesses.

- Both malignant and benign neoplasms can arise from the periurethral tissues. The combination of an enlarging periurethral mass and bloody urethral discharge should raise the concern for malignancy.

- Both transvaginal ultrasonography and MRI are superior to voiding cystourethrography in diagnosing the etiology of periurethral masses.

- Periurethral leiomyomas are a rare but recognized unusual location to find extrauterine fibroids. Their treatment entails surgical excision with layered closure. Care must be taken to avoid urethrovaginal fistulas and urethral stricture following excision.

References

1. Blaivas JG, Flisser AJ, Bleustein CB, Panagopoulos G. Periurethral masses: Etiology and diagnosis in a large series of women. *Obstet Gynecol* 2004; 103(5 Pt 1):842–7.

2. Dmochowski RR, Ganabathi K, Zimmern PE, Leach GE. Benign female periurethral masses. *J Urol* 1994; 152(6 Pt 1):1943–51.

3. Golomb J, Leibovitch I, Mor Y, Morag B, Ramon J. Comparison of voiding cystourethrography and double-balloon urethrography in the diagnosis of complex female urethral diverticula. *Eur Radiol* 2003; 13(3):536–42.

4. Jacoby K, Rowbotham RK. Double balloon positive pressure urethrography is a more sensitive test than voiding cystourethrography for diagnosing urethral diverticulum in women. *J Urol* 1999;162(6):2066–9.

5. Lee JW, Fynes MM. Female urethral diverticula. *Best Pract Res Clin Obstet Gynaecol* 2005;19(6):875–93.

6. Siegel CL, Middleton WD, Teefey SA, et al. Sonography of the female urethra. *Am J Roentgenol* 1998;170(5): 1269–74.

7. Shadbolt CL, Coakley FV, Qayyum A, Donat SM. MRI of vaginal leiomyomas. *J Comput Assist Tomogr* 2011;25(3): 355–7.

8. Fasih N, Shanbhogue A, Macdonald DB, et al. Leiomyomas beyond the uterus: Unusual locations, rare manifestations. *RadioGraphics* 2008;28:1931–48.

9. Quade BJ, Robboy SJ. Uterine smooth muscle tumors. In Robboy SJ, Mutter GL, Prat J, et al., eds. *Robboy's Pathology of the Female Reproductive Tract*, 2nd edn. Oxford, Churchill Livingstone Elsevier, 2009, p. 474.

New-onset incontinence in a 42-year-old woman

Tanaz R. Ferzandi

History of present illness

A 42-year-old, premenopausal, healthy woman presents with new-onset urinary incontinence that has lasted for a week. She also complains of burning and irritation in the vagina and has used over-the-counter anti-fungal cream for a presumed yeast infection. She feels that the symptoms are getting worse and it is painful to urinate. She has some urinary urgency and suprapubic tenderness, but denies any other discomfort. She denies any fever, chills, nausea, vomiting, or back pain. She has been recently reunited with her husband who has been overseas for the past two months on a job assignment. She has no other medical problems and her only prior surgery was a postpartum tubal ligation.

Physical examination

General appearance: Well-developed woman in no acute distress

Vital signs:

Pulse: 67 beats/min
Blood pressure: 130/60 mmHg
Respiratory rate: 16 breaths/min
BMI: 25 kg/m^2

Abdomen: Soft, nontender, nondistended, no palpable masses

Back: No costo-vertebral tenderness

Pelvic:

No lesions on external genitalia
No discharge or cervical lesions noted on speculum exam
Normal uterus and adnexa with no tenderness

Laboratory studies:

Urine dipstick: ++ Nitrites, ++ leukocyte esterase, + blood

How would you manage this patient?

This patient has a urinary tract infection (UTI) based on her symptoms and the urine dipstick results obtained in clinic. Per current guidelines, she was given a prescription for nitrofurantoin monohydrate 100 mg BID for 7 days [1]. As this was her first UTI, a urine culture was not sent and the patient was instructed to follow-up in 48–72 hours if her symptoms were not improved. She was also provided a urinary analgesic (phenazopyridine hydrochloride) to aid in symptom relief.

Urinary tract infections

More than half of all women will have at least one UTI in their lifetime, while 3–5% of women will have multiple recurrences. The cost is staggering, if office visits are taken into account, with an estimated 3.5 billion dollars for evaluation and treatment in 2000 [2]. Risk factors include, but are not limited to, young age at first UTI, prior history of UTI, frequent or recent sexual activity, new sexual partner, use of diaphragm as contraception, use of spermicidal agents, increasing parity, diabetes mellitus, obesity, and urinary tract calculi [1]. UTIs typically involve fecal flora with the most common pathogens being *Escherichia coli* (75–95% of all infections), *Staphylococcus saprophyticus*, *Klebsiella pneumonia*, *Enterococcus faecalis*, *Streptococcus agalactiae* (group B streptococcus), and *Proteus mirabilis*. In essence, these pathogens colonize the vagina and cause an ascending infection in the bladder via the urethra.

A UTI is considered uncomplicated if it occurs in a healthy premenopausal woman who is not pregnant and does not have a history of an anatomic abnormality of the urinary tract. Cystitis is the term that captures an infection limited to the lower urinary tract, with symptoms of dysuria and urinary urgency. Asymptomatic bacteruria refers to the case of significant bacteruria without symptoms of infection. UTIs can be relapsing, meaning that the patient has an infection with the same organism after adequate therapy. Reinfection is defined as a UTI that occurs after the patient has cleared the initial infection with the previously isolated bacteria. Recurrent UTIs are defined as more than three UTIs in one year or more than two UTIs in six months.

Clinical presentation and symptomatology is important in the diagnosis of an uncomplicated case of acute cystitis. Common symptoms include dysuria, urinary frequency and urgency, suprapubic pain, and hematuria. It is prudent to keep in mind that the differential diagnosis might include acute urethritis due to infections caused by *Neisseria gonorrhoeae* and *Chlamydia trachomatis*, which also present with dysuria; pain secondary to genital herpex simplex virus (type 1, type 2) can also cause similar symptoms. Therefore, patients with additional complaints of a vaginal discharge warrant a pelvic examination to rule out vaginitis or urethritis. A common office test helpful for diagnosis includes a clean-voided midstream urine sample and urinalysis by dipstick. Urine dipstick testing for leukocyte esterase or nitrite is a rapid and inexpensive method with a sensitivity of 75% and specificity of 82%; however, the use of the dipstick as a surrogate has also come into question [3]. In cases where there is a high suspicion for a UTI based on history and a negative dipstick, further testing is warranted as negative dipstick testing does not reliably rule out infection. Additional testing includes formal urinalysis and urine culture.

Formal urinalysis testing with microscopic identification of white blood cell count greater than or equal to $10/\mu L$ (pyuria) along with the presence of bacteria is highly suggestive of infection. Urine culture is very helpful in the diagnosis as well as antibiotic selection. The basic criterion of greater than or equal to 100 000 colony-forming units per millilitre (CFU/mL) of clean-catch urine for the diagnosis of UTI has been validated repeatedly. Bacterial counts greater than or equal to 100 000 CFU/mL in two consecutive clean-catch urine samples allows differentiation between asymptomatic UTI and contamination ($<100 000$ CFU/mL). For infections with *S. saprophyticus* and *Candida* sp., the lower cut-off level of greater than or equal to 10 000 CFU/mL is commonly accepted. Contamination is sometimes unavoidable and remains a pitfall in the diagnosis of UTI. Contamination is likely if only small numbers of bacteria or several bacterial species grow in urinary cultures. *Lactobacilli*, *Corynebacteria* sp., *Gardnerella*, alpha-haemolytic streptococci, and aerobes are considered urethral and vaginal contaminants. The presence of true infection can be confirmed by urethral catheterization or more accurately by suprapubic aspiration [4]. Urine culture is not required for the diagnosis of uncomplicated cystitis, but is helpful in cases where the diagnosis is unclear or in situations where a patient has failed standard treatment.

Acute uncomplicated cystitis is a benign condition, and early resolution of symptoms is observed in 25–42% of women [2]. However, UTIs are one of the most common reasons for prescription of antimicrobials to otherwise healthy young women. In spite of study guidelines that are specific to the condition, selection of antimicrobials varies greatly, in the setting of greater resistance. Specific guidelines have focused on the treatment of premenopausal, nonpregnant women with no known urological abnormalities or comorbidities. Leading societies such as the American College of Obstetricians and Gynecologists (ACOG) and the Infectious Diseases Society of America (IDSA) have updated their guidelines in an effort to standardize and help prevent ongoing resistance. Below is a summary of those guidelines and the references are listed for further study [1,5].

First-line therapy

First-line therapy includes the following:

- Nitrofurantoin monohydrate/macrocrystals 100 mg BID × 5–7 days, or:
- Trimethoprim–sulfamethoxazole 160/800 mg (one DS tablet) BID × 3 days (avoid if resistance prevalence is known to be >20% or if used for UTI in past 3 months), or:
- Fosfomycin trometamol 3 g single dose (lower efficacy than for those listed above), or:

- Pivmecillinam 400 mg BID × 5 days (currently not available in the United States).

Second-line therapy

Second-line therapy is as follows:

- Fluoroquinolones (resistance prevalence high in some areas), or:
- Beta-lactams (avoid ampicillin or amoxicillin alone; lower efficacy).

Continuous antimicrobial prophylaxis

A daily bedtime dose (except for fosfomycin) as follows:

- Nitrofurantoin: 50–100 mg.
- Trimethoprim–sulfamethoxazole: 40 mg and 200 mg.
- Cephalexin: 124–250 mg.
- Fosfomycin: 3 g sachet every 10 days.

Nitrofurantoin monohydrate/macrocrystals and trimethoprim-sulfamethoxazole 160/800 mg are the preferred drugs of choice in young, healthy women as empiric treatment. The former has a low resistance profile, while the latter is higher. Clinicians should be aware of their particular geographic regions' susceptibilities. Additionally, nitrofurantoin monohydrate/ macrocrystals should be used with caution in patients with known glucose-6-phosphate dehydrogenase deficiency, as it can induce hemolytic anemia in rare instances.

Some guidelines, such as those proposed by the American Urological Association and the IDSA recommend that fluoroquinolones be avoided due to the dramatic emergence of antibiotic resistance. In an era of greater antibiotic resistance, it is recommended that not all patients get empiric treatment routinely. For patients without a prior laboratory confirmed UTI, an office visit for urinalysis is appropriate prior to initiation of antibiotics. In patients with atypical symptoms or those who have had a recurrence of a UTI, treatment should be based on obtaining a urine culture. For those patients with recent treatment failures or re-infections, it is also recommended to obtain a follow-up culture within two weeks of completion of antibiotics to confirm resolution.

In patients with recurrent UTIs, the need for continuous antibiotic prophylaxis or postcoital prophylaxis should be assessed. Daily antibiotic prophylaxis for 6–12 months has been proved to be effective in the prevention of recurrent UTIs, even reducing the risk of recurrence by 95%, when compared with placebo [6]. The issue of prevention should also be discussed with patients, including hygiene practices. Interestingly, case control studies have shown no clear, significant associations between recurrent UTIs and precoital or postcoital voiding patterns, daily beverage consumption, frequency of urination, delayed voiding habits, wiping patterns, tampon use, douching, use of hot tubs, types of underwear, or body mass index [2]. Many patients use cranberry supplements in a variety of formulations, with mixed evidence to support its use. The theory behind cranberry use is that it keeps the bacteria from adhering to the urothelium, due to its fructose and proanthocyanidins [5]. One study randomized patients who had recurrent UTIs to a combination of tablets, juice, and placebo. The conclusion of the study was that cranberry tablets were the best in reduction of UTIs, followed by cranberry juice, and, lastly, placebo ($P < 0.05$) [7].

Key teaching points

- Patients with a first presentation of a urinary tract infection should have an office evaluation with urinalysis to confirm diagnosis prior to initiating antibiotics.

- Nitrofurantoin monohydrate/macrocrystals and trimethoprim–sulfamethoxazole 160/800 mg are the preferred drugs of choice in young, healthy women as empiric treatment.
- Fluoroquinolones should be avoided as a first-line therapy for acute uncomplicated cystitis.
- Daily antibiotic prophylaxis for 6–12 months has been proved to be effective in the prevention of recurrent UTIs.
- Urine culture is not required for the diagnosis of uncomplicated cystitis, but is helpful in cases where the diagnosis is unclear or in situations where a patient has failed standard treatment.

References

1. American College of Obstetricians and Gynecologists. Treatment of urinary tract infections in nonpregnant women. Practice Bulletin, No. 91. *Obstet Gynecol* 2008;111(3):785–94.

2. Hooton TM. Uncomplicated urinary tract infection. *N Engl J Med* 2012;366:1028–37.

3. Khasriya R, Khan S, Lunawat R, et al. The inadequacy of urinary dipstick and microscopy as surrogate markets of urinary tract infection in urological outpatients with lower urinary tract symptoms without acute frequency and dysuria. *J Urol* 2010:183;1843–7.

4. Franz M, Hörl WH. Common errors in diagnosis and management of urinary tract infection. I: Pathophysiology and diagnostic techniques. *Nephrol Dial Transplant* 1999;14(11):2746–53.

5. Gupta K, Hooton TM, Naber KG, et al. International Clinical Practice Guidelines for the treatment of acute uncomplicated cystitis and pyelonephritis in women: A 2010 Update by the Infectious Diseases Society of America and the European Society for Microbiology and Infectious Diseases. *Clin Infect Dis* 2011;52(5): e103–20.

6. Hooton TM. Recurrent urinary tract infection in women. *Int J Antimicrob Agents* 2001:17(4):259–68.

7. Jepson RG, Craig JC. Cranberries for preventing urinary tract infections. *Cochrane Database Syst Rev* 2008, Issue 1. Art. No.: CD001321. DOI: 10.1002/14651858.CD001321.pub5.

Urinary leakage following hysterectomy

Edward J. Gill

History of present illness

A 47-year-old gravida 4, para 2-0-2-2 woman presents on postoperative day 9 from a laparoscopic-assisted vaginal hysterectomy with a complaint of watery vaginal discharge. The discharge is constant throughout the day and she is now wearing a pad daily. She denies dysuria or urinary urgency. The indication for surgery was a history of pelvic pain, irregular bleeding and fibroids. Her surgery was uncomplicated as she was discharged home on postoperative day 1. She is a smoker and has had diabetes mellitus for 18 years. The preoperative evaluation included a transvaginal ultrasound, which showed an $11.0 \times 8.3 \times 6.6$ cm uterus with several fibroids, the largest measuring 4.1 cm. Ovaries appeared normal with no other pathology seen. Her past history is significant for two Cesarean section deliveries. Preoperative laboratory evaluation included Hb 10.2 g/dL and a HbA1c of 7.7.

Physical examination

General appearance: Well-appearing woman in no distress

Vital signs:

Temperature: 37.0°C
Pulse: 95 beats/min
Blood pressure: 132/78 mmHg
Respiratory rate: 16 breaths/min
Oxygen saturation: 100% on room air
BMI: 38.8 kg/m^2

Abdomen: Soft, nontender, incisions healing well, normoactive bowel sounds

External genitalia: Unremarkable

Vagina: Vaginal cuff healing well, small amount of watery fluid pooled in vault

Cervix: Absent

Uterus: Absent

Adnexa: Nontender, without masses

Laboratory studies:

Urine analysis: pH 5.5; specific gravity 1.010; WBCs 20–40/high power field; RBCs 10–20/high power field
Hb: 9.8 g/dL (normal 12.1–15.1 g/dL)
WBCs: 12 000/μL (normal 4500–10 000/μL)
Glucose: 208 mg/dL

How would you manage this patient?

Due to the symptoms of a persistent watery vaginal discharge and examination findings of fluid-filling the vaginal vault, there is a high suspicion for a post-hysterectomy vesicovaginal fistula (VVF). A CT urogram was ordered and the diagnosis was confirmed (Fig. 86.1). A 4 mm VVF was identified at the superior portion of the vagina just left of the midline. She was initially managed with continuous bladder drainage with an indwelling transurethral Foley catheter for four weeks; however, this failed to resolve the fistula. She then underwent surgical repair via a vaginal approach with a Latzko partial colpocleises. This surgery was uncomplicated and she was managed postoperatively with continuous bladder drainage via a transurethral Foley catheter for 10 days along with daily antibiotic suppression while the catheter remained in place. A cystogram was performed to confirm integrity of the repair prior to catheter removal. At her six-week postoperative visit, her symptoms had completely resolved.

Post-hysterectomy vesicovaginal fistula

A vesicovaginal fistula (VVF) is an abnormal connection between the bladder and vagina that causes persistent and involuntary leakage of urine into the vagina. VVFs are the most common urogenital fistula encountered. Other less common types of urogenital fistula include ureterovaginal, urethrovaginal, vesicocervical, and vesicouterine fistulas. In developing countries VVF are most commonly caused by obstructed labor and obstetrical trauma. However, in developed areas such as the United States and Europe, over 90% of VVFs are caused by bladder injury at the time of hysterectomy. A majority of these bladder injuries are unrecognized at the time of surgery and lead to poor healing and fistula formation.

Performing a hysterectomy usually requires at least some dissection of the bladder off of the upper vagina and lower uterus to complete the procedure. In addition, the ureters run in close proximity to the lateral borders of the lower uterus and cervix and are at risk of injury during hysterectomy. Recent reports on the overall incidence of lower urinary tract (LUT) injury after hysterectomy range from 0.23 [1] to 4.8% [2]. Most series report that laparoscopic hysterectomy has the highest rate of LUT and subtotal (supracervical) and vaginal hysterectomies have the lowest reported rate of injury. However, Vakili and colleagues reported a trend toward a higher

Acute Care and Emergency Gynecology, ed. David Chelmow, Christine R. Isaacs and Ashley Carroll. Published by Cambridge University Press. © Cambridge University Press 2015.

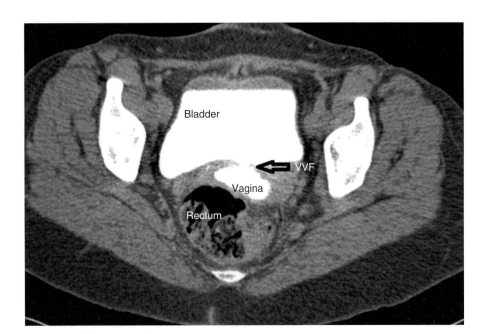

Fig. 86.1 Superiorly located vesicovaginal fistula with a 4 mm neck just left of the midline with contrast filling the bladder and vagina.

rate of bladder injury with vaginal hysterectomy with a rate of 6.3%, which is higher than previously reported [2]. Supracervical hysterectomy limits the amount of bladder dissection required and may explain the lower rate of injury to the LUT. It is unclear what effect the newer robotic approach to hysterectomy will have on LUT injury.

All hysterectomies have an inherent risk of LUT injury, but some conditions increase that risk. Ischemia, tissue hypoxia, infection, diabetes, prior pelvic radiation, and smoking are known risk factors for poorer healing. In patients with these conditions small injuries or needle injuries of the bladder are more likely to heal poorly and progress to fistula formation. Any conditions that disrupt normal anatomy predispose to injury at the time of surgery and increase the risk of fistula formations. These conditions include leiomyomata (myomas or fibroids), endometriosis, prior pelvic infections, including pelvic inflammatory disease (PID), and prior pelvic surgery, especially prior Cesarean section(s) since this common operation usually requires a similar bladder dissection as hysterectomy and can result in scar tissue formation in the direct path of hysterectomy surgery. Cesarean section was the most common identifiable risk factor associated with injury occurring in Tancer's review [3].

VVF can present any time after surgery and depends on the size, location, and etiology of the fistula. Large anterior vaginal wall lacerations can present immediately postoperatively, while devascularization injuries can take up to 30 days to present. Fistulas after pelvic radiation may not emerge for one year or longer. The most common symptom is leakage of urine or thin watery vaginal discharge. Leakage can be intermittent or continuous. The patient may still retain normal voiding patterns in the face of a genitourinary (GU) fistula and this cannot be relied on to eliminate the possibility of a GU fistula. In addition, the patient may have dysuria, hematuria, cystitis, abdominal, or flank pain. Some patients with a VVF will have no leakage of fluid from the vagina.

The evaluation of VVF after hysterectomy requires a speculum examination looking for abnormal fluid in the vagina and a thorough search for a fistula opening. Posthysterectomy VVF are often very small and can be difficult to visualize. Creatinine, blood urea nitrogen, and electrolytes can be ordered on any collected vaginal fluid to see if it consistent with urine. The urine analysis may show hematuria and/or pyuria. This may be from a UTI or from inflammation or bleeding at the site of injury. Urine culture is required to distinguish the two. In addition to urine analysis, consideration should be given to imaging both upper and LUT. A CT urogram with intravenous contrast is the preferred imaging modality as it can also detect unrecognized ureteric injury which can happen concomitantly in up to 12% of cases [4]. Cystourethroscopic examination will also eventually be required but is not mandatory in the initial evaluation and management of a postoperative GU fistula. Other tests that can be done in the outpatient setting to help identify a fistula include placing a pad or tampon in the vagina followed by maneuvers to color the urine to make it easier to identify and visualize any fluid leaking into the vagina. Examples include oral phenazopyridine hydrochloride (Pyridium®) (orange-red), intravesical administration of methylene blue via transurethral catheter or intravenous indigo carmine dye. Under normal circumstances no colored fluid should be seen on the vaginally placed tampon. Discoloration of the tampon vaginally should prompt a further search for urogenital fistula.

Conservative treatment of a postoperative VVF includes treating any concurrent UTI and placement of an indwelling catheter to continually drain the bladder. With small fistulas, conservative treatment with continuous bladder drainage has been curative without the need for surgery [5]. The outcomes of this treatment are variable and success rates have been found to be highest when the fistula is identified in the first few days following the surgical injury. Injuries that are identified weeks following surgery, those with larger fistulous openings or in women with risk factors for poor healing are less likely to resolve with continuous bladder drainage. At least 30 days of continuous bladder drainage is recommended for optimal healing and consideration of low-dose antibiotic prophylaxis with nitrofurantoin or trimethoprim should be given to prevent catheter-associated infection.

For those who fail continuous bladder drainage or are poor candidates for conservative management, surgical revision is necessary. Occasionally, when larger fistulas are recognized immediately and there is limited inflammation, they can be surgically repaired without delay. More commonly, surgery is delayed for at least six weeks when most inflammation has resolved. Surgical repair of fistulas associated with pelvic radiation may not be repaired for up to one year. Any fistula associated with pelvic malignancy will require a biopsy of the fistula tract. The surgical approach to fistula repair depends on location, size, and surrounding tissue quality of the fistula. When possible, a vaginal approach to repair offers a low morbidity and shorter recovery option compared to an abdominal approach. Consultation with Urogynecolgy or Urology would be appropriate for recommendations on surgical approach and repair.

Following surgical repair, continuous bladder drainage for 7–14 days with a transurethral or suprapubic catheter is recommended to promote healing. A cystogram is typically performed to ensure integrity of the repair prior to catheter removal. For postmenopausal women, vaginal estrogen treatment may promote vaginal healing and by improving tissue vascularization. Patients are counseled to strictly adhere to pelvic rest with nothing inserted into the vagina for at least six weeks following surgical repair.

Key teaching points

- Risk factors for vesicovaginal fistula (VVF) after hysterectomy includes conditions that predispose to poor healing, including diabetes mellitus, smoking, prior pelvic radiation, and tissue hyopoxia. In addition, conditions that disrupt the anatomy, including leiomyomata, prior pelvic surgery, a history of prior pelvic infection including pelvic inflammatory disease, and endometriosis, also increase the risk of VVF.

- The diagnosis of VVF requires a high index of suspicion in patients complaining of vaginal discharge after hysterectomy and a thorough examination to investigate this complaint, including a speculum examination to search for a fistula opening.

- A CT urogram with intravenous contrast is the preferred imaging modality as it can also detect unrecognized ureteric injury which has been reported to occur in up to 12% of cases of VVF.

- Smaller fistulas may respond to conservative treatment with an indwelling catheter, but larger fistulas and those with other risk factors will often require surgical repair.

References

1. Harkki-Siren P, Sjoberg J, Titner A. Urinary tract injury after hysterectomy. *Obstet Gynecol* 1998;92(1)113–18.

2. Vakili B, Chesson RR, Kyle BL, et al. The incidence of urinary tract injury after hysterectomy: A prospective analysis based on universal cystoscopy. *Am J Obstet Gynecol* 2005;192(5):1599–604.

3. Tancer ML. Observations on prevalence and management of vesicovaginal fistulas after total hysterectomy. *Surg Gynecol Obstet* 1992;175(6):501–6.

4. Goodwin WE, Scardino PT. Vesicovaginal and ureterovaginal fistulas: A summary of 25 years of experience. *J Urol* 1980;123(3): 370–4.

5. Davits RJ, Miranda SI. Conservative treatment of vesicovaginal fistulas by bladder drainage alone. *Br J Urol* 1991;68(2):155–6.

Urinary retention following urethral sling surgery

Edward J. Gill

History of present illness

A 56-year-old postmenopausal woman, with a history of hypertension and Pelvic Organ Prolapse Quantification system (POP-Q) stage II pelvic organ prolapse with cystocele and stress urinary incontinence, underwent a tension-free vaginal tape midurethral sling (MUS), repair of cystocele, and postoperative cystoscopy one week ago. She now presents with the inability to empty her bladder for the last 16 hours. She has the urge to urinate but cannot empty well. She had been discharged home on the evening of surgery in good condition. Since then, she was describes her urination as frequent, intermittent, and with a slow stream, and she described a feeling of not being able to empty her bladder completely. She has no back pain, and no nausea or vomiting. Her bowel function has been normal. She has no vaginal bleeding.

Physical examination

General appearance: Well-appearing woman in no distress
Vital signs:

Temperature: 37.0°C
Pulse: 88 beats/min
Blood pressure: 110/68 mmHg
Respiratory rate: 14 breaths/min
Oxygen saturation: 100% on room air
BMI: 28 kg/m^2

Back: No costovertebral angle (CVA) tenderness
Abdomen: Soft, mildly tender over suprapubic area, no guarding or rebound
Pelvic: Normal external genitalia
Vagina: No discharge, no fluid leak, anterior wall incision difficult to visualize under urethra, but appears to be healing well without signs of infection. No mesh exposure
Imaging: Bedside bladder ultrasound scan shows a volume of 1200 cc

How would you manage this patient?

The patient has voiding dysfunction (VD) after recent MUS surgery for stress urinary incontinence. She is suffering from urethral obstruction from the recent surgery. A transurethral catheter was placed with the return of 1300 cc of clear urine with immediate relief of her symptoms. The urine analysis was normal. She was discharged home with the catheter on prophylactic nitrofurantoin and returned to the office in seven days. The Foley catheter was discontinued after voiding trials in the office demonstrated marked improvement in bladder emptying with a post-void residual volume of 70 cc. A follow-up visit at four weeks revealed normal voiding function and no urinary leakage.

Voiding dysfunction following midurethral sling surgery

Today, midurethral sling (MUS) surgery is the most common treatment in the world for stress urinary incontinence (SUI) and has reported success rates of 80–100%. It is performed through a small midline anterior vaginal wall incision and involves the placement of a small piece of polypropylene mesh under the midurethral. There are two main routes of MUS surgery (which refer to the route the arms of the slings take anatomically): the retropubic and trans-obturator. In both types, the sling rests in tissue tunnels created by introducer trocars specific for the procedure, and is not sutured in to place. If no operative report is available, they may be distinguished at the bedside by the small exit incisions made at the time of surgery. These are small (<1 cm) incisions and are located on the lower abdomen just above the pubic bone approximately 6 cm apart and centered on the midline in the retropubic approach, and one on each side in the labio-crural folds in the trans-obturator approach. In addition, there is more recent version of "mini-slings," which have no external excisions.

Voiding dysfunction (VD) after anti-incontinence surgery for stress urinary incontinence is a well-known complication. Although MUSs have a lower incidence of VD than previous procedures like the Burch retropubic urethropexy, which is performed abdominally, and the more surgically involved pubovaginal slings, voiding difficulties still occur. The retropubic MUSs have a higher likelihood of VD than the trans-obturator slings [1]. VD describes problems with either bladder emptying or storage, or both. Lower urinary tract symptoms typically associated with storage problems include daytime urinary frequency, urgency, nocturia, and overactive bladder syndrome. Symptoms of problems with emptying include slow stream, hesitancy, intermittency, straining to void, spraying of the stream, and either incomplete emptying or complete inability to empty. These problems with storage and emptying can further be divided into arising from the bladder or from the outlet. It is useful to approach any problems with VD by considering these etiologies.

Acute Care and Emergency Gynecology, ed. David Chelmow, Christine R. Isaacs and Ashley Carroll. Published by Cambridge University Press. © Cambridge University Press 2015.

This patient has difficulty with emptying. This can result from a hypoactive or acontractile detrusor muscle of the bladder or from obstruction at the bladder outlet. In this patient, who is in the recent postoperative period, the etiology is likely outlet obstruction from the MUS. Other postoperative causes of obstruction after MUS surgery include postoperative edema, hematoma, or infection with abscess. Cystitis can mimic many of these symptoms and must be considered in this patient. Cystitis is relatively common after MUS surgery occurring in up to 12.7% of patients [2]. Delayed return of voiding from a transient neuropathy can occur after any pelvic surgery including MUS surgery, hysterectomy, or surgery for pelvic organ prolapse (POP). This usually resolves within several months. Decreased urine production in the postoperative period is less likely but possible, and can result from hypovolemia, occult blood loss, or from failure to restart a diuretic medication that had been used preoperatively.

The evaluation of postoperative VD after MUS begins with a thorough history and physical examination. This should include inquiry into fluid intake, fever, abdominal and/or back pain, medication use, especially hypertension medications and diuretics that could affect renal function. In addition, it is important to note any preoperative problems with VD or history of urinary tract infections (UTIs). An operative report from the recent surgery also provides valuable information as it will document which type of MUS was performed. Physical examination should include a thorough abdominal and pelvic examination including assessment of costovertebral angle tenderness. Vaginal examination should assess wound healing including signs of infection or hematoma formation, a check for mesh exposure or extrusion, and examination for urine pooling in vagina. Overcorrection of the urethrovesical angle with kinking of the urethra may or may not be apparent on vaginal inspection. A urine analysis should be obtained and UTI ruled out. Bladder volume should be assessed by bedside ultrasound/bladder scan if available or by transurethral catheterization. Most adults feel the normal urge to void at a bladder volume of approximately $250–300 \, cm^2$. A bladder volume of more than $500 \, cm^2$ often causes extreme urgency and discomfort. Most adults empty almost all the bladder volume with voiding and a post-void residual greater than $50–100 \, cm^2$ may be pathologic, although there is no clearly defined volume in the literature at which a diagnosis of urinary retention can be made. Large bladder volume requires immediate drainage to relieve symptoms, prevent neuropraxis type injury with resultant neuropathy, and protect the upper urinary tract from the effects of prolonged increased pressure. Further evaluation with urodynamic testing and cystourethroscopy may be indicated for those patients when the diagnosis is unclear or for those who fail to respond to conservative treatment measures. Referal to an Urogynecologist or Urologist with expertise in management of sling complications is advised.

After a presumptive diagnosis of VD after MUS from outlet obstruction has been made, the immediate treatment is for catheter drainage of the bladder. This may be accomplished with clean intermittent self-catheterization by the patient or a trained assistant. This may be useful in a motivated patient with less severe obstruction and dysfunction. Many patients in this situation, however, will require an indwelling transurethral catheter. The length of catheterization is variable and controversial, but many surgeons will leave the catheter in place and recheck in a week. Patients with indwelling catheters may benefit from low-dose antibiotic prophylaxis with nitrofurantoin or trimethoprim.

Some of the causes of VD after MUS surgery like postoperative edema will resolve with time; however, physical obstruction from the sling may require further surgery to relieve the obstruction. Some experts feel that urinary retention that persists greater than one week requires surgical release of the sling, whereas others will not surgically intervene until the patient has been catheter dependent for greater than four weeks. The argument for earlier intervention is a concern for irreversible bladder dysfunction that may occur with prolonged bladder outlet obstruction. Further surgery is required for VD in 1.3–3.0% of patients [3,4]. Jonsson and colleagues recently reported the largest series to date, involving over 188 000 women from 2001 to 2010, and showed a 1.3% rate of reoperation for urinary retention [5]. Surgical interventions include early release of tension on the sling by downward traction, incision of the sling to release tension, urethrolysis, or removal of part or all of the sling.

Key teaching points

- Midurethral sling (MUS) surgery is the most common surgical treatment for stress urinary incontinence in females.
- Voiding dysfunction (VD) is a well-known complication of surgery for urinary incontinence. It is less common with the current use of MUSs, but it can still occur.
- Any complaint consistent with VD after surgery for urinary incontinence should prompt an evaluation for residual bladder volume with either bedside ultrasound if available, or by transurethral catheterization.
- Large residual bladder volumes and/or the inability to urinate require catheter drainage of the bladder to prevent neuropathy of the bladder and to protect the upper tract from the effects of prolonged increased pressure.
- VD after MUS surgery will often resolve with bladder drainage, but requires close follow-up with a physician with expertise in the complications of incontinence surgery.

References

1. Ogah J, Cody DJ, Rogerson L. Minimally invasive synthetic suburethral sling operations for stress urinary incontinence in women: A short version Cochrane review. *Neurourol Urodyn* 2011;30: 284–91.

2. Barber MD, Gustillo-Ashby AM, Chen CC, et al. Perioperative complications and adverse events of the MONARCH transobturator tape, compared with the tension free vaginal tape. *Am J Obstet Gynecol* 2006;195:1820–5.

3. Nguyen JN, Jakus-Waldman SM, Walter AJ, et al. Perioperative complications and reoperations after incontinence and prolapse surgeries using prosthetic implants. *Obstet Gynecol* 2012;119:539–46.

4. Brubaker L, Norton PA, Albo ME, et al. Adverse events over two years after retropubic or transobturator midurethral sling surgery: Findings from the Trial of Midurethral Slings (TOMUS) study. *Am J Obstet Gynecol* 2011;205: 498e1–e6.

5. Jonsson Funk M, Siddiqui NY, Pate V, et al. Sling revision/removal for mesh erosion and urinary retention: Long-term risk and predictors. *Am J Obstet Gynecol* 2013;2089(1):73 e1–7.

A urethral mass in a postmenopausal woman

Audra Jolyn Hill

History of present illness

A 58-year-old gravida 4, para 4 African-American woman presented to an urgent care clinic because of a new mass on her urethra. She noticed a nontender protrusion coming from her urethra while doing routine hygiene earlier that day. She was very concerned that it could be a cancer. She denied pelvic pain, bleeding, or vaginal discharge. The remainder of her review of systems was negative. Her past medical history included hypertension and obesity and she had no prior surgeries. Her gynecologic history was significant for menopause at age 49, normal cervical cytology and human papillomavirus (HPV) test within the past year, no history of sexually transmitted infections, and four spontaneous vaginal deliveries. She had not been sexually active for over a year.

Physical examination

General appearance: Healthy-appearing woman in no acute distress
Vital signs:

Temperature: 37.2°C
Pulse: 88 beats/min
Blood pressure: 146/84 mmHg
Respiratory rate: 16 breaths/min

Abdomen: Soft, nontender
External genitalia: Friable 1 cm circumferential violet-colored, nontender mass protruding from the urethra (Fig. 88.1)
Vagina: Mucosa consistent with vaginal atrophy
Uterus: Anteverted, 8–10 weeks' size, mobile, nontender
Adnexa: No palpable masses, nontender

What is the diagnosis?

This patient has a urethral prolapse and can be reassured that this is an uncommon but benign finding. This diagnosis requires no further imaging or workup and can be initially managed with a topical estrogen cream. If first-line management is not successful, the patient would benefit from referral to a specialist for follow-up care. In unusual circumstances where the prolapse does not resolve with conservative medical management, surgical revision may be appropriate.

Urethral prolapse

Urethral prolapse, an eversion of the urethral mucosa through the distal urethra, is a rare condition typically seen in postmenopausal women and prepubescent African-American women [1]. The exact etiology of urethral prolapse is unknown. The female urethra is approximately 4 cm in length and is composed of two layers of muscular fibers, an inner longitudinal layer surrounded by an outer circumferential layer. One theory suggests that prolapse of the mucosa occurs when these two layers separate, either from damaged muscular attachments or increased intra-abdominal pressure [2]. Another proposed theory is that decreased estrogen levels and resultant atrophy may retract the epithelial edge of the external urethral meatus. This may explain why the distribution of urethral

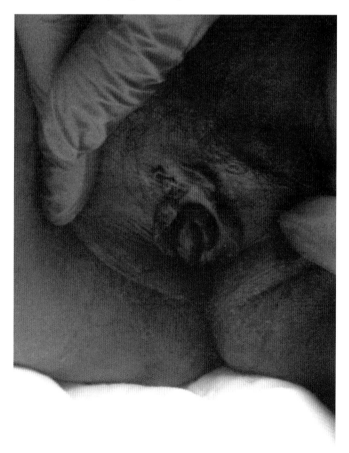

Fig. 88.1 Friable 1 cm circumferential violet-colored, nontender mass protruding from the urethra.

Acute Care and Emergency Gynecology, ed. David Chelmow, Christine R. Isaacs and Ashley Carroll. Published by Cambridge University Press. © Cambridge University Press 2015.

Table 88.1 The differential diagnosis of peri-urethral masses

Urethral diverticulum
Vaginal cyst
Leiomyoma
Urethral prolapse
Urethral caruncle
Skene's gland abscess/cyst
Gartner's duct cyst
Ectopic ureterocele
Malignancy

prolapse is bimodal, occurring in prepubescent and postmenopausal women [3], and why mild urethral prolapse may resolve with the use of topical vaginal estrogen. Depending on the extent of prolapse, tissue swelling and venous congestion may lead to the protrusion of a friable doughnut-shaped mass that is routinely described in urethral prolapse.

Diagnosis should be routinely made by physical examination and typically does not require additional diagnostic imaging. The most common presenting symptom is vaginal bleeding. Other symptoms may include complaints of vaginal mass, dysuria, or abnormal voiding [4]. A circumferential urethral mass is identified on vaginal examination (Fig. 88.1). The differential diagnosis of peri-urethral masses is listed in Table 88.1 with urethral diverticula being the most common [5].

Determining the location of the mass, identifying if there is a central opening leading to the urethra, and review of the patient's symptoms are important to accurately diagnose peri-urethral masses. Urethral caruncles and urethral prolapse are commonly mistaken for one another. A urethral caruncle differs from urethral prolapse in that it is usually less than 1 cm in diameter and is noncircumferential. It is usually pedunculated or sessile and typically arises from the posterior aspect of the urethral meatus [6]. A urethral prolapse has a central opening in the circumferential prolapsed tissue leading to the urethral meatus. This can be confirmed by catheterization, which is often not necessary. Urethral diverticula are distinguished from urethral prolapse by characteristically being a spherical tender mass usually located along the anterior vaginal wall near the urethra with associated symptoms such as dysuria, post-void dribbling, dyspareunia, and recurrent urinary tract infections [7].

Because urethral prolapse is rare, there is limited evidence to guide treatment. Conservative management is usually the first step in the treatment of uncomplicated mild urethral prolapse if no signs of vascular compromise are present. Conservative management consists of topical estrogen therapy two to three times daily for two to four weeks along with periodic sitz baths. Addition of an antibiotic, such as sulfamethoxazole and trimethoprim, is recommended if infection is present. If symptoms initially improve, long-term vaginal estrogen cream with twice weekly application may prevent recurrence. If vascular compromise is noted or if symptoms are refractory to medical management, referral to a specialist with expertise in surgical excision is appropriate. Multiple surgical procedures have been described for the management of urethral prolapse. All involve a variation of excising the prolapsed urethral tissue and re-approximating the two muscular layers of the urethra. Multiple studies describe both conservative [3,8] and surgical management [4,9] as first-line treatment in young females with urethral prolapse, however limited data exists for preferred management of postmenopausal women. Each case should be evaluated individually with respect to medical history, surgical morbidity, and severity of symptoms when deciding between medical or surgical management.

Key teaching points

- Urethral prolapse is a rare condition typically seen in prepubescent and postmenopausal women.
- Urethral prolapse is a circumferential lesion originating from the distal urethra usually presenting as asymptomatic vaginal bleeding.
- Conservative management is indicated for cases of mild urethral prolapse and includes application of topical estrogen cream.
- Surgical management should be considered in cases of vascular compromise or failed medical management.

References

1. Richardson DA, Hajj SN, Herbst AL. Medical treatment of urethral prolapse in children. *Obstet Gynecol* 1982; 59(1):69–74.

2. Lowe FC, Hill GS, Jeffs RD, Brendler CB. Urethral prolapse in children: Insights into etiology and management. *J Urol* 1986;135(1):100–3.

3. Holbrook C, Misra D. Surgical management of urethral prolapse in girls: 13 years' experience. *BJU Int* 2012;110(1):132–4.

4. Hillyer S, Mooppan U, Kim H, Gulmi F. Diagnosis and treatment of urethral prolapse in children: Experience with 34 cases. *Urology* 2009;73(5):1008–11.

5. Blaivas JG, Flisser AJ, Bleustein CB, Panagopoulos G. Periurethral masses: Etiology and diagnosis in a large series of women. *Obstet Gynecol* 2004; 103(5 Pt 1):842–7.

6. Conces MR, Williamson SR, Montironi R, et al. Urethral caruncle: Clinicopathologic features of 41 cases. *Hum Pathol* 2012;43(9):1400–4.

7. Romanzi LJ, Groutz A, Blaivas JG. Urethral diverticulum in women: Diverse presentations resulting in diagnostic delay and mismanagement. *J Urol* 2000;164(2):428–33.

8. Rudin JE, Geldt VG, Alecseev EB. Prolapse of urethral mucosa in white female children: Experience with 58 cases. *J Pediatr Surg* 1997;32(3):423–5.

9. Valerie E, Gilchrist BF, Frischer J, et al. Diagnosis and treatment of urethral prolapse in children. *Urology* 1999; 54(6):1082–4.

A 70-year-old woman with a new vulvar mass

Weldon Chafe

History of present illness

A 70-year-old gravida 3, para 3 white woman presents on referral from her primary care physician for a new growth on her vulva. She first noticed the growth about four months ago. At first it appeared to be a small skin "mole," but it has continued to grow in size and now gets caught in her underwear causing discomfort with walking and sitting. She denies bleeding from the growth. She has been menopausal for over 20 years with no postmenopausal hormone usage. She admits to problems with her Pap smear in her mid-forties and had a "freezing" procedure to get rid of the abnormal cells. Her last Pap was three years ago and was normal by her report.

Her past history includes smoking a pack of cigarettes a day for the last 50 years. She is currently being treated for chronic obstructive lung disease. She has hypertension. She has never had any surgery and her last mammogram was three years ago and normal by patient report.

Physical examination

Vital signs:

Blood pressure: 130/80 mmHg
BMI: 25 kg/m^2

Pain: 2 out of 10 on the pain scale

Palpation of all nodal bearing areas: Negative – including the groins

Chest: Clear to auscultation bilaterally

Cardiovascular: Normal heart rate and rhythm, no murmur elicited

Abdomen: Soft, no tenderness or masses

Genitourinary: There is a 4-cm raised and centrally grooved verruciform lesion present on the left labia that is tender to touch, the base is indurated, and the central portion of the lesion is infiltrative and appears to invade into the subcutaneous fat (Fig. 89.1)

Speculum and bimanual examination: Within normal limits

Rectal examination: Negative

How would you manage this patient?

After discussion with the patient about the findings on her physical examination it is recommended to her that a biopsy of this lesion be obtained during this office visit. After infiltration of the edge of the lesion with local anesthesia, a punch biopsy is obtained from the leading lateral edge, where there appears to be local invasion into the subcutaneous tissue. Hemostasis at the biopsy site is controlled with silver nitrate application. The patient is instructed to return in one week for biopsy results and management planning. She is counseled about the importance of smoking cessation and a preliminary discussion about the diagnosis of invasive vulvar cancer is carried out with her prior to departure. She is provided a prescription for topical lidocaine cream to be applied three to four times per day to her vulvar lesion to help alleviate her discomfort. Local hygiene is discussed as well.

On returning to the office one week later the biopsy results are reviewed with the patient and the diagnosis of invasive squamous cell carcinoma of the vulva is confirmed. Surgical treatment is recommended and she underwent a hemivulvectomy on her left side with ipsilateral surgical excision of superficial and deep inguinal and femoral lymph nodes. All nodes removed were negative for metastatic disease and the surgical margins around the primary tumor were negative by at least 2 cm. The depth of invasion was measured at 1 cm.

Final staging for her vulvar cancer is stage IB (lesion >2 cm in size with stromal invasion of >1.0 mm, confined to the vulva). Her surgical course was uneventful and she was discharged from hospital on postoperative day 2. Follow-up three weeks later showed complete healing of all surgical sites. Her prognosis is considered excellent given the fact that all surgical margins were negative and nodes excised were histologically negative. No additional therapy is recommended. Patient counseling on smoking cessation continues to be emphasized.

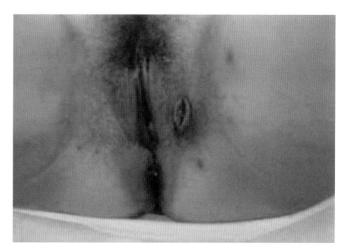

Fig. 89.1 External genitalia.

Acute Care and Emergency Gynecology, ed. David Chelmow, Christine R. Isaacs and Ashley Carroll. Published by Cambridge University Press.
© Cambridge University Press 2015.

Vulvar cancer

Vulvar cancer accounts for about 5% of the gynecologic malignancies with an increasing incidence with advancing age; however, there is a recent increase in younger patients due to human papillomavirus (HPV) infections. About 40–60% of vulvar cancers are due to HPV infections, and typically present in more than one location and may be associated with other HPV genital lesions such as cervical, vaginal, and anal neoplasias. The other type of vulvar cancer is thought to be associated with chronic inflammatory or autoimmune processes. This type presents typically in the seventh or eighth decade and is often seen with lichen sclerosis [1].

Risk factors for vulvar cancer include smoking, infection with HPV, immunosuppressive diseases, and chronic skin diseases such as lichen sclerosis [2]. Diagnosis of vulvar cancer can be delayed often due to nonspecific symptoms, such as itching and burning sensation. Most patients will present with a lesion on the labia that may be a raised plaque that is often discolored. Lesions may also be ulcerative or exophytic and may be multifocal; thus, evaluation of the remaining vulvar, vaginal, cervical, and perianal epithelium should be carefully performed.

Providers should have a low threshold for performing a biopsy of any suspicious lesion. All areas that appear abnormal should be biopsied in cases of multifocal disease. Biopsy can easily be performed in the office with a 3–5 mm Keyes punch biopsy. For ulcerative areas, the edge of the lesion should be biopsied, while hyperpigmented lesions should be sampled in the thickest region [3]. Topical and/or local anesthesic, such as lidocaine, is recommended prior to biopsy. Hemostasis can be achieved by applying pressure or use of silver nitrate sticks.

Prior to 1988 the staging system for vulvar cancer was based on the clinical examination to include size of lesion, spread to adjacent structures, and presence of palpable and suspicious groin nodes. There was a significant error rate in predicting positive nodes and so in 1988 the International Federation of Gynecology and Obstetrics (FIGO) adopted a surgical staging system for the staging of vulvar cancer. This would allow histologic assessment of regional lymph nodes in the staging of this disease. It was felt that the surgical staging system of 1988 did not adequately reflect the prognosis in some groups of women with this disease. In 2009 FIGO amended its surgical staging system to include the size of lesion, the involvement of adjacent structures, and the number and size of nodal metastases [4] (Table 89.1).

Table 89.1 International Federation of Gynecology and Obstetrics (FIGO) classification of carcinoma of the vulva

IA. Tumor confined to the vulva or perineum, ≤2 cm in size with stromal invasion ≤1 mm, negative nodes

IB. Tumor confined to the vulva or perineum, >2 cm in size or with stromal invasion >1 mm, negative nodes

II. Tumor of any size with adjacent spread (1/3 lower urethra, 1/3 lower vagina, anus), negative nodes

IIIA. Tumor of any size with positive inguinal-femoral lymph nodes
 (i) 1 lymph node metastasis ≥5 mm
 (ii) 1–2 lymph node metastases of <5 mm

IIIB. (i) 2 or more lymph nodes metastases ≥5 mm
 (ii) 3 or more lymph nodes metastases <5 mm

IIIC. Positive node(s) with extra-capsular spread

IVA. (i) Tumor invades other regional structures (2/3 upper urethra, 2/3 upper vagina), bladder mucosa, rectal mucosa, or fixed to pelvic bone
 (ii) Fixed or ulcerated inguinal-femoral lymph nodes

IVB. Any distant metastasis including pelvic lymph nodes

Current surgical staging consists of excision of the primary lesion by vulvectomy or radical local excision and removal of lymph nodes. In the patient above, although there are no clinical suspicious or palpable lymph nodes in her groin, surgical excision of ipsilateral nodes is recommended due to a lateralized vulvar lesion. Bilateral nodal excision is recommended for midline vulvar lesions. This is necessary to treat the primary disease and to effectively stage her cancer. For patients with more extensive disease, as in the case with stage IV vulvar cancers, chemoradiation is often used as a primary treatment modality prior to surgical management.

Key teaching points

- Office-based biopsies are safe, accurate, and diagnostic for vulvar cutaneous lesions.
- Physical examination is not reliable in staging vulvar cancer.
- The treatment and staging of vulvar cancer is accomplished by surgical removal of the lesion and careful assessment of regional lymph nodes.
- The number and size of nodal metastases seem to be prognostic in vulvar cancer, and this was separated in the staging system of 2009.

References

1. Dittmer C, Fischer D, Diedrich K, Thill M. Diagnosis and treatment options of vulvar cancer: a review. *Arch Gynecol Obstet* 2012;285:183–93.

2. Madsen B, Jensen H, van den Brule A, et al. Risk factors for invasive squamous cell carcinoma of the vulva and vagina – population-based case-control study in Denmark. *Int J Cancer* 2008; 122:2827–34.

3. American College of Obstetricians and Gynecologists. Diagnosis and management of vulvar skin disorders. Practice Bulletin No. 93. *Obstet Gynecol* 2008;11:1243–53.

4. Mutch DG. The new FIGO staging system for cancers of the vulva, cervix, endometrium and sarcomas. *Gynecol Oncol* 2009;115: 325–8.

A 45-year-old woman with a fungating cervical mass

Jori S. Carter

History of present illness

A 45-year-old gravida 3, para 3 woman presents to the emergency room with heavy post-coital vaginal bleeding. This is the first time she has been sexually active in six months. She usually has regular monthly menses and has not had irregular bleeding before. She has vague lower abdominal pain that has been present for the last several months. She has not received gynecologic care since the birth of her youngest child 20 years ago.

Her medical history is unremarkable, but she does not receive regular checkups. She is a 30 pack-year cigarette smoker, and occasionally drinks alcohol. Upon further questioning, she states that she has some occasional foul-smelling vaginal discharge. Aside from intermittent cramping lower abdominal pain, the remainder of her review of systems is negative.

Physical examination

General appearance: Well-nourished woman who is alert and oriented and in no apparent distress
Vital signs:

Temperature: 37.0°C
Pulse: 100 beats/min
Blood pressure: 110/60 mmHg
Respiratory rate: 16 breaths/min
Oxygen saturation: 97% on room air
BMI: 25 kg/m^2

HEENT: Normal
Neck: Supple, no lymphadenopathy
Chest: Clear to auscultation in all four quadrants
Cardiac: Regular rate and rhythm
Abdomen: Soft, nondistended, minimal tenderness across the lower abdomen, greater on the left than right, without rebound or guarding
External genitalia: Unremarkable
Speculum examination: Vagina with a large amount of blood in the vaginal vault. The cervix is replaced by a 7 cm friable, fungating cervical mass deviated to the left (Fig. 90.1)
Bimanual examination: A 7-cm fixed mass deviating to the left that obliterates the left vaginal fornix, but otherwise no extension to the vagina
Rectovaginal examination: A 7-cm cervical mass that is fixed to the left pelvic sidewall and with right parametrial involvement not extending to the pelvic sidewall. No invasion of the rectal mucosa

How would you manage this patient?

This patient has a large, friable, bleeding cervical mass. She is presumed to have cervical cancer until proven otherwise. Her history of heavy smoking and a lack of gynecologic care are risk factors for this diagnosis. She will need a biopsy for a tissue diagnosis; however, she is currently having heavy vaginal bleeding, which should be managed acutely with the placement of vaginal packing. Referral to a gynecologic oncologist is recommended for the staging and workup.

Cervical cancer

Cervical cancer is the most common gynecologic cancer in women worldwide and it is overall the third most common cancer and the fourth leading cause of death in women. An

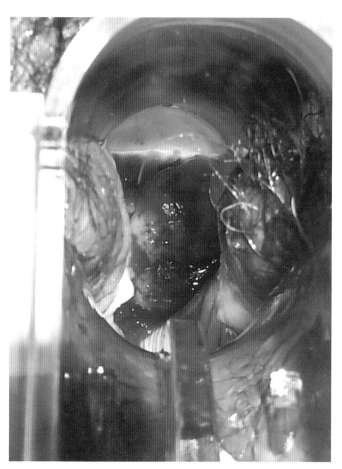

Fig. 90.1 Fungating cervical mass.

Acute Care and Emergency Gynecology, ed. David Chelmow, Christine R. Isaacs and Ashley Carroll. Published by Cambridge University Press. © Cambridge University Press 2015.

Table 90.1 International Federation of Obstetricians and Gynaecologists (FIGO) staging for cervical cancer

Stage I			The carcinoma is strictly confined to the cervix (extension to the corpus would be disregarded).
	IA		Invasive carcinoma which can be diagnosed only by microscopy, with deepest invasion ≤5 mm and largest extension ≤7 mm
		IA1	Measured stromal invasion of ≤3 mm in depth and extension of ≤7 mm
		IA2	Measured stromal invasion of >3 mm and not >5 mm with an extension of not >7 mm
	IB		Clinically visible lesions limited to the cervix uteri or preclinical cancers greater than stage IA
		IB1	Clinically visible lesion ≤4 cm in greatest dimension
		IB2	Clinically visible lesion >4 cm in greatest dimension
Stage II			Cervical carcinoma invades beyond the uterus, but not to the pelvic wall or to the lower third of the vagina
	IIA		Without parametrial invasion
		IIA1	Clinically visible lesion ≤4 cm in greatest dimension
		IIA2	Clinically visible lesion >4 cm in greatest dimension
	IIB		With obvious parametrial invasion
Stage III			The tumor extends to the pelvic wall and/or involves lower third of the vagina and/or causes hydronephrosis or nonfunctioning kidney
	IIIA		Tumor involves lower third of the vagina, with no extension to the pelvic wall
	IIIB		Extension to the pelvic wall and/or hydronephrosis or nonfunctioning kidney
Stage IV			The carcinoma has extended beyond the true pelvis or has involved (biopsy proven) the mucosa of the bladder or rectum. A bullous edema, as such, does not permit a case to be allotted to stage IV
	IVA		Spread of the growth to adjacent organs
	IVB		Spread to distant organs

estimated 12 340 new cases of cervical cancer will be diagnosed in the United States in 2013, accounting for 4030 deaths [1].

Most cases of cervical cancer occur in women who were inadequately or never screened. The most important risk factor is human papilloma virus (HPV) infection (especially the high-risk types 16, 18, 31, 33, and 45). Risk factors also include cigarette smoking, immunosuppression, high parity, increased number of sexual partners, young age at first intercourse, low socioeconomic status, and (while the mechanism is unclear) combination oral contraceptive pill use [2]. HPV infection is essential for malignant transformation leading to the development of cervical cancer, and can be identified in 99% of cervical cancer cases. The high-risk subtypes of HPV are more strongly linked to cervical cancer, with HPV 16 and 18 accounting for 70% of cervical cancer cases in the United States [3]. While most HPV infections are transient, when they are persistent, it takes over 15 years from initial infection to the development of cervical intraepithelial neoplasia (CIN) and then to invasive cervical cancer. The implementation of the HPV vaccine promises to reduce the incidence of cervical cancer when widely administered, and is most effective when given in sexually naïve people. The vaccine is approved for administration between the ages of 9 and 26 years of age [4].

Cervical cancer is staged clinically after tissue diagnosis is obtained. A thorough gynecologic examination, including external genitalia and vagina, should be performed. Visible cancer may appear ulcerated, papillary, exophytic, polypoid, or barrel-shaped. If the lesion is large, such as in this case, it can become friable or necrotic and give off a foul odor with discharge that is bloody, watery, or purulent. A rectovaginal examination is performed to evaluate for spread into the parametria that may feel firm and irregular resulting in less mobility of the uterus. Vaginal involvement is present when there is obliteration of the vaginal fornices or a thick rectovaginal septum. Often exams are performed under anesthesia to achieve a thorough evaluation along with cystoscopy and proctoscopy to evaluate for regional spread to the rectum or bladder.

Renal function is taken into consideration in the staging of cervical cancer and can be evaluated with serum creatinine and/or intravenous pyelogram to assess for the presence of hydronephrosis. Generally in developed countries a CT scan is performed, which can add information about the tumor size, extent of disease spread, lymph node involvement, and hydronephrosis. Information gathered from CT is not included in the International Federation of Gynecology and Obstetrics (FIGO) staging parameters however, because the purpose is to have a unified international staging system that is feasible in resource-rich and resource-poor countries, which allows for consistent data for research and comparability.

Stage I cervical cancer is diagnosed after screening (by cytology and/or positive high-risk HPV testing) leads to colposcopy and cervical biopsy. Screening guidelines can detect preinvasive dysplasia, but also can detects early stage, asymptomatic disease. The implementation of cervical screening has decreased the incidence of cervical cancer by 75% over the last three decades in the United States [5]. Advanced stage cervical cancer (as in the case of this patient) often presents with physical findings of irregular bleeding, malodorous vaginal discharge, vaginal or abdominal pain, and dysuria. Stage II cancer can involve the upper vagina or extend into the parametria (but not to the pelvic sidewall). Patients with stage III (or greater) disease may present with acute renal failure or with hydronephrosis. Patients with stage IVA disease may have hematuria, hematochezia, or changes in bowel movements as the tumor burden extends to the bladder or rectum. Palpable inguinal or supraclavicular lymphadenopathy can be indicative of widespread metastases present in stage IVB disease.

Cervical cancer is clinically staged as opposed to surgically staged (Table 90.1). FIGO clinical staging allows inclusion of physical examination, colposcopy, cervical biopsy, endocervical curettage, conization, hysteroscopy, cystoscopy, proctoscopy, x-ray of the chest, skeleton, and intravenous pyelogram to determine the proper stage [6]. The earliest stages IA1 and IA2 are distinguished using an excisional cervical biopsy to evaluate the depth and width of invasion. Any stage higher usually has a visible lesion, and requires only a direct biopsy. The patient in this scenario has a large 7-cm visible lesion, which makes her at least a stage IB. Because the tumor extends to the left pelvic sidewall, she becomes a stage IIIB.

The treatment of stage IA1 cervical cancer is with either a simple hysterectomy or cone biopsy (loop electrosurgical excisional procedure [LEEP] or cold knife) and is associated with a 99% 5-year overall survival rate [7]. Stage IA2 lesions have a 7% risk of lymph node metastases and are treated with radical hysterectomy (or radical trachelectomy for fertility-sparing in young women [8]) and pelvic lymphadenectomy. Stage IB–IIA1 tumors can be treated by radical hysterectomy (or radical trachelectomy for stage IB) or receive primary radiation therapy with similar 5-year overall survival rates of 83% and 74%,

respectively [9]. Stages IIA2–IVA generally have a 5-year survival rate of less than 50% and are treated with a combination of primary radiation therapy (external beam and brachytherapy) and cisplatin-based chemotherapy, based on five randomized phase III trials showing that the use of concurrent chemoradiation decreased the risk of death by 30–50% [10]. Treatment for stage IVB cervical cancer is individualized, and can include multiagent systemic chemotherapy for disseminated disease, radiation therapy for pain or bleeding, and an emphasis on clinical trials and palliative care [11], with consideration that the 5-year overall survival is 15%.

The patient in this case presented with common symptoms of locally advanced cervical cancer. When women present with symptoms of pain and bleeding it is essential that they undergo a thorough pelvic examination with visualization of the cervix. If a cervical mass is identified in the acute care setting, biopsies should be obtained and if a cervical cancer is confirmed, follow-up with gynecologic oncology is recommended to perform accurate staging and for coordination of future care.

Key teaching points

- A thorough pelvic examination should be performed in any women presenting with abnormal bleeding, vaginal/abdominal pain, or malodorous discharge.
- Risk factors for cervical cancer include: women without regular cervical cancer screening, human papilloma virus (HPV) infection, cigarette smoking, immunosuppression, high parity, increased number of sexual partners, young age at first intercourse, low socioeconomic status, and oral contraceptive pill use.
- Cervical cancer is staged clinically and treatment is dependent on the stage at diagnosis.
- Cervical cancer can be prevented or detected at an early stage with regular cervical cancer screening with cytology and HPV testing.

References

1. American Cancer Society. *Cervical Cancer*. Last revised 1/31/2014. Available at http://www.cancer.org/acs/groups/cid/documents/webcontent/003094-pdf.pdf.

2. Moreno V, Bosch FX, Munoz N, et al. Effect of oral contraceptives on risk of cervical cancer in women with human papillomavirus infection: The IARC multicentric case-control study. *Lancet* 2002;359:1085–92.

3. de Sanjose S, Quint WG, Alemany L, et al. Human papillomavirus genotype attribution in invasive cervical cancer: A retrospective cross-sectional worldwide study. *Lancet Oncol* 2010;11:1048–56.

4. American College of Obstetricians and Gynecologists. Human papillomavirus

vaccination. Committee Opinion No. 467. *Obstet Gynecol* 2010;116:800–3.

5. American College of Obstetricians and Gynecologists. Screening for cervical cancer. Practice Bulletin No. 131. *Obstet Gynecol* 2012;120:1222–38.

6. Lea JS, Lin KY. Cervical cancer. *Obstet Gynecol Clin N Am* 2012;39:233–53.

7. Ostor AG, Rome RM. Micro-invasive squamous cell carcinoma of the cervix: A clinico-pathologic study of 200 cases with long-term follow-up. *Int J Gynecol Cancer* 1994;4:257–64.

8. Wethington SL, Cibula D, Duska LR, et al. An international series on abdominal radical trachelectomy: 101 patients and 28 pregnancies. *Int J Gynecol Cancer* 2012;22:1251–7.

9. Landoni F, Maneo A, Colombo A, et al. Randomised study of radical surgery versus radiotherapy for stage IB-IIA cervical cancer. *Lancet* 1997;350:535–40.

10. National Institutes of Health. *NCI issues Clinical Announcement on Cervical Cancer: Chemotherapy Plus Radiation Improves Survival*. Released Feb 22, 1999. Available at http://www.nih.gov/news/pr/feb99/nci-22.htm.

11. Scatchard K, Forrest JL, Flubacher M, Cornes P, Williams C. Chemotherapy for metastatic and recurrent cervical cancer. *Cochrane Database Syst Rev* 2012, Issue 1. Art. No.: CD006469. DOI: 10.1002/14651858.CD006469.pub2.

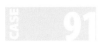

A 48-year-old woman with a 4-month history of intermittent abdominal pain and urinary frequency

Kirk J. Matthews and Jori S. Carter

History of present illness

A 48-year-old woman presents to clinic after being seen in a local emergency department for recurrence of a nagging abdominal and pelvic pain that has been bothering her intermittently for 3–4 months. Her symptoms have not been severe enough to require pain medications, but she is becoming increasingly worried about them. She reports increasing urinary frequency. An abdominal examination revealed no focal pain or peritoneal signs. Laboratory studies from her emergency department visit included a urinalysis, which revealed small leukocytes and blood. A urine culture was obtained and she was treated empirically for a urinary tract infection with trimethoprim/sulfamethoxazole 160 mg/800 mg BID for 3 days. Several days later, when her symptoms persisted and a final report of her urine culture was negative, she was referred to you.

Today she describes her abdominal pain as a "bloating" that is rather uncomfortable, but she is still able to go about her day as usual. On the days with worst symptoms, she has trouble fitting into most of her pants. Her increasing urinary frequency is not associated with dysuria, hematuria, or urinary incontinence. She usually has regular bowel movements, but occasionally has bouts of constipation that are very uncomfortable and usually resolve with over-the-counter laxatives and stool softeners.

Her past medical history is positive for mild hypertension, which is controlled with 25 mg of atenolol daily. Her only surgery was a postpartum bilateral tubal ligation after the birth of her second child at the age of 30. Her menstrual periods are noted to be quite regular, every four weeks, and associated with typical cramping and bloating that she has always had. This is usually treated with over-the-counter nonsteroidal anti-inflammatory drugs and hot packs. Her last Pap test was last year, and she has never had an abnormal smear. Her family history is notable only for hypertension. She denies tobacco use, but does report drinking 2–3 glasses of wine per week.

Physical examination

General appearance: Well-dressed, well-groomed woman with no apparent disease

Vital signs:

Temperature: 36.8°C

Pulse: 85 beats/min

Blood pressure: 132/90 mmHg

Respiratory rate: 16 breaths/min

Oxygen saturation: 100% on room air

BMI: 27.3 kg/m^2

HEENT: Moist mucous membranes, no neck lymphadenopathy, normal palpating thyroid

Chest: Clear to auscultation bilaterally, no adventitious breath sounds noted. Heart is noted to have normal rate and rhythm. S1 and S2 noted

Abdomen: Soft, minimally distended, no masses palpated, no rebound or tenderness. The patient appears slightly uncomfortable with the abdominal exam

Lymphatics: No inguinal lymphadenopathy noted. No lower extremity edema

External genitalia/vagina: Normal appearing genitalia for age. No urethral irritation or erythema noted. Normal appearing vaginal mucosa and cervix without masses or lesions

Bimanual examination: Reveals a small uterus, but with limited mobility. Slightly tender fullness noted in the posterior cul-de-sac

Rectovaginal examination: Reveals similar fullness, which is also mildly uncomfortable to the patient. Stool obtained with rectal finger has no occult blood

How would you manage this patient?

Given the patient's complaints and examination findings above, a differential diagnosis should include: endometriosis, endometrioma, uterine fibroids, functional ovarian cysts, pelvic inflammatory disease (PID), and ovarian and colon malignancies.

PID is less likely given that the patient has no cervical motion tenderness or mucopurulent discharge from the external cervical os. However, sexually transmitted infections can easily be detected with quick and inexpensive nucleic acid amplification tests (NAATs) obtained from cervix or urine. Information about the other possible diagnoses can be obtained from ultrasonographic imaging.

A colonoscopy and transvaginal ultrasound (TVUS) were both ordered as was a complete blood count (CBC). The CBC showed a hemoglobin level of 10.9 mg/dL with a normal mean corpuscular volume (MCV) of 92 fL. While the uterus

---

Acute Care and Emergency Gynecology, ed. David Chelmow, Christine R. Isaacs and Ashley Carroll. Published by Cambridge University Press. © Cambridge University Press 2015.

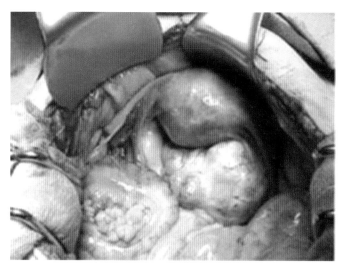

Fig. 91.1 Intraoperative findings of ovarian carcinoma arising from right ovary. The normal appearing uterus and contralateral adnexal structures suggest the early stage of disease at time of surgery. (Courtesy of Weldon Chafe, MD.)

appeared to be of normal size and shape, the ultrasound revealed the right ovary to be posterior to the uterus, measuring 77 mm × 56 mm with several solid and cystic septations. There was a small amount of posterior cul-de-sac fluid noted as well. Upon movement of the ultrasound probe, the ovary did not appear to be mobile at all. A colonoscopy revealed no abnormal findings.

The ultrasonographic findings were concerning for malignancy, so a CA-125 was drawn, which returned only slightly elevated at 82 U/mL. The patient was referred to a gynecologic oncologist, who recommended an exploratory laparotomy.

Intraoperative findings included a frozen section of the right ovary, which showed evidence of an adenocarcinoma (Fig. 91.1). The gynecologic oncologist, after having counseled the patient in the preoperative setting that it may be necessary, proceeded with a full-staging procedure including a total hysterectomy, bilateral salpingo-oophorectomy, omentectomy, and pelvic and para-aortic lymph node dissection and pelvic washings to definitively stage the patient. There was no overt evidence of intraperitoneal disease and the pelvic and para-aortic lymph nodes palpated normally.

The final pathology showed a well-differentiated serous cystadenocarcinoma of ovarian origin. The right ovarian capsule was felt to be intact. The only evidence of malignant spread was a focus of tumor involving the right fallopian tube, giving the patient an International Federation of Gynecology and Obstetrics (FIGO) stage of 2A. Given that the malignancy in question was found at a relatively early stage, the patient's prognosis is also proportionately good with an expected 5-year survival rate of approximately 76% [1]. The gynecologic oncologist made plans to start a course of platinum-based chemotherapy with plans for six cycles. This will be followed by CT scans and CA-125 measurements to evaluate response.

Detection of ovarian cancer

Ovarian cancer has, for many years, been the most catastrophic gynecologic malignancy for women. Ovarian cancer is estimated to cause 14 030 deaths in the United States in 2013, more than cervical and uterine cancer combined [1]. The main reason that this malignancy can be so lethal is due to the usual advanced stages at which it is usually diagnosed. While stage I disease has a 90% 5-year survival rate, stage III or IV has only an 18–34% 5-year survival rate [1]. It has been reported many times that ovarian cancer is a "silent killer." However, when looking retrospectively, ovarian cancer patients often exhibit signs and symptoms, which may aid in an early diagnosis of this lethal disease.

Currently, there is no good screening test available for ovarian cancer. As the overall prevalence of ovarian cancer diagnoses is very low (only 22 240 estimated new diagnoses in 2013 [1]), any future screening test would be very difficult to implement. As would be true of any disease with a low prevalence, a theoretical screening examination with 100% sensitivity and 99% specificity would only have a very low positive predictive value, resulting in many false positives. In the case of ovarian cancer screening, such a high false positive rate would result in many unnecessary surgeries. In support of this, several large randomized controlled trials comparing screening with TVUS and CA-125 with usual care have not demonstrated a proven benefit [2,3,4]. At this time, it is not recommended that physicians routinely screen for ovarian cancer in asymptomatic, low risk women with either CA-125 or transvaginal ultrasound. However, women who exhibit symptoms of possible ovarian malignancy should receive further workup, as this patient did.

While early stage ovarian cancer is a difficult diagnosis to make, ovarian cancer patients oftentimes exhibit a number of signs and symptoms. The majority of ovarian cancer patients (95%) develop symptoms several months prior to seeing a physician. The most common symptoms are increased abdominal size, bloating, fatigue, abdominal pain, indigestion, urinary frequency, pelvic pain, constipation, back pain, and pain with intercourse (Table 91.1) [5]. The majority of symptoms are not gynecologic. Many of the most common symptoms are abdominal, gastrointestinal, pain, or constitutional in nature, so it is quite common for providers to incorrectly diagnose a patient with irritable bowel syndrome, gastritis, or depression several months before the correct diagnosis can be made [6]. It is incumbent upon both the physician and patient to have a high index of suspicion for ovarian cancer when presented with these nonspecific symptoms.

A thorough physical exam, including a pelvic and rectovaginal examination, is of paramount importance in the evaluation of a patient with these symptoms. Any adnexal masses, posterior cul-de-sac fullness, or nodularity should prompt imaging studies. While slightly invasive, transvaginal ultrasonography is quite sensitive for detecting ovarian abnormalities, oftentimes before symptoms may fully arise.

Table 91.1 Frequency of symptoms in ovarian cancer

Symptom	Frequency (%)
Increased abdominal size	61
Bloating	57
Fatigue	47
Abdominal pain	36
Indigestion	31
Urinary frequency	27
Pelvic pain	26
Constipation	25
Back pain	23
Pain with intercourse	17
Unable to eat normally	16
Palpable mass	14
Vaginal bleeding	13
Weight loss	11
Nausea	9
Bleeding with intercourse	3
Diarrhea	1
Deep venous thrombosis	1
None	5

The upper limit of normal for a nonpregnant premenopausal ovary is approximately 20 cm^3, and is only 10 cm^3 in a postmenopausal ovary. The ultrasound also provides other information, such as cyst wall characteristics, presence or absence of septae, or Doppler blood flow studies, which may be of use in detecting malignant lesions [7].

According to the American College of Obstetricians and Gynecologists (ACOG), a CA-125 may be helpful in the further evaluation of suspicious ovarian lesions. In the premenopausal woman, a mildly elevated CA-125 has low specificity for an ovarian malignancy, however severely elevated levels may be useful. In contrast, for the postmenopausal women with a pelvic mass, a CA-125 is helpful in predicting the likelihood of a malignancy [7]. However, a normal CA-125 may be found in up to 50% of early stage ovarian cancer and 25% of advanced stage cancers. For this reason, it may be better to order an ultrasound study prior to a CA-125, as was done in this patient.

If ovarian cancer is likely, a gynecologic oncologist should perform the surgery in a facility that has a pathology department prepared to perform intraoperative surgical frozen sections. According to ACOG, patients who receive a comprehensive staging procedure have better outcomes than those who do not [7]. Patients with ovarian cancer who have surgery done by gynecologic oncologists have improved overall survival [8].

Full staging includes peritoneal cytology and complete inspection of the abdominal and pelvic organs. Any adnexal masses should be removed intact where possible and complete staging should include a hysterectomy, bilateral salpingo-oophorectomy, omentectomy, bilateral pelvic and paraaortic lymphadenectomy, and peritoneal biopsies. It may be appropriate to preserve the uterus and contralateral ovary and fallopian tube in a younger woman with limited disease who wishes to retain her fertility.

For many years, ovarian cancer has been seen as "the silent killer." However, patients diagnosed with ovarian cancer often exhibit symptoms prior to seeking medical evaluation, and often receive an initial incorrect diagnosis. While a difficult diagnosis to make, early stage ovarian cancer has much better five-year survival rates than advanced stage cancers. Currently, the best detection strategy for ovarian malignancies is for the treating provider to have a high index of suspicion. A complete evaluation of the symptomatic patient always includes a thorough physical examination and may include transvaginal ultrasonography and CA-125 measurement.

Key teaching points

- At this time, there is no effective screening test for ovarian cancer and screening for ovarian cancer in women of average risk is not recommended.
- Most women with ovarian cancer exhibit symptoms prior to their diagnosis and this malignancy should no longer be considered a "silent killer." The best detection tool currently available is physician and patient awareness, and suspicion of ovarian malignancy in women with symptoms.
- The most common symptoms of ovarian cancer include abdominal or pelvic pain, gastrointestinal issues, early satiety, or urinary issues.
- Further workup for an ovarian malignancy should include transvaginal ultrasonography. Consideration may also be given to a CA-125 measurement.

References

1. American Cancer Society. *Cancer Facts and Figures 2013*. Atlanta, American Cancer Society, 2013.

2. Buys SS, Partridge E, Greene M, et al. Ovarian cancer screening in the prostate, lung, colorectal and ovarian (PLCO) cancer screening trial: Findings from the initial screen of a randomized trial. *Am J Obstet Gynecol* 2005;193(5): 1630–9.

3. Kobayashi H, Yamada Y, Sado T, et al. A randomized study of screening for ovarian cancer: A multicenter study in

Japan. *Int J Gynecol Cancer* 2008; 18(3):414–20.

4. Menon U, Gentry-Maharaj A, Hallett R, et al. Sensitivity and specificity of multimodal and ultrasound screening for ovarian cancer, and stage distribution of detected cancers: Results of the prevalence screen of the UK Collaborative Trial of Ovarian Cancer Screening (UKCTOCS). *Lancet Oncol* 2009;10(4):327–40.

5. Goff, BA. Ovarian cancer: Screening and early detection. *Obstet Gynecol Clin North Am* 2012;39(2): 183–94.

6. Goff BA, Mandel L, Muntz HG, et al. Ovarian carcinoma diagnosis. *Cancer* 2000;89:2068–75.

7. American College of Obstetricians and Gynecologists. The role of the obstetrician/gynecologist in early detection of epithelial ovarian cancer. Committee Opinion Number 477. *Obstet Gynecol* 2011;117(3): 742–6.

8. Chan J, Sherman AE, Kapp DS, et al. Influence of gynecologic oncologists on the survival of patients with endometrial cancer. *Obstet Gynecol* 2007;109(6): 1342–50.

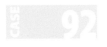

A 65-year-old woman with profuse vaginal bleeding

Amy Hempel and Jori S. Carter

History of present illness

A 65-year-old postmenopausal white woman with a past medical history significant for hypertension, diabetes, and hypercholesterolemia presents urgently to your office with profuse vaginal bleeding. The patient states she began to notice intermittent, dark spotting about one month ago. At that time, she used one panty-liner daily. About two weeks later, she began noting bright red blood for one to two days, which she described as "heavy as her prior periods." Today she presents saying her bleeding has worsened. The patient is nulliparous and reports menopause was at age 55. She is sexually active with her husband and denies any history of sexually transmitted diseases. She has no significant surgical history. Her medications include an angiotensin-converting enzyme (ACE) inhibitor, a statin, and metformin. She does not smoke or drink. She is a retired teacher. Review of symptoms is negative for fever, chills, weight loss, vaginal discharge, or dysuria.

Physical examination

General appearance: Pleasant, well-groomed woman who is in no acute distress

Vital signs:

Temperature: 36.4°C

Pulse: 78 beats/min

Blood pressure: 134/89

Respiratory rate: 16 breaths/min

BMI: 40 kg/m^2

HEENT: Normal

Cardiovascular: Regular rate, regular rhythm without murmurs

Respiratory: Clear to auscultation bilaterally

Abdominal: Soft, nontender, obese, normal bowel sounds

Genitourinary: Normal appearing external genitalia; vaginal vault with one scopette of brown blood. No obvious active bleeding from the cervical os, which was noted to be stenotic. On bimanual examination the uterus was anteverted without obvious masses. Ovaries were not palpated

Laboratory studies:

Comprehensive metabolic panel: Normal

Leukocyte count and platelet count: Normal

Hb: 11 g/dL (normal 12–16 g/dL)

Imaging: Transvaginal ultrasound is performed (Fig. 92.1)

How would you manage this patient?

This patient is a postmenopausal woman with abnormal vaginal bleeding. The most common differential diagnosis of postmenopausal bleeding in this age group includes vaginal trauma, atrophy, uterine and cervical polyps, and endometrial hyperplasia or neoplasia. In this case, a pelvic ultrasound was performed revealing a thickened endometrial stripe of 20 mm. An endometrial biopsy was performed in the office after gently dilating the cervix, and pathology revealed an endometrial adenocarcinoma. The patient was referred to a gynecologic oncologist for further surgical management. She ultimately underwent a robotic-assisted laparoscopic total hysterectomy, bilateral salpingo-oophorectomy, pelvic washings, and lymph-node dissection. She was diagnosed with stage IB, grade 1, endometrioid adenocarcinoma of the endometrium and did not require any additional treatment (Fig. 92.2).

She follows up with her gynecologic oncologist every three months.

Endometrial cancer

Endometrial cancer is the most common malignancy of the female genital tract in the United States [1] and is the fourth most common cancer in women after breast, lung, and colorectal cancers [2]. More than 90% of patients with endometrial cancer will present with abnormal vaginal bleeding or discharge, allowing for 72% of endometrial cancers to be diagnosed as stage I [1]. Risk factors for developing endometrial cancer include increased age, white race, nulliparity, history of infertility, late age of menopause and early age of menarche, obesity, diabetes, hypertension, gallbladder disease, and thyroid disease. Ninety percent of cases occur in women over the age of 50, and 70% of patients with early-stage endometrial cancer are obese [2]. The lifetime endometrial cancer mortality risk is 0.5%, translating into over 7310 deaths each year. The 5-year survival rate is 80.8% for white females and 53.3% for black females with the cause of the discrepancy being unclear, although it is known that black women are diagnosed more commonly at advanced stages and get more aggressive histologic types of endometrial cancer [1,3]. Hypotheses that account for the racial discrepancy include lack of access to care, delay in treatments, and more advanced stages of cancer identified at diagnosis. Only 52% of black women over the age of 50 have disease confined to the uterus at diagnosis compared to 73% of white women in the same age group. Curiously, the death rate per 100 000 population has soared

---

Acute Care and Emergency Gynecology, ed. David Chelmow, Christine R. Isaacs and Ashley Carroll. Published by Cambridge University Press. © Cambridge University Press 2015.

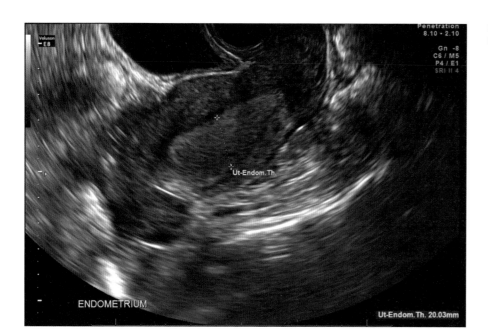

Fig. 92.1 Transvaginal ultrasound of uterine endometrial thickness at 20 mm.

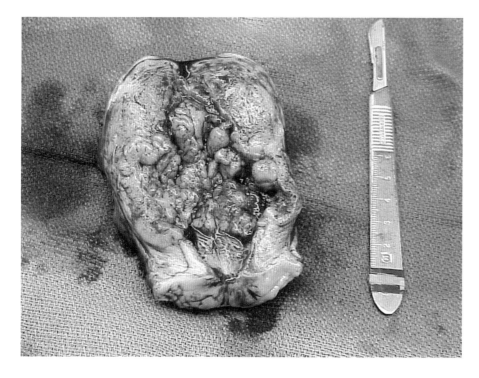

Fig. 92.2 Excised adenocarcinoma of the endometrium. (Image courtesy of Stephen Cohen, MD.)

more than 100% during the past 20 years, likely secondary to longer life spans and medical comorbidities [2].

The most common etiology of endometrial cancer is an excess of endogenous or exogenous estrogen with a lack of opposing progesterone. Two classifications of endometrial cancer exist: type I, or estrogen dependent, and type II, which is not related to estrogen status. The former is more common and confers a relatively good prognosis while type II is a more lethal type. Despite type II being the more lethal form, carcinosarcoma is the most aggressive form of endometrial cancer. Carcinosarcomas possess cancerous cells both originating from epithelial and connective tissue cells and are not estrogen dependent.

To make the diagnosis of endometrial cancer, tissue sampling of the endometrium (via endometrial biopsy or sharp curettage) must be obtained. Premenopausal patients being evaluated for abnormal uterine bleeding should have negative pregnancy testing prior to sampling the endometrium. While office endometrial biopsy is the preferred first-line approach to obtain endometrial tissue sampling due to the fact that is less expensive and less invasive than dilation and curettage under anesthesia, an endometrial biopsy will not adequately characterize lesions in terms of extent of involvement within the uterus. Meta-analyses have showed that the sensitivity of endometrial biopsy to diagnose endometrial hyperplasia or cancer is 68% when compared to surgical pathology obtained at hysterectomy, while the sensitivity of dilation and curettage is 78%. [4].

While tissue sampling is the gold standard to rule out endometrial cancer, other options to characterize the uterine anatomy in an effort to diagnose the etiology of postmenopausal bleeding include hysteroscopy and transvaginal ultrasound. Hysteroscopy allows one to directly visualize the uterine cavity, which aids in identifying a focal lesion, as well as allows one to biopsy such a lesion under direct visualization, and assess for other sources of uterine bleeding including polyps and leiomyomas. When hysteroscopy is negative, the likelihood of actual endometrial cancer existing is 0.4–0.5% [4]. Transvaginal ultrasound can also be used to identify the thickness of the endometrial lining, which is related to the amount of estrogen exposure at the endometrium. When the endometrial thickness measures less than 5 mm, a 99% negative predictive value exists for the diagnosis of endometrial cancer [2]. Similarly, 96% of women with endometrial cancer have an endometrial stripe of greater than 5 mm [2]. The patient in this case was found to have an endometrial stripe of 20 mm on ultrasound prompting an endometrial biopsy and, thus, the diagnosis.

Once endometrial cancer is diagnosed, the patient should be referred to a gynecologic oncologist. A physical examination and chest radiograph are the only components of preoperative staging, and a physical examination specifically provides information regarding the most beneficial surgical approach and planning for removal of the uterus. MRI and CT are not routinely required preoperatively.

Endometrial cancer is surgically staged by performing a total hysterectomy with bilateral salpingo-oophorectomy with pelvic washings for cytology and bilateral pelvic and para-aortic lymph node dissection. Staging of endometrial cancer includes assessments of histologic grade by the International Federation of Gynecology and Obstetrics (FIGO) system, nuclear grade, myometrial depth of invasion, stromal involvement of the cervix, and assessments of metastasis to the vagina or ovaries, as well as spread to the lymph nodes, other components of the abdomen, or distant structures (Table 92.1 [5]). The staging of the disease guides prognosis as well as treatment. Site of metastasis is the primary indicator of prognosis, and therapy including radiation and chemotherapy will depend on the surgical stage at time of diagnosis. When stage I endometrial carcinoma is diagnosed, about 75% of women are cured with total hysterectomy, bilateral salpingo-oophorectomy, and lymph node dissection alone [2]. Multiple randomized trials have shown no survival benefit to adjuvant radiation for stage I disease despite better local control of recurrence. Adjuvant radiation may be offered for patients if they have high risk factors including serous or clear cell cancer; or if they have intermediate- to high-risk factors at

Table 92.1 International Federation of Gynecology and Obstetrics (FIGO) staging of endometrial cancer as defined by surgical and pathologic findings*

FIGO stage	Surgical/pathologic findings
I	Tumor confined to corpus uteri
IA	No or less than half myometrial invasion
IB	Invasion equal to or more than half of the myometrium
II	Tumor invades cervical stroma, but does not extend beyond the uterus.
III	Local and/or regional spread of the tumor.
IIIA	Tumor invades the serosa of the corpus uteri and/or adnexa
IIIB	Vaginal and/or parametrial involvement
IIIC	Metastases to pelvic and/or para-aortic lymph nodes
IIIC1	Positive pelvic nodes
IIIC2	Positive para-aortic lymph nodes with or without positive pelvic lymph nodes
IV	Tumor invades bladder and/or bowel mucosa, and/or distant metastases
IVA	Tumor invasion of bladder and/or bowel mucosa
IVB	Distant metastases, including intra-abdominal metastases and/or inguinal lymph nodes

* From Pecorelli [5].

specific ages. Intermediate-risk factors include FIGO grade 2 or 3, outer half of myometrial invasion, and lymphovascular space invasion. Patients at any age with all 3 risk factors qualify for radiation, as well as patients between the ages of 50 and 69 with 2 risk factors, or patients 70 years or older with 1 risk-factor. [6] If stage II–IV endometrial cancer is diagnosed, attention is turned to radiation of affected areas. Extrauterine disease requires pelvic radiation and considerations are made for systemic therapy including chemotherapy especially in cases of intraperitoneal disease. After completion of recommended therapy, most patients should be followed clinically every 3–4 months for 2–3 years, then twice yearly thereafter to monitor for any signs of recurrence on speculum or rectovaginal exam, as up to 70% of recurrences are detected within 3 years [1].

Key teaching points

- Any patient with postmenopausal bleeding must be evaluated as to the etiology and ruled out for endometrial cancer.
- A diagnosis of endometrial cancer requires tissue histology obtained from the endometrium by office endometrial biopsy or by sharp curettage in the operating room.

- When pelvic ultrasound is used in the diagnostic workup of postmenopausal bleeding, an endometrial stripe measuring greater than 5 mm requires follow-up tissue sampling.

- Endometrial cancer is surgically staged and requires a total hysterectomy, bilateral salpingo-oophorectomy, pelvic washings, and bilateral pelvic/para-aortic lymph-node dissection by a surgical specialist.

References

1. American College of Obstetricians and Gynecologists. Management of endometrial cancer. Practice Bulletin No. 65. *Obstet Gynecol* 2005;106: 413–25.

2. Sorosky, J. Endometrial cancer. *Obstet Gynecol* 2012;120:383–97.

3. Long, B; Liu, FW; Bristow, RE. Disparities in uterine cancer epidemiology, treatment, and survival among African Americans in the United States. *Gynecol Oncol* 2013;130:652–9.

4. American College of Obstetricians and Gynecologists. Management of abnormal uterine bleeding associated with ovulatory dysfunction. Practice Bulletin No. 136. *Obstet Gynecol* 2013;122: 176–85.

5. Pecorelli, S. Revised FIGO staging for carcinoma of the vulva, cervix, and endometrium. *Int J Gynaecol Obstet* 2009;105:103–4.

6. Keys, H; Roberts, J; Bruno, V; et al. A phase III trial of surgery with or without adjuvant external pelvic radiation therapy in intermediate risk endometrial adenocarcinoma: A Gynecologic Oncology Group study. *Gynecol Oncol* 2004;92:744–51.

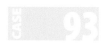

A 38-year-old woman with heavy vaginal bleeding 6 months after D&C for complete mole

Emily E. Landers and Warner K. Huh

History of present illness

A 38-year-old gravida 4, para 3–0–1–3 woman presents to the emergency department complaining of heavy vaginal bleeding for the past 2 days. Six months prior to presentation she had undergone a dilation and curettage (D&C) for a complete molar pregnancy. She reports that she has not kept any of her follow-up appointments since surgery. Over the past few months, she has developed irregular, heavy menses, and now reports that her bleeding is so heavy it often soaks through her clothing. She also reports nausea and mild lower abdominal cramping. She recently developed a persistent cough with blood-streaked sputum, which seems to be worsening. She otherwise denies fever, chills, dizziness, palpitations, chest pain, or shortness of breath.

She has no other medical problems and has never had abdominal surgery. She is on no medication and her husband plans a vasectomy for contraception. She is a stay-at-home mother who doesn't smoke and reports having one glass of wine each evening.

Physical examination

General appearance: Well-nourished woman in no acute distress

Vital signs:

Temperature: 36.9°C
Pulse: 102 beats/min
Blood pressure: 118/76 mmHg
Respiratory rate: 18 breaths/min
Oxygen saturation: 97% on room air

HEENT: Unremarkable

Cardiovascular: Regular rhythm, mild tachycardia; no rubs, murmurs, or gallops

Lungs: Mild diffuse crackles bilaterally

Abdomen: Soft, nontender, nondistended, active bowel sounds present. Firm uterine fundus palpated 3–4 cm below umbilicus

Rectal: Normal tone, no masses; brown stool noted; hemoccult negative

Pelvic: Active bleeding from the cervical os, with blood pooling in vaginal vault; cervix closed; uterus mobile and enlarged, approximately 16-weeks' size; enlarged adnexa bilaterally. No cervical motion or adnexal tenderness

Extremities: No clubbing, cyanosis, or edema
Neurologic: Alert and oriented × 4. No focal deficits
Laboratory studies:

Urine pregnancy test: Positive
Quantitative beta-hCG: 376 524 mIU/mL (normal nonpregnant <5 mIU/mL)
Ht: 21% (normal 34.9–44.5%)
Blood type: B positive
Hepatic function panel, thyroid function tests, and metabolic panel were all within normal limits

Imaging:

Transvaginal ultrasound: Demonstrated an enlarged uterus with a 5.5 cm well-circumscribed, heterogeneous mass and bilateral enlarged ovaries with multiple theca lutein cysts. There was no evidence of an intrauterine or ectopic pregnancy
Chest x-ray: Showed multiple, diffuse opacities bilaterally (Fig. 93.1)

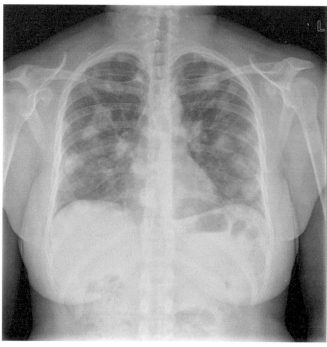

Fig. 93.1 Chest x-ray.

Acute Care and Emergency Gynecology, ed. David Chelmow, Christine R. Isaacs and Ashley Carroll. Published by Cambridge University Press.
© Cambridge University Press 2015.

How would you manage this patient?

The patient's diagnosis is suspicious for choriocarcinoma. Due to persistent heavy vaginal bleeding and severe anemia, the patient was counseled on the need for surgical intervention with repeat D&C versus hysterectomy. The patient had no desire for future childbearing and, thus, elected hysterectomy for definitive management.

Intraoperative findings included an enlarged uterus and enlarged multicystic ovaries bilaterally. No other abnormalities were noted in the abdomen or pelvis.

The patient had an uncomplicated postoperative course and was discharged home on postoperative day 3. Surgical pathology demonstrated abnormal trophoblastic hyperplasia and anaplasia, hemorrhage, necrosis, and no chorionic villi. Findings were consistent with choriocarcinoma (Fig. 93.2).

Given the findings on chest x-ray, a metastatic workup was performed with a CT scan of the head and chest. The CT scan confirmed numerous pulmonary metastases. The patient was referred to a gynecologic oncologist and was treated with adjuvant multi-agent chemotherapy. Beta-human chorionic gonadotropin (beta-hCG) levels were monitored weekly until undetectable for 3 weeks, and then followed monthly for 24 months to monitor for potential recurrence. She remains healthy to date.

Choriocarcinoma

Choriocarcinoma is a rapidly growing malignant tumor of placental origin, characterized by invasion into the myometrium and vasculature [1,2]. It is the most aggressive form of gestational trophoblastic neoplasia (GTN). This describes a spectrum of malignancies that arise from placental tissue, which include invasive hydatidiform mole, placental site trophoblastic tumor, epithelioid trophoblastic tumor, and choriocarcinoma [3]. Choriocarcinoma accounts for approximately 10% of all GTNs. The incidence of

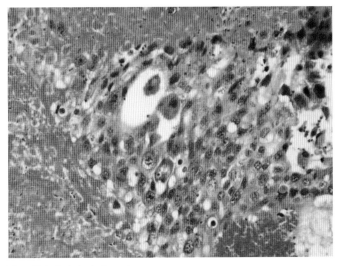

Fig. 93.2 Pathological specimen.

choriocarcinoma is approximately 1 in 40 000 pregnancies, and 1 in 40 hydatidiform moles [2]. GTN most commonly develops following a molar pregnancy, but can occur after any type of pregnancy including a term gestation or spontaneous miscarriage. After treatment of a molar pregnancy (partial or complete), beta-hCG levels usually normalize within two months [2]. If serum beta-hCG levels plateau, increase, or persist for more than six months after molar evacuation, persistent GTN needs to be considered [4]. Clinical characteristics associated with an increased risk of developing GTN after treatment of molar pregnancies includes age greater than 40 years, previous GTN, initial beta-hCG greater than 100 000 mIU/mL, and the presence of cytologic atypia or hyperplasia on histology of the evacuated molar tissue [5].

Patients with choriocarcinoma typically present with postpartum bleeding longer than six to eight weeks following delivery or uterine evacuation, as was the case in this patient [4]. They may also present with respiratory complaints such as cough, chest pain, hemoptysis, or signs of gastrointestinal, urologic, or intracerebral bleeding, which is likely indicative of metastatic disease. One of the hallmarks of choriocarcinoma is its ability to directly invade into the uterine myometrium and vasculature with rapid, hematogenous spread to distant sites (lungs, vagina, pelvis, liver, and brain) [3,6].

The diagnosis of choriocarcinoma is made by obtaining information regarding a patient's pregnancy history, in addition to laboratory and radiographic studies. Beta-hCG levels can vary widely with this malignancy, though they are always elevated above normal nonpregnant levels. Transvaginal ultrasound images often demonstrate a uterine mass. Bilateral enlarged ovaries with multiple theca lutein cysts are also a common finding with this diagnosis, which results from a hypersensitive response of the ovaries to high levels of circulating beta-hCG [3]. A chest x-ray should be performed to evaluate for evidence of pulmonary metastatic disease [3]. If there is suspicion for metastasis, a CT scan of the head, chest, abdomen and pelvis should also be obtained [3]. Choriocarcioma is generally a biopsy-proven diagnosis, in most circumstances. Treatment, however, is sometimes initiated without a definitive pathologic diagnosis given the risk of massive hemorrhage following biopsy or endometrial curettage [2]. Hysterectomy is not always necessary in the treatment of choriocarcinoma; however, it may be necessary for the management of uterine hemorrhage. Key histopathologic features of choriocarcinoma include abnormal trophoblastic hyperplasia, hemorrhage, necrosis, and the absence of chorionic villi [2].

Prognosis of choriocarcinoma is good even in cases of distant metastatic disease, given the sensitivity of these tumors to chemotherapy [3]. A scoring system developed by the World Health Organization (WHO) is used to determine prognostic risk (low vs. high) of disease. This scoring system is based on patient age, ABO blood type, extent of spread, largest tumor size, beta-hCG level, duration of disease from initial pregnancy event to start of treatment, number and specific sites of metastases, nature of preceding pregnancy, and extent of prior treatment [6]. Additionally, an anatomical staging system developed by the International Federation of Gynecology and Obstetrics (FIGO) is used to further categorize disease status and aid in determining the appropriate treatment and surveillance strategies. Stage I includes disease confined to the uterus, stage II includes disease extending beyond the uterus but limited to genital structures, stage III includes disease extending to the lungs, and stage IV includes metastatic disease involving other sites [6]. With low risk or stage I–III disease, single-agent chemotherapy with either methotrexate or dactinomycin is generally sufficient. With high-risk or stage IV disease, alternating cycles of etoposide, methotrexate, and dactinomycin with cyclophosphamide and vincristine are indicated [1,4,6]. Radiation therapy is a rarely used treatment option for choriocarcinoma, and is often reserved for patients with metastatic disease to the central nervous system or those who require treatment in addition to surgery for persistence of disease despite appropriate chemotherapy. Fortunately, beta-hCG levels are a highly sensitive marker for tracking disease progression or resolution [3]. Monitoring generally consists of weekly measurement of quantitative beta-hCG until levels are undetectable for three consecutive weeks. This is followed by monthly measurements for 12 months (stage I–III disease) or 24 months (stage IV disease) [6]. Overall cure rates for choriocarcinoma are greater than 90% [3].

Key teaching points

- Choriocarcinoma is a rapidly growing malignant tumor of placental tissue origin, characterized by invasion into the myometrium and vasculature.
- Patients most commonly present with vaginal bleeding longer than six to eight weeks after the preceding pregnancy event.
- Gestational trophoblastic neoplasia (GTN) most commonly develops following a molar pregnancy, but can occur after any type of pregnancy including a term gestation or spontaneous miscarriage.
- The diagnosis of choriocarcinoma is made from the patient's clinical history, elevated beta-human chorionic gonadotropin (beta-hCG) levels, ultrasound imaging (which confirms no identifiable current pregnancy despite a likely uterine mass), chest x-ray, and, ideally, a biopsy confirmation.
- Treatment with chemotherapy is associated with an excellent prognosis and overall cure rates greater than 90%.

References

1. Deng L, Zhang J, Wu T, Lawrie TA. Combination chemotherapy for primary treatment of high-risk gestational trophoblastic tumor. *Cochrane Database Syst Rev* 2013, Issue 1. Art. No.: CD005196. DOI:10.1002/14651858.CD005196.pub4.

2. Lurain JR. Gestational trophoblastic disease I: Epidemiology, pathology, clinical presentation and diagnosis of gestational trophoblastic disease, and management of hydatidiform mole. *Am J Obstet Gynecol* 2010;203(6): 531–9.

3. Goldstein DP, Berkowitz RS. Current management of gestational trophoblastic neoplasia. *Hematol Oncol Clin North Am* 2012;26(1): 111–31.

4. Soper JT, Mutch DG, Schink JC. Diagnosis and treatment of gestational trophoblastic disease: ACOG Practice Bulletin No. 53. *Gynecol Oncol* 2004; 93(3):575–85.

5. Ayhan A, Tuncer ZS, Halilzade H, Kucukali T. Predictors of persistent disease in women with complete hydatidiform mole. *J Reprod Med* 1996;41(8):591–4.

6. Berkowitz RS, Goldstein DP. Chorionic tumors. *N Engl J Med* 1996;335(23): 1740–8.

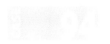

A 62-year-old woman with a vulvar lesion

Megan M. Shine and Warner K. Huh

History of present illness

A 62-year-old gravida 4, para 4 woman presents to her gynecologist complaining of new itching and irritation of her vulva. The patient reports noticing multiple "bumps" approximately 10 months earlier but thought this could be normal in menopause. She is sexually active with one male partner and does not use condoms. She has not seen a gynecologist in many years but notes a remote history of chlamydia, and has a history of multiple abnormal Pap tests in the past with "multiple biopsies" done.

Her past medical history is notable for chronic hypertension controlled on an angiotensin-converting enzyme (ACE) inhibitor. The patient denies alcohol or illicit drug use, but does report a 1 pack per day smoking history for 40 years.

Physical examination

General appearance: Thin woman in no acute distress
Vital signs:

Temperature: 36.8°C
Pulse: 86 beats/min
Blood pressure: 120/82 mmHg
Respiratory rate: 16 breaths/min
Oxygen saturation: 99% on room air
BMI: 21 kg/m^2

HEENT: Unremarkable
Neck: Supple
Cardiovascular: Regular rate, regular rhythm without rubs, murmurs, or gallops
Lungs: Clear to auscultation bilaterally
Abdomen: Soft, nontender, nondistended, active bowel sounds present
Rectal: Normal tone, no masses, brown stool
Pelvic:

External genitalia revealed flat, rough white lesions on the left labia measuring 1.5 × 2 cm, with no areas of ulceration (Fig. 94.1). No tenderness to touch with a probe.
Speculum exam: Vaginal mucosa and cervix without gross lesions
Bimanual exam: No cervical motion tenderness.
The uterus was normal postmenopausal size and the adnexa were without masses or tenderness to palpation

Lymphatics: No inguinal lymphadenopathy
Extremities: Negative
Neurologic: Nonfocal

How would you manage this patient?

A colposcopic examination of the vulva was performed with the lesion revealing profound acetowhite changes. Biopsies were obtained. Pathologic examination showed vulvar intraepithelial neoplasia (VIN).

The patient was counseled on the results and treatment options. She underwent a surgical excision as an outpatient. Final pathology of the excisional biopsy was consistent with VIN, differentiated type, with negative margins. The patient was seen back in six weeks for a postoperative appointment. All surgical sites were noted to be well healed. The patient was counseled on the need for close surveillance with colposcopy every six months, as well as smoking cessation.

Vulvar intraepithelial neoplasia

The International Society for the Study of Vulvovaginal Disease (ISSVD) introduced the term vulvar intraepithelial neoplasia (VIN) in 1986 [1]. VIN is recognized as the precursor to squamous cell carcinoma (SCC) of the vulva. SCC accounts for 5% of all malignant tumors of the female genital tract, but 95% of vulvar tumors [2]. Recently, there has been an increase in the incidence of VIN, particularly in younger women, possibly due to improved surveillance [1]. Currently, the median age for diagnosing VIN is 35.8 years [3].

The ISSVD recognizes two types of VIN: usual and differentiated. These two groups carry different pathogenesis,

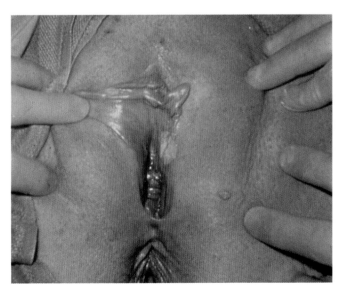

Fig. 94.1 External genitalia. (Image courtesy of Weldon Chafe, MD.)

Acute Care and Emergency Gynecology, ed. David Chelmow, Christine R. Isaacs and Ashley Carroll. Published by Cambridge University Press.
© Cambridge University Press 2015.

clinical features, and risk of progression to squamous carcinoma [1]. The more common **usual** type is associated with HPV infection and is typically seen in younger women, while the **differentiated** type is associated with lichen sclerosus and is typically seen in elderly women [1]. It is important for clinicians to recognize these two subtypes of VIN, because the risk of progression to SCC is dramatically different.

Usual type VIN (the more common type of VIN) is associated with high-risk types of HPV, with HPV 16 being the most common [1]. Usual type VIN is often multifocal and has an association with other lower genital tract neoplasias such as cervical intraepithelial neoplasia (CIN), vaginal intraepithelial neoplasia (VAIN), and anal intraepithelial neoplasia (AIN). Usual type VIN is divided into warty and basaloid subtypes [1]. The clinical presentation of usual type VIN can range from white to red lesions, and symptoms may range from no complaints to intense pruritus [2]. The progression of usual type VIN to SCC is low, occurring in 9–16% of untreated cases and 3% of treated cases [1]. Differentiated VIN (the less common type VIN) comprises only 2–10% of VIN cases [1]. Differentiated is a high-grade VIN that is often diagnosed in elderly patients with lichen sclerous and vulvar dystrophy [1]. The chronic inflammation can make the clinical diagnosis of differentiated VIN challenging [2]. There is a significant risk of progression to SCC with differentiated type VIN, and VIN can often be found at the periphery of invasive SCC [1]. The patient in this case has differentiated VIN, which was also suggested by her age and clinical findings.

Biopsy is the gold standard for diagnosis and is recommended in all postmenopausal patients presenting with a vulvar lesion. After histologic diagnosis is made, patients with VIN can be treated with surgical excision, carbon dioxide laser ablation, or imiquimod cream. Surgical excision with 5 mm margins is the gold standard of treatment, allowing for histologic examination and assurance of no concurrent invasive disease [3]. Carbon-dioxide laser ablation is also an acceptable treatment modality and can better preserve the appearance and function of external genitalia, but does not provide a pathology specimen [3]. The efficacy of imiquimod cream is debatable. Frega and colleagues evaluated the use of imiquimod 5% cream compared to surgical excision and found surgical excision to be superior in terms of overall response and a lower risk of recurrence at 5-years of follow-up [4]. In comparison, Wallbillich and colleagues conducted a retrospective chart review and found imiquimod cream to have the lowest recurrence rate (13.6%) compared to surgical excision (26.4%) and carbon-dioxide laser ablation (41.9%), with an average follow-up of 21 months [5].

Regardless of treatment modality, patients should be followed closely with examination/colposcopy every six months for five years, and then annually for recurrence. Historically, 30% of patients will have recurrence of disease [5] and Fehr and colleagues found 34.9% of patients had recurrence of disease after 5 years [6]. Risk factors associated with recurrence include: multifocal disease, smoking, larger lesions, and positive margins upon surgical exision [5]. Clinical examination and biopsy of any suspicious lesions, as well as smoking cessation are the current means for follow-up for patients after treatment for VIN. Current research is investigating other methods for follow-up with promising results. In regards to usual type VIN, one study found that human papillomavirus (HPV) testing in combination with a clinical examination can improve the efficacy of follow-up surveillance [3]. In patients with lichen sclerosus, the development of a vulvar brush for cytology has demonstrated promising results for the detection of premalignant lesions, with a sensitivity of 97% and a negative predictive value of 88% [7].

Key teaching points

- Vulvar intraepithelial neoplasia is divided into two subgroups: usual type VIN and differentiated VIN.
- Usual type VIN is associated with human papillomavirus (HPV) infection and affects younger women, with a low risk of progression to squamous cell carcinoma. Differentiated VIN is associated with lichen sclerosus and typically presents in older women, with a higher risk for progression to squamous cell carcinoma.
- Biopsy is the gold standard for diagnosis and is recommended in all postmenopausal patients presenting with a vulvar lesion.
- Current treatment options include surgical excision, carbon-dioxide laser ablation, and imiquimod cream.
- VIN has a high recurrence rate; thus, patients will need close and prolonged follow-up after treatment for VIN.

References

1. McCluggage WG. Premalignant lesions of the lower female genital tract: Cervix, vagina and vulva. *Pathology* 2013;45:214–28.

2. Ueda T, Enomoto T, Kimura T, et al. Two distinct pathways to development of squamous cell carcinoma of the vulva. *J Skin Cancer* 2011;2011:951250.

3. Frega A, Sopracordevole F, Scirpa P, et al. The re-infection rate of high-risk HPV and the recurrence rate of vulvar intraepithelial neoplasia (VIN) usual type after surgical treatment. *Med Sci Monit* 2011;17:532–5.

4. Frega A, Sesti F, Sopracordevole F, et al. Imiquimod 5% cream versus cold knife excision for treatment of VIN 2/3: a five-year follow-up. *Eur Rev Med Pharmacol Sci* 2013;17:936–40.

5. Wallbillich JJ, Rhodes HE, Millbourne AM, et al. Vulvar intraepithelial neoplasia (VIN 2/3): Comparing clinical outcomes and evaluating the risk factors for recurrence. *Gynecol Oncol* 2012;127:312–15.

6. Fehr MK, Baumann M, Mueller M, et al. Disease progression and recurrence in women treated for vulvovaginal intraepithelial neoplasia. *J Gynecol Oncol* 2013;24:236–41.

7. van den Eiden LCG, Grefte JMM, van der Avoort IAM, et al. Cytology of the vulva: Feasibility and preliminary results of a new brush. *Br J Cancer* 2012;6:269–73.

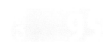

A 62-year-old woman with ovarian cancer and new-onset pelvic and right-leg pain

Kirk J. Matthews

History of present illness

A 62-year-old postmenopausal white woman, who is currently being treated for stage IIa ovarian adenocarcinoma, presents to the emergency department with severe pain in the right side of her pelvis that radiates down into her right lower extremity. Her symptoms started one day prior and are constant in nature. She reports no alleviating or exacerbating factors. She has a small amount of associated lower extremity swelling and denies any trauma to the affected area.

Her ovarian adenocarcinoma was treated with an initial staging procedure consisting of a total abdominal hysterectomy, bilateral salpingo-oophrectomy, omentectomy, and pelvic and para-aortic lymph-node dissection approximately four months ago. She finished her second cycle of adjuvant chemotherapy, with carboplatinum and taxol, two weeks ago. She has tolerated these treatments well with the exception of nausea and vomiting, which are well managed with ondansetron.

The patient's past medical history is otherwise benign. She is a gravida 3, para 3 woman who has been postmenopausal for 10 years. She denies previous sexually transmitted infections or abnormal cervical screening. Her family history is notable for adult-onset diabetes mellitus. She denies tobacco use and reports drinking two to three glasses of wine per week. She is a retired accountant who has been married for 35 years.

Physical examination

General appearance: Well-developed, well-groomed woman who appears anxious and unable to get comfortable on the hospital bed

Vital signs:

Temperature: 37.9°C
Pulse: 106 beats/min
Blood pressure: 135/88 mmHg
Respiratory rate: 18 breaths/min
Oxygen saturation: 96% on room air
BMI: 36 kg/m^2
Weight: 198 lb

HEENT: Moist mucous membranes; no jugular venous distention or carotid bruit appreciated

Chest: Lungs are clear to auscultation

Cardiac: Examination reveals a mild sinus tachycardia

Abdomen: Soft, no abnormal masses, nontender, nondistended. A midline vertical surgical incision appears well healed and without signs of infection

Lymphatics: No lymphadenopathy noted in the bilateral groins

External genitalia/vagina: Unremarkable with no discharge or bleeding noted; normal appearing vaginal mucosa; well-healed vaginal cuff

Extremities: +1 Edema noted in the right lower extremity to the upper calf. Tenderness in the right calf noted with palpation. The pain is exacerbated by dorsiflexion of the patient's foot

Laboratory studies:

WBCs: 6000/μL (normal 4000–12 000/μL)
Hb: 9.8 g/dL (normal 12.0–15.0)
Platelets: 215 000/μL (normal 172 000–440 000/μL)
Electrolytes are within normal limits
Urinalysis reveals no evidence of infection

How would you manage this patient?

Given this patients symptoms in the setting of ongoing treatment for an ovarian malignancy, a deep venous thrombosis (DVT) should be high on the differential diagnosis and requires further assessment. DVTs may present with a wide range of clinical signs and symptoms including pain, erythema, unilateral swelling, or warmth of the affected extremity. The history and medical context should raise suspicion for a DVT, which requires diagnostic confirmation.

Doppler ultrasonography of the right lower extremity was performed and was found to be positive for a large DVT in the right popliteal vein. The patient was promptly started on low-molecular-weight heparin (LMWH) and she was admitted to the hospital for initial monitoring. After initiating LMWH anticoagulation at 90 mg subcutaneously every 12 hours, she was also started on an oral vitamin K antagonist (warfarin), which was titrated until an international normalized ratio (INR) was in the therapeutic range of 2.0–3.0. The patient felt she was able to comply with oral therapy better than subcutaneous injections for her follow-up. Her anticoagulation treatment will be continued for a minimum of six months while she continues her chemotherapy.

Acute Care and Emergency Gynecology, ed. David Chelmow, Christine R. Isaacs and Ashley Carroll. Published by Cambridge University Press. © Cambridge University Press 2015.

Venous thromboembolism in cancer patients

There are numerous environmental, inherited, and acquired risk factors that influence a hypercoaguable state. Chief among these, however, are patients with an active malignancy. Venous thromboembolism (VTE) includes both deep venous thrombosis (DVT) and pulmonary embolism (PE) and is a major complication of cancer, occurring in anywhere from 4 to 20% of patients. Hospitalized patients with cancer and those receiving active therapy seem to be at the greatest risk for development of VTE. In a population-based study, cancer was associated with a 4.1-fold greater risk of thrombosis, whereas the use of chemotherapy increased the risk 6.5-fold [1].

Increasing the risk for VTE formation amongst patients with malignancy include higher stages of cancer at time of diagnosis, intervals less than six months since the time of diagnosis (as in the case of this patient), current treatment with chemotherapeutic agents or radiation, and indwelling venous access catheters [1].

Symptoms that commonly arise during DVT formation are swelling of the affected extremity, pain or tenderness (oftentimes only felt when provoked with standing or walking), increased warmth in the area of the extremity that is swollen or painful, and erythema or discoloration of the skin on the affected extremity. A common physical examination finding as was found in our patient is that of Homan's sign. A positive Homan's sign occurs when there is pain elicited in the calf on dorsiflexion of the patient's foot at the ankle joint while the knee is fully extended.

When clinical suspicion for a DVT exists, radiologic confirmation is required to make the diagnosis. Historically, CT contrast venography was the "gold standard" for confirming the diagnosis of a DVT. Unless a DVT needs to be identified deep within the pelvis however, today it is rarely used as venography is invasive, expensive, and has been shown to cause thrombosis on its own. By contrast, Doppler ultrasonography is noninvasive, inexpensive and typically readily available. Doppler ultrasound is the diagnostic test of choice with a mean sensitivity and specificity for the diagnosis of symptomatic proximal DVT at 97% and 94%, respectively. Laboratory assessment with D-dimer levels should not be obtained as patients with cancer will often have an elevated D-dimer even in the absence of a VTE. Using D-dimer levels may be helpful in excluding VTE in patients with a low pretest probability, but it certainly would not be useful in the case of this patient given the context of her malignancy and current chemotherapy treatment.

According to the American Society of Clinical Oncology (ASCO), 2013 guideline updates for VTE prophylaxis and treatment, treatment with LMWH is preferred over unfractionated heparin (UFH) for the initial 5–10 days of anticoagulation for the cancer patient with a newly diagnosed VTE (as long as no renal impairment exists defined as creatinine clearance <30 mL/min) [2]. These recommendations are due in part to a recent Cochrane meta-analysis, which found improved survival rates in cancer patients who were treated with LMWH over

Table 95.1 Dosing regimens for treatment of VTE in patients with cancer

Treatment of established DVT		
Clinical setting	Drug	Regimen*
Initial		
	UFH	80 U/kg IV bolus, then 18 U/kg per hour IV. Adjust dose based on aPTT
	Dalteparin	100 U/kg once every 12 hours or 200 U/kg once daily
	Enoxaparin	1 mg/kg once every 12 hours or 1.5 mg/kg once daily
	Tinzaparin	175 U/kg once per day
	Fondaparinux	<50 kg, 5.0 mg once daily 50–100 kg, 7.5 mg once daily >100 kg, 10 mg once daily
Long-term		
	Dalteparin	200 U/kg once daily for 1 month, then 150 U/kg once daily
	Enoxaparin	1.5 mg/kg once daily or 1 mg/kg once every 12 hours
	Tinzaparin	175 U/kg once daily
	Warfarin	Adjust dose to maintain INR 2–3

* All doses are given as subcutaneous doses except as indicated.
aPTT, activated partial thromboplastin time; DVT, deep venous thrombosis; INR, international normalized ratio; IV, intravenous; UFH, unfractionated heparin; VTE, venous thromboembolism.

UFH [3]. Dosing should be weight-based for treatment (Table 95.1) and can be administered as a twice-daily or once-daily regimen [2].

The 2013 ASCO guidelines recommend treatment regimens should be continued for a period of at least six months in the oncology patient with a VTE [2]. For this treatment duration, LMWH is still preferred over vitamin K antagonists (warfarin) due to improved efficacy and ease of administration. In addition, LMWH carries the added benefit of not requiring any laboratory monitoring to follow clotting factor levels such as prothrombin time (PT), INR, or factor Xa levels. In contrast, however, vitamin K antagonists are much less costly, can be administered orally, and are an acceptable alternative for long-term therapy if LMWH is not feasible. If vitamin K antagonists are chosen for long-term use, they should be started while the patient is being treated concurrently with LMWH as "bridge therapy" until an INR of 2–3 is achieved. In the outpatient setting, INRs must be also checked frequently to ensure adequate dosing, and the practitioner must be mindful of other medications and dietary influences that may interact with vitamin K antagonists and, thus, alter INR levels.

At this time, no published studies address the need for further treatment of VTE beyond six months. However,

Table 95.2 Dosing regimens for prophylaxis of VTE in patients with cancer

Prophlaxis of VTE		
Clinical setting	Drug	Regimen*
Hospitalized		
	UFH	5000 U once every 8 hours
	Dalteparin	5000 U once daily
	Enoxaparin	40 mg once daily
	Fondaparinux	2.5 mg once daily
Surgical patients		
	UFH	5000 U 2–4 hours preop. and then once every 8 hours thereafter
	Dalteparin	2500 U 2–4 hours preop. and then once daily thereafter
	Enoxaparin	20 mg 2–4 hours preop. and 40 mg once daily thereafter
	Fondaparinux	2.5 mg once daily beginning 6–8 hours postop.

* All doses are given as subcutaneous doses except as indicated.
UFH, unfractionated heparin; VTE, venous thromboembolism.

certain experts agree that continuing anticoagulation beyond six months should be considered for selected patients who continue to have high-risk factors for recurrent VTEs. This decision must be balanced against the inherent risk of bleeding while on anticoagulation, costs, and patient compliance [2].

Contraindications to therapeutic anticoagulation include severe platelet dysfunction, active peptic or other gastrointestinal ulceration at risk of bleeding, major surgery or serious bleeding within the preceding 2 weeks, or persistent thrombocytopenia (platelets <50 000/μL). In these instances, the insertion of a vena cava filter is often indicated. Vena cava filters may also be considered as additional therapy in patients with progression of thrombosis despite treatment therapy with LMWH or warfarin.

Since cancer patients have such a dramatic overall increased risk of VTE formation, questions often arise as to whether VTE prophylaxis is indicated in this population. For this reason, ASCO recommends that hospitalized patients who have an active malignancy with an acute medical illness or reduced mobility should receive pharmacologic thromboprophylaxis, assuming no active bleeding is observed. As with treatment-dosing regimens, there are several regimens available for prophylaxis dosing (Table 95.2). For active, ambulatory cancer patients not admitted to the hospital, current recommendations do not include routine pharmacologic thromboprophylaxis in patients who are undergoing short chemotherapy infusions in the outpatient setting. Anticoagulants are not recommended to improve survival in cancer patients without a VTE [1].

Over the years, there have been several attempts to construct predictive models to aid in the identification of cancer patients who are at heightened risk for the development of VTE in the outpatient setting. The risks versus benefits of medical thromboprophylaxis in such patients are still being studied and as such, routine thromoboprophylaxis is not currently recommended.

Key teaching points

- Clinicians should have high suspicion for deep venous thrombosis (DVT) in an oncology patient presenting with any new-onset symptoms of unilateral lower extremity pain, erythema, swelling, or tenderness.
- A D-dimer is not a helpful diagnostic laboratory value in the cancer patient.
- Doppler ultrasound is the diagnostic test of choice with high sensitivity and specificity for diagnosing a DVT.
- Treatment for a DVT in the cancer patient should begin with low-molecular-weight heparin, ideally for a minimum of six months. Other treatment regimens can be considered.
- While the cancer patient is considered high risk for development of a VTE, current recommendations do include thromboprophylactic therapy for an ambulatory patient in the outpatient setting.

References

1. American Society of Clinical Oncology. Recommendations for venous thromboembolism prophylaxis and treatment in patients with cancer: practice guideline. *Jour Clin Oncol* 2007;25:5490–505.

2. American Society of Clinical Oncology. Venous thromboembolism prophylaxis and treatment in patients with cancer: practice guideline update. *Jour Clin Oncol* 2013;31:2189–204.

3. Akl EA, Vasireddi SR, Gunukula S, et al. Anticoagulation for the initial treatment of venous thromboembolism in patients with cancer. *Cochrane Database Syst Rev* 2011, Issue 2. Art. No.: CD006649. DOI: 10.1002/14651858.

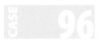

A 64-year-old woman with ovarian cancer, emesis, and abdominal pain

Nguyet A. Nguyen and Warner K. Huh

History of present illness

A 64-year-old white woman with stage IIIC ovarian cancer presents to the emergency room with the chief complaint of abdominal pain. She reports acute onset of moderate-to-severe diffuse abdominal pain as well as progressive nausea and vomiting over the past three days. The emesis is nonbloody but bilious. The patient reports that she has not been able to tolerate any oral intake, including fluids or anti-emetics, for the past 24 hours. Her last bowel movement four days ago was loose and watery, although she reports flatus. She was diagnosed with ovarian cancer one year ago and was treated with complete surgical cytoreduction followed by six cycles of platinum- and taxane-based chemotherapy. Her medical history is otherwise unremarkable, and her surgical history is significant for a laparoscopic cholecystectomy as well as a complete hysterectomy and staging procedure as above.

She was recently seen in clinic and was noted to have a rising CA-125 and underwent a CT scan that demonstrated recurrence with diffuse intrabdominal disease including peritoneal implants.

Physical examination

General appearance: Well-dressed thin woman in mild distress

Vital signs:

Temperature: 37.0°C
Pulse: 116 beats/min
Blood pressure: 108/61 mmHg
Respiratory rate: 22 breaths/min
Oxygen saturation: 99% on room air

HEENT: Dry mucous membranes
Cardiovascular: Regular rhythm, tachycardia, no murmurs, rubs, or gallops
Pulmonary: Symmetric chest expansion, clear to auscultation bilaterally
Abdomen: Well-healed midline scar; high-pitched bowel sounds heard in bilateral upper quadrants; moderately distended abdomen tympanic to percussion with mild tenderness diffusely; no palpable masses; no rebound or guarding
Genitourinary: Normal external female genitalia; bimanual examination reveals an intact vaginal cuff; no adnexal masses; cervix is surgically absent

Rectal: Normal sphincter tone, hemoccult negative, no masses palpated
Neurologic: Alert and oriented × 4
Laboratory studies: The patient had blood drawn for laboratory tests. A peripheral intravenous line was placed, and the patient was given a 1 L bolus of lactated Ringer's solution, intravenous ondansetron for nausea, and intravenous morphine for pain. Laboratory results were:

Leukocyte count: 11 300/µL (normal 3500–12 500/µL)
Hb: 10.2 g/dL (normal 12.0–15.5 g/dL)
Ht: 31% (normal 38–46%)
Platelets: 170 000/µL (normal 150 000–400 000/µL)
Sodium (Na): 131 mEq/L (normal 135–145 mEq/L)
Potassium: 3.0 mEq/L (normal 3.7–5.2 mEq/L)
Chloride: 92 mmol/L (normal 96–106 mmol/L)
Bicarbonate: 22 mmol/L (normal 20–29 mmol/L)
BUN: 30 mg/dL (normal 7–20 mg/dL)
Creatinine: 1.4 mg/dL (baseline in clinic visit 1.0 mg/dL)
Calcium: 7.8 mg/dL (normal 8.4–10.2 mg/dL)
Magnesium: 1.3 mg/dL (normal 1.8–2.5 mg/dL)
Phosphorus: 2.2 mg/dL (normal 2.4–5.0 mg/dL)

Imaging: Abdominal radiographs (KUB [kidney, ureter, bladder x-ray]) were obtained (Fig. 96.1a,b)

How would you manage this patient?

The diagnosis is a partial small bowel obstruction (SBO). The KUB shows dilated loops of small bowel (Fig. 96.1a) with multiple air-fluid levels in a "step-ladder" pattern and small amount of gas noted in colon (Fig. 96.1b). A nasogastric tube (NGT) was placed and 1300 mL of bilious output was immediately noted. On hospital day 2, the patient reported persistent nausea; the NGT had an additional 1200 mL of bilious output. On examination, her abdomen remained moderately distended with high-pitched bowel sounds and absent peritoneal signs (i.e. guarding and/or rebound). She underwent a repeat KUB with diatrizoic acid (Gastrograffin®) contrast that showed a transition point in LLQ (Fig. 96.2), with a small amount of contrast beyond the transition point. By hospital day 3, the patient began to have watery bowel movements, and her abdominal distension and pain improved. Her NGT was removed. The patient's diet was advanced as tolerated, and by hospital day 5 she was discharged home on a low-residue diet.

Acute Care and Emergency Gynecology, ed. David Chelmow, Christine R. Isaacs and Ashley Carroll. Published by Cambridge University Press.
© Cambridge University Press 2015.

(a)

(b)

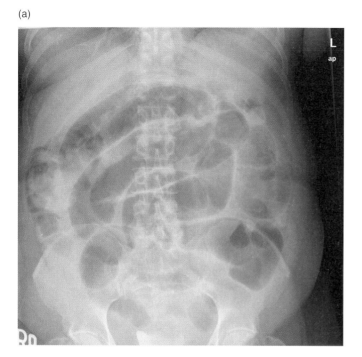

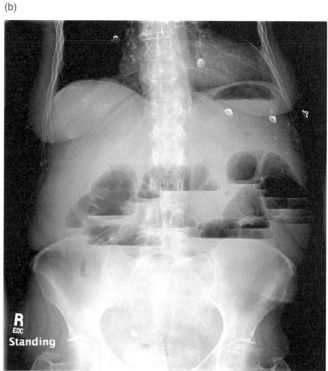

Fig. 96.1 KUB supine (a); KUB upright (b). (Images courtesy of University of Alabama at Birmingham, Department of Radiology.)

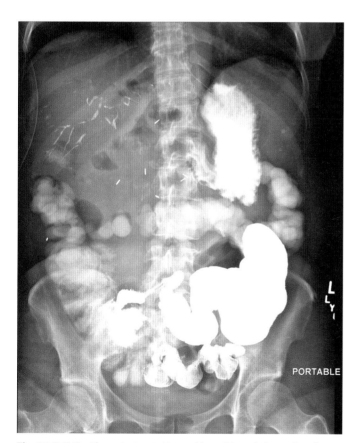

Fig. 96.2 KUB with contrast noted in partial small bowel obstruction. (Image courtesy of University of Alabama at Birmingham, Department of Radiology.)

Small bowel obstruction

The most common causes of SBO are adhesions, malignancy, and hernias. About 80% of SBO are due to adhesions from previous surgeries and carcinomatosis or peritoneal implants from metastatic malignancies [1,2]. About 20–50% of ovarian cancer patients will develop a SBO during their disease course [1]. SBO is commonly encountered in advanced-stage or recurrent ovarian cancer patients due to their diffuse intra-abdominal disease and history of previous surgery.

Patients usually present with the classic triad of symptoms: abdominal pain, distension, and nausea and vomiting. Patients may experience loose, watery stool due to gastrointestinal contents distal to the obstruction or may report no bowel function subsequent to the onset of symptoms. Clinical signs can include dehydration, abdominal distension, and metabolic alkalosis [1,2] with electrolyte abnormalities due to persistent emesis.

SBOs may be due to mechanical or malignant causes. Mechanical SBO occurs when the intestinal lumen is either partially or completely obstructed by either extrinsic or intrinsic factors such as compression by adhesions or intra-luminal masses, respectively. When the lumen is obstructed, the proximal bowel becomes distended with air and fluid due to the inability of bowel contents to pass distally. Malignant SBOs occur due to dysfunctional bowel motility due to carcinomatosis or tumor implants that cause abnormal bowel peristalsis leading to accumulation of bowel contents and obstructive symptoms. In both cases, distension of the bowel lumen causes a positive feedback mechanism thereby increasing intestinal peristalsis, circulation, and hormone release to aid in digestion and absorption of bowel contents. As such, fluid accumulates from this physiologic response causing the bowel lumen to become more distended. The distension leads to retrograde flow that manifests as nausea and vomiting [2].

The severity and timing of symptoms may aid in differentiating between partial and complete SBO. Partial SBOs may have a more indolent course with progressive nausea and vomiting. Up to 80% resolve with conservative management [2]. Patients with complete obstructions tend to have shorter onset of symptoms and may also have symptoms related to obstipation. Pain may be more acute and localized to one area. Complete SBOs may also be managed conservatively; however, it is imperative to recognize signs of bowel strangulation or compromise such as fever, peritoneal signs, leucocytosis, or lactic acidosis. Expeditious surgical management may be required to avoid significant morbidity and even mortality. Unfortunately, the clinical signs and symptoms of bowel strangulation often do not occur until there is irreversible bowel injury [3]. The morbidity and mortality of SBO significantly increases with bowel ischemia.

KUB films are helpful in the initial workup for SBO and can diagnose up to 66% of SBOs [1,2]. Supine KUBs will show distended bowel lumen proximal to the obstruction and may identify a transition point, while upright radiographs will illustrate air-fluid levels in a "step-ladder" pattern (Fig. 96.1a,b). A KUB may not differentiate between a partial versus complete SBO; however, the presence or absence of colonic gas may aid in the diagnosis [4]. In complete SBO, there is no passage of stool or gas beyond the obstruction resulting in the absence of colonic gas. More importantly, the presence of gas in the colon does not rule out a complete SBO; however, the absence of colonic gas is more specific and suggests the obstruction is less likely to be partial. If the clinical picture is unclear, a CT of the abdomen and pelvis with contrast may be obtained. CT is more sensitive in diagnosing partial versus complete SBO. It may also help elucidate a transition point, identify bowel wall thickening or pneumatosis intestinalis. Bowel wall thickening occurs due to vascular congestion resulting from the transition point. As the SBO progresses, intraluminal gas may enter the injured mucosal wall leading to pneumatosis intestinalis – a late finding in bowel ischemia. Evidence of these serious findings on CT may assist in surgical decision-making [5]. Although modern imaging techniques are extremely sensitive, a patient's clinical presentation and physician's judgment should dictate management.

Resuscitation and intestinal decompression are the most important treatment goals in patients with SBOs. Patients will require intravenous access, isotonic fluid resuscitation with lactated Ringer's or normal saline, intravenous anti-emetics and pain medication. Electrolyte repletion with sodium, potassium, and magnesium is usually required due to gastric and intestinal losses. NGT or long nasointestinal tube decompression are used in SBO treatment to relieve bowel distension, improve nausea and vomiting, decrease risk of aspiration and also to prepare the bowel for surgery, if needed [6]. In patients who do not require surgical intervention, studies have shown that about 88% of patients have resolution of their SBO in the first 48 hours, and the remaining resolve within 72 hours [7].

A large systematic review has shown that the use of water-soluble contrast such as diatrizoic acid (DA) accurately predicts the need for surgical intervention and reduces the patient's hospital stay [8]. DA is hyperosmolar and induces water-reuptake by the intestinal lumen, leading to a change in consistency and aiding in the passage of bowel contents through the partial obstruction. The advantage of using DA for radiographic contrast is due to its water solubility. If there is any bowel compromise and contrast is leaked intra-abdominally, DA may cause less damage to intraperitoneal tissue surfaces. It does not reduce the patients' need for surgery if it is clinically indicated; however, in those who may be conservatively managed, DA significantly decreases hospital stay and interval time to surgical intervention [8]. In our case, DA was not given during the patient's initial diagnostic KUB as the etiology and severity of the SBO is unknown and contrast may worsen a patient's clinical status depending on severity of the SBO. Once the etiology is known, a repeat KUB with DA may be performed for therapeutic purposes. If successful, a patient may avoid surgery; however, if no contrast is seen past the transition point, then the likelihood the SBO will resolve without surgery is low. Therefore, if a patient's clinical presentation suggests bowel compromise or if medical management fails, then surgery is indicated for possible adhesiolysis or bowel resection if necessary.

Surgery is necessary in a majority of cases of SBO that fail conservative management. In malignant SBO, the decision to proceed with surgery is individualized. Life expectancy, performance status, and disease state should be taken into consideration prior to surgery, as the risk of recurrent SBO ranges from 10 to 50% [9]. A large systematic review showed no compelling evidence to support or refute surgery in patients with malignant SBO. Patients who were managed surgically generally had a better performance status and prognosis than those managed conservatively; however, surgery did not change overall survival [9]. In patients with advanced stage cancers with refractory SBO, palliative interventions including hospice and venting gastrostomy tubes may be indicated for symptomatic relief.

Key teaching points
- Bowel obstructions usually present with the classic symptom triad of abdominal pain, distension, and nausea and vomiting.
- Up to 80% of small bowel obstructions (SBOs) are due to adhesions and malignancy. A KUB is a simple

yet prompt diagnostic test that can aid in diagnosing SBOs; CT may aid in diagnosis if the KUB is unclear.

- Patients who present with fever, leukocytosis, lactic acidosis, or signs of an acute abdomen may have bowel compromise and surgical intervention should not be delayed.

- The mainstay of SBO treatment is symptom relief, fluid resuscitation, and bowel decompression. Frequent evaluations are necessary to identify patients with bowel ischemia requiring surgery.

- Complete or partial SBOs that fail conservative management usually require surgery; however, patients with malignant SBO require individualized management. Quality of life, performance status, and prognosis may dictate whether palliative interventions should be considered in lieu of surgery.

References

1. Hayanga AJ, Bass-Wilkins K, Bulkley GB. Current management of small-bowel obstruction. *Adv Surg* 2005; 39:1–33.

2. Soybel DI, Landman WB. Ileus and bowel obstruction. In Mulholland MW, Lillemoe KD, Doherty GM, et al., eds. *Greenfield's Surgery: Scientific Principles and Practice*, 5th edn. Philadelphia, Lippincott, Williams and Wilkins. 2010. Available at Surgical Council on Resident Education (SCORE): http://www.surgicalcore.org/chapter/46224.

3. Sarr MG, Bulkley GB, Zuidema GD. Preoperative recognition of intestinal strangulation obstruction. Prospective evaluation of diagnostic capability. *Am J Surg* 1983;145(1):176–82.

4. Brolin RE, Krasna MJ, Mast BA. Use of tubes and radiographs in the management of small bowel obstruction. *Ann Surg* 1987;206(2): 126–33.

5. Balthazar EJ. CT of small-bowel obstruction. *Am J Roentgenol* 1994;162:255–61.

6. Fleshner PR, Siegman MG, Slater GI, et al. A prospective, randomized trial of short versus long tubes in adhesive small-bowel obstruction. *Am J Surg* 1995;170(4):366–70.

7. Cox MR, Gunn IF, Eastman MC, et al. The safety and duration of nonoperative treatment for adhesive small bowel obstruction. *Aust N Z J Med* 1993;63:367–71.

8. Abbas S, Bissett IP, Parry BR. Oral water soluble contrast for the management of adhesive small bowel obstruction. *Cochrane Database Syst Rev* 2008, Issue 3. Art. No.: CD004651.

9. Kucukmetin A, Naik R, Galaal K, Bryant A, Dickinson HO. Palliative surgery versus medical management for bowel obstruction in ovarian cancer. *Cochrane Database Syst Rev* 2010, Issue 7. Art. No.:CD007792.pub2.

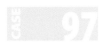

A 65-year-old woman with new-onset fatigue, parasthesias, and muscle cramps after chemotherapy for ovarian cancer

Haller J. Smith and Warner K. Huh

History of present illness

A 65-year-old white woman with stage IIIC papillary serous ovarian carcinoma presents with complaints of numbness and muscle cramps. She is currently undergoing chemotherapy with paclitaxel and carboplatin. She completed her fourth cycle three days ago. For the past two days, she has noted numbness around her mouth and a tingling sensation in her hands and feet. Last night, she was unable to sleep due to cramps in her legs. She reports that she has never had symptoms like this before, and she is anxious about what could be causing them.

Her past medical history is significant only for mild hypertension and hyperlipidemia, for which she takes hydrochlorothiazide 25 mg daily and atorvastatin 40 mg nightly. Her other home medications include a daily multivitamin and hydrocodone/acetaminophen 5 mg/325 mg as needed for pain.

Physical examination

General appearance: Well-developed white woman in no acute distress

Vital signs:

Temperature: 98.3°C
Pulse: 71 beats/min
Blood pressure: 134/82 mmHg
Respiratory rate: 14 breaths/min
BMI: 24 kg/m^2

Neurologic: Alert and oriented to person, place, time, and situation; 5/5 strength in all extremities; decreased sensation to pinprick, temperature, and vibration in distal extremities. Twitching of the left side of the mouth elicited by tapping just anterior to the patient's left ear. When a blood pressure cuff was inflated to 160 mmHg and left in place, flexion of the wrist and metacarpophalangeal joints, as well as extension and adduction of the fingers, were noted

Laboratory studies:

Serum calcium: 6.3 mg/dL (normal 8.4–10.2 mg/dL)
Ionized calcium: 3.8 mg/dL (normal 4.4–5.3 mg/dL)
Serum magnesium: 1.3 mg/dL (normal 1.8–2.5 mg/dL)
Serum albumin: 2.9 g/dL (normal 3.4–5.0 g/dL)
The remainder of her basic metabolic panel, CBC, and hepatic function panel were within normal limits

Imaging: ECG showed a prolonged QT interval

How would you manage this patient?

The patient was admitted to the hospital with the diagnosis of acute hypocalcemia. She was placed on telemetry monitoring. She was given one ampule of calcium gluconate as a slow intravenous push. She was then started on a continuous calcium gluconate infusion, and her magnesium was repleted with intravenous magnesium sulfate. Halfway through the calcium gluconate infusion, the patient reported resolution of her leg cramps and improvement in her paresthesias. Repeat labs showed a serum calcium level of 8.1 mg/dL, an ionized calcium of 4.6 mg/dL, and a serum magnesium level of 1.9 mg/dL. The patient was started on oral calcium carbonate, 1000 mg BID, along with vitamin D supplementation, and was discharged home in stable condition.

Hypocalcemia

In the setting of chemotherapy, her neurologic symptoms likely stem from electrolyte imbalance or paclitaxel toxicity. Electrolyte abnormalities, particularly hyper- or hypokalemia, hypomagnesemia, and hyper- or hypocalcemia are common in cancer patients undergoing chemotherapy. These electrolyte imbalances can be a consequence of the mechanism of action of the chemotherapy or related to side effects, such as renal toxicity, nausea, vomiting, or diarrhea [1]. When patients present with unusual complaints that raise suspicion for an electrolyte imbalance, they should be promptly evaluated, as many of these conditions can be life-threatening if not addressed appropriately. Initial evaluation should include a thorough physical examination, a complete blood count, and a basic metabolic panel. Many electrolyte disorders can be associated with cardiac arrhythmias, so an ECG should also be obtained in any patient in whom a significant electrolyte imbalance is suspected. This patient has several symptoms that could be attributed to paclitaxel-induced peripheral neuropathy; however, the presence of neuromuscular irritability in combination with her laboratory findings makes hypocalcemia the correct diagnosis.

The symptoms of hypocalcemia are typically a result of increased excitability of the nervous system and can range from mild to life-threatening (Table 97.1) [2,3]. The most common symptoms are those of neuromuscular irritability, commonly manifested as fasciculations, cramps, and paresthesias. Tetany

Acute Care and Emergency Gynecology, ed. David Chelmow, Christine R. Isaacs and Ashley Carroll. Published by Cambridge University Press. © Cambridge University Press 2015.

Table 97.1 Clinical manifestations of hypocalcemia [2,3]

Neurologic manifestations	Neuromuscular manifestations
Seizures	Paresthesias of distal limbs and perioral region
Dementia*	Muscle cramps
Movement disorders*	Fasiculations
Cardiac manifestations	Tetany
Prolonged QT interval	Other manifestations
Hypotension	Laryngospasm
	Bronchospasm
	Cataracts*

* Develops with long-standing hypocalcemia.

is less common. The classic neuromuscular manifestations of hypocalcemia are Chvostek's and Trousseau's signs, which are both described in the patient in this case. Chvostek's sign is twitching of the face elicited by tapping over the facial nerve, while Trousseau's sign involves carpal spasm produced by inducing distal hypoxia with a blood pressure cuff [4,5].

Hypocalcemia is defined as serum calcium of less than 8.8 mg/dL (or 2.2 mmol) and is a common laboratory finding. Extracellular calcium concentration is predominantly regulated by parathyroid hormone (PTH) and its subsequent effects on target organs such as the kidneys, bone, and gastrointestinal tract. A decrease in serum calcium leads to increased release of PTH, which increases osteoclastic bone resorption, stimulates absorption of calcium in the renal tubule, and signals the kidneys to increase production of 1,25 dihydroxy-vitamin D (calcitriol), which in turn stimulates increased absorption of calcium from the gastrointestinal tract [2,3,4,6]. Of the calcium in the extracellular compartment, approximately 50% exists as the biologically active ionized form, while the remainder is either protein-bound (40%), predominantly to albumin, or complexed to anions [2,3,5].

When measuring calcium levels, the most accurate method is to directly measure the ionized calcium (normal 4.5–5.0 mg/dL); however, the total serum calcium is more frequently encountered [6]. One of the most common causes of a low total serum calcium concentration is hypoalbuminemia. While not as accurate as measuring ionized calcium directly, correcting the total serum calcium for the serum albumin can assist with interpretation of laboratory values and ensure that the total serum calcium level has not been falsely lowered by hypoalbuminemia. The most common formula for correction is 0.8 (4 − measured serum albumin) added to the measured total serum calcium [2,3]. If applied to the case above, the corrected total serum calcium is 6.3 + 0.8 (4–2.9) = 7.18 mg/dL. In this case, the patient still has significant hypocalcemia even after correction for her hypoalbuminemia.

pH also can also significantly effect serum calcium concentrations. Increased pH causes increased binding affinity of calcium, thus decreasing the concentration of ionized calcium [4]. Patients with either a metabolic or a respiratory alkalosis will often be hypocalcemic [6].

There are multiple causes of hypocalcemia. After excluding issues such as hypoalbuminemia, steps should be taken to identify the cause of the hypocalcemia. The most common culprits are hypoparathyroidism, vitamin D deficiency, acute or chronic kidney disease, and hypomagnesemia; however, there are a host of other causes, including certain drugs, malignancy, and sepsis or other critical illness [2].

The hypocalcemia in this patient is likely related to her chemotherapy regimen. First-line chemotherapy for ovarian cancer includes a combination of a platinum and a taxane, such as the carboplatin and paclitaxel that this patient is receiving. The platinum chemotherapy agents, especially cisplatin, are nephrotoxic and have been shown to cause significant renal magnesium wasting [7,8]. Hypomagnesemia interferes with PTH secretion and may affect its peripheral action, thereby leading to hypocalcemia [3].

The management of hypocalcemia depends on whether it is acute or chronic, the severity of the hypocalcemia, and whether the patient is symptomatic. In general, patients with symptomatic or severe hypocalcemia (serum calcium <7.6 mg/dL) should be hospitalized for parenteral treatment [2,3]. As the patient in this case has neuromuscular irritability, evidence of cardiovascular effects, and severe hypocalcemia, she meets the criteria for inpatient management and treatment with intravenous calcium. There are several calcium-containing compounds that are suitable for use; however, the most common is intravenous calcium gluconate as it causes the least local irritation. One ampule of calcium gluconate contains 90 mg of elemental calcium. Recommended treatment involves giving one ampule of calcium gluconate by slow intravenous push followed by a continuous calcium gluconate infusion as described in the clinical case. An infusion of 15 mg/kg over a 4–6 hour period can be expected to raise the serum calcium by 2–3 mg/dL [2,3]. Calcium gluceptate and calcium chloride can also be used for acute therapy [3]. It is important to note that if the patient has concurrent hypomagnesemia, correction of the serum magnesium concentration is imperative for adequate treatment of hypocalcemia. Following correction of serum calcium levels and resolution of symptoms, the patient can be transitioned to an oral calcium regimen, typically either calcium citrate or calcium carbonate. Concurrent vitamin D supplementation is also recommended [6].

Key teaching points

- Electrolyte disturbances are common in cancer patients receiving chemotherapy and can be life-threatening. A high index of suspicion should be maintained in order to diagnose and treat electrolyte imbalances.

- The most common presenting symptoms of hypocalcemia are related to neuromuscular irritability and can include muscle cramps, fasciculations, and tetany.
- The total serum calcium level is inaccurate and can be affected by many factors, such as pH and albumin concentration. Whenever possible, an ionized calcium level should be obtained to assess the true degree of hypocalcemia.

- All patients with severe hypocalcemia should be hospitalized for intravenous repletion. Telemetry monitoring is important given the risk of prolonged QT interval and resultant cardiac arrhythmias.
- In patients with concurrent hypomagnesemia, serum magnesium must be repleted in order to adequately correct hypocalcemia.

References

1. Lamiere N, Van Biesen W, Vanholder R. Electrolyte disturbance and acute kidney injury in patients with cancer. *Semin Nephrol* 2010;30:534–47.

2. Thakker RV. Hypocalcemia: Pathogenesis, differential diagnosis, and management. In Favus MJ, ed. *Primer on the Metabolic Bone Diseases and Disorders of Mineral Metabolism.* Washington, DC, American Society for Bone and Mineral Research, 2006.

3. Bushinsky DA, Monk RD. Calcium. *Lancet* 1998;352:306–11.

4. Reber PO, Heath H. Hypocalcemic emergencies. *Med Clin North Am* 1995;79:93–106.

5. Cooper MS, Gittoes NJ. Diagnosis and management of hypocalcemia. *BMJ* 2008;336:1298–302.

6. Ariyan CE, Sosa JA. Assessment and management of patients with abnormal calcium. *Crit Care Med* 2004;32: S146–54.

7. Ariceta G, Rodriguez-Soriano J, Vallo A, Navajas A. Acute and chronic effects of cisplatin therapy on renal magnesium homeostasis. *Med Pediatr Oncol* 1997;28:35–40.

8. Schilsky RL, Anderson T. Hypomagnesemia and renal magnesium wasting in patients receiving cisplatin. *Ann Intern Med* 1979;90:929–31.

Index

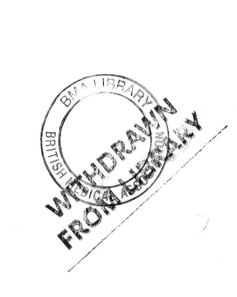